DRY SKIN and MOISTURIZERS

Chemistry and Function

DERMATOLOGY: CLINICAL AND BASIC SCIENCE SERIES

Edited by Howard I. Maibach, M.D.

Published Titles:

Bioengineering of the Skin: Cutaneous Blood Flow and Erythema
Enzo Berardesca, Peter Elsner, and Howard I. Maibach

Bioengineering of the Skin: Water and the Stratum Corneum
Peter Elsner, Enzo Berardesca, and Howard I. Maibach

Bioengineering of the Skin: Methods and Instrumentation
Enzo Berardesca, Peter Elsner, Klaus P. Wilhelm, and Howard I. Maibach

Bioengineering of the Skin: Skin Surface, Imaging, and Analysis
Klaus P. Wilhelm, Peter Elsner, Enzo Berardesca, and Howard I. Maibach

Dermatologic Research Techniques
Howard I. Maibach

Hand Eczema
Torkil Menne and Howard I. Maibach

Health Risk Assessment: Dermal and Inhalation Exposure and Absorption of Toxicants
Rhoda G. M. Wang, James B. Knaak, and Howard I. Maibach

Pigmentation and Pigmentary Disorders
Norman Levine

Protective Gloves for Occupational Use
Gunh Mellström, J.E. Walhberg, and Howard I. Maibach

Skin Cancer: Mechanisms and Human Relevance
Hasan Mukhtar

Human Papillomavirus Infections in Dermatovenereology
Gerd Gross and Geo von Krogh

Contact Urticaria Syndrome
Smita Amin, Arto Lahti, and Howard I. Maibach

Skin Reactions to Drugs
Kirsti Kauppinen, Kristiina Alanko, Matti Hannuksela, and Howard I. Maibach

Dermatologic Botany
Javier Avalos and Howard I. Maibach

DERMATOLOGY: CLINICAL & BASIC SCIENCE SERIES

DRY SKIN and MOISTURIZERS

Chemistry and Function

Edited by

Marie Lodén, Dr. Med. Sci.

Howard I. Maibach, M.D.

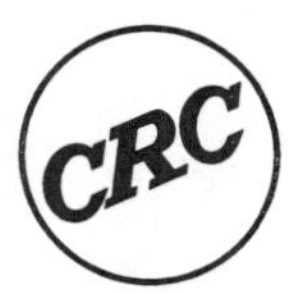

CRC Press

Boca Raton London New York Washington, D.C.

Library of Congress Cataloging-in-Publication Data

Dry skin and moisturizers : chemistry and function / edited by Marie Lodén and Howard I. Maibach.
p. cm. -- (CRC series in dermatology)
Includes bibliographical references and index.
ISBN 0-8493-7520-7 (alk. paper)
1. Dermatologic agents. 2. Skin--Diseases. 3. Barrier creams. 4. Wetting agents. I. Loden, Marie. II. Maibach, Howard I. III. Series
[DNLM: 1. Skin Diseases--drug therapy. 2. Emollients--pharmacokinetics. 3. Emollients--therapeutic use. 4. Skin Diseases--physiopathology. WR 650 D798 1999]
RL801.D79 1999
616.5′061--dc21
DNLM/DLC
for Library of Congress 99-38984
CIP

International Standard Book Number 0-8493-7520-7
Library of Congress Card Number 99-38984
Printed in the United States of America 1 2 3 4 5 6 7 8 9 0
Printed on acid-free paper

Series Preface

Our goal in creating the "Dermatology: Clinical and Basic Science Series" is to present the insights of experts on emerging applied and experimental techniques and theoretical concepts that are, or will be, at the vanguard of dermatology. The books cover new and exciting multidisciplinary areas of cutaneous research. We want these to be the books every physician will use in order to get acquainted with new methodologies in skin research. These books can be given to graduate students and postdoctoral fellows when they are looking for guidance to start a new line of research.

The series consists of books that are edited by experts and consist of chapters written by the leaders in a particular field. The books are richly illustrated and contain comprehensive bibliographies. Each chapter provides substantial background material relevant to the particular subject. These books contain detailed "tricks of the trade" and information as to where the methods presented can be safely applied. In addition, information on where to buy equipment and Web sites that will be helpful in solving both practical and theoretical problems are included.

We are working with these goals in mind and hope that as the books become available, the effort put in by the publisher, the book editors, and individual authors will contribute to the further development of dermatology research and clinical practice. The extent that we achieve this goal will be determined by the utility of these books.

Howard I. Maibach, M.D.
Series Editor

Preface

During the past decade there has been an explosion in new information relating to the biochemistry and pathology of the skin. As a result we are now beginning to understand the defects underlying some dry skin disorders and to recognize the complex interactions occurring between topically applied substances and the skin. Both the chemistry and the function of the skin are affected by vehicle ingredients in moisturizers, incorporated mainly due to their stability and viscosity-improving effects. Likewise, ordinary humectants exhibit other properties than just water binding and lipids may also affect skin barrier homeostasis. The new information opens up possibilities for further improvement of treatment of different dry skin disorders.

In this book the pharmaceutical and cosmetic industry will find important information for tailoring of moisturizers according to the underlying skin abnormality, rather than just aiming at a general increase of water content by occlusion or addition of humectants. Safety issues are also covered. Moreover, the book delivers information to dermatologists who would like to broaden and deepen their knowledge about dry skin and learn more about the effects of constituents in moisturizing creams and pharmaceutical preparations. Furthermore, experienced researchers will get inspiring and fruitful ideas due to the easily accessible information about neighboring research areas, which will promote new discoveries. Readers who wish to go deeper into topics in which they have a special interest are able to do so via the numerous references provided.

We are indebted to the 47 renowned international specialists who have contributed excellent chapters for the book. We sincerely hope that you will enjoy reading the book as much as we have enjoyed planning and receiving the chapters from these authors. Suggestions for improvements for a proposed second edition are appreciated.

We also wish to express our appreciation to Ms. Barbara Norwitz and Ms. Naomi Lynch at CRC Press for accelerating the editorial process.

Marie Lodén
Howard I. Maibach

The Editors

Marie Lodén, Pharm. Dr. Med. Sc., is Research Manager of the dermatological company ACO Hud AB, Stockholm, Sweden. She obtained her pharmacist degree in 1980 from Uppsala University and received her doctoral degree in Medical Science in 1995. She started her dermatological research with chemical warfare agents at the National Defense Research Institute and continued with development of topical products at a pharmaceutical company in Sweden. In 1992 she assumed her present position.

Dr. Lodén is a member of several national and international societies, such as the International Society for Bioengineering and the Skin, acts in the committee of the European Group of Efficacy Measurements of Cosmetics and Other Topical Products (EEMCO), and is President of the Scandinavian Society of Cosmetic Chemists (SCANCOS).

Dr. Lodén's major research interests are skin barrier function, contact dermatitis, skin care, biophysical measurements, and toxicology. She has published about 30 papers and book chapters.

Howard I. Maibach, M.D., is Professor of Dermatology, School of Medicine, University of California, San Francisco. Dr. Maibach graduated from Tulane University, New Orleans, LA (A.B. and M.D.), and received his research and clinical training at the University of Pennsylvania, Philadelphia. He received an honorary doctorate from the University of Paris Sud in 1988.

He has long had a laboratory and clinical interest in the effects of chemicals — including moisturizers — on normal and abnormal skin.

Dr. Maibach is a member of the International Contact Dermatitis Research Group, the North American Contact Dermatitis Group, and the European Environmental Contact Dermatitis Group. He is the author, co-author, and/or editor of 1600 publications and 60 volumes.

Contributors

Patricia A. Aikens
ICI Surfactants
Wilmington, DE

Yohini Appa, Ph.D.
Neutrogena Corporation
Los Angeles, CA

Bruce J. Aungst, Ph.D.
DuPont Pharmaceuticals
Wilmington, DE

Ebba Bárány, M.Sc. Pharm.
ACO HUD AB
Danderyd, Sweden

John Bartolone, Ph.D.
Department of Cell Biology and Physiology
Unilever Research
Colworth Laboratory
Sharnbrook, Bedford, U.K.

Martin Behne, M.D.
Departments of Medicine (Metabolism Section) and Dermatology
University of California, San Francisco
Medical and Dermatology Services
Department of Veterans Affairs Medical Center
San Francisco, CA

Enzo Berardesca, M.D.
Clinica Dermatologica
Mattéo Pavia, Italy

Ying Liu Boissy
Miami Valley Laboratories
Procter and Gamble
Cincinnati, OH

Barbara E. Brown, B.S.
Departments of Medicine (Metabolism Section) and Dermatology
University of California, San Francisco
Medical and Dermatology Services
Department of Veterans Affairs Medical Center
San Francisco, CA

Cornelia J. Calhoun, Ph.D.
Departments of Medicine (Metabolism Section) and Dermatology
University of California, San Francisco
Medical and Dermatology Services
Department of Veterans Affairs Medical Center
San Francisco, CA

Ai-Lean Chew, M.B., Ch.B.
Department of Dermatology
University of California
San Francisco, CA

Anton C. de Groot, M.D., Ph.D.
Department of Dermatology Carolus
'‘s-Hertogenbosch, the Netherlands

Mitsuhiro Denda, Ph.D.
Shiseido Research Center
Yokohama, Japan

Donald T. Downing, Ph.D.
Professor of Dermatology
Marshall Research Dermatology Laboratories
College of Medicine
University of Iowa
Iowa City, IA

Torbjörn Egelrud, M.D.
Professor
Department of Dermatology
University Hospital
Umeå, Sweden

Peter M. Elias, M.D.
Departments of Medicine (Metabolism Section) and Dermatology
University of California, San Francisco
Medical and Dermatology Services
Department of Veterans Affairs Medical Center
San Francisco, CA

Kenneth R. Feingold, M.D.
Departments of Medicine (Metabolism Section) and Dermatology
University of California, San Francisco
Medical and Dermatology Services
Department of Veterans Affairs Medical Center
San Francisco, CA

Eleanor J. Fendler
GoJo Industries, Inc.
Akron, OH

Joachim W. Fluhr, Dr. Med.
Department of Dermatology
Klinikum Karlsruhe
Karlsruhe, Germany

Bo Forslind, M.D., Ph.D.
Professor
Experimental Dermatology Research Group
Medical Biophysics, MBB
Karolinska Institute
Stockholm, Sweden

Stig E. Friberg, Ph.D.
Professor
Department of Chemistry
Clarkson University
Potsdam, NY

Bernard Gabard, Ph.D.
Department of Biopharmacy
Spirig Ltd. Pharmaceuticals
Egerkingen, Switzerland

Matti Hannuksela, M.D., Ph.D.
Director of Medical Services
South Karelia Central Hospital
Lappeenranta, Finland

Clive R. Harding, B.Sc.
Department of Cell Biology and Physiology
Unilever Research
Colworth Laboratory
Sharnbrook Bedford, U.K.

Ian Harris, Ph.D.
Beiersdorf AG
Hamburg, Germany

Walter M. Holleran, Pharm. D.
Departments of Medicine (Metabolism Section) and Dermatology
University of California, San Francisco
Medical and Dermatology Services
Department of Veterans Affairs Medical Center
San Francisco, CA

Udo Hoppe, Ph.D.
Professor
Beiersdorf AG
Hamburg, Germany

Zenro Ikezawa, M.D.
Yokohama City University
Urfune Hospital
Yokohama, Japan

Genji Imokawa, Ph.D.
Institute for Fundamental Research
Kao Corporation
Haga, Tochigi, Japan

Albert Kligman, M.D., Ph.D.
Department of Dermatology
University of Pennsylvania
Philadelphia, PA

Ludger Kolbe, Ph.D.
Paul Gerson Unna Research Center
Hamburg, Germany

Noel D. Lazo, Ph.D.
Marshall Research Dermatology Laboratories
College of Medicine
University of Iowa
Iowa City, IA

Magnus Lindberg, M.D., Ph.D.
Associate Professor
Experimental Dermatology Research Group
Department of Dermatology
University Hospital
Stockholm, Sweden

Marie Lodén, Dr. Med. Sci.
ACO HUD AB
Research and Development
Danderyd, Sweden

Howard I. Maibach, M.D.
Professor
University of California Hospital
San Francisco, CA

David S. Morrison, Ph.D.
Penreco Technology Center
Woodlands, TX

Donald S. Orth, Ph.D.
Neutrogena Corporation
Los Angeles, CA

Jan Pallon, Ph.D.
Associate Professor
Department of Nuclear Physics
Lund University
Stockholm, Sweden

Danielle Quiec, Ph.D.
Departments of Medicine (Metabolism Section) and Dermatology
University of California, San Francisco
Medical and Dermatology Services
Department of Veterans Affairs Medical Center
San Francisco, CA

Anthony V. Rawlings, Ph.D.
Department of Cell Biology and Physiology
Unilever Research
Colworth Laboratory
Sharnbrook Bedford, U.K.

Lesley E. Rhodes, Ph.D.
Dermatology Unit
Department of Medicine
Liverpool, U.K.

Donald Rudikoff, M.D.
The Mount Sinai Medical Center
Department of Dermatology
The Mount Sinai Hospital
New York, NY

David Salter, M.A., M.Sc.
Professor
Cussons (International) Limited
Stockport, U.K.

Mary Ellen Stewart, Ph.D.
Associate Research Scientist
Marshall Research Dermatology Laboratories
College of Medicine
University of Iowa
Iowa City, IA

Christian Surber
Department of Biopharmacy
Spirig Ltd. Pharmaceuticals
Egerkingen, Switzerland

Motoji Takahashi, Ph.D.
Shiseido Research Center
Yokohama, Japan

Monica Tammela, Ph.D.
Medical Products Agency
Uppsala, Sweden

Carl Thornfeldt, M.D.
Cellegy Pharmaceuticals Inc.
Foster City, CA

Anders Vahlquist, M.D., Ph.D.
Professor
Department of Dermatology and Venereology
University Hospital
Uppsala, Sweden

Hisashi Wakita, M.D.
Department of Dermatology
Hamamatsu University
School of Medicine
Hamamatsu, Japan

Ronald R. Warner, Ph.D.
Miami Valley Laboratories
Procter and Gamble
Cincinnati, OH

Contents

PART 3
DRY SKIN AND HYPERKERATOTIC CONDITIONS

PART 4
FORMULATIONS AND INTERACTIONS WITH THE SKIN

Part 1

Dry Skin and Moisturizers

1 Introduction

Albert Kligman

CONTENTS

The intent of this preview is to present a general background for the detailed accounts which follow. These perspectives derive from a long-term involvement with a rapidly developing field, in which the marketplace has created a cornucopia of products which largely lack scientific support. Controversies abound making it extremely difficult to separate the wheat from the chaff. This volume comprehensively summarizes current knowledge of the field of moisturization, covering all aspects from basic science to clinical practice. This voluminous text is indispensable for the diverse players in the lively field of skin care: the cadre of scientists who specialize in the biology of skin whether in industry or in academia, various breeds of clinicians (especially dermatologists), merchandizers of skin care products, governmental regulators, etc.

A great majority of women apply moisturizers to their hands and faces daily for what amounts to their adult lifetime. It thus behooves skin care specialists of all stripes to possess a comprehensive knowledge of the diverse effects of these multitudinous products, good and bad, short and long term.

This volume is the first of its kind covering all aspects of moisturizers, a subject which receives short shrift in dermatologic texts. Evidently moisturizers are deemed to be beneath the notice of serious scholars and are downgraded to the category of cosmeceuticals, slightly above the vulgar level of cosmetics. This is an egregious disservice to an important subject in the broad field of skin care and provides a fertile ground for the unscrupulous to promote products based on consumer appeal and not on scientific substantiation of safety and efficacy. Products that feel good and look good are often not good for skin health. There is an urgent need to make consumers aware of these quandaries.

An authoritative volume is long overdue to bring up to date the impressive advances in our knowledge of the stratum corneum. The contributors are mostly world class scientists, recognized internationally in their field of expertise. This is a magnum opus which will enable the parvenu to get a firm grasp of a complex and fascinating subject.

1.1 WHAT IS A MOISTURIZER?

Curiously, no consensus exists regarding the definition of a *moisturizer*. The term itself is a neologism coined by Madison Avenue marketers, promoting the facile idea that moisturizers moisten the skin and thereby keep it soft and supple. But wetting the skin only transiently relieves dryness. Showering 15 times daily or immersion of dry legs in water for ten 5-minute exposures is *not* only not beneficial, but may be harmful by removing water-binding soluble substances which make up the natural moisturizing factor. We learn from this that for moisturizers to be effective they must

0-8493-7520-7/00/$0.00+$.50

do a good deal more than moisten. In fact, we are confronted with unsolved complexities in explaining how moisturizers work. Surprisingly, there is no internationally accepted definition of what constitutes dry skin. This is a troublesome question because dry skin may lack water only in the two or three superficial desquamating layers but may be normally hydrated in the coherent portion below. Then, too, the surface may look soft and smooth but actually be dry, a paradox often seen on the face where sebum conceals scales. There is also a widespread misconception that dryness is the opposite of oiliness. In fact, dryness comprises a spectrum ranging from dry to non-dry, whereas oiliness depicts oily vs. non-oily. These are not semantic squabblings, but they can cause considerable confusion in the minds of consumers. Then, too, patients and doctors often disagree regarding the degree of dryness or oiliness. A predominance of women think they have dry skin because of a lack of natural oil; however, measurements of sebum production do not confirm this widespread estimate. Given these misperceptions how can manufacturers rationally target the consumers of their specialty products.

Those who work in this area often use an operational definition which states that "moisturizers are substances used to reduce the signs and symptoms of dry, scaly skin, making the rough surface soft and smooth." This definition lacks specificity and includes "barrier" creams which are used to prevent the development of chronic dermatoses usually in occupational settings.

Barrier creams also are not exempt from controversy. They are praised by some and condemned by others, depending upon whether the exposure is to water-soluble irritants or oil-soluble ones. This is certainly an area where the knowledge contained in this volume will lead to improved products.

Dry, xerotic states of skin are often denigrated as merely cosmetic nuisances, disagreeable but without medical significance. In the elderly, however, dry skin is ubiquitous and often associated with pruritus. Itching by itself is serious because it disturbs sleep, becoming a preoccupation which adversely affects the quality of life, leading to testiness and even depression. In addition, scratching breaks the barrier, sometimes followed by infection with pyogenic organisms, especially b-hemolytic streptococci. This is largely subclinical and usually goes unrecognized because of the absence of fever and suppuration. Such patients are unwell, fatigued, and listless. The sad consequence is that the antibiotic which would promptly lead to a cure is not prescribed. In nursing homes, in particular, these misdiagnosed patients are treated with whatever topical creams happen to be in the supply room, often free samples that are not only worthless but potentially harmful. Scratching leads to more pruritus owing to implantation into the dermis of fragments of stratum corneum which is rich in pro-inflammatory cytokines. This culminates in the dreaded itch–scratch–itch cycle, a vicious despoiler of equanimity.

Attention is called to another situation in which dry skin turns out to be very serious, even life-threatening. Epidemiologists have established beyond doubt that dry skin is a precursor to decubitus ulcers (pressure sores) in immobilized patients. Only a handful of geriatricians know that cracked, dry skin is a major risk factor for the development of pressure sores in hospitalized, motionless, bedridden patients who cannot be turned frequently. These patients are routinely not treated with an appropriate moisturizer, such as petrolatum which could help prevent friction, thus reducing the likelihood of cracks in the stratum corneum barrier.

Another serious but unrecognized problem, amenable to moisturizers, is the fragility of the skin of the hands and forearms of elderly women, especially those with strong signs of photodamage. In these thin-skinned women minor traumas lead to bursts of purpura in which erythrocytes escape into the skin producing long-lasting bruises. The tendency of this skin to tear and rupture after minor trauma leads to unsightly white stellate scars. These events are certainly not trivial cosmetic complaints.

The simple fact is that moisturizers do a good deal more than moisten dry skin. Their effects are multifunctional and cannot always be explained by current scientific knowledge. Clinicians have long recognized that traditional emollients have an important place in the treatment of chronic dermatoses, such as atopic dermatitis and psoriasis, where their beneficial effects may be due in part to restoration of an impaired barrier. Emollients may also function as adjuncts to anti-inflammatory drugs such as corticosteroids or in conjunction with phototherapy such as PUVA. This is an appropriate place to point out that controlled clinical trials often refer to the unmedicated emollient vehicle as the "placebo." This is incorrect. All emollients have some measurable effect on the structure and the function of the stratum corneum and are not inert placebos used to please the patient.

Moisturizers used daily for 6 months or more are also surprisingly effective for the treatment of photodamaged facial skin. Of course, this skin is also dry. It is not so surprising to learn that old-fashioned moisturizers such as lanolin and petrolatum or emulsions containing these can moderately efface fine lines, overcome dryness, reduce mottling, make the surface smoother, and improve texture.

1.2 THE MOISTURIZER MARKETPLACE

The marketplace is awash with a flood of brand-name moisturizers which crowd the shelves of supermarkets. Each one is touted for its peerless beneficial effects. Manufacturers have added a great variety of "actives" to basic emulsions, raising these up to the level of functional cosmeceuticals. This tactic expands the indications for the use of moisturizers to various categories of common conditions such as eczemas, photoaging, and "sensitive skin," another mystery area where basic knowledge is soon to bring enlightenment. It is current dogma that patients with "sensitive" skin have defective barriers, but the evidence so far is unconvincing.

It must always be remembered that xerotic skin is not a single diagnostic entity. Indeed, dry skin syndromes encompass a large family of unrelated disorders such as hereditary ichthyosis, winter xerosis, chronic irritant and allergic dermatitis, chronic endogenous dermatoses, photoaged skin, etc. Xerotic skin is a reaction pattern to a variety of disorders which have in common abnormalities of desquamation; namely, the tendency for corneocytes to be shed as large scales made up of many thousands of corneocytes instead of as tiny clusters, an invisible process. Scales make the surface look and feel dry, obscuring the glyphic patterns and replacing smooth-textured skin with a roughened, flaky appearance. The clinical manifestations of ichthyotic and dry, xerotic states are mainly expressed as abnormalities of the stratum corneum; the common pathological feature is abnormal desquamation. However, it is naive to suppose that the deficit is localized to the stratum corneum. A defective horny layer ineluctably reflects earlier changes in the viable epidermis below involving disturbances in the pattern of differentiation as keratinocytes become cornified and make their way to the surface to be shed. An abnormal horny layer is always subtended by an abnormal epidermis. In the end one is not simply treating the visibly abnormal horny layer, but more fundamentally the abnormalities below.

It is important for the clinician to diagnose the underlying condition in order to select the appropriate moisturizer. No single formulation can be effective against the diverse family of xerotic disorders. For example, the treatment of the various familial ichthyoses requires exfoliating agents, often wrongly called keratolytics, aimed at removing excessive horn. These include α-hydroxy acids, salicylic acid, propylene glycol, urea, and mixtures of these. These same agents may be harmful on the dry face, often causing neurosensory reactions such as itching, burning, and stinging as well as scaling and redness.

It is all but impossible for the consumer, or for that matter the generalist, to select the optimal moisturizer from the huge inventory of products sold at cosmetic counters and supermarkets. The marketplace for moisturizers is highly competitive, forcing producers to create a steady stream of new products to obtain market share, usually accompanied by exorbitant claims. Newness often resides in nothing more than adding trendy ingredients. Fueling this rushing stream of novel products is the current consumer preference for "naturals," meaning no synthetic chemicals. Consumers are susceptible to the totally irrational bias that *natural* is somehow fundamentally safe and desirable. The idea has become entrenched that we are living in a world where toxic chemicals are everywhere and threaten our well-being. This universal chemophobia extends to skin care products, encouraging some unscrupulous marketers to take out full page ads showing how dangerous, even lethal, are products produced by leading cosmetic companies! The "natural" craze is nonsense. Nature abounds in harmful materials. For example, heavy metals such as lead, mercury, and arsenic are completely natural but have caused severe toxicity, even deaths, when incorporated into topicals. Poison ivy plants are also natural, though capable of causing a maddening, pruritic dermatitis. A huge number of botanicals, originating from ancient folklore remedies, especially Chinese, are now appearing in myriads of products. For the most effective way to ruin the skin in early life, nothing matches excessive exposure to sunlight, which many people worship with religious zeal. Is anything more natural than sunlight?

The numbers game has added an element of craziness to the frenetic marketplace of moisturizers. This game is predicated on the spurious belief that more is better. The ingredients are not only increasingly numerous but more diverse, satisfying the popular desire for more "actives." New terms such as *dermaceuticals* and *neutraceuticals* add medical glamour to such multi-ingredient products. So we find moisturizers containing vitamins A, B, C, D, and E, a melange of anti-oxidants, minerals (selenium, copper), various micronutrients, exfoliating enzymes (papain), humectants (urea, glycerin), ad infinitum. In no case has it been demonstrated that the removal of any one of the many ingredients making up these preposterous cocktails would lessen efficacy. It is commonplace for moisturizers to contain 2 to 3 dozen or more "active" ingredients which are intended to seduce consumers into pricey purchases while avoiding the regulatory snare of being classified as drugs.

Despite all this commercial hawking, there is no doubt that the major skin care companies in Europe, Japan, and the U.S. have produced a variety of effective products whose benefits have been reasonably well substantiated. Large international companies have too much at stake to sell ineffective or hazardous products. Lacking reliable guidelines for choosing the optimal moisturizer, the intelligent consumer would be well advised to avoid unknown fly-by-night companies which promise fantastic benefits.

1.3 HOW DO MOISTURIZERS WORK?

This is not only the most exciting area in the whole field, but also the one in which basic scientists have made the most progress, giving us deeper insights all the way down to the molecular level.

Because the xerotic states are expressed in a deranged stratum corneum, major effects have been made, using advanced technologies, to better understand the structure and function of the horny layer barrier. In this volume, such masters as Elias, Downing, Imokawa, Rawling, and their many colleagues present detailed accounts of a multiplicity of new findings regarding the formation of the horny layer.

Until recently the stratum corneum was thought to have a single function, a protective one; namely, its remarkable ability to retard the diffusion of substance into and out of the skin. Without a barrier we would all dry out and life on earth would be impossible. The barrier was viewed as a passive membrane which acted as a kind of impermeable plastic wrap to keep vital substances from leaking into the environment while preventing noxious exogenous materials from penetrating to living tissue. Suddenly the quite dead stratum corneum has come very much alive. Without nuclei and DNA, corneocytes cannot synthesize anything. Nonetheless, corneocytes undergo dramatic transformations when first formed until they complete their argosy to the surface where they are shed.

The stratum corneum is metabolically very much alive. A great array of studies dealing with the biochemistry of lipids, enzymes, keratin filaments, the cornified envelope, and filaggrin, abetted by studies of ultrastructure, has begun to reveal the long-hidden mysteries of how the stratum corneum actually functions. Powerful new tools, such as electron probes, freeze fracture, nuclear magnetic resonance, X-ray crystallography, and post-osmium ruthenium staining, have made it possible to study the most intricate, hitherto invisible anatomical features of this remarkable tissue. For clinicians, the chapters describing the minute findings of these new technologies will make for daunting reading. Still, nowhere else can one find in one place studies of such depth, clarity, and comprehensiveness. As a reference source this volume has no equal and will not soon be outdated.

In addition to its essential role as a "barrier" and protective membrane against chemical, physical, and mechanical insults, a multitude of other complementary functions of the stratum corneum have come to light. These include regulation of homeostatic mechanisms to assure steady-state conditions in the face of an ever-changing environment, mechanisms of repair after disruption of the barrier by disease or exogenous insults, the presence of antibacterial substances (defenses) which protect against infection by the enormous number and variety of potential pathogens in our microbe-infested environment, a depot of pro-inflammatory cytokines which serve as early warning systems to mobilize appropriate adaptive reactions against external threats, and a semiotic signaling device for sensing changes which are then transmitted to the tissue below. The stratum corneum even serves as a depot for the storage of lipophilic drugs such as corticosteroids, which now explains why once-daily applications with potent steroids are therapeutically equivalent to twice- or thrice-daily applications.

With this still unfolding exciting background, we can return to the question "How do moisturizers work?" The subject could be quickly dispatched by the bold statement that we really do not know, and much of what we think we know is wrong. The fact is that the customary explanations in the trade literature are too simplistic.

For example, manufacturers instinctively put various humectants into their formulations because these are thought to be capable of picking up and holding water, without which the horny layer would become dry and brittle, subject to cracking. The well-known humectants include urea, propylene glycol, glycerin, and hydroxy-acids (especially lactic), all of which take up water in a humid atmosphere. But where does this water come from in the real world where in the winter months, low humidities prevail over the dry skin season? It turns out that humectants are beneficial at low humidities. In the worst case scenario, one could imagine that humectants would have to draw water from the wet tissue down below, thus depleting the water level in the lower stratum corneum.

The so-called natural moisturizing factors (NMF) which are assigned the function of keeping the horny layer hydrated and flexible are made up of a mix of low molecular weight soluble hygroscopic substances, including lactic acid, pyrollidone-carboxylic acid, and amino acids. But including these humectants in moisturizers is not always salutary. High concentrations of propylene glycol and urea can be irritating and cause a variety of subjective and objective signs of irritation. Then, too, it does not necessarily follow that external applications of components of the NMF will be effective, because water-soluble substances are notoriously incapable of penetrating into the barrier. Pure mixtures of amino acids are useless as moisturizers. Pure solutions of the most celebrated humectants, such as glycerin, are ineffective, and propylene glycol by itself may be harmful.

The point here is that other mechanisms are at play and are probably more influential than mere humectancy. For example, propylene glycol and lactic acid promote detachment of superficial corneocytes, acting as exfoliants that remove loose surface scales, immediately making the surface smoother. This explains the phenomenal success of the α-hydroxy acids in the marketplace. Consumers immediately recognize that the surface has become smoother and less scaly. A completely different story applies to glycerin, a long-time star in the firmament of moisturizers. It, too, promotes desquamation but by an entirely unexpected mechanism; namely, by enhancing the action of chymotrypsin-like proteases which attack the corneodesmosomes that rivet corneocytes together. This could not have been imagined a few years ago.

Urea, in addition to humectancy, causes unfolding and denaturation of proteins leading to dehiscence of corneocytes. Nails immersed in 40% urea literally dissolve into a soft mush. In fact, the actions of urea on the stratum corneum are in dispute. Some think that urea enhances penetration by making the barrier more permeable. Others deny that urea can diffuse into the horny layer and give no credence to its supposed role as a penetration enhancer. An unheralded benefit of urea is its ability to deodorize smelly, suppurating lesions, because of its broad-spectrum antibacterial actions.

The message here is that our concept of humectants falls far short of explaining how they work. It is worth repeating that used alone they are not much good. It is when they are properly formulated with other ingredients that their potential benefits are realized. Other factors such as pH also have to be taken into account, because the proteases which lead to orderly desquamation of horny cells within the stratum corneum are activated only at acid pHs of 4 to 5. Interestingly, the renowned acid mantle hypothesis seems at last to have been validated! Also the various hydrolytic enzymes, which are found in the stratum corneum and which are essential to the formation of the intercorneocyte lipids that establish the impermeability of the barrier, are activated only at acid pHs. All these insights represent triumphs of biochemistry.

1.4 HYDROPHOBIC GREASES

The prototypes in this category of moisturizers are lanolin, petrolatum, and various vegetable oils. As usual, the accounts of their modes of action are incomplete, simplistic, and often downright wrong.

Lanolin is the grandfather of all of these, having been used for centuries to protect the hands of wool gatherers. According to standard teaching anhydrous lanolin forms an occlusive film on the surface preventing the loss of water, enabling it to accumulate and hydrate the horny layer. This is simply not true. After liberal applications, 3.5 mg/cm^2, transepidermal water loss measured by evaporimetry decreases moderately for up to 10 to 15 minutes and then normalizes rather rapidly.

The fact is that lanolin is a good emulsifier which forms stable emulsions in the presence of water. USP hydrous lanolin is an oil-in-water emulsion which is quite effective in various xerotic states. Moreover, there is evidence from tracer studies that lanolin penetrates into the horny layer, via the lipophilic intercellular spaces.

Lanolin is a complex mixture of sterols, sterol esters, and alcohols which probably act in different ways to relieve the signs and symptoms of dry skin. One can theorize that certain constituents, such as cholesterol, might traverse the horny layer and reach the viable granular layer where they might be endocytosed and secreted by exocytosis into the intercellular space. They might even be metabolized in the granular layer to effect the lipid synthesis of cholesterol, fatty acids, and ceramides. We know nothing about these possibilities. Theoretically, lanolin could work exogenously and endogenously, if it reaches the cellular epidermis. Perhaps it is not too fanciful to think of finding the skin with precursor lipids which would become incorporated into lamellar bodies with subsequent metabolic processing ending up in the intercellular spaces along with endogenous lipids, resulting in an improved barrier.

Regrettably dermatologists at large look with disfavor on lanolin and its derivatives, because they are victims of the delusion that these are strong contact allergens. Lanolin is one of the best of the moisturizers, and one can hope that knowledge of its multifarious effects on skin will not only reinstate lanolin but provide us with useful insights regarding the biology of the horny layer.

Petrolatum is an altogether different case, a mixture of hydrocarbons deriving from the fractional distillation of petrolatum. After application, it strongly inhibits transepidermal water loss for 2 to 3 hours; hence, it does form an occlusive film. But again, this does not fully explain its beneficial effects as a moisturizer. Tracer studies show that petrolatum enters the intercellular lipid-filled spaces throughout the entire width of the horny layer, obscuring the stacks of lipid bilayers which comprise the actual barrier to the penetration of exogenous materials. Its physical presence throughout the intercellular lipid pathways should fortify the barrier and further limit water loss. It does not reach the viable layers and so cannot be metabolized. Here again we know all too little about this complex material and the specific effects which have enabled it to acquire its reputation as the paterfamilias of moisturizers. Calling it occlusive (which then occludes further thought) causes us to ignore lesser known effects, such as its ability to prevent the formation of ultraviolet-induced tumors in the skin of hairless mice, even though it is not a sunscreen. It also seems to possess some nonspecific, anti-inflammatory activity, for which there is no adequate explanation.

It is worth noting that some of the best of the old-fashioned, venerable moisturizers are mixtures of lanolin and petrolatum, a powerful duo which acting in different ways could complement each other to enhance the beneficial effect. It cannot be too strongly emphasized that the best moisturizers are artful compositions containing a complex mixture of ingredients that work well together.

Finally, many dermatologists, having been badly misled by their mentors who hand down therapeutic secrets which they have gleaned from clinical practice, recommend a melange of vegetable oils including olive oil, safflower oil, Crisco, cocoa butter, and many others derived from the annals of folklore. None of these has been validated by controlled studies.

These are not completely worthless since all oils, regardless of origin, can moderate the appearance of dry, rough, scaly skin. Comparative studies in our laboratories always end in the judgment that these are marginally beneficial, especially in comparison to modern moisturizers. Some sadistic dermatologists opine that lard is an effective moisturizer!

Clinicians are not in a good position to make sound judgments regarding the efficacy of moisturizers, a task that is not so easy as it seems.

1.5 EPILOGUE

The past two decades have witnessed brilliant discoveries regarding the structure and functions of the stratum corneum. Scientists from diverse disciplines have converged upon the stratum corneum as a new territory whose exploration has yielded exciting insights, promising novel therapeutic possibilities.

The dramatic story of the rebirth of the stratum corneum as a homeostatic membrane signaling and responding to external changes is by no means nearing a final act. New revelations appear monthly; these are not merely academic abstractions. They pave the way for new opportunities to improve the therapeutic efficacy of topical drugs and cosmeceuticals. With the power of modern technology, the fabled barrier might become selectively permeable to a great variety of potentially useful substances, including proteins, cytokines, immunomodulators, enzymes, and a host of other substances now excluded from entry into living tissue. New physical tools will make it possible to drive a wide variety of substances into skin by temporarily altering the barrier. Reaching the level of practicality are such techniques as electroporation, sonophoresis, iontophoresis, and high voltage single pulses.

The most stunning revelation may be that of Pfeiffer's group in Hamburg whose findings not only are revolutionary, but well-nigh incredible. They proclaim that our present concepts of the structure of the stratum corneum are mainly artifacts of fixation. Through ultrastructural studies we think we have a good idea of the subcellular features of keratinocytes, but we may be sizing what is actually there in the native state. Using high-pressure cryofixation, they boldly suggest that our fabled granular layer with its distinctive keratohyaline granules is fiction, due to a violent assault on native structures resulting from our current methods of fixation. For example, organelles may not be distributed throughout the entoplasm as currently believed but may be localized in special domains. Is it possible that almost everything we have painfully learned is an artifact of processing?

So, welcome to the wonderful world of the stratum corneum, whose once sturdy walls, like medieval castles, are crumbling under the irresistible armaments of high technology.

Part 2

Biochemistry and Function of the Skin

2 Epidermal Composition

Donald T. Downing and Mary Ellen Stewart

CONTENTS

2.1 INTRODUCTION

The structure and composition of the epidermis are of interest to those who wish to understand how the barrier function of mammalian skin resists the transpiration of water through the skin. The barrier property is also of obvious interest to those who wish to provide cosmetic or pharmaceutical treatment through application to the skin surface. This introductory chapter aims to provide a brief overview of the structure and function of the epidermis as they relate to these barrier properties.

0-8493-7520-7/00/$0.00+$.50

2.2 STRUCTURE AND FUNCTION OF THE EPIDERMIS

2.2.1 Anatomy of the Epidermis

Detailed knowledge of the structure of mammalian epidermis began with the examination of histologically prepared sections using the light microscope. Much of what is known of the general organization of the epidermis was learned with this technique, including observations of cell division in the innermost, basal layer; the spiny appearance of several layers of cells above the basal layer; the granular appearance of several more layers of cells above the spiny layer; and many layers of flattened, apparently disjunctive cells in the outer, cornified layer.

More details have emerged from subsequent studies of the epidermis using the electron microscope,[1,2] including the presence of the lamellar granules in the spinous and granular cells; the abundance of cytoplasmic filaments within all of the viable cells,[1,3] the organization of desmosomes (Chapter 9 by Egelrud); and the presence of lipid lamellae between the cells of the cornified layer.[4,5] Perhaps most significant for theories of epidermal barrier function was the electron microscopic observation that the cells of the cornified layer are closely adherent to each other, rather than having a disjunctive, basketweave appearance as seen in light micrographs. Some of the principal anatomical features of the epidermis are shown in Figure 1.

2.2.1.1 Basal Cells

This innermost layer is responsible for the generation of new tissue by cell division.[1,6] Each cell is attached to its neighbors by desmosomes and to the basement membrane, adjacent to the dermis, by hemidesmosomes. On the dermal side of the basement membrane, anchoring fibrils aid in adherence of the basal cells to the dermis.

2.2.1.2 Spinous Cells

Daughter cells produced by cell division move away from the basal layer to become spinous cells, the spiny appearance of which is due to the strains of cell-to-cell attachment through desmosomes. Bundles of keratin fibers stream throughout each cell to produce a strengthening framework of attachments between the desmosomes and the nucleus.[3] Displaced by the continual cell division in the basal layer, cells move upward through the spinous layer.

As the spinous cells mature, they accumulate the specialized organelles named variously as Odland bodies, membrane-coating granules, lamellar bodies, granular bodies, and lamellar granules, the general appearance of which is indicated in Figure 2.

2.2.1.3 Granular Cells

The description of the cells in this layer results from the granular appearance produced by deposits of keratohyalin, which were seen in early investigations using the light microscope, and not from the appearance of the lamellar granules, which are much smaller and are only observed with the electron microscope.[1] Usually, there are two to four layers of cells in the granular layer, and the keratohyalin granules increase in size in the outer granular cells. The numbers of lamellar granules increase as the granular cells move toward the skin surface, and these granules tend to accumulate in the outer (apical) side of the cytoplasm in each cell.

2.2.1.4 Transition Cells

The outermost cells of the granular layer become transformed into the dead, flattened cells of the cornified layer. However, cells in the process of this transition can be observed to gradually lose their subcellular organelles, including the nucleus and cytoplasmic membrane structures.[8] During this process, the keratohyalin granules begin to fuse with the keratin filament bundles, with a

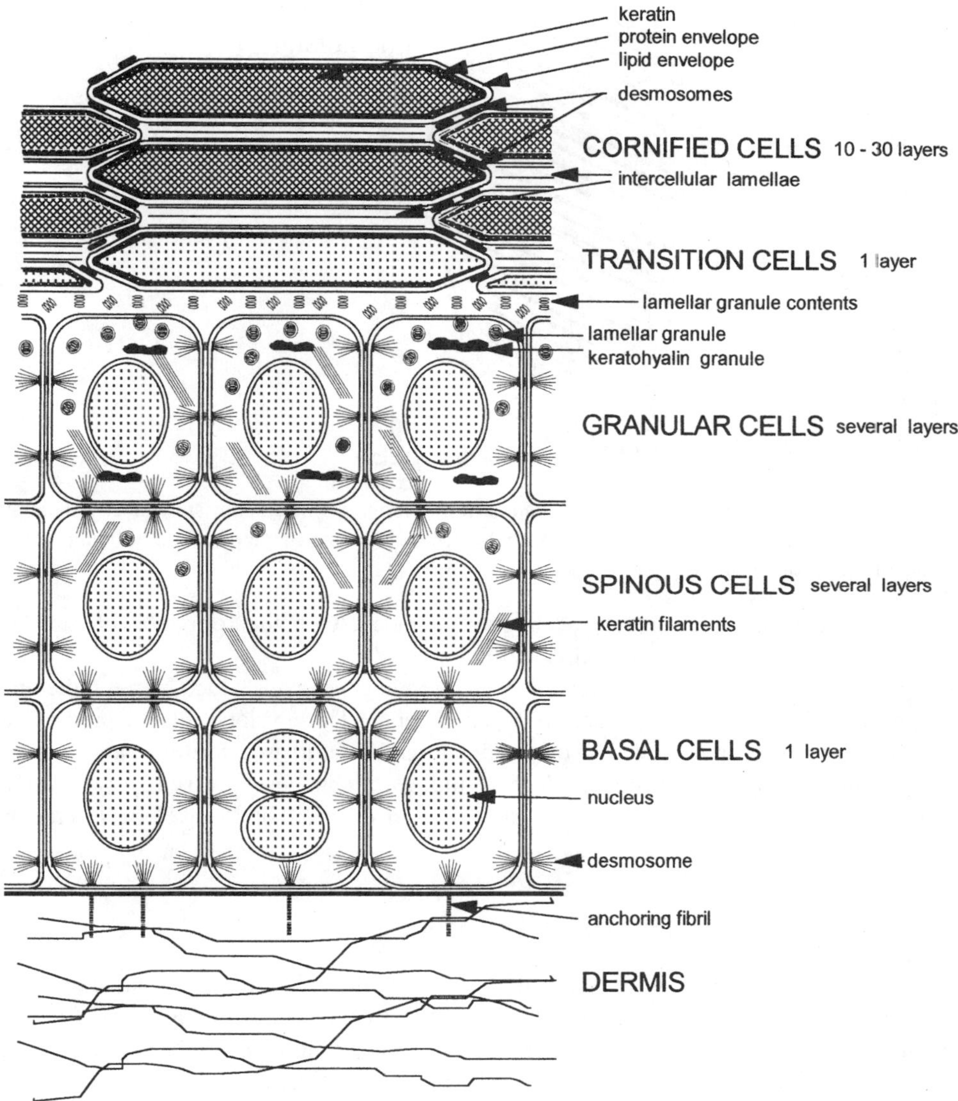

FIGURE 1 Some of the changes occurring during epidermal differentiation that are relevant to development of the lipid structures involved in the permeability barrier which resides in the stratum corneum intercellular lamellae.

consequent loss of the granular appearance of the cell.[1,8] In addition, the lamellar granule contents are discharged from the cells into the intercellular space above the cell by fusion of the bounding membrane of each lamellar body with the cell membrane, followed by the extrusion of the granule's content of lamellar disks.[1,7,8]

2.2.1.5 Cornified Cells

Following discharge of the lamellar granule contents into the intercellular space, the transition cell completes its transformation into the flat, keratin-filled cell of the stratum corneum.[8] This process entails the complete digestion of all subcellular organelles so that all that remains within the cell is the tightly packed raft of keratin fibrils that are oriented roughly parallel to the long dimension of the cell.[1] Between the keratin fibers is a matrix consisting of the remains of the keratohyalin.

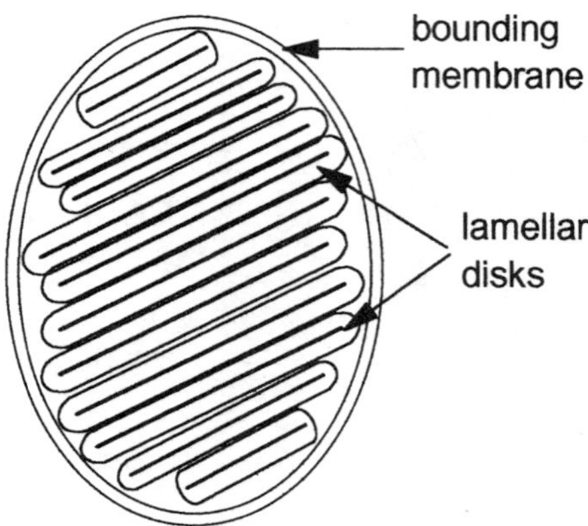

FIGURE 2 The lamellar granule is a roughly ovoid body 100 nm in diameter, consisting of a lipid membrane surrounding one or more stacks of circular disks, with each disk having the appearance of being formed by the collapse of a liposome, as indicated in Figure 4.

The protein of this matrix appears to be largely degraded, with the formation of mostly low molecular weight material, including individual amino acids.

During the cornification process, the corneocyte protein envelope is added between the internal surface of the cell membrane and the stacks of keratin fibers.[1,9] The envelope consists predominantly of proteins that have been cross-linked by the action of transglutaminases, forming isopeptide bonds between glutamine and lysine residues.[9] The resulting protein envelope is highly resistant to digestion by enzymes and is the substrate to which an external lipid envelope is chemically attached[10-12] (Chapter 4).

2.3 LIPID STRUCTURES IN THE EPIDERMIS

Lipids are involved in a number of anatomical structures in the epidermal cells that are significant in the structure and function of the tissue.[13] These include the plasma membranes of the individual cells; a variety of internal cytoplasmic cell membranes,[1] including the endoplasmic reticulum, the Golgi bodies, and the bounding membranes of the lamellar granules in the living cells; and the lipids which constitute the intercellular lamellae between the cornified cells. The composition of the lipids in these structures have, for the most part, been established by isolation of material from the respective cell layers and, in some cases, individual organelles, followed by extraction and analysis of the constituent lipids.

2.3.1 LIPIDS OF THE LIVING CELLS

Early investigations aimed at the isolation and lipid analysis of specific cell layers in the epidermis were of limited success and, for the most part, were conducted before knowledge of the unique chemical structures of the epidermal lipids were known. After the lipid structures had been determined, an analysis of the total lipid composition of the viable cells of the epidermis was obtained through isolation of full thickness epidermis of pigs using heat separation, followed by trypsin digestion of the uncornified cells. The digest was then freeze dried, and the lipids were extracted with chloroform/methanol mixtures. The extracted lipids consisted principally of phospholipids, cholesterol, and glucosylceramides, with trace amounts of free fatty acids, triglycerides,

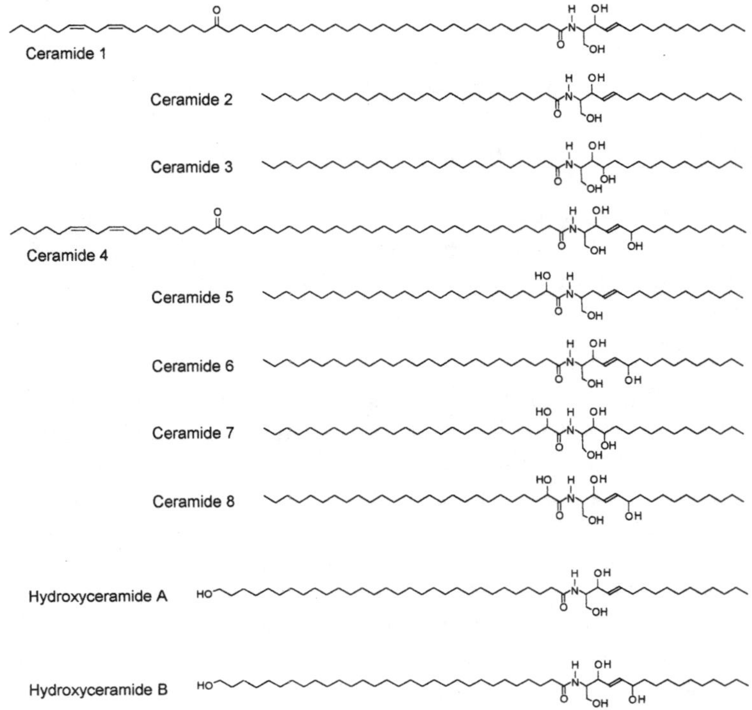

FIGURE 3 Chemical structures of the ceramides of human stratum corneum.

and ceramides.[14] From this, it can be deduced that the living cells of the epidermis are quite similar in lipid composition to cells in other mammalian tissues, in that the membranes are composed predominantly of phospholipids and cholesterol. It has further been assumed that the high content of glucosylceramides in the trypsin-digested cells are derived from the lamellar granules of the spinous and granular cells. This is supported by the observation that the trypsin digest contains many intact lamellar granules and by the analysis of lipids extracted from isolated lamellar granules, which were found to be rich in glucosylceramides.[15] It seems likely that the membranes of the living cells of the epidermis contain mostly phospholipids and cholesterol, while the lamellar granules contain mainly glucosylceramides.

2.3.2 Lipids of the Cornified Cells

2.3.2.1 Solvent-Extractable Lipids

After trypsin digestion of the living cells of full thickness epidermis, the cornified layer remains as an intact sheet that can be extracted with chloroform/methanol to obtain the free lipids of the horny layer. Electron micrographs show that these lipids reside principally in the intercellular spaces between the cornified cells,[4,16] with no evidence of lipids within the cells. The extracted lipids of pig stratum corneum were found to consist mainly of ceramides (45%); cholesterol (25%); free fatty acids (15%); and 2 to 3% each of triglycerides, cholesterol sulfate, sphingosine, and phospholipids.[5,17]

The free lipids extractable from human stratum corneum contain a mixture of ceramides similar to those in pig epidermis, but they also contain a unique series of ceramides in which the sphingoid base is 6-hydroxysphingosine.[18,19] The structures of the ceramides from human epidermis are shown in Figure 3.

2.3.2.2 Protein-Bound Lipids

After exhaustive extraction of the free lipids from isolated pig stratum corneum, mild alkaline hydrolysis liberates additional lipids consisting mostly of ceramides formed from very long chain (C_{30}-C_{34}) ω-hydroxyacids in amide linkage with sphingosine.[10,12] Electron micrographs show that these bound lipids of the stratum corneum form a lipid envelope on the exterior of the protein envelope.[11,14,16,20]

In human stratum corneum, the protein-bound lipids include a second hydroxyceramide in which the base is the novel 6-hydroxysphingosine.[18] The structures of the two protein-bound hydroxyceramides of human stratum corneum are included in Figure 3.

2.3.3 Extraneous Lipids

Attempts to analyze the composition of epidermal lipids, especially those of the surface layers, should always take into account the likelihood of contamination by lipids from the environment and also by lipids produced by the sebaceous glands in the skin. In most species, including humans, copious amounts of sebaceous lipids anoint the skin surface, even in those areas that may be free of sebaceous glands, such as the palms and soles. It should also be noted that the palms and soles contain a much smaller proportion of lipids than other areas of the skin and have a much poorer barrier function. To obtain an analysis of human epidermal lipid uncontaminated by sebum, it was necessary to resort to extraction of the lipids from excised epidermal cysts.[21] The cyst contents contained no wax esters or squalene (markers of human sebum) and therefore can be accepted as being free from sebaceous lipids.

Extraneous lipids in human epidermal lipids which have been traced to the environment include the paraffin hydrocarbons that are ubiquitous in human epidermis. Gas chromatographic analyses of these hydrocarbons show that they are similar in composition to those in higher boiling petroleum distillates such as petrolatum.[22] To establish that the paraffin hydrocarbons in human epidermis are derived from petroleum rather than from biosynthesis in the epidermis, we isolated these hydrocarbons and had them examined by tandem accelerator mass spectrometry to determine the ratio of carbon isotopes. The absence of any significant amount of the carbon-14 radioisotope showed that the hydrocarbon sample was more than 36,000 years old (the practical limit of carbon dating), so that the possibility of endogenous biosynthesis was eliminated.[22] The inference is that avoidance of environmental contamination may be impractical and that reported variations in the epidermal content of paraffin hydrocarbons have no clinical significance.

2.4 EPIDERMAL LIPID BIOSYNTHESIS

During the 2 to 3 weeks that elapse between cell division in the basal layer and eventual loss of the daughter cell from the skin surface, the overall composition of the lipids in full-thickness epidermis remains constant. Nevertheless, biosynthesis, transformation, and translocation of the epidermal lipids within each cell continue and change with time. To track the resulting changes in the composition and the location of the epidermal lipids during the differentiation of each cell requires a study of the time course of lipid biosynthesis and composition. Such studies have been carried out mostly in pigs using radiolabeling techniques. The results have allowed deductions to be made regarding the anatomical locations of epidermal lipid biosynthesis, translocation, and tranformation.[5,23-25]

2.4.1 Lipid Biosynthesis in the Viable Cells

Electron micrographs indicate that the epidermal basal cells contain little lipid other than that contained in the membranes of the cell surface and the cytoplasm. The lipids extractable from trypsin-digested viable cells of pig epidermis contain mainly phospholipids and cholesterol, presumably derived from cellular membranes. The phospholipids contain a high proportion of linoleic acid,[25] so it can be inferred that the membranes are likely to have been constructed from preformed lipids obtained from the blood. However, there is evidence that cells that have migrated from the basal layer are no longer able to absorb lipids from the circulation[26] and must synthesize *de novo* any additional lipids using low molecular weight precursors. It has usually been assumed that the water-soluble precursor for skin lipids is glucose, but there is some evidence to the contrary. For example, the biosynthesis of squalene, the characteristic human sebaceous lipid, continued unabated during total starvation.[27,28] It is likely, and perhaps biologically imperative, that lipid biosynthesis in the epidermis is also independent of the availability of glucose from the circulation. An alternative substrate is always available, even during starvation, in the form of circulating acetate. This immediate precursor in lipid biosynthesis is present in blood at a concentration, and at a turnover rate, that is adequate for the amounts of lipid that must be synthesized to maintain the epidermal structure.

As the epidermal cells differentiate, significant amounts of lipid must be synthesized to construct the lamellar granules that accumulate in the spinous and granular cells. The ceramides and free fatty acids that constitute these structures consist almost exclusively of straight chain saturated and monounsaturated fatty acids, and they contain very little linoleic acid other than that esterified to the very long chain ω-hydroxyacid ceramides.[5,29,30] These observations support the idea that the differentiating epidermal cells are able to accomplish *de novo* biosynthesis of most of the lipids that they accumulate and are highly specialized in the types of lipids they produce.

Radiolabel time course studies have shown that the lipids synthesized initially in the epidermis are phospholipids and that these are transformed first to glucosylceramides and then to ceramides and free fatty acids over a period of weeks.[23,24] Nevertheless, the total level of lipid radioactivity does not diminish during the first week after labeling, which demonstrates that the lipid contents of the differentiated epidermal cells do not exchange with the circulation. Subsequent decline in total radioactivity appears to result from the loss of cells from the surface of the stratum corneum. These chemical transformations of lipids may be interpreted in relation to the translocations of lipid structures that are observable in the electron microscope.

2.4.2 Biochemical Transformations and Translocation of Lipids During Epidermal Differentiation

Electron micrographs show that the lamellar granules are discharged from the granular cells immediately before the cells become cornified.[1,2,7,8] Chemical analyses of extracted lipids show that the viable cells contain only glucosylceramides, while the cornified layer contains only ceramides.[14] It must be inferred that some time after their discharge from the granular cells, the glucosylceramides become deglycosylated to form ceramides. As part of the discharge process, the bounding membrane of the lamellar granule attaches to, and becomes part of, the cell membrane. It seems reasonable to infer that this process results in delivery of the very long chain ω-hydroxyceramides to the cell envelope immediately prior to formation of the cross-linked protein envelope. The ω-hydroxyceramides thereby arrive at the location where they become attached to the protein envelope.

2.4.2.1 The Intercellular Lamellae

Following discharge of the lamellar disk contents from the lamellar granules, the stacks of disks slowly disperse in the intercellular space, rearrange edge-to-edge, and then fuse to form continuous intercellular lamellae. Because of the way in which the lamellar disks are believed to be formed by the flattening of liposomes, the resulting lamellar disks (and, consequently, the intercellular lamellar sheets) are double lipid bilayers.[5,13,31-37] This process of double-bilayer formation is illustrated in Figure 4.

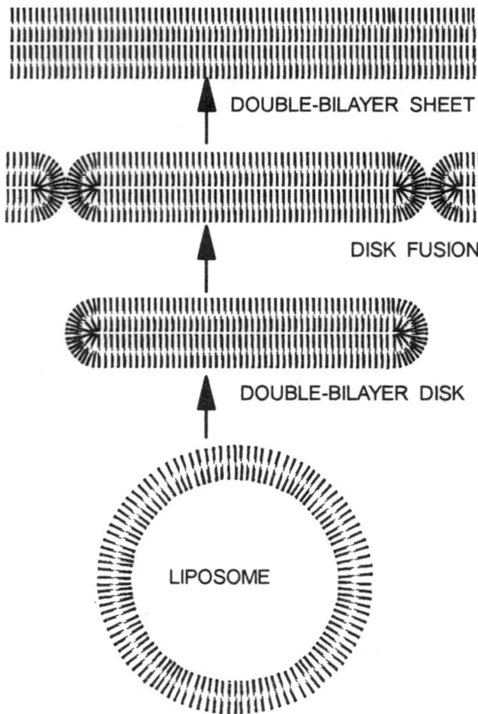

FIGURE 4 Hypothetical scheme for the formation of the double lipid bilayers observed in the lamellar disks in lamellar granules and in the intercellular lamellae of the stratum corneum.

After their formation by fusing of the lipid disks, the intercellular lipid lamellae have a unique structure, seen in electron micrographs of stratum corneum that has been fixed with ruthenium tetroxide.[4,5,13,16] In sections of tissue that have been treated only with the conventional osmium tetroxide fixative, the intercellular spaces throughout most of the stratum corneum appear to be empty.[1,2] This led earlier investigators to believe that the epidermal barrier existed only in the lowest layers of the stratum corneum, while the upper layers were irrelevant to the barrier function. However, the introduction of ruthenium tetroxide fixation of epidermal specimens showed that competent intercellular lamellae exist throughout the depth of the stratum corneum.[4,5,16]

The ruthenium tetroxide-fixed specimens show a unique pattern of lucent lipid bands in the intercellular lamellae which has been described as $(broad\text{-}narrow\text{-}broad)_n$, where n is usually 1, 2, or 3.[11,16] This pattern of lipid lamellae has been attributed to the formation of mutual monolayers between the adjacent double bilayer sheets formed by fusing of the lamellar disks.[16] Lipid monolayers are also postulated to form between the outermost double bilayer and the lipid envelope of the adjacent cell.[16] This hypothesis is illustrated in Figure 5. The lipid monolayers would be formed by interdigitation of the chains of sphingosine moieties in touching bilayer pairs, while the pairs of bilayers are bound to each other by the ability of ceramide 1 molecules to span one bilayer and extend into another. Some investigators have attributed the *broad-narrow-broad* pattern to the influence of protein constituents in the intercellular lamellae, but X-ray diffraction studies of reconstituted mixtures of purified lipids have shown that the pattern can be induced by low concentrations of ceramide 1 molecules.[38,39] The effect of ceramide 1 in binding pairs of lipid bilayers together results in a structure that is highly resistant to dispersion by heat or detergents.[16] However, even in the absence of ceramide 1, liposomes formed from reconstituted mixtures of epidermal lipids are resistant to dispersion.[40]

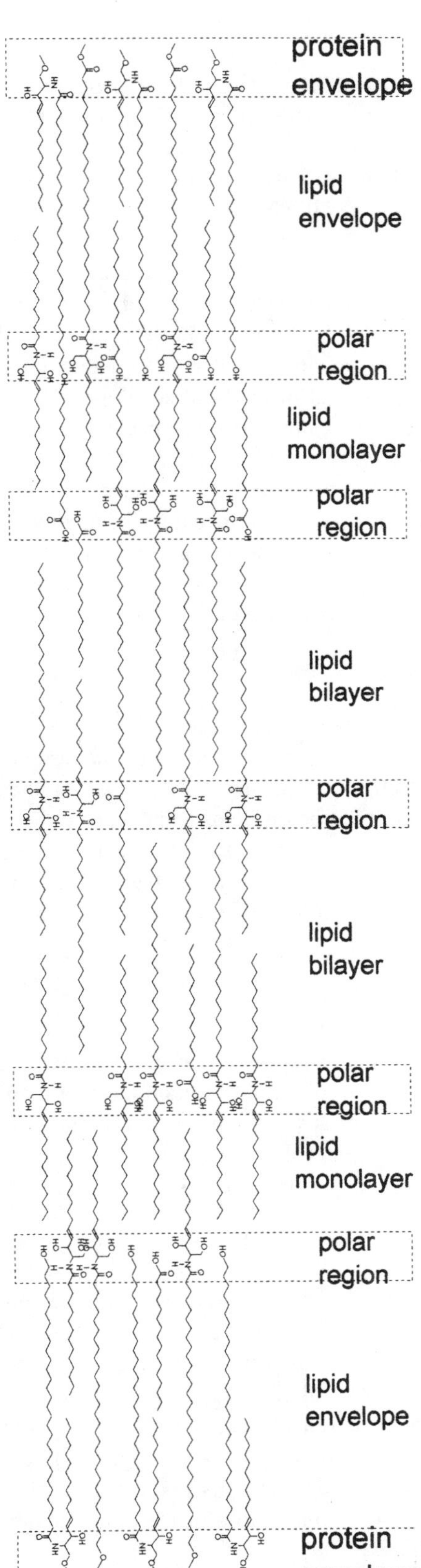

FIGURE 5 An interpretation of the lipid orientations and interactions that might produce the unique lamellar patterns of stratum corneum intercellular lamellae seen in ruthenium tetroxide-fixed mammalian epidermis.

2.4.2.2 The Corneocyte Lipid Envelope

ω-Hydroxyceramides amounting to 2% of the weight of solvent-extracted stratum corneum are chemically linked to the corneocyte protein envelope.[10-14] Calculations show that this amount of lipid is sufficient to provide a monomolecular layer of lipid over the entire surface of the cornified cell. Electron micrographs of ruthenium tetroxide-fixed stratum corneum confirm these deductions by revealing an electron-lucent envelope on the exterior of each cell[11,16] and verify the removal of the lipid envelope by mild alkaline hydrolysis.[11]

After the corneocyte lipid envelope was discovered, it became apparent that the chemically bound lipid molecules, which have hydroxyls as the only functional groups by which they could be linked, must be esterified to carboxyl side chains of the protein envelope. The ease of removal by alkaline hydrolysis[10-12] indicated an ester linkage rather than an amide. It was soon realized that quite an unusual protein substrate would be required for attachment of the lipid envelope, since a very high concentration of carboxyl groups would be needed for binding the close-packed palisade of lipid molecules.[13,16] It was also realized that the protein involucrin, which has 20% of glutamate residues in its amino acid sequence, is present in the corneocyte envelope and is a likely candidate as the substrate for attachment of the lipid envelope.[13] It remains to be determined how the involucrin molecule might be folded in order to present its glutamate residues in a concentrated, planar array for attachment of the lipid envelope ω-hydroxyceramides. Molecular modeling has suggested a conformation of the involucrin that could perform this function, as described in Chapter 4.

2.4.3 Lipid Transformations in the Stratum Corneum

Because the cornified cells were regarded as metabolically inactive and incapable of enzymic transformations, it has long been assumed that the lipid structures incorporated into the stratum corneum would persist until the eventual loss of the cell from the skin surface. However, studies have shown that some enzymatic transformations of the stratum corneum lipids can occur throughout the cornified layer. The first of these to be observed was the replacement of cholesterol sulfate with free cholesterol at the surface of the stratum corneum. Recently, it has been shown that the tissue can hydrolyze ceramides to produce free sphingosine. These transformations may have significant structural and physiological significance.

2.4.3.1 Cholesterol Sulfate Hydrolysis

Elevated cholesterol sulfate concentration at the skin surface is correlated with a severe skin disease, recessive X-linked lamellar ichthyosis.[41] In this disease, the level of cholesterol sulfate is greatly increased, and the stratum corneum becomes thickened and scaly. It was found that desquamation is correlated with conversion of cholesterol sulfate to free cholesterol,[42,43] but it remains unclear why the failure to hydrolyze the cholesterol sulfate results in such a devastating disease.

2.4.3.2 Ceramide Hydrolysis

Stratum corneum lipids have been found to contain 2 to 3% of free sphingosine,[44-46] and it was subsequently demonstrated that the stratum corneum can provide this material by enzymatic hydrolysis of ceramides.[47] Free sphingosine is widely recognized as a potent biological agent, especially as an inhibitor of protein kinase C and in its effects on cell division and differentiation. Particularly surprising was the observation that the concentration of free sphingosine in the stratum corneum is roughly a thousand times greater than that required for its biological effects in other tissues. Therefore, it was unclear how the epidermis must deal with its vast concentration of free sphingosine. The answer appears to lie in discovery of an interaction of free sphingosine with cholesterol sulfate.

2.4.3.3 Cholesterol Sulfate–Sphingosine Interaction

Thin layer chromatograms of stratum corneum lipids often reveal two cholesterol sulfate-containing spots, identifiable by their pink coloration produced during charring of the chromatograms with sulfuric acid. Explanation of this observation came with the discovery that cholesterol sulfate and sphingosine form an adduct that migrates on thin layer chromatograms like a single compound,[48] even in the presence of acetic acid, although the effect is eliminated by ammonia. One of the spots on the chromatograms is produced by the adduct, and the second is produced by excess cholesterol sulfate.

It was speculated that adduct formation between these two biologically active compounds may explain the ability of the epidermis to tolerate the high concentrations of free sphingosine. This idea was supported when it was shown that the toxicity of sphingosine toward microorganisms is eliminated by an equimolar amount of cholesterol sulfate.[49] However, the hydrolysis of cholesterol sulfate at the skin surface liberates free sphingosine, which may act to inhibit the colonization of the skin surface by fungi and bacteria.

It was also speculated that the sphingosine that is liberated at the skin surface may permeate into the living layers of the epidermis to regulate cell division and differentiation.

2.5 EPIDERMAL LIPIDS AND BARRIER FUNCTION

The lipids that are found in the stratum corneum are ideally suited to the formation of a permeability barrier because of their high melting point and polarity, which result in the formation of water-resistant lipid bilayers. However, additional factors in the intercellular lamellae and the corneocyte lipid envelopes serve to increase the inherent effectiveness of the barrier lipids.

2.5.1 The Intercellular Lamellae

The effectiveness of a lipid bilayer depends to a significant extent on the physical state of the lipid phase and also on the coherence of the polar head groups. Lipids in the crystalline or gel phase are far less permeable to water than those in the liquid phase. The resistance to water permeation is also increased if hydrogen bonding between adjacent polar head groups stabilizes their association. Both of these factors favor the function of the stratum corneum intercellular lamellae as a barrier to water and other polar molecules.

There undoubtedly is also a significant enhancement of epidermal barrier function by the existence of multiple lipid lamellae within each intercellular space, especially since most of the lamellae are tightly bound to each other without intervening spaces in which water molecules could accumulate in staging points across the barrier.

2.5.2 The Corneocyte Lipid Envelopes

The bound lipids of the corneocyte lipid envelopes, like the lipids of the intercellular lamellae, are largely saturated high melting compounds[10,12] and most likely function as a permeability barrier around each cornified cell. This function is quite unlike that of the plasma membrane of conventional living cells, in which the membrane lipids are liquid and highly permeable to water. The barrier function of the corneocyte lipid envelope explains how the stratum corneum cells can retain the low molecular weight amino acids that appear to contribute to the properties of the epidermis.

The corneocyte lipid envelope also contributes to the formation and maintenance of the intercellular lipid lamellae by acting as a substrate to which the unbound lipids may adhere and adopt their lamellar organization.[5,13,16,20] This effect has been demonstrated in experiments in which solvent-extracted corneocytes were immersed in liposomal dispersions of reconstituted stratum corneum lipids, resulting in the adherence and accumulation of lipid lamellae.[50]

2.5.3 Maintenance of the Epidermal Barrier

Biological and biochemical processes are required for the generation, modification, and translocation of the epidermal lipids that are involved in formation of the permeability barrier. However, purely physical properties govern the association of the lipids and the adoption of specific macroscopic conformations. As a result, reconstituted mixtures of specific lipids can adopt conformations that resemble the native lamellae and function as efficient barriers to water permeation in entirely synthetic constructions.[35,36,39,40,50]

These observations also imply that lipid lamellae in the stratum corneum, *in vivo* and *in vitro*, have the capacity to reform their barrier conformations after physical disturbances, such as heat, abrasion, or solvent exposure. This capability would have clear biological importance, but it also suggests that topical applications of synthetic lipid mixtures may have unsuspected roles in the treatment of deficiencies in epidermal barrier function.

REFERENCES

1. Matoltsy, A. G., Structure and function of the mammalian epidermis, in *Biology of the Integument. 2. Vertebrates,* Bereiter-Hahn, J., Matoltsy, A. G., and Richards, K. S., Eds., Springer-Verlag, New York, 1986, 255.
2. Odland, G. F., Structure of the skin, in *Physiology, Biochemistry and Molecular Biology of the Skin,* 2nd Edition, Goldsmith, L. A., Ed., Oxford University Press, New York, 1991, 3.
3. Steinert, P. M., and Freedberg, I. M., Epidermal structural proteins, in *Physiology, Biochemistry and Molecular Biology of the Skin,* 2nd Edition, Goldsmith, L. A., Ed., Oxford University Press, New York, 1991, 113.
4. Madison, K. C., Swartzendruber, D. C., Wertz, P. W., and Downing, D. T., Presence of intact intercellular lamellae in the upper layers of the stratum corneum, *J. Invest. Dermatol.*, 88, 714, 1987.
5. Wertz, P. W., and Downing, D. T., Epidermal lipids, in *Physiology, Biochemistry and Molecular Biology of the Skin,* 2nd Edition, Goldsmith, L. A., Ed., Oxford University Press, New York, 1991, 205.
6. Dover, R., and Wright, N. A., The cell proliferation kinetics of the epidermis, in *Physiology, Biochemistry and Molecular Biology of the Skin,* 2nd Edition, Goldsmith, L. A., Ed., Oxford University Press, New York, 1991, 239.
7. Lavker, R. L., Membrane coating granules: The fate of the discharged lamellae, *J. Ultrastruct. Res.*, 55, 79, 1970.
8. Lavker, R. M., and Matoltsy, A. G., Formation of horny cells. The fate of organelles and differentiation products in ruminal epithelium, *J. Cell Biol.*, 44, 501, 1970.
9. Polakowska, R. R., and Goldsmith, L. A., The cell envelope and transglutaminases, in *Physiology, Biochemistry and Molecular Biology of the Skin,* 2nd Edition, Goldsmith, L. A., Ed., Oxford University Press, New York, 1991, 168.
10. Wertz, P. W., and Downing, D. T., Covalently bound ω-hydroxyacylsphingosine in the stratum corneum, *Biochim. Biophys. Acta*, 917, 108, 1987.
11. Swartzendruber, D. C., Wertz, P. W., Madison, K. C., and Downing, D. T., Evidence that the corneocyte has a chemically bound lipid envelope, *J. Invest. Dermatol.*, 88, 709, 1987.
12. Wertz, P. W., Madison, K. C., and Downing, D. T., Covalently bound lipids of human stratum corneum, *J. Invest. Dermatol.*, 92, 109, 1989.
13. Downing, D. T., Lipid and protein structures in the permeability barrier of mammalian epidermis, *J. Lipid Res.*, 33, 301, 1992.
14. Swartzendruber, D. C., Kitko, D. J., Wertz, P. W., and Downing, D. T., Isolation of corneocyte envelopes from porcine epidermis, *Arch. Dermatol. Res.*, 123, 1538, 1988.
15. Wertz, P. W., Downing, D. T., Freinkel, R. K., and Traczyk, T. N., Sphingolipids of the stratum corneum and lamellar granules of fetal rat epidermis, *J. Invest. Dermatol.*, 83, 193, 1984.
16. Swartzendruber, D. C., Wertz, P. W., Kitko, D. J., Madison, K. C., and Downing, D. T., Molecular models of the intercellular lipid lamellae in mammalian stratum corneum, *J. Invest. Dermatol.*, 92, 251, 1989.

17. Yardley, H. J., Epidermal lipids, in *Biochemistry and Physiology of the Skin*, Goldsmith, L. A., Ed., Oxford University Press, New York, 1991, 363.
18. Robson, K. J., Stewart, M. E., Michelsen, S., Lazo, N. D., and Downing, D. T., 6-Hydroxysphingosine in human epidermal ceramides, *J. Lipid Res.*, 35, 2060, 1994.
19. Stewart, M. E., and Downing, D. T., A new 6-hydroxy-4-sphingenine-containing ceramide in human skin, *J. Lipid Res.*, 40, 1434, 1999.
20. Wertz, P. W., Swartzendruber, D. C., Kitko, D. J., Madison, K. C., and Downing, D. T., The role of the corneocyte lipid envelope in cohesion of the stratum corneum, *J. Invest. Dermatol.*, 93, 169, 1989.
21. Wertz, P. W., Swartzendruber, D. C., Madison, K. C., and Downing, D. T., Composition and morphology of epidermal cyst lipids, *J. Invest. Dermatol.*, 89, 419, 1987.
22. Bortz, J. T., Wertz, P. W., and Downing, D. T., The origin of alkanes found in human skin surface lipids, *J. Invest. Dermatol.*, 93, 723, 1989.
23. Hedberg, C. L., Wertz, P. W., and Downing, D. T., The time course of lipid biosynthesis in pig epidermis, *J. Invest. Dermatol.*, 91, 169, 1988.
24. Downing, D. T., *In vivo* studies of cutaneous lipid biosynthesis, *Semin. Dermatol.*, 11, 162, 1992.
25. Downing, D. T., Metabolism of linoleate in the epidermis, in *Essential Fatty Acids and Prostaglandins*, Sinclair, A., and Gibson, R., Eds., American Oil Chemists Society, Champaign, IL, 1993, 433.
26. Ponec, M., Havekes, L., Kempenaar, J., Lavrijsen, S., Wijsman, M., Boonstra, J., and Vermeer, B. J., Calcium-mediated regulation of the low density lipoprotein receptor and intracellular cholesterol synthesis in human epidermal keratinocytes, *J. Cell. Physiol.*, 125, 98, 1985.
27. Pochi, P. E., Downing, D. T., and Strauss, J. S., Sebaceous gland response in man to prolonged total caloric deprivation, *J. Invest. Dermatol.*, 55, 303, 1970.
28. Downing, D. T., Strauss, J. S., and Pochi, P. E., Changes in skin surface lipid composition induced by severe caloric restriction in man, *Am. J. Clin. Nutr.*, 25, 365 1972.
29. Wertz, P. W., and Downing, D. T., Ceramides of pig epidermis, *J. Lipid Res.*, 24, 759, 1983.
30. Wertz, P. W., Miethke, M. C., Long, S. A., Strauss, J. S., and Downing, D. T., The composition of the ceramides from human stratum corneum and from comedones, *J. Invest. Dermatol.*, 84, 410, 1985.
31. Landmann, L., Epidermal permeability barrier: transformation of lamellar granule disks into intercellular sheets by a membrane fusion process, *J. Invest. Dermatol.*, 87, 202, 1986.
32. Landmann, L., Wertz, P. W., and Downing, D. T., Acylglucosylcermide causes flattening and stacking of liposomes: an analogy for assembly of the epidermal permeability barrier, *Biochim. Biophys. Acta*, 778, 412, 1984.
33. Abraham, W., Wertz, P. W., and Downing, D. T., Effect of epidermal acylglucosylceramides and acylceramides on the morphology of liposomes prepared from stratum corneum lipids, *Biochim. Biophys. Acta*, 939, 403, 1988.
34. Abraham, W., Wertz, P. W., and Downing, D. T., Fusion patterns of liposomes formed from stratum corneum lipids, *J. Invest. Dermatol.*, 90, 259, 1988.
35. Abraham, W., and Downing, D. T., Preparation of model membranes for skin permability studies using stratum corneum lipids, *J. Invest Dermatol.*, 93, 809, 1989.
36. Abraham, W., and Downing, D. T., Factors affecting the formation, morphology, and permeability of stratum corneum lipid bilayers *in vitro*, in *Prediction of Percutaneous Penetration*, Scott, R. C., Guy, R. H., and Hadgraft, J., Eds., IBC Technical Services, London, 110, 1990.
37. Downing, D. T., Lipids: their role in epidermal structure and function, *Cosmet. Toiletries*, 106, 63, 1991.
38. Bouwstra, J. A., Gooris, G. S., Bras, W., and Downing, D. T., Lipid organization in pig stratum corneum, *J. Lipid Res.,* 36, 685, 1995.
39. McIntosh, T. J., Stewart, M. E., and Downing, D. T., X-ray diffraction analysis of isolated skin lipids: Reconstitution of intercellular lipid domains, *Biochemistry,* 35, 3649, 1996.
40. Downing, D. T., Abraham, W., Wegner, B. K., Willman, K. W., and Marshall, J. L., Partition of sodium dodecyl sulfate into stratum corneum lipid liposomes, *Arch. Dermatol. Res.*, 285, 151, 1993.
41. Shapiro, L. J., Weiss, R., Webster, D., and France, J. T., Enzymatic basis of typical x-linked ichthyosis, *Lancet*, 1, 70, 1978.
42. Long, S. A., Wertz, P. W., Strauss, J. S., and Downing, D. T., Human stratum corneum polar lipids and desquamation, *Arch. Dermatol. Res.,* 277, 284, 1985.

43. Ranasinghe, A. W., Wertz, P. W., Downing, D. T., and Mackenzie, I. C., Lipid composition of cohesive and desquamated corneocytes from mouse ear skin, *J. Invest. Dermatol.*, 86, 187, 1986.
44. Wertz, P. W., and Downing, D. T., Free sphingosines in porcine epidermis, *Biochim. Biophys. Acta*, 1002, 213, 1989.
45. Wertz, P. W., and Downing, D. T., Free sphingosine in human epidermis, *J. Invest. Dermatol.*, 94, 159, 1990.
46. Stewart, M. E., and Downing, D. T., Free sphingosines of human skin include 6-hydroxysphingosine and unusually long-chain dihydrosphingosines, *J. Invest. Dermatol.*, 105, 613, 1995.
47. Wertz, P. W., and Downing, D. T., Ceramidase activity in porcine epidermis, *FEBS Letts.*, 268, 110, 1990.
48. Downing, D. T., Dose, R. W., and Abraham, W., Interaction between sphingosine and cholesterol sulfate in epidermal lipids, *J. Lipid Res.*, 34, 563, 1993.
49. Payne, C. D., Ray, T. L., and Downing, D. T., Cholesteryl sulfate protects *Candida albicans* from inhibition by sphingosine *in vitro*, *J. Invest. Dermatol.*, 106, 549, 1996.
50. Abraham, W., and Downing, D. T., Interaction between corneocytes and stratum corneum lipid liposomes, *Biochim. Biophys. Acta*, 1021, 119, 1990.

3 The Skin as a Barrier

Magnus Lindberg and Bo Forslind

CONTENTS

3.1 INTRODUCTION

This chapter will deal with the stratum corneum barrier with a special focus on structure–function relationships. For this reason our approach has been to describe some details of the epidermal physiology that have a bearing on upholding the barrier function. We see it as important that skin barrier function is regarded as part of the dynamic processes of cellular transformation during the differentiation of epidermal keratinocytes, hence dependent on the status of the skin.

It is taken for granted that the skin barrier prevents foreign material from entering the system. But, a deeper insight into the barrier function of the integument makes it clear that the primary function of the barrier is to prevent water loss, and the barrier toward environmental factors is only of secondary importance, albeit very important.[1] The water homeostasis is absolutely necessary for normal physiology, and the role of the kidneys is to maintain that homeostasis. Therefore, the integument should represent a water-impermeable "bag." However, we have to account for the *perspiratio insensibilis* which obviously has its origin in the need for a hydration of the corneocytes. Water acts as a plasticizer on the corneocyte keratin, giving the cells the necessary elastic properties. If deprived of water, a dry skin is prone to crack open at mechanical stress. Since the relative humidity of the environment varies enormously, the corneocytes have to be hydrated from a permanent water source, the body. The fact that the *perspiratio insensibilis* is markedly constant reveals that this water leakage is not a defect in the barrier, but an inbuilt factor with a required function.

3.2 THE CORNEOCYTES CONSTITUTE A SCAFFOLD FOR THE BARRIER LIPIDS

The entire horny layer, the stratum corneum, can be regarded as the outer barrier of the skin. The horny layer is continuously exposed to contact with the environment and suffers from the effects of chemical and physical agents which will cause a continuous loss of material. We can assume

0-8493-7520-7/00/$0.00+$.50

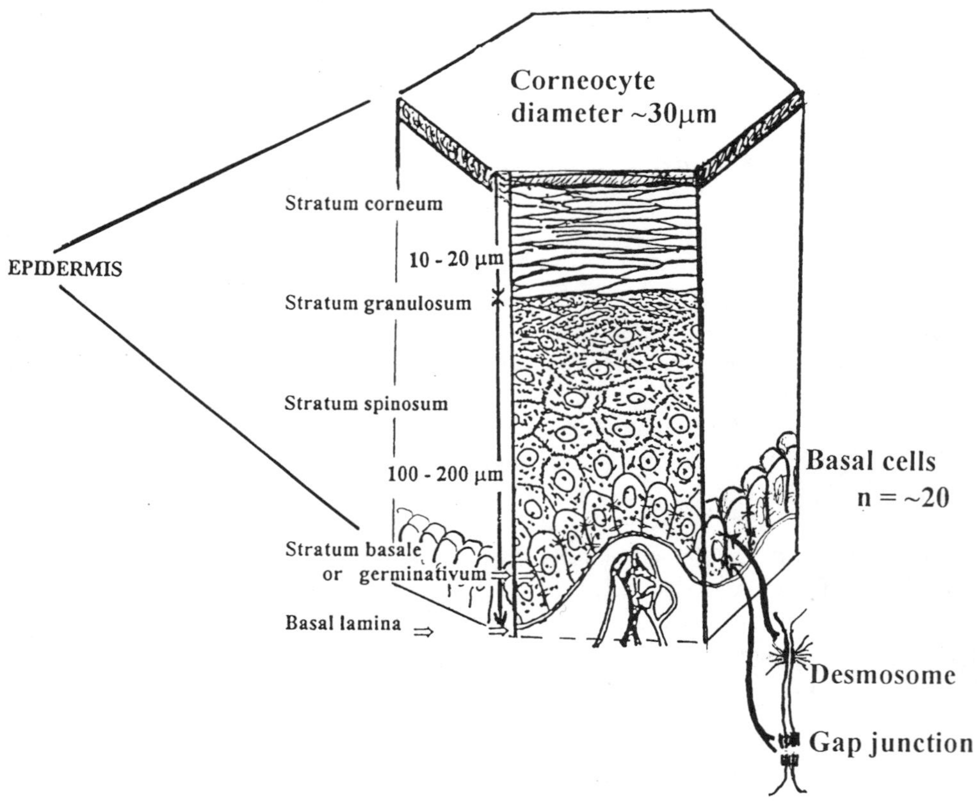

FIGURE 1 The proliferative unit as deduced from Potten.[2]

that the loss of material over the entire body surface (~1.8 m^2) corresponds to a "film," the thickness of which is at least that of a corneocyte. Assuming that the surface of a corneocyte is approximately 1000 μm^2, this surface "film" corresponds roughly to 1.8×10^9 cells. The thickness of a corneocyte is ~0.3 µm, and with a specific weight of 0.75 kg m^{-3} (= protein) these data can be used to calculate a daily loss of about 40 mg of horny cells, most likely an underestimation. Thus, the total amount of material in this turnover is not negligible. This continuous renewal of cells is a prerequisite for keeping the thickness of stratum corneum approximately constant and thus the barrier intact in all its aspects.

Through autoradiographic investigations it has beeen shown that a corneocyte stems from 1 of about 20 basal cells under the projected area of a corneocyte.[2] This is the so-called *proliferative unit* (Figure 1). The cells on the basal lamina communicate via gap junctions, and through this means a regulation of cell division is possible within the proliferative unit controlling the progeny travel from the stratum basale to the stratum corneum at a pace that ensures a smooth surface.[3] An additional controlling mechanism may be the shift in the Na/K ratio that occurs as the cells move into the stratum spinosum.[4] Thus, higher than normal Na and lower than normal K concentrations within the cell of the upper stratum will effectively hinder the cell to enter the cell division cycle.

3.3 CORNEOCYTE STRUCTURE

A corneocyte can be described as a very flat cell, about 30 µm in diameter and approximately 0.3 µm thick, filled with keratin inside a protein envelope. Keratin is a highly hydrophilic material that can bind substantial amounts of water, and we discern a fibrous component as well an an

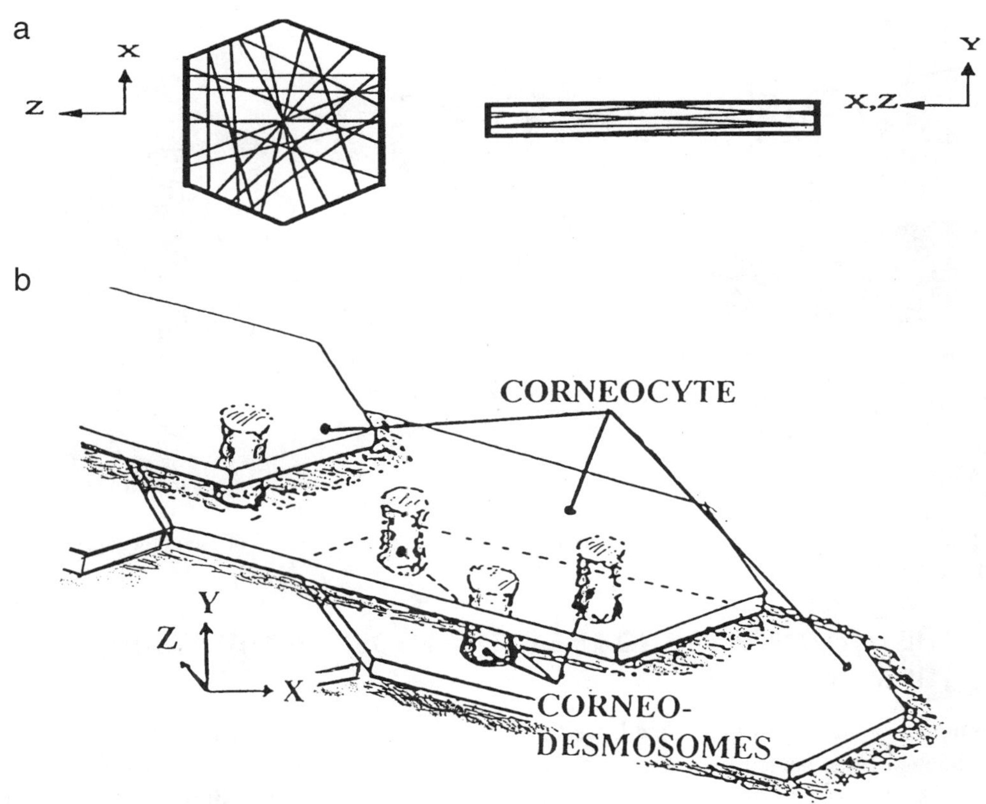

FIGURE 2 (a) The corneocyte is a flat, hexagonal-like structure with a surface area of about 1000 μm^2 and a thickness of 0.3 μm. A protein envelope encloses a cell compartment containing only fibrous and amorphous keratin. The keratin fibrils inside the cell are randomly oriented in the plane of the cell and constitute an internal reinforcement that ensures that the cell form in the plane of the skin is preserved within very narrow limits. (b) The corneocytes are coupled to each other through protein "rivets," corneodesmosomes. This arrangement makes a mechanically rigid scaffold. The lipid bilayers, which are separated by thin water sheaths and are mechanically very soft, are protected from sliding relative to each other and being directly exposed to mechanical shear that would break up the structure.

amorphous one. The fibrils, 8 nm in diameter, span the inside of the corneocyte and thus constitute an internal reinforcement ensuring that the cell form in the plane of the skin remains virtually unchanged even at long exposures to water. This is achieved by an orientation of the fibrils in the plane of the cell (Figure 2a). In the vertical dimension there are virtually no reinforcement fibrils, and thus the cells have more freedom to swell in this direction. Norlén et al.[5] have actually shown that the swelling is less than 5% in the horizontal dimension, but can be more than 25% in the vertical dimension. This ensures a minimal roughness of the skin surface even at maximal swelling, thus minimizing the risk of surface breaks at mechanical stress on wet skin. The conspicuously thicker stratum corneum of the palms and foot soles do indeed become wrinkled at maximal swelling, but here a conspicuous thickness of the stratum corneum compensates for this roughness.

The corneocytes are mutually joined by desmosome rivets that effectively hinder the cells to move in relation to each other in the plane of the skin (Figure 2b). This prevents shearing forces from disrupting the stacked bilamellar lipid structures in the extracellular space (Figure 3). The desmosome "rivets" also prevent this space from being increased due to mechanical forces imposed on the skin.

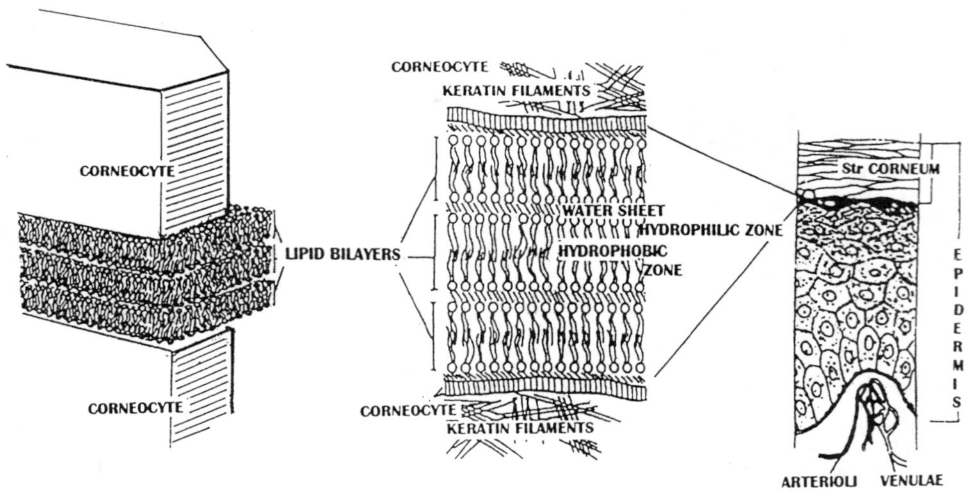

FIGURE 3 Stacked bilayers of lipids are inserted into the extracellular space of the corneocyte scaffold to form the lipid barrier of the skin.

3.4 THE HYDROPHILIC AND THE HYDROPHOBIC PATHWAYS THROUGH THE SKIN BARRIER

Looking at the barrier in more detail, we find that it can be described as composed of two main components. Interspersed between the corneocytes we find the "hydrophobic" (water-repellent) substance, the barrier lipids. The keratinized corneocytes containing fibrous and amorphous proteins represent a "hydrophilic" (water-attracting) component. Neutral lipids (fatty acids, cholesterol) and ceramides dominate the lipid phase, and it is mainly these lipids that are responsible for the control and limitation of water transport through the skin. Visualization of the penetration pathway through the skin by tracer methods has demonstrated that the extracellular pathway is likely to be the only route through the barrier for substances other than water.[6] Water diffusion through the keratinocytes is not expected to occur freely due to the fact that keratin will adsorb water. The bound water is likely to take on a certain degree of structured organization; hence the amount of freely diffusible water will be comparatively small. Consequently, the water transport through the keratinocytes will be impeded. Norlén et al.[7] have shown that water permeation through lipid-extracted stratum corneum membranes is only about three times higher than through a nonextracted stratum corneum membrane.

3.5 THE PHYSICAL STATE OF THE LIPIDS DETERMINES THE PROPERTIES OF A LIPID MEMBRANE OR BARRIER

Lipids that can form biological membranes are characterized by a hydrophilic head group and a hydrophobic part, usually a carbon chain (cf. fatty acids vs. cholesterol). From physical, thermodynamic considerations it can be shown that it takes a lot of energy to keep the hydrophobic part of a lipid dissolved in a water solution.[8] For this reason lipids tend to aggregate in micelles or bilayers. This means that they form a hydrophobic compartment (or phase) which encloses the carbon chains that separates them from the water. The hydrophilic head groups face the water and thus constitute a border between a hydrophobic phase and the water (Figure 4). A number of factors determine how stable such aggregates are.[9] These include temperature, the length of the hydrophobic carbon chain, their degree of unsaturation (double bonds), the temperature, the presence of divalent ions, etc.

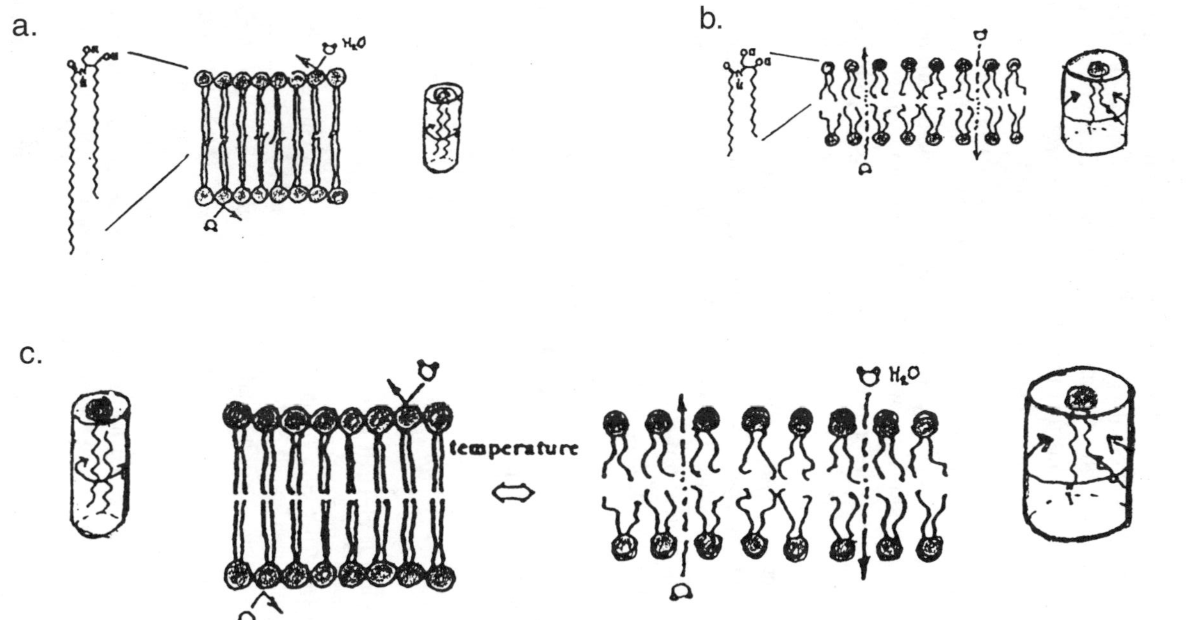

FIGURE 4 (a) Long, saturated carbon chains can attract each other through van der Waal's forces, and this causes a tight, close-packed crystalline structure that is impermeable to water. Straight (saturated) carbon chains demand less space than kinked (unsaturated) chains. Saturated long aliphatic chains (C > 20 carbons) tend to pack close at skin temperatures (26 to 32°C). When associated with water, there may still be a freedom of rotation along the carbon chain axis and the structure is sometimes denoted *gel phase*. (b) Short carbon chains and carbon chains with a double bond form liquid crystalline structures, where the chains of the bilayer show high degrees of freedom to diffuse in the plane of the bilayer. The liquid crystalline state thus becomes favored if one of the carbon chains is unsaturated. (c) The transition temperature of bilamellar lipid structures. Long, saturated carbon chains (left), tightly close packed form a crystalline structure that is impermeable to water. Short carbon chains (right) form liquid crystalline structures where the chains of the bilayer show high degrees of freedom to diffuse in the plane of the bilayer. The transition between these two states is dependent on temperature, chain length, and degree of unsaturation of the chain. If the temperature is lowered, the thermal movements of the chains decrease and van der Waal's attraction forces become operative; the structure becomes crystalline and impermeable to water. Thus, the transition between these two states depends on the parameters of temperature, chain length, and degree of unsaturation of the chain. Saturated, long aliphatic chains (C > 20 carbons) tend to pack close at skin temperatures (26 to 32°C).

In general, the most important factor is the temperature. It has been demonstrated that lipid membranes exist in two main physical states: one extremely close packed, the crystalline state (Figure 4a), and the other, the liquid crystalline state (see Figure 4b). In the latter state the structure is more open, and the lipid units are free to diffuse in the plane of the membrane. This actually allows water molecules to pass right through the membrane. The transition between these two main states is determined by the so-called transition temperature, and this is in turn dependent on the particular properties of the lipids forming the membrane[8] (Figure 4c). Lipids with short chains and lipids that are unsaturated have their transition temperature at lower temperatures than long-chain and saturated lipids. Biological membranes (bilayers) are generally complex mixtures of different lipid species, and the transition temperature for such a structure is expected to vary with the actual proportions of the lipid components. This also means that the transition occurs within a comparatively broad temperature interval compared to the corresponding sharply defined interval of a single lipid species.[8]

As a generalization, we may be allowed to state that the transition temperature for cell membranes in biological living systems is found between 0 to 40°C and the chain lengths are between 16 and 18 carbons. This is in conspicuous contrast to the lipids of the stratum corneum barrier where chain lengths up to and over 30 carbons have been demonstrated.[10] From such facts we expect the transition temperature of the skin barrier lipids to be around 40°C, and this has also been substantiated in a number of investigations.[11-13] This means that under normal conditions with a skin temperature about 30°C the barrier will essentially be impermeable to water.

Straight carbon chains can be housed in comparatively small volumes and allow van der Waal's forces to act and cause a close packing (Figure 4a). The van der Waal's forces are not effective if the distance between the atoms is several atoms in diameter.[9] Double bonds tend to create kinks on the carbon chains, preventing them from close apposition with neighbor chains, which is a prerequisite for allowing the weak van der Waal's forces to contribute to a close packing of the chains. Thus, kinked carbon chains hinder close packing of the lipid chains and promote a liquid crystalline state of the bilayer where the lipid units are allowed to diffuse in the plane of the bilayer[14] (see Figure 4b). A cell membrane is actually this kind of structure and therefore allows almost free passage of water in both directions over the membrane. The important message here is that the cell membrane is not a water barrier!

3.6 FREE FATTY ACIDS AND CHOLESTEROL

As a consequence of these facts, we expect the bulk of lipids that form the skin barrier to be in a crystalline (gel) state, i.e., to be long chain (C > 20:0) to comply with the physical requirement that the transition temperature should be higher than normal skin temperature (>35°C). The recent data of Norlén et al.[7,15] actually demonstrate that the free fatty acids (FFA) retrieved from stripped lower arm skin (and therefore essentially uncontaminated by sebum lipids) are all saturated and long-chain species (C > 20). This harmonizes with lipid data from epidermal cysts, which are virtually free from triglycerides of sebum origin.[16] Furthermore, the ceramides of the barrier lipids are all long-chain species and therefore also comply with the requirement set up for a water-impermeable barrier.

The third class of lipids found in stratum corneum extracts is represented by cholesterol and cholesteryl esters. The actual role of cholesterol remains enigmatic, and no clear reason for its role in the barrier function has been proposed so far. However, it has been suggested that contrary to what is the role in cell membranes where cholesterol increases close packing of phospholipids, it acts as kind of a detergent in lipid bilayers of long-chain, saturated lipids (Prof. Stig Friberg, Prof. Håkan Wennerström, personal communication). This would allow some fraction of the barrier to be in a liquid crystalline state, hence water permeable in spite of the fact that not only ceramides, but also fatty acids found in the barrier are saturated, long-chain species.[15,17]

3.7 THE CERAMIDES OF THE HUMAN SKIN BARRIER

At physiological pH the long-chain ceramides of the horny layer barrier in the presence of cholesterol and fatty acids have been shown to have equal capacity to form lamellar lipid structures as have phospholipids.[18,19] The chain length of the ceramides is to a great extent longer than 18 carbons, even up to 34 carbons in one of the chains, and this suggests close packing of the crystalline type at normal skin temperatures.

There is still controversy regarding the actual role of the ceramides in the stratum corneum barrier. It has been suggested that lower amounts of ceramides are related to the increased transepidermal water loss of dry atopic skin, but since no fully quantitative lipid analysis of this skin type is available this relation remains tentative.

In this context it is of special interest to note data that indicate that part of the long-chain ceramides of the horny layer are covalently bound to the proteins forming the corneocyte envelope.[19] This suggests that such lipids constitute anchors of the hydrophobic phase to the corneocytes and thereby add to the cohesion of the cells of the horny layer.*

3.8 THE DOMAIN MOSAIC MODEL

With the background given previously, the requirements on the stratum corneum barrier can be summarized. From a functional point of view the barrier should be watertight but still allow a small, controlled amount of water to leak from the system in order to keep the corneocyte keratin hydrated.

From these requirements we may infer a structure where the bulk of intercorneocyte lipids exist in the crystalline, close-packed state in stacked bilayer structures (Figure 5) due to the large amounts of long-chain saturated species. However, circumstantial evidence, e.g., transepidermal water loss, indicates that a fraction of the lipid compartment should be in the liquid crystalline state, but as yet we do not know the composition of this fraction. Again the role of cholesterol may be crucial, as mentioned earlier.

Accepting that the bulk of barrier lipids are in the watertight crystalline state we may depict the bilayers as composed of crystalline domains separated by lipids in the liquid crystalline state.[20,21] The cross section of a domain can tentatively be assumed to be of the same size as the cross section of a lamellar granule, the structure from which the lipids are extruded into the extracellular space of the stratum corneum, i.e., ~200 nm. Several bilayers are stacked on top of each other and separated by a thin film of water adherent to the hydrophilic head groups (Figure 3). Since it is unlikely that the crystalline domains are exactly uniform in size and form, we do not expect the fluid crystalline interdomain areas to overlap precisely. A water molecule leaving the body via the stratum corneum on a downhill diffusion gradient will therefore have to suffer a tortuous, meandering way through the lipid barrier[22,23] (Figure 5). In the water sheath separating the bilayers the water molecule will diffuse randomly until it finds a "hole-in-the-roof," i.e., a liquid crystalline phase through which it can tunnel into the next, overlaying water sheath. Considering the fact that it, in addition a number of water molecules, will have to circumvent water-saturated corneocytes shows us that the path out to the environment will be extremely long, hence the actual low value of the transepidermal water loss!

3.9 PROPERTIES OF THE LAMELLAR BARRIER — EFFECTS OF PENETRATION ENHANCERS

Based on the concept of the domain mosaic model and the Fick model for downhill gradients over a barrier, Engström[24] has presented arguments to show that only a fraction of the total lipid mass of the barrier has to be involved in structural changes that will open up or prevent barrier passage.

* Interestingly, swelling of lipid-extracted stratum corneum is almost nil compared to nonextracted.

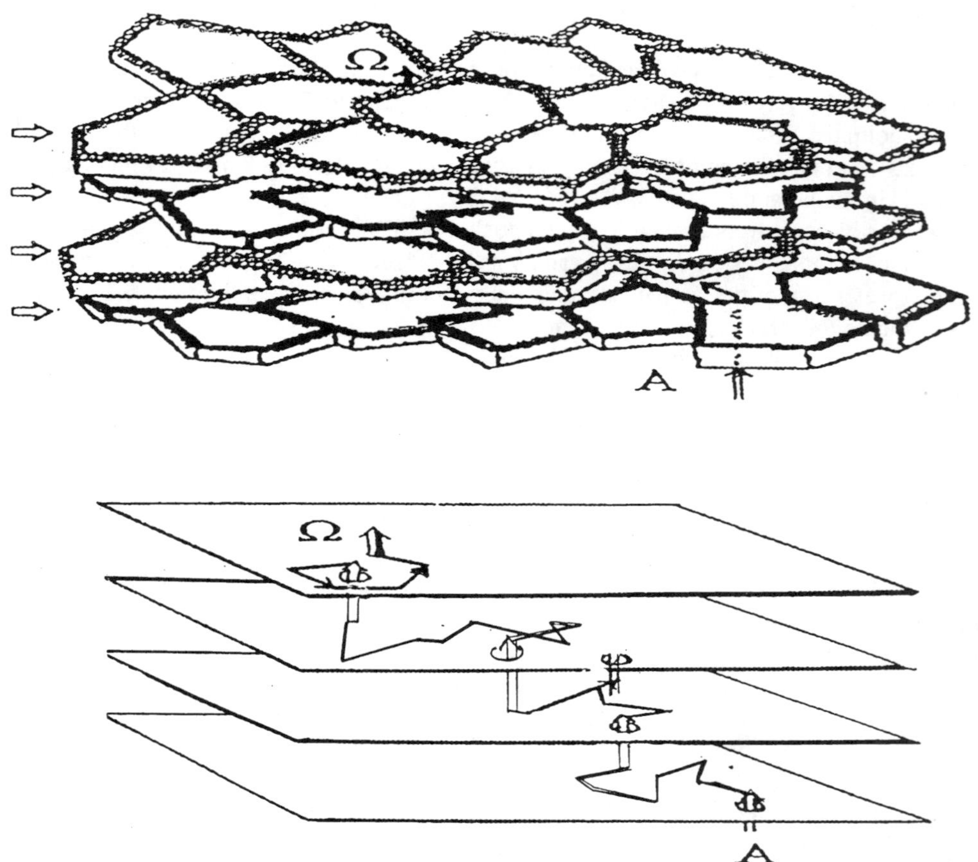

FIGURE 5 The stacked bilayers of the skin barrier are envisioned as composed of crystalline domains separated by fringes of lipids in the liquid crystalline state.[21] The fringe zones may actually oscillate in a very small time scale between a liquid crystalline state and a crystalline (gel) state. Such a tentative idea would mean that the barrier is open just temporarily at a certain location since penetration must occur in the liquid crystalline areas. Thus, the action of a penetration enhancer would be to "stabilize" a liquid crystalline state or transform it into another type of structure, e.g., a cubic phase.

These ideas were more extensively presented in a sequel publication which demonstrated that enhancement factors for barrier penetration of the order of 100 could easily be obtained for substances with partition coefficients far from one.[22] This is true even if the fraction of the extracellular bilayer that has undergone structural transformation, e.g., to a hexagonal or cubic phase, is small, i.e., 1 to 10% (Figure 6). It is to be noted that the structural transformations, e.g., conversion of a lamellar phase into a hexagonal phase, a bicontinuous cubic phase, or a sponge phase, are expected to occur only in the liquid crystalline phase regions between the crystalline domains, hence only a very small part of the total barrier is involved in the process.

It must be realized that structural changes of these kinds are local phenomena. This reasoning implies that a penetration enhancer introduced into the lipid barrier is expected to diffuse in the liquid crystalline phase and exert its structure transformation effects more or less exclusively there. Within a relatively short time it will also be diluted through this diffusion process and then the bilayer structure will be restored and the normal barrier function will be regained.

A problem which is rarely taken into account is related to the fact that the water concentration shows a conspicuous gradient within the stratum corneum thickness. These factors are likely to influence the physical state of lipids in bilayer formations, and therefore we expect lipid barrier

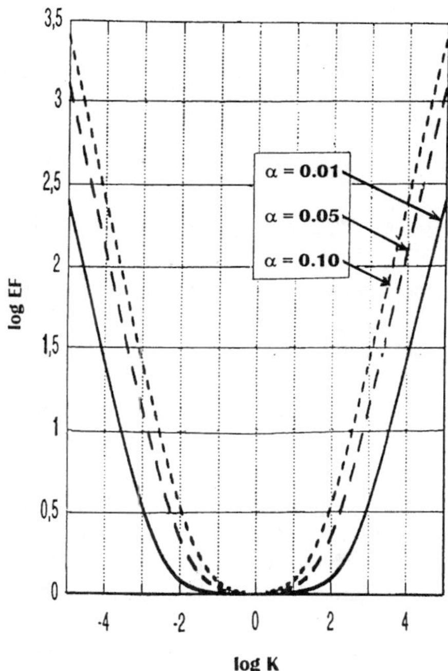

FIGURE 6 The enhancement factor EF (log EF) plotted vs. the partition coefficient (log K) demonstrates that small changes in the fraction α of the liquid crystalline phase of the barrier that undergoes a structural transformation from lamellar to cubic, hexagonal, etc. phase causes vast changes in the EF.[24]

structure to vary within the thickness of the stratum corneum. This problem will be addressed shortly.[26]

3.10 CONCLUSIONS — BARRIER PENETRATION IN A FUNCTIONAL PERSPECTIVE

In the past, barrier research for the most part had the character of "black box" descriptions of the dynamics of substance penetration through the skin. Today, skin barrier research is oriented toward an understanding of the molecular structures of penetrants and the lipid bilayers including processes and structural events occurring at penetration. Yet, we have only fragmentary knowledge of the actual lipid barrier structure(s) and its detailed function. Biophysical techniques such as X-ray diffraction, NMR, and FTIR have confirmed that a large part of the barrier lipids are in a crystalline state.[27-29] This is supported by lipid analyses of stripped human skin extracted *in vivo*, which has demonstrated that the free fatty acids (FFA) and the ceramides are long-chain species ($C > 22$) and hence should pack in crystalline (gel) structures at skin temperature. The role of cholesterol remains enigmatic, but is likely to influence the structural organization of the FFA and ceramides. The lipid bilayers of the stratum corneum not only constitute a barrier, but may also function as a pool from which substances can slowly penetrate into the system on a downhill gradient. The actual effect of solvents and detergents on barrier lipid structure is not known in any satisfactory detail. Likewise, we are only starting to understand how different moisturizers might influence the structure and function of the barrier. We still lack an understanding of how the composition of the ceramide, FFA, and cholesterol influences the defect barrier in some pathological disorders, e.g., dry atopic skin.

The answers to these and other questions not mentioned here relating to the human skin barrier function cannot be found by "black box" investigations, but must be sought in relation to the structural organization of the barrier lipids. The unique character and the particular composition of the human skin barrier lipids call for investigations on human skin, possibly pig skin, and to a great extent preclude rodents as models for barrier function in penetration studies.

REFERENCES

1. Forslind, B., The skin: upholder of physiological homeostasis. A physiological and biophysical study program. *Thromb Res* 80:1–22, 1995.
2. Potten, C.S., Cell replacement in epidermis [keratopoesis] via discrete units of proliferation. *Int Rev Cytol* 69:272–317, 1981.
3. Caputo, R. and Peluchetti, D., The junctions of normal human epidermis. A freeze-fracture study. *J Ultrastruct Res* 61:44–61, 1977.
4. Wei, X., Roomans, G.M., and Forslind, B., Elemental distribution in the guinea-pig skin revealed by X-ray microanalysis in the scanning transmission electron microscope. *J Invest Dermatol* 79:167–169, 1982.
5. Norlén, L., Emilson, A., and Forslind, B., Stratum corneum swelling. Biophysical and computer assisted quantitative assessments. *Arch. Exp Dermatol* 289:506–513, 1997.
6. Boddé, H., van den Brink, I., Koerten, H.K., and de Haan, F.H.N., Visualisation of in vitro penetration of mercuric chloride: transport through intercellular space vs. cellular uptake through desmosomes. *J Controlled Release* 15:227–236, 1990.
7. Norlén, L., Engblom, J., Andersson, M., and Forslind, B., A new computer based system for rapid measurement of water diffusion through stratum corneum in vitro. Submitted to *J Invest Dermatol* Vol. 113, 1999.
8. Larsson, K., Lipids — molecular organisation, physical function and technical applications. Vol 5. In *Oily Press Lipid Library,* Oily Press, Dundee, U.K., 1994.
9. Iraelachvili, J.N., Marcelja, S., and Horn, R.G., Physical principles of membrane organisation. *Q Rev Biophys* 13:121–200, 1980.
10. Gray, G.M. and Yardley, H.J., Lipid compositions of cells isolated from pig, human, and rat epidermis. *J Lipid Res* 16:434–440, 1975.
11. Bowstra, J.A., de Vries, M.A., Gooris, G.S., Bras, W., Brusse, J., and Ponec, M., Thermodynamic and structural aspects of the skin barrier. *J Controlled Release* 15:209–220, 1991.
12. Guy, C.L., Guy, R.H., Golden, G.M., Mak, V.H.W., and Francoeur, M.L., Characterisation of low-temperature [i.e., <65°C] lipid transitions in human stratum corneum. *J Invest Dermatol* 103:233–239, 1994.
13. Ongpipanattanakul, B., Francoeur, M.L., and Potts, R.O., Polymorphism in stratum corneum lipids. *Biochem Biophys Acta* 1190:115–122, 1994.
14. Singer, S.J. and Nicholson, G.L., The fluid mosaic model of the structure of cell membranes. *Science* 175:720–731, 1972.
15. Norlén, L., Nicander, I., Lundh Rozell, B., Ollmar, S., and Forslind, B., Differences in human stratum corneum lipid content related to physical parameters of skin barrier function in vivo. *J Invest Dermatol* 112:72–77, 1999.
16. Wertz, P.W., Schwartzendruber, D.C., Madison, K.C., and Downing, D.T., Composition and morphology of epidermal cyst lipids. *J Invest Dermatol* 89:419–4125, 1987.
17. Norlén, L., Nicander, I., Lundsjö, A., Cronholm, T., and Forslind, B., A new HPLC-based method for the quantitative analysis of inner stratum corneum lipids invivo with special reference to the free fatty acid fraction. *Arch Dermatol Res* 290:508–516, 1998.
18. Gray, G.M. and White, R.J., Epidermal lipid liposomes. A novel non-phospholipid membrane system. *Biochem Soc Trans* 7:1129–1131, 1979.
19. Wertz, P.W. and Downing, D.T., Epidermal lipids. Chap. 6. In LA Goldsmith, (ed), *Physiology, Biochemistry, and Molecular Biology of the Skin,* Oxford University Press, New York, pp. 205–236, 1991.
20. Fartasch, M., Bassuskas, I.D., and Diepgen, T.L., Structural relationship between epidermal lipid lamellae, lamellar bodies and desmosomes in humans epidermis: an unltrastructural study. *Br J Dermatol* 128:1–9, 1993

21. Forslind, B., A domain mosaic model of the skin barrier. *Acta Derm Venereol* 74:1–6, 1994.
22. Forslind, B., Engström, S., Engblom, J., and Norlén, L., A novel approach to the understanding of human skin barrier function. *J Derm Sci* 14:115–125, 1997.
23. Forslind, B., Norlén, L., and Engblom, J., A structural model for the human skin barrier. In Colloid Science of Lipids. New Paradigms for self-assembly in Science and Technology. *Prog Colloid Polym Sci* 108:40–46, 1998.
24. Engström, S., Engblom, J., and Forslind, B., Lipid polymorphism — a key to the understanding of skin penetration. K.R. Brain, V.J. James, and K.A. Walters (eds). In *Proceedings of Prediction of Percutaneous Penetration.* Vol 4b, STS Publishing Ltd, Cardiff C59, U.K., 1995.
25. Engblom, J., On the Phase Behaviour of Lipids with Respect to Skin Barrier Function. Thesis, Lund University, Sweden, 1996.
26. Norlén, L.P.O., The Skin Barrier. Structure and Physical Function. Thesis, Karolinska Institutet, Stockholm, Sweden, 1999.
27. Bouwstra, J.A., Gooris, G.S., Bras, W., and Downing, D.T., Lipid organization in pig stratum corneum. *J Lipid Res* 36:685–695, 1995.
28. Thewalt, J., Kitson, N., Araujo, C., MacKay, A., and Bloom, M., Models of stratum corneum intercellular membranes: the sphingolipid headgroup is a determinant of phase behaviour in mixed lipid dispersions. *Biochem Biophys Res Commun* 188:1247–1252, 1992.
29. Moore, D.J., Rerek, M.E., and Mendelsohn, R., Lipid domains and orthorhombic phases in model stratum corneum: evidence from Fourier transform infrared spectroscopy studies. *Biochem Biophys Res Commun* 231:797–801, 1997.

4 Lipid and Protein Structures in the Permeability Barrier

Donald T. Downing and Noel D. Lazo

CONTENTS

4.1 INTRODUCTION

While it is well established that the epidermal permeability barrier depends primarily on lipid structures, there are instances where proteins are inherent partners in the formation and maintenance of the necessary biological structures.

4.2 LIPIDS AND PROTEINS OF THE CORNEOCYTE ENVELOPE

The corneocyte envelope forms a vital part of the permeability barrier of the epidermis. This elaborate structure consists of two parts: (1) a thick layer (~15 nm) adjacent to the cytoplasm which is composed of structural proteins and (2) a thin layer (~4 nm) on the exterior of the protein part which is composed of lipids. The protein layer is highly insoluble, due to the extensive cross-linking of several proteins by disulfide and ε-(γ-glutamyl)lysine isopeptide bonds. Table 1 shows some of the cross-linked components of human epidermal corneocyte envelopes as well as the secondary structures present in the isolated proteins.

The existence of a lipid envelope on the exterior of the corneocyte is a relatively recent discovery,[1-3] and the molecular structure of the lipid/protein interface remains under investigation.[4,5] As described in Chapter 2, the chemical structures of the lipids that constitute the corneocyte lipid envelope are well established, and the fact that the lipids are ester linked to the protein involucrin in the corneocyte envelope is generally accepted. It is clear that attachment of the ceramide molecules requires that the protein substrate provide a surface rich in carboxylic acid side chains. A diagrammatic representation of the lipid/protein compound envelope of the mammalian cornified cell is shown in Figure 1.

What remains to be determined is how involucrin is arranged in the envelope so as to present the planar array of glutamate side chains that is required as a support for the lipid envelope. The

0-8493-7520-7/00/$0.00+$.50

TABLE 1
Cross-Linked Protein Components of Human Epidermal Corneocyte Envelopes

Protein	Structures Present in Isolated Protein
Involucrin[21]	α-Helix and random coil[9,22]
Elafin[23]	β-Sheet, random coil, and β-turn[24]
Small, proline-rich proteins[25]	Random coil, no α-/β-structures[26]
Loricrin[27]	Glycine-rich loops interrupted by Q/K-rich regions[28]
Filaggrin[29]	Random coil[30]
Keratin intermediate filaments[29]	α-Helix, β-helix, and random coil[31]

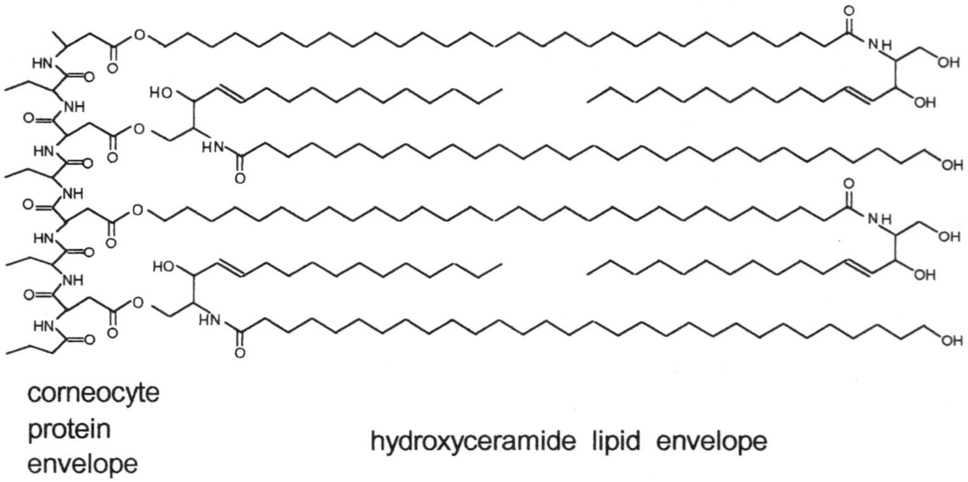

corneocyte protein envelope

hydroxyceramide lipid envelope

FIGURE 1 A representation of the attachment of hydroxyceramide molecules to a glutamate-rich protein substrate to form the compound lipid-protein envelope of the epidermal corneocyte. Spatial requirements dictate the alternation in orientation of the hydroxyceramide molecules, which is supported by the demonstration that roughly half of the lipid molecules are bound by their ω-hydroxyl group and half by the sphingosine head group.[2]

answer to this question is being sought in some instances by the isolation of the stratum corneum and chemical investigation of the sites of attachment of lipids to protein.[5] In the authors' laboratory, molecular modeling is being used in attempts to predict plausible protein conformations that could support the lipids, and potential conformations are being verified by the synthesis of model peptides that might adopt the conformation of the native protein.

4.2.1 Molecular Modeling of Involucrin

While involucrin is most likely the protein to which the corneocyte lipid envelope is attached, it is a curious fact that the involucrin of human epidermis is a distinctly different protein from that in the epidermis of mammals other than the anthropoids.[6,7] Therefore, care must be taken in extrapolation of results with lower mammals to humans.

In studies of human involucrin, attempts have been made to predict the likely molecular conformation, based on the spatial requirements for the attachment of lipids and the known conformational predilections of specific amino-acid sequences. Initially, we predicted that involucrin

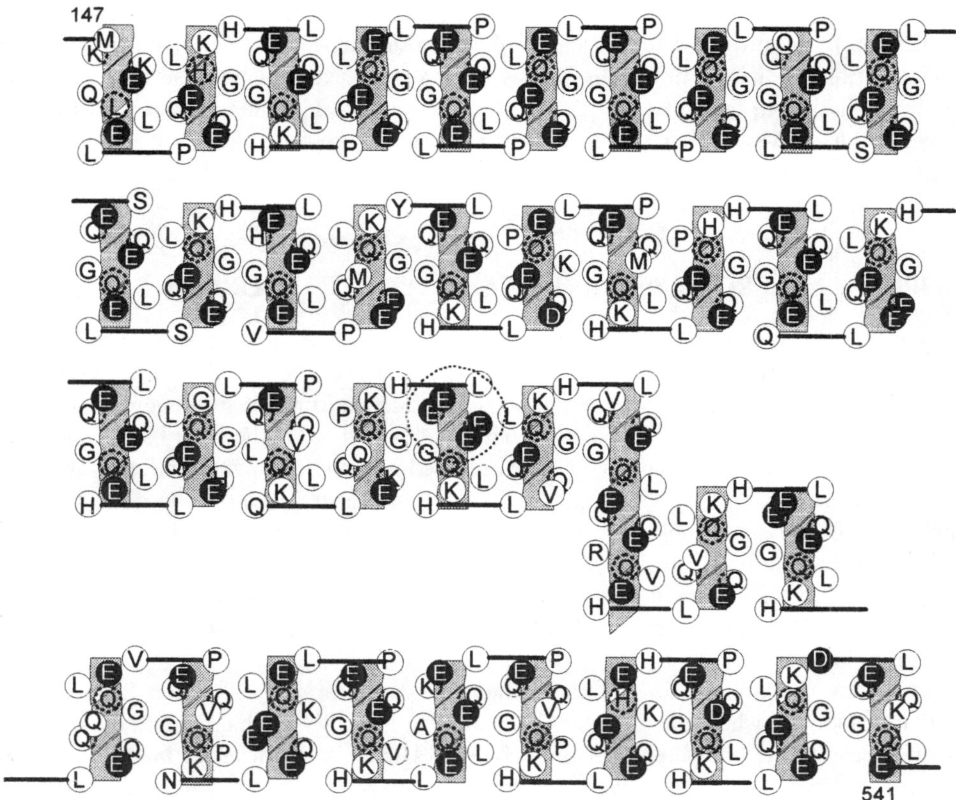

FIGURE 2 Involucrin, the protein to which the epidermal lipid envelope is believed to be attached, is shown in an α-helical conformation in which the glutamate side chains could be arrayed in a dense surface sheet. A demonstrated point of attachment of a hydroxyceramide molecule[5] is circled.

might adopt the β-sheet conformation,[8] since this could provide the required surface density of glutamate residues. This concept was supported by solid-state NMR studies of corneocyte envelopes isolated from pig epidermis, which indicated that the cross-linked proteins are predominantly in the β-conformation.[4] Recently, we have observed that a conventional α-helical conformation of human involucrin could provide the necessary surface concentration of glutamate side chains, as illustrated in Figure 2.

4.2.2 Peptide Analogues

To evaluate the conformation of involucrin, peptides representing 1, 2, and 3 of the 10-residue repeat motifs of involucrin (PEQQEGQLEL) were synthesized. Circular dichroic spectra of the 20- and 30-residue peptides in phosphate buffered saline solutions at various pH levels showed only random coil conformations, but in solutions containing 50% or more of trifluoroethanol, spectra indicative of a predominantly α-helical conformation were obtained.[9] This indicates that in a relatively nonpolar environment, involucrin may spontaneously adopt the α-helical conformation.

4.2.3 Direct Studies of the Corneocyte Envelope Structure

Marekov and Steinert obtained solvent-extracted corneocyte envelope preparations from human epidermis and, after partial removal of bound lipids with alkali, digested the tissue with proteases.[5] Subsequent analysis of lipid-bearing peptide fragments indicated sites in the native involucrin to which hydroxyceramides were attached. All but one of these sites was in the less organized region of the protein, proximal to the region of 10-residue repeats. The one attachment point in the repeat region (indicated in Figure 2) may have been identified because it is one that has limited cross-linking to the substrate protein through isopeptide bonds, which are formed from glutamine residues. Most other potential fragments in the repeat region have more than one glutamine residue available for attachment and are therefore less likely to become detached from the tissue by proteolysis.

4.3 LIPIDS AND PROTEINS IN THE CORNEOCYTE INTERIOR

It has frequently been speculated whether the barrier function of the epidermis is augmented by the contents of the corneocytes and whether this might be enhanced by the presence of lipids in the interior of the cornified cell. However, there is no evidence from electron microscopy that lipid structures exist in significant amounts in mammalian corneocytes. On the other hand, lipid lamellae have been observed in large amounts within the cornified cells in birds[10] and reptiles.[11] This appears to be a normal process in these vertebrates in which lamellar granules tend to remain within the cell during cornification and subsequently adopt the lamellar structure inside the corneocyte. It has been proposed that the extent to which the lamellar granules are discharged in avian epidermis may be governed by variations in relative humidity and water availability.[10] Whether there is any specific interaction between the retained lipids and the keratin filaments within the avian or reptilian corneocytes is unclear.

No mechanism involving the retention of lamellar granules appears to have been detected in mammalian epidermis, where the granules seem always to be fully discharged into the intercellular spaces regardless of the competence of the epidermal barrier or the level of humidity. The rapid restoration of barrier function following experimental abrogation of the barrier may result from redistribution and reorientation of lipids remaining in the intercellular spaces, rather than increased discharge of lamellar granules, since this is complete even when the barrier is adequate.

4.4 LIPIDS AND PROTEINS IN THE INTERCELLULAR LAMELLAE

The striking pattern of the intercellular lamellae in mammalian stratum corneum, as revealed by ruthenium tetroxide fixation and electron microscopic examination,[12-14] has led some investigators to speculate that proteins may contribute to the observed structures. The absence of relevant intercellular structures in electron micrographs of osmium tetroxide-fixed stratum corneum argues against a significant role or presence of protein, since this would be visualized by the conventional fixative.

It has been argued that the unusual spacings of intercellular lamellae, as observed with X-ray diffraction,[15-17] also indicate a role for proteins in the lamellar sheets. The prominent 13-nm spacing, which is equivalent to three lipid bilayers, has not been observed in lipid lamellae from other sources and seems to originate from the *broad-narrow-broad* repeat structure that is a distinctive feature of the intercellular lipids.[12-14] In recrystallized stratum corneum lipids,[13] a similar repeat distance is observed, but the *broad-narrow-broad* repeat is replaced by a *broad-broad-broad* pattern, where the appearance of the electron-opaque polar regions can be described as $(\textit{dense-light-light})_n$. The spacing of this repeat is similar to that of the native lipids and is not differentiated by X-ray diffraction. Nevertheless, the 13-nm X-ray spacing is absent in reconstituted mixtures of pure stratum corneum lipids unless a small proportion of acylceramide (ceramide 1) is included in the mixture.[17] The restoration of the 13-nm X-ray spacing on addition of 8% ceramide 1 shows that a protein component is unnecessary for producing the unique appearance of lipid lamellae formed from stratum corneum lipids.

4.5 LIPIDS AND PROTEINS IN HAIR

Although unrelated to the barrier function of the epidermis itself, it is interesting to note that mammalian hair also possesses a protein-bound lipid barrier in the cuticle cells of the hair shaft. This lipid envelope is chemically quite unlike that of the corneocyte, consisting almost exclusively of saturated fatty acids, more than half of which were shown to be the unusual, branched chain compound 18-methyl-eicosanoic acid and its longer-chain homologues.[18,19] As diagrammed in Figure 3, the fatty acids are attached to the protein through thioester bonds, unlike the epidermal lipid envelope which is linked through conventional ester bonds. The unusual fatty acid composition of the hair cuticle lipid envelope occurs throughout the many mammalian species that have been studied,[18-20] regardless of whether the sebum of an individual species contains branched-chain fatty acids, as in sheep, or if it is entirely derived from straight-chain fatty acids, as in cattle.

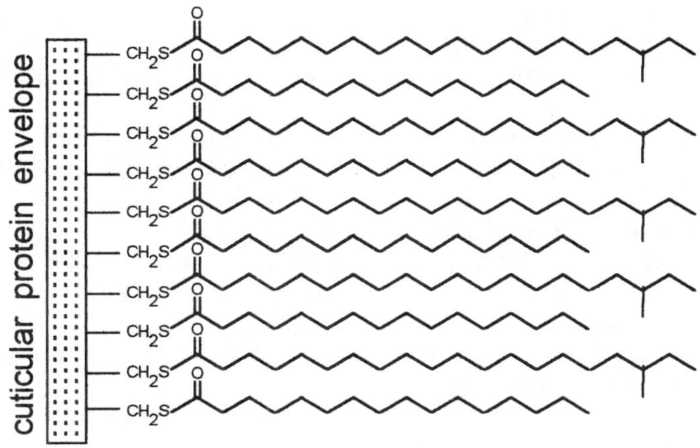

FIGURE 3 A postulated arrangement of the straight-chain and branched-chain (18-methyl-eicosanoic acid) fatty acids attached to the cuticular surface of mammalian hair.[18-20]

REFERENCES

1. Wertz, P. W. and Downing, D. T., Covalent attachment of ω-hydroxyacid derivatives to epidermal macromolecules: a preliminary characterization, *Biochem. Biophys. Res. Commun.*, 137, 992, 1986.
2. Wertz, P. W. and Downing, D. T., Covalently bound ω-hydroxyacylsphingosine in the stratum corneum, *Biochim. Biophys. Acta*, 917, 108, 1987.
3. Swartzendruber, D. C., Wertz, P. W., Madison, K. C., and Downing, D. T., Evidence that the corneocyte has a chemically bound lipid envelope, *J. Invest. Dermatol.*, 88, 709, 1987.
4. Lazo, N. D., Meine, J. G., and Downing, D. T., Lipids are covalently attached to rigid corneocyte protein envelopes existing predominantly as β-sheets: a solid-state nuclear magnetic resonance study, *J. Invest. Dermatol.*, 105, 296, 1995.
5. Marekov, L. N. and Steinert, P. M., Ceramides are bound to structural proteins of the human foreskin epidermal cornified cell envelope, *J. Biol. Chem.*, 273, 17763, 1998.
6. Eckert, R. L. and Green, H., Structure and evolution of the human involucrin gene, *Cell*, 46, 583, 1986.
7. Tseng, H. and Green, H., The involucrin genes of pig and dog: comparison of their segments of repeats with those of prosimians and higher primates, *Mol. Biol. Evol.*, 7, 293, 1990.
8. Downing, D. T., Lipid and protein structures in the permeability barrier of mammalian epidermis, *J. Lipid Res.*, 33, 301, 1992.
9. Lazo, N. D. and Downing, D. T., unpublished results, 1999.
10. Menon, G. K., Baptista, L. F., Brown, B. E., and Elias, P. M., Avian epidermal differentiation II: adaptive response of permeability barrier to water deprivation and replenishment, *Tissue Cell*, 21, 83, 1989.

11. Matoltsy, A. G. and Bednarz, J. A., Lamellar bodies of the turtle epidermis, *J. Ultrastruct. Res.*, 53, 128, 1975.
12. Madison, K. C., Swartzendruber, D. C., Wertz, P. W., and Downing, D. T., Presence of intact intercellular lamellae in the upper layers of the stratum corneum, *J. Invest. Dermatol.*, 88, 714, 1987.
13. Swartzendruber, D. C., Wertz, P. W., Kitko, D. J., Madison, K. C., and Downing, D. T., Molecular models of the intercellular lipid lamellae in mammalian stratum corneum, *J. Invest. Dermatol.*, 92, 251, 1989.
14. Wertz, P. W. and Downing, D. T., Epidermal lipids, in *Physiology, Biochemistry, and Molecular Biology of the Skin,* 2nd ed., Goldsmith, L. A., Ed., Oxford University Press, New York, 1991, 205.
15. White, S. H., Mirejovsky, D., and King, G. I., Structure of lamellar lipid domains and corneocyte envelopes of murine stratum corneum: an X-ray diffraction study, *Biochemistry*, 27, 3725, 1988.
16. Bouwstra, J. A., Gooris, G. S., Bras, W., and Downing, D. T., Lipid organization in pig stratum corneum, *J. Lipid Res.*, 36, 685, 1995.
17. McIntosh, T. J., Stewart, M. E., and Downing, D. T., X-ray diffraction analysis of isolated skin lipids: reconstitution of intercellular lipid domains, *Biochemistry*, 35, 3649, 1996.
18. Wertz, P. W. and Downing, D. T., Integral lipids of human hair, *Lipids*, 23, 878, 1988.
19. Wertz, P. W. and Downing, D. T., Integral lipids of mammalian hair, *Comp. Biochem. Physiol.*, 92B, 759, 1989.
20. Peet, D. J., Wettenhall, R. E. H., Rivett, D. E., and Allen, A. K., A comparative study of covalently bound fatty acids in keratinized tissues, *Comp. Biochem. Physiol.*, 102B, 363, 1992.
21. Rice, R. H. and Green, H., The cornified envelope of terminally differentiated human epidermal keratinocytes consists of cross-linked protein, *Cell*, 11, 417, 1977.
22. Yaffe, M. B., Beegen, H., and Eckert, R. L., Biophysical characterization of involucrin reveals a molecule ideally suited to function as an intermolecular cross-bridge of the keratinocyte cornified envelope, *J. Biol. Chem.*, 267, 12233, 1992.
23. Tezuka, T. and Takahashi, M., The cystine-rich envelope protein from human epidermal stratum corneum cells, *J. Invest. Dermatol.,* 88, 47, 1987.
24. Francart, C., Dauchez, M., Alix, A. J. P., and Lippens, G., Solution structure of R-elafin, a specific inhibitor of elastase, *J. Mol. Biol.*, 268, 666, 1997.
25. Kartasova, T., Cornelissen, B. J., Belt, P., and Van Du Putte, P., Effects of UV, 4-NQO and TPA on gene expression in cultured human epidermal keratinocytes, *Nucleic Acids Res.*, 15, 5945, 1987.
26. Tarcsa, E., Candi, E., Kartasova, T., Idler, W. E., Marekov, L. N., and Steinert, P. M., Structural and transglutaminase substrate properties of the small proline-rich 2 family of cornified cell envelope proteins, *J. Biol. Chem.*, 273, 23297, 1998.
27. Mehrel, T., Hohl, D., Rothnagel, J. A., Longley, M. A., Bundman, D., Cheng, C., Lichti, U., Bisher, M. E., Steven, A. C., Steinert, P. M., Yuspa, S. H., and Roop, D. R., Identification of a major keratinocyte cell envelope protein, loricrin, *Cell*, 61, 1103, 1990.
28. Hohl, D., Mehrel, T., Lichti, U., Turner, M. L., Roop, D. R., and Steinert, P. M., Characterization of human loricrin: structure and function of a new class of epidermal cell envelope proteins, *J. Biol. Chem.,* 266, 6626, 1991.
29. Steinert, P. M. and Marekov, L. N., The proteins elafin, filaggrin, keratin intermediate filaments, loricrin, and small proline-rich proteins 1 and 2 are isodipeptide cross-linked components of the human epidermal cornified cell envelope, *J. Biol. Chem.*, 270, 17702, 1995.
30. Tarcsa, E., Marekov, L. N., Giampiero, M., Melino, G., Lee, S.-C., and Steinert, P. M., Protein unfolding by peptidylarginine deiminase: substrate specificity and structural relationships of the natural substrates trichohyalin and filaggrin, *J. Biol. Chem.*, 271, 30709, 1996.
31. Downing, D. T., Molecular modeling indicates that homodimers form the basis for intermediate filament assembly from human and mouse epidermal keratins, *Proteins: Struct. Func., Genet.*, 23, 204, 1995.

5 The Environmental Interface: Regulation of Permeability Barrier Homeostasis

Kenneth R. Feingold and Peter M. Elias

CONTENTS

5.1 INTRODUCTION

The cutaneous permeability barrier is required for territorial existence. Moreover, disruptions of this barrier are seen in a number of cutaneous diseases such as psoriasis and atopic dermatitis, and abnormalities of barrier homeostasis occur with normal aging.[1,2] Additionally, disruption of the barrier is associated with increased keratinocyte proliferation which may lead to epidermal hyperplasia[3,4] and increased production and secretion of cytokines which may lead to cutaneous inflammation.[5-8] Thus, abnormalities of the barrier are seen in a variety of cutaneous disorders and may play a role in the pathogenesis of some of these disorders, either as an initiating factor or as a mechanism that sustains and exacerbates the cutaneous condition. In this chapter we will describe our laboratory efforts in elucidating the mechanisms and regulatory factors that form and maintain the permeability barrier.

0-8493-7520-7/00/$0.00+$.50

5.2 CUTANEOUS PERMEABILITY BARRIER

The cutaneous barrier resides in the stratum corneum (SC) layer of the epidermis, which is composed of two components: protein enriched nonviable corneocytes and lipid laden intercellular domains.[9,10] Based on abundant experimental data obtained by a variety of different avenues of investigation, it is now widely accepted that the lipids within the intercellular domains are crucial in providing the barrier to water loss.[9,10]

The lipid composition of the SC differs greatly from the other layers of the epidermis and other tissues.[11,12] The SC is composed primarily of three classes of lipids: free sterols, free fatty acids, and ceramides. Ceramides contain unusually long chained, fully saturated fatty acids, and some species contain linoleic acid esterified to the terminus of the N-acyl fatty acid, forming an extremely long hydrophobic structure potentially capable of linking two or more adjacent bilayers.[10,12] The importance of this molecule is underscored by the fact that deficiency of the essential fatty acid, linoleic acid, results in abnormalities in membrane structure leading to defective barrier function.[9-12]

The lipids in the intercellular spaces of the SC are derived primarily from the exocytosis of lamellar bodies (LB).[9,12] LB first appear in the upper spinous layer, and in the SG cells they are displaced apically and laterally, i.e., close to the SG–SC interface. LB are enriched in lipids — mostly free sterols, sphingolipids, phospholipids and hydrolytic enzymes, and sugars linked to lipid and/or protein.[9,12] The exocytosis of LB provides a pathway by which the cells of the epidermis transfer lipids to the intercellular spaces of the SC.

5.3 CHOICE OF EXPERIMENTAL MODELS

The central aim of our research has been to elucidate how the epidermal permeability barrier is formed and maintained. To accomplish this goal we have utilized several experimental models in which barrier function is disrupted, allowing us to characterize the response of the epidermis to these perturbations. By "stressing" the system, we have been able to elucidate a number of the key pathways required for barrier homeostasis. The first model of barrier disruption involves wiping the skin of hairless mice with acetone or SDS, which extracts SC lipids, thereby disrupting barrier function.[13] The second model uses cellophane tape stripping of hairless mice, which mechanically removes the SC, including intercellular lipids, thereby disrupting the barrier. In both of these acute models of barrier perturbation, changes in lipid metabolism within the nucleated layers of the epidermis rapidly lead to the return of lipids to the SC and the restoration of barrier function.[14,15] The third model involves feeding an essential fatty acid deficient (EFAD) diet to hairless mice, which results in a chronic disruption of barrier function.[16] By employing several different approaches to disrupt the barrier (solvent or detergent extraction, mechanical, dietary), we avoid the potential pitfall of a single manipulation artifactually causing a change in epidermal metabolism that might be unrelated to alterations in barrier function. Finally, in each of these models we have also demonstrated the link to barrier function by applying a water-impermeable membrane (Latex or plastic wrap) which instantly restores barrier function.[14,15] If a change in epidermal metabolism is seen in response to a variety of different methods of disrupting the barrier, and if it is normalized or prevented following application of a water-impermeable membrane, then the metabolic alteration is very likely to be due to barrier dysfunction rather than a nonspecific response to a toxic insult.

5.4 EFFECT OF BARRIER DISRUPTION ON LAMELLAR BODY SECRETION AND REFORMATION

Either acetone or tape stripping of hairless mice disrupts the barrier, causing a marked increase in transepidermal water loss (TEWL) (>3 $g/M^2/h$). Very rapidly, lipid is replenished in the SC, and barrier function improves (by 360 min, TEWL is approximately 50% of that seen immediately after disruption).[14,15,17] In humans the time course of recovery of barrier function is slower than in hairless mice but the shape of the recovery curve is very similar.[2] The first step identified in the repair process following acute disruption of the barrier with either acetone or tape stripping is the secretion (within 15 min) of preformed LB contents by cells of the upper SG, which leaves the cytosol of these cells largely devoid of LB.[18] Newly formed LB then begin to reappear in the SG cells at 30 to 60 min, and by 3 to 6 h these cells have a full complement of normal appearing LB.[18] Moreover, between 60 and 360 min the quantity of secreted LB contents at the SG–SC interface increases.[18] New lamellar bilayer units begin to appear in the lower SC between 30 min and 2 h.[18] Thus, acute barrier disruption in hairless mice leads to the rapid secretion of preformed LB followed by the formation and continued secretion of LB, which lead to the appearance of new lamellar bilayers in the SC. This progressive return of lamellar bilayers to the lower SC is associated with the restoration of barrier function. Occlusion with an impermeable membrane prevents the formation and secretion of nascent LB by the SG cells and prevents barrier repair.[18] These morphological changes in response to barrier disruption are localized to the upper epidermis (SG cells and SC).

5.5 IMPORTANCE OF LAMELLAR BODY SECRETION AND REFORMATION

Our studies have demonstrated that the topical application of nontoxic doses of monensin, which affects multiple steps in the assembly and exocytosis of secretory vesicles, delays barrier repair by inhibiting the generation and secretion of LB.[19] Similarly, topical application of nontoxic doses of brefeldin A, which blocks the anterograde movement of newly synthesized protein and lipid from the endoplasmic reticulum to the Golgi apparatus, also prevents the formation of LB in SG cells and delays barrier recovery.[19] These results demonstrate the essential role of the formation and secretion of LB in the repair of the barrier.

5.6 THE EFFECT OF BARRIER DISRUPTION ON LIPID SYNTHESIS

As discussed previously, SG cells rapidly form a large number of LB following barrier disruption. The major lipid components of LB are cholesterol, glucosylceramides (precursor of ceramides), and phospholipids (precursor of fatty acids). The epidermis is a very active site of lipid synthesis, and lipid synthesis occurs in all layers of the epidermis.[14,20] As will be detailed below, the increase in epidermal lipid synthesis that follows barrier disruption plays an important role in providing the lipid building blocks necessary to form new LB.

5.6.1 Cholesterol Synthesis

Both acute and chronic disruption of the barrier increase epidermal cholesterol synthesis two- to threefold without altering synthesis in the dermis.[21,22] The increase in cholesterol synthesis occurs almost immediately after barrier disruption and returns toward normal in parallel with barrier recovery.[21] Additionally, the increase in cholesterol synthesis directly correlates with the extent of damage to the barrier. Moreover, in both the acute and chronic models, the increase in epidermal cholesterol synthesis can be completely inhibited by occlusion with an impermeable membrane.[21,22] The increase in epidermal cholesterol synthesis is associated with an increase in the activity of HMG-CoA reductase, the rate-limiting enzyme in cholesterogenesis.[23] This increase in activity can be explained by an increase in the mass of HMG-CoA reductase protein and an increase in epidermal HMG-CoA reductase mRNA levels.[24] In addition to increasing enzyme mass, barrier disruption also produces an increase in the activation state of HMG-CoA reductase.[23] The extent of the increase in enzyme content and activation state correlates directly with the degree of disruption of the barrier and can be attenuated by occlusion with an impermeable membrane.[23] Thus, barrier disruption increases HMG-CoA reductase activity by activating the enzyme and by increasing enzyme mass (and mRNA levels), which together result in an increase in cholesterol synthesis in the epidermis.

In recent studies we have shown that other key enzymes in the cholesterol synthetic pathway (HMG-CoA synthase, farnsyl pyrophosphate synthase [FPPS], and squalene synthase) are also increased by barrier disruption.[25]

Separation of the epidermis into upper and lower epidermis using either the staphylococcal epidermolytic toxin or DTT separation has permitted localization of epidermal cholesterol synthesis and HMG-CoA reductase activity.[26,27] Under basal conditions almost 70% of cholesterol synthesis occurs in the basal layer.[26] Following acute barrier disruption, HMG-CoA reductase activity increases in both the upper and lower epidermis, but quantitatively the increase is greater in the basal layer.[27] Moreover, the mechanism accounting for the increase in HMG-CoA reductase activity following barrier disruption differs in the upper and lower epidermis. In the lower epidermis the increase is due to both an increase in enzyme content and activation state, while in the upper epidermis the increase is due to an increase in activation state.[27] Whereas the increase in the activation state of HMG-CoA reductase could provide an immediate source of cholesterol for the early formation of LB in the upper epidermis, the large increase in enzyme activity in the lower epidermis could provide cholesterol either for cell proliferation and/or for transport to SG cells for further LB formation. Whether lipids are transported from the lower epidermis to the upper epidermis for the purpose of barrier repair is unknown.

5.6.2 Fatty Acid Synthesis

In addition to cholesterol synthesis, both acute and chronic disruption of the barrier increase fatty acid synthesis in the epidermis.[28] Similar to cholesterol synthesis, the increase in fatty acid synthesis occurs almost immediately after barrier disruption and returns toward normal in parallel with barrier recovery.[28] Likewise, occlusion with an impermeable membrane prevents the characteristic increase in epidermal fatty acid synthesis.[28] The increase in epidermal fatty acid synthesis is due to an increase in both of the key enzymes of fatty acid synthesis, acetyl-CoA carboxylase and fatty acid synthase activities.[29] In recent studies we have shown that disruption of the barrier increases acetyl-CoA carboxylase and fatty acid synthase mRNA levels in the epidermis.[25] The location of the increase in epidermal fatty acid synthesis that occurs in response to barrier disruption has not yet been addressed, but in normal animals the majority of fatty acid synthesis is localized to the lower epidermis.[30]

5.6.3 Sphingolipid Synthesis

We have also demonstrated that sphingolipid synthesis increases following either acute or chronic disruption of the barrier.[31] However, in contrast to cholesterol and fatty acid synthesis, the increase in sphingolipid synthesis is delayed, first being observed 6 to 7 h following acute barrier disruption.[31] The stimulation of sphingolipid synthesis is due to an increase in the activity of serine palmitoyl transferase (SPT), the enzyme that catalyzes the initial and first committed step in sphingolipid synthesis.[31] Moreover, similar to cholesterol and fatty acid synthesis, artificial restoration of the barrier with an impermeable membrane prevents the increase in both sphingolipid synthesis and SPT activity.[31] Furthermore, recent studies have shown that the increase in sphingolipid synthesis and SPT activity in response to barrier disruption occurs to a similar degree in both the upper and lower epidermis.[32] Recently, we have shown that SPT mRNA levels increase following barrier disruption.

Glucosylceramide is the predominant ceramide in lamellar bodies and is synthesized by the enzyme UDP:glucose:ceramide D-glucosyl transferase (glucosylceramide synthase, GC synthase). GC synthase activity in the epidermis is predominantly localized to the outer epidermis.[33] However, barrier disruption does not effect the activity of GC synthase, indicating that there is sufficient enzyme present to allow for the large increase in glucosylceramide formation required for the marked increase in LB formation that occurs following barrier disruption.[33]

5.7 REGULATION OF LIPID SYNTHESIS

The regulation of the expression of many of the genes involved in cholesterol metabolism is coordinately regulated. For example, under most conditions the mRNA levels of HMG-CoA reductase, HMG-CoA synthase, farnesyl pyrophosphate synthase, squalene synthase, and the LDL receptor are coordinately increased or decreased.[34-39] 25OH cholesterol is a very potent inhibitor of the expression of these genes.[34-39] Of course there are exceptions, and recently our laboratory has reported that in the liver of hamsters, LPS or cytokine treatment results in discordant regulation producing an isolated increase in the transcription and mRNA levels of HMG-CoA reductase without affecting HMG-CoA synthase, farnesyl pyrophosphate synthase, or the LDL receptor.[40] The basis for the usual coordinate regulation is that the genes involved in cholesterol metabolism all have a similar approximately 10-base-pair response element in the 5′ flanking region which has been called the sterol regulatory element (in some genes more than one sterol regulatory element is present).

Recent studies by the laboratory of Brown, Goldstein, and co-workers have further defined the mechanisms underlying coordinate regulation.[39] They isolated, sequenced, and cloned two proteins that both bind to sterol regulatory elements and stimulate gene transcription (sterol regulatory element binding proteins, SREBP-1, SREBP-2).[41,42] The SREBPs are synthesized as 125-kD proteins which attach to the endoplasmic reticulum and nuclear membranes by means of hydrophobic sequences.[43] Under conditions of sterol deficiency (and perhaps other factors), two proteases cleave the SREBPs, releasing the amino terminal portion which is 68 kD on SDS gels. 25OH cholesterol is a very potent inhibitor of the formation of mature active SREBP.[43] The mature active amino terminal peptide contains a basic-helix-loop-helix leucine zipper motif that allows for the formation of homodimers and binding to sterol regulatory elements. Additionally, this amino terminal domain contains an acidic region that acts as a transcriptional activator. The activation of SREBPs is analogous to the activation of NF-κB, which coordinately stimulates the expression of a wide variety of genes involved in the inflammatory response.[44]

Many cells in culture express both SREBP-1 and SREBP-2. In these cells the processing of both proteins is regulated coordinately, and either protein by itself is capable of regulating gene transcription.[43,45] There is no evidence for the formation of heterodimers. Recent studies in intact animals have demonstrated a greater degree of complexity with discordant regulation of SREBP-1 and SREBP-2. In hamster liver in the basal state, mature active SREBP-1 was present, but no mature SREBP-2 was found.[46] However, sterol depletion led to a marked increase in mature SREBP-2 and a reciprocal decline in SREBP-1.[46] Additionally, SREBP-2 mRNA levels increase, while no change was seen in SREBP-1 mRNA. These results indicate that in liver SREBP-1 is responsible for basal transcription, while SREBP-2 is responsible for the increase in transcription that occurs following sterol depletion.

Over the years it has been frequently noted that cholesterol synthesis and fatty acid synthesis are coordinately regulated.[47] For example, in the liver many physiological (i.e., diurnal rhythm, increased food intake, starvation) and pathological (i.e., nephrotic syndrome, insulin-resistant diabetes) conditions result in a coordinate increase or decrease in cholesterol and fatty acid synthesis.[47] Moreover, as noted earlier, barrier disruption stimulates both cholesterol and fatty acid synthesis in the epidermis. Additionally, we have also shown that chronic treatment with lovastatin, which inhibits cholesterol synthesis, leads to a marked increase in the enzymes involved in cholesterol synthesis (up-regulation by absence of feedback inhibition), while also markedly stimulating fatty acid synthesis, providing further evidence that these pathways are coordinately regulated in the epidermis.[48] A possible basis for this linkage has recently been elucidated by studies demonstrating, first, that fatty acid synthase has a regulatory element that binds SREBPs[49,50] and, more recently, by studies demonstrating that SREBPs regulate the transcription of fatty acid synthase mRNA.[51] Additionally, recent studies have shown that the transcription of acetyl-CoA carboxylase mRNA is also regulated by SREBPs.[52]

We recently demonstrated that SREBP-2 is the predominant SREBP in human keratinocytes and murine epidermis, while SREBP-1 is not detected.[53] Sterols regulate SREBP-2 mRNA levels in keratinocytes and the epidermis and the proteolytic cleavage of SREBP-2 to the mature active form in keratinocytes.[53] In parallel to the increase in mature active SREBP, there is a coordinate increase in mRNA levels for cholesterol (HMG-CoA reductase, HMG-CoA synthase, farnesyl diphosphate synthase, and squalene synthase) and fatty acid (acetyl-CoA carboxylase, fatty acid synthase) synthetic enzymes.[53] However, mRNA levels for SPT, the first committed step for ceramide synthesis, do not increase in parallel.[53] The increase of mRNA for enzymes required for epidermal cholesterol and fatty acid synthesis is consistent with both the previously described early increase of cholesterol and fatty acid synthesis after barrier disruption and a role for SREBP-2 in the regulation of cholesterol and fatty acid synthesis for epidermal barrier homeostasis. In contrast, SPT appears to be regulated by different mechanisms, consistent with the different time course of its stimulation after barrier disruption.

5.8 REQUIREMENT OF LIPID SYNTHESIS FOR BARRIER REPAIR

To demonstrate the specific requirements for cholesterol, fatty acid, and sphingolipid synthesis for barrier formation, we performed a series of studies with specific pharmacological inhibitors of the key enzymes in the biosynthetic pathways of each of these lipids. Blocking the synthesis of cholesterol with inhibitors of HMG-CoA reductase, such as lovastatin or fluvastatin, delays the early phase (1 to 6 h) of barrier recovery.[54] This inhibition of barrier recovery is associated with a selective decrease in the return of cholesterol to the SC.[54] Also, LB formed in the presence of lovastatin display an abnormal appearing internal membrane structure, presumably secondary to a deficiency in cholesterol content.[54] That the inhibition of barrier recovery by HMG-CoA reductase inhibitors is due to a specific block in cholesterol synthesis and not to nonspecific toxicity is shown by the reversal of the pharmacologic blockade by simultaneous topical treatment with either mevalonate (the immediate product of HMG-CoA reductase) or cholesterol (the final end product of the biosynthetic pathway).[54] Moreover, co-application of cholesterol with HMG-CoA reductase inhibitors also normalizes the appearance of nascent LB.[54] These results provide direct evidence that epidermal cholesterol synthesis is required for barrier homeostasis.

We have also examined the effects of 5-(tetradecyloxy)-2-furancarboxylic acid (TOFA), a drug that inhibits acetyl-CoA carboxylase (ACC), one of the rate-limiting enzymes of fatty acid synthesis, on barrier repair.[55] Topical TOFA treatment inhibits fatty acid synthesis in the epidermis by approximately 50%.[55] Moreover, as with HMG-CoA reductase inhibitors, TOFA treatment inhibits the early phase (1 to 6 h) of barrier repair following disruption of the barrier and is associated with abnormal appearing LB.[55] Most importantly, the inhibition of barrier repair produced by TOFA can be overcome by topical co-applications of free fatty acids, again demonstrating the specificity of the inhibitor effect.[55] These results indicate that epidermal fatty acid synthesis also is required for barrier homeostasis.

Analogous studies have been carried out using topically applied β-chloroalanine, a selective inhibitor of SPT activity and sphingolipid synthesis.[56] Inhibition of sphingolipid synthesis with β-chloroalanine also delays barrier recovery after acute barrier disruption, but in contrast to the effects of topical HMG-CoA reductase and fatty acid synthesis inhibitors, this inhibition occurs during the late phases of barrier repair (12 to 24 h).[56] These findings are consistent with our data showing that the increase in sphingolipid synthesis following barrier disruption occurs at a later time than the increase in cholesterol and fatty acid synthesis.[31] Moreover, the delay in barrier repair in the β-chloroalanine-treated animals is associated with both a decrease in the return of sphingolipids to the SC and abnormal appearing LB.[56] Finally, β-chloroalanine inhibition of barrier repair can be overcome by providing exogenous sphingolipids, demonstrating that the effect of β-chloroalanine on barrier repair is not a nonspecific or toxic effect.[56] These results provide direct evidence that epidermal sphingolipid synthesis is required for barrier homeostasis.

While our studies have shown that GC synthase activity is not regulated by barrier disruption, recent studies have shown that inhibition of GC synthase activity by topical applications of d,1-threo-1-phenyl-2-hexadecanoylamino-3-pyrrolidino-1-propanol (PPPP) delays barrier recovery following barrier perturbation.[33] The delay in barrier recovery was present as early as 2 h, persisted for 6 h, but by 24 h barrier recovery was normal in PPPP-treated animals.[33] Additionally, PPPP-treated epidermis displayed abnormal LB contents at 2 and 4 h.[33] These results indicate that the synthesis of glucosylceramides is required for normal LB formation and barrier homeostasis.

Thus, the epidermal synthesis of all three of the major classes of lipids that are contained in LB increases following barrier disruption and is required for barrier homeostasis.

5.9 EXTRACUTANEOUS ORIGIN OF EPIDERMAL LIPIDS

While the previously described studies indicate that local epidermal lipid synthesis plays an important role in barrier repair, a number of lines of evidence suggest that extracutaneously derived lipids may also make a significant contribution to maintaining epidermal barrier function. First, in the inhibitor studies described earlier, despite blocking lipid synthesis to a large extent (in the lovastatin studies cholesterol synthesis was decreased by 95+%), the effect on barrier repair was only modest.[54-56] This discrepancy suggests that alternate sources of lipid are available for regeneration of the SC barrier. Second, studies by our laboratory have shown that systemically administered, labeled cholesterol and fatty acids are delivered to the epidermis.[21,28] Third, essential fatty acids are present in the SC in large quantities and are required for the maintenance of a competent barrier.[11,12,16] By definition, these essential fatty acid are only derived from dietary sources. Fourth, the epidermis lacks Δ^6 and Δ^5 desaturase activity and, therefore, the epidermis presumably must obtain arachidonic acid from other sites.[57] Finally, plant-derived fatty acids accumulate in the epidermis in certain disease states, such as Refsum's disease.[58,59] Taken together, these observations indicate that extracutaneous sources can contribute to the epidermal lipid pool.

5.10 EXTRACELLULAR LIPID PROCESSING

Whereas the intercellular lipid membranes in the SC contain primarily cholesterol, free fatty acids, and ceramides, the principle source of these lipids, the LB, contains cholesterol, phospholipids, and glucosylceramides.[11,12] These chemical differences suggest that the extracellular processing of secreted LB lipid precursors into more hydrophobic lipid products occurs during barrier formation. Moreover, LB are known to be enriched in a number of hydrolytic enzymes, including proteases, glycosidases, and a family of lipases which could be involved in extracellular processing.[9]

Barrier disruption increases the activity of β-glucocerebrosidase, the enzyme which hydrolyzes glucosylceramides to ceramides, by increasing epidermal β-glucocerebrosidase mRNA levels.[60] Recent studies have shown that inhibition of β-glucocerebrosidase activity by the topical application of bromo-condritol-B-epoxide (Br-CBE) delays barrier repair.[61] Associated with this defect in barrier repair, electron microscopic studies revealed immature lamellar membranes in the intercellular spaces of the SC.[61] A similar barrier defect and altered ultrastructure are evident in patients and transgenic mice with severe β-glucocerebrosidase deficiency (Gauchers disease Type II).[62,63] Moreover, studies have shown that inhibition of secretory (Type I) phospholipase A_2 ($_SPLA_2$), which converts extracellular phospholipids to free fatty acids by either bromophenacylbromide (BPB) or MJ33, also inhibits barrier repair.[64] Inhibition of PLA_2 also results in the formation and persistence of abnormal, immature lamellar bilayers in the SC interstices.[64] Normal barrier recovery and the appearance of normal intercellular lamellar structures could be induced by the topical co-application of nonessential free fatty acid (palmitate) with either BPB or MJ33, indicating that these effects were not due to nonspecific toxicity.[64] Whether the activity or synthesis of $_{S}PLA_2$ is regulated by barrier status has not yet been directly addressed. These studies indicate that the extracellular processing of lipids plays an important role in the formation of normal lamellar membranes in the SC and that interference with the formation of these membranes adversely affect barrier homeostasis.

5.10.1 Effect of pH

The epidermal surface has been known for many years to be acidic, but the role of this acidic pH of the stratum corneum in barrier homeostasis was unknown. It is well recognized that β-glucocerebrosidase is most active at pH 5.5. Recently, we have examined barrier recovery at an acidic vs. neutral pH. Barrier recovery proceeded normally when acetone-treated skin was exposed to solutions buffered to an acidic pH.[65] In contrast, barrier recovery was delayed when treated skin was exposed to neutral or alkaline pH regardless of buffer composition.[65] The formation and secretion of LB proceeded comparably at pH 5.5 and 7.4.[65] However, exposure to pH 7.4, not 5.5, resulted in both the persistence of immature extracellular lamellar membranes and a marked decrease in the *in situ* activity of β-glucocerebrosidase.[65] These results indicate that an acidic extracellular pH in the SC is required for normal extracellular lipid processing and normal barrier homeostasis.

5.11 IONIC SIGNALS FOR BARRIER REPAIR

The signals that initiate barrier restoration following barrier disruption are unknown, but our studies suggest that specific ions, particularly Ca^{2+}, may be crucial.[66-70] Cytochemical studies have demonstrated a Ca^{2+} gradient in the epidermis *in vivo* with low Ca^{2+} concentrations in the basal, proliferating layers and progressively higher concentrations as one proceeds to the outer differentiated layers.[71] A comparable Ca^{2+} gradient has been demonstrated in the epidermis using both energy dispersive X-ray microanalysis, proton probe, or PIXE techniques.[72-74] Recently, we have demonstrated that disruption of the barrier depletes Ca^{2+} from the upper epidermis, resulting in the loss of the Ca^{2+} gradient.[67,74,75] The Ca^{2+} gradient disappears after disrupting the barrier with acetone treatment or tape stripping due to accelerated water transit which leads to the increased passive loss of Ca^{2+} into and through the SC.[67,74,75] Accordingly, providing exogenous Ca^{2+} by immersion in a solution containing Ca^{2+} maintains the Ca^{2+} content in the upper epidermis and inhibits barrier repair.[66,67,75] In contrast, loss of Ca^{2+} from the upper epidermis is associated with the rapid secretion of LB.[66,67]

To further determine whether Ca^{2+} plays a crucial role in regulating LB secretion independent of barrier repair requirements, we have used a second model, high frequency sonophoresis, to selectively alter the Ca^{2+} content in the SG layer.[68] At the frequencies employed, sonophoresis enhances transepidermal penetration of Ca^{2+} without disrupting the permeability barrier, thereby allowing for the bulk movement of fluid into the epidermis (hydrokinesis).[68] Sonophoresis of Ca^{2+}-free solutions results in a marked decrease in Ca^{2+} content in the upper epidermis and the loss of the Ca^{2+} gradient.[68] In support of our hypothesis, the decrease in Ca^{2+} content in the upper epidermis caused by the sonophoresis of Ca^{2+}-free solutions is accompanied by accelerated LB secretion.[68] In contrast, sonophoresis of Ca^{2+}-containing solutions results in the addition of large quantities of Ca^{2+} to the upper epidermis, and LB secretion is not altered from basal rates.[68] Finally, both positive and negative iontophoresis, which did not affect barrier function, caused the disappearance of the epidermal calcium gradient with a marked decrease in calcium content in the upper epidermis.[76] Positive iontophoresis was associated with increased calcium in the stratum basale and dermis, whereas negative iontophoresis increased calcium in the SC.[6] Most importantly, the decrease in calcium content in the upper epidermis was associated with increased LB secretion and the build-up of lamellar material at the SC–SG interface.[76] These results demonstrate that epidermal Ca^{2+}

content can be manipulated by sonophoresis or iontophoresis without prior barrier disruption and that changes in the Ca^{2+} gradient induce LB secretion independent of barrier disruption. While in many tissues increases in Ca^{2+} are usually associated with increased secretion, there are other situations, comparable to the epidermis, where decreases in Ca^{2+} also stimulate secretion (e.g., parathyroid hormone secretion by the parathyroid gland).[77] Thus, water loss may induce a decrease in the concentration of Ca^{2+} in the upper epidermis, which in turn may stimulate LB secretion and barrier repair.

Both verapamil and nifedipine, which inhibit Ca^{2+} transport into cells via L channels, reverse the Ca^{2+}-induced inhibition of barrier repair, i.e., they normalize barrier recovery.[66] This finding suggests that changes in intracellular Ca^{2+} levels are important in mediating the inhibition of barrier repair. Moreover, both trifluoperazine and W7, two calmodulin inhibitors, also normalize barrier repair, even in the presence of high extracellular Ca^{2+} concentrations.[66] Taken together, these results indicate that Ca^{2+} enters the cells via L channels, binds to calmodulin in the cytosol, and then, by mechanisms yet to be elucidated, inhibits LB secretion and barrier repair.[66]

While Ca^{2+} is the most effective inhibitor of barrier repair, potassium, phosphate, and magnesium also modestly inhibit barrier repair. As with Ca^{2+}, it is likely that increased water transit after barrier disruption decreases the concentrations of a variety of epidermal ions due to increased passive ion loss. Indeed, others have demonstrated increased potassium flux following disruption of the barrier.[78]

5.12 EFFECT OF BARRIER DISRUPTION ON EPIDERMAL DNA SYNTHESIS

Although the epidermis is a rapidly replicating tissue, the factors that regulate epidermal DNA synthesis are not completely resolved. Our studies have demonstrated that both acute and chronic perturbations of barrier function increase epidermal DNA synthesis.[3] This increase in DNA synthesis is localized to the basal layer of the epidermis.[3] Moreover, the magnitude of the increase in epidermal DNA synthesis directly correlates with the degree of barrier disruption.[3] Furthermore, occlusion with an impermeable membrane largely inhibits the increase in DNA synthesis, while vapor-permeable membranes permit the increase in DNA synthesis to occur in proportion to their degree of vapor permeability.[3] Since the complete repair process requires 24 to 36 h, this increase in cell proliferation 16 to 20 h following barrier disruption could provide additional cells which could contribute to the final restoration of barrier function.

5.13 CONCLUSION

While many of the biosynthetic pathways and some of the regulatory factors involved in maintaining barrier homeostasis have been elucidated, many factors remain to be described. Our correct understanding is summarized in Figure 1. Hopefully understanding the mechanisms and regulatory factors responsible for barrier homeostasis will allow us to repair barrier defects and perhaps ameliorate or improve certain cutaneous diseases.

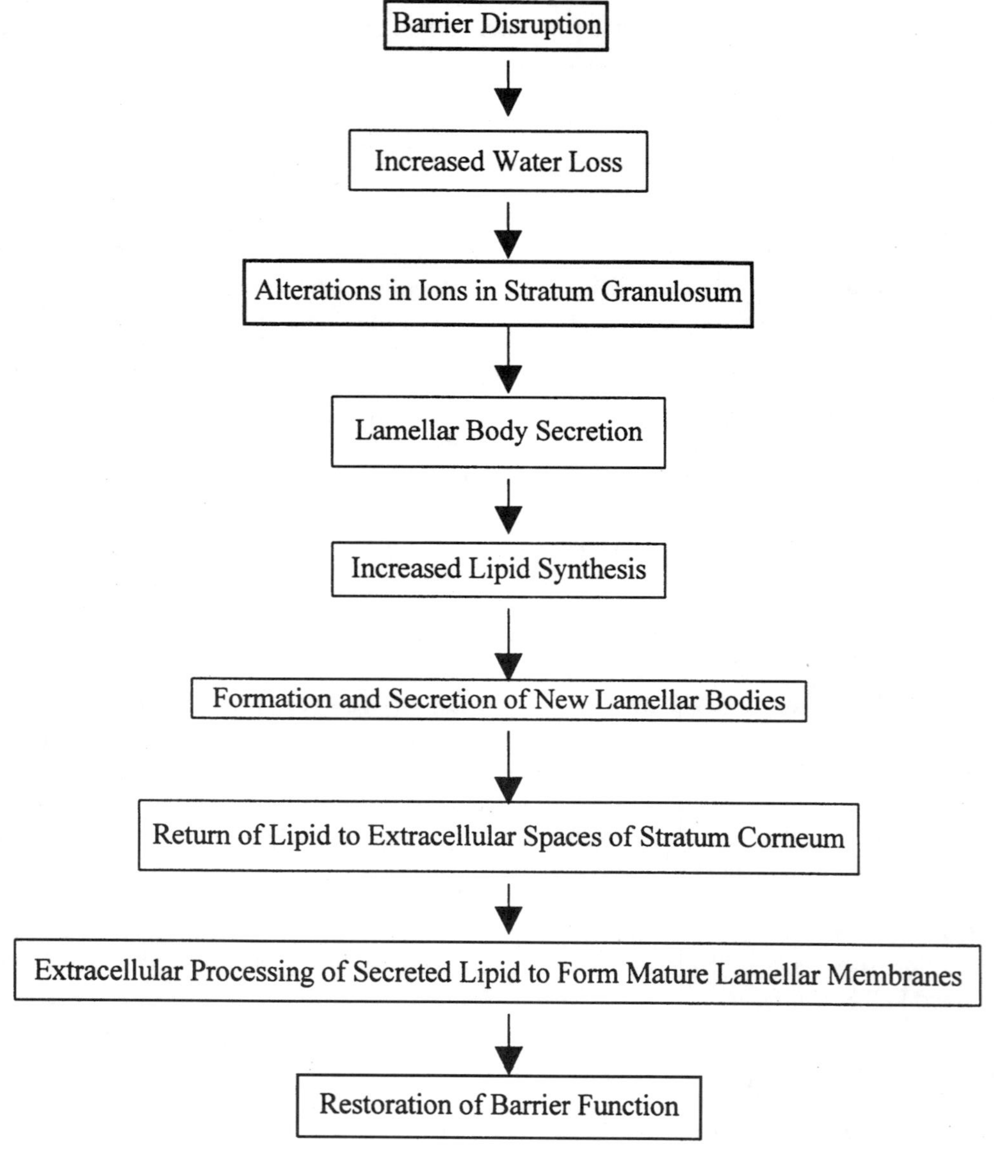

FIGURE 1 Diagram of the mechanisms and regulatory factors responsible for maintaining barrier homeostasis.

REFERENCES

1. Grice, K.A. Transepidermal water loss in pathologic skin. In: *The Physiology and Pathophysiology of the Skin,* Jarrett, A. (ed.), Academic Press, London, pp. 2147–2153, 1980.
2. Ghadially, R., Brown, B.E., Sequeria-Martin, S.M., Feingold, K.R. and Elias, P.M. The aged epidermis permeability barrier. *J. Clin. Invest.* 95:2281–2290, 1993.
3. Proksch, E., Feingold, K.R., Man, M.Q. and Elias, P.M. Barrier function regulates epidermal DNA synthesis. *J. Clin. Invest.* 87:1668–1673, 1991.
4. Denda, M., Wood, L.C., Emami, S., Calhoun, C., Brown, B.E., Elias, P.M. and Feingold, K.R. Epidermal hyperplasia associated with repeated barrier disruption by acetone treatment or tape stripping cannot be attributed to increase water loss. *Arch. Dermatol. Res.* 288:230–238, 1996.
5. Wood, L.C., Jackson, S.M., Elias, P.M., Grunfeld, C. and Feingold, K.R. Cutaneous barrier perturbation stimulates cytokine production in the epidermis of mice. *J. Clin. Invest.* 90:482–487, 1992.
6. Wood, L.C., Feingold, K.R., Sequeira-Martin, S.M., Elias, P.M. and Grunfeld, C. Barrier function coordinately regulates epidermal IL-1 and IL-1 receptor antagonist mRNA levels. *Exp. Dermatol.* 3:56–60, 1994.
7. Tsai, J.C., Feingold, K.R., Crumrine, D., Wood, L.C., Grunfeld, C. and Elias, P.M. Permeability barrier disruption alters the localization and expression of TNFa protein in the epidermis. *Arch. Dermatol. Res.* 286:242–248, 1994.
8. Wood, L.C., Elias, P.M., Calhoun, C., Tsai, J.C., Grunfeld, C. and Feingold, K.R. Barrier disruption stimulates interleukin-1 alpha expression and release from a pre-formed pool in murine epidermis. *J. Invest. Dermatol.* 106:397–403, 1996.
9. Elias, P.M. and Menon, G.K. Structural and lipid biochemical correlates of the epidermal permeability barrier. *Adv. Lipid Res.* 24:1–26, 1991.
10. Downing, D.T. Lipid and protein structures in the permeability barrier of mammalian epidermis. *J. Lipid Res.* 33:301–313, 1992.
11. Yardley, H.J. and Summerly, R. Lipid composition and metabolism in normal and diseased epidermis. *Pharmacol. Ther.* 13:357–383, 1991.
12. Schurer, N.Y. and Elias, P.M. The biochemistry and function of stratum corneum lipids. *Adv. Lipid Res.* 24:27–56, 1991.
13. Grubauer, G., Feingold, K.R., Harris, R.M. and Elias, P.M. Lipid content and lipid type as determinants of the epidermal permeability barrier. *J. Lipid Res.* 30:89–96, 1989.
14. Feingold, K.R. The regulation and role of epidermal lipid synthesis. *Adv. Lipid Res.* 24:57–82, 1991.
15. Proksch, E., Holleran, W.M., Menon, G.K., Elias, P.M. and Feingold, K.R. Barrier function regulates epidermal lipid and DNA synthesis. *Br. J. Dermatol.* 128:473–482, 1993.
16. Prottey, C. Essential fatty acids and the skin. *Br. J. Dermatol.* 94:579–587, 1976.
17. Elias, P.M. and Feingold, K.R. Lipids and the epidermal water barrier: metabolism regulation and pathophysiology. *Semin. Dermatol.* 11:176–182, 1992.
18. Menon, G.K., Feingold, K.R. and Elias, P.M. The lamellar body secretory response to barrier disruption. *J. Invest. Dermatol.* 98:279–289, 1992.
19. Man, M.Q., Brown, B.E., Wu-Pong, S., Feingold, K.R. and Elias, P.M. Exogenous inert vs. physiological lipids: divergent mechanisms for correction of permeability barrier function. *Arch. Dermatol.* 131:809–816, 1995.
20. Feingold, K.R. The regulation of epidermal lipid synthesis by permeability barrier requirements. *Crit. Rev. Ther. Drug Carrier Syst.*, 8:193–210, 1991.
21. Menon, G.K., Feingold, K.R., Moser, A.H., Brown, B.E. and Elias, P.M. De novo sterologenesis in the skin: Fate and function of newly synthesized lipids. *J. Lipid Res.* 26:418–427, 1985.
22. Feingold, K.R., Brown, B.E., Lear, S.R., Moser, A.H. and Elias, P.M. The effect of essential fatty acid deficiency on cutaneous sterol synthesis. *J. Invest. Dermatol.* 87:588–591, 1986.
23. Proksch, E., Elias, P.M. and Feingold, K.R. Regulation of 3-hydroxy-3-methylglutaryl-coenzyme A reductase activity in murine epidermis: modulation of enzyme content and activation state by barrier requirements. *J. Clin. Invest.* 85:874–882, 1990.
24. Jackson, S.M., Wood, L.C., Lauer, S., Taylor, J.M., Cooper, A.D., Elias, P.M. and Feingold, K.R. Effect of cutaneous permeability barrier disruption on HMG CoA reductase, LDL receptor and apoprotein E mRNA levels in the epidermis of hairless mice. *J. Lipid Res.* 33:1307–1314, 1992.

25. Harris, I.R., Farrell, A.M., Grunfeld, C., Holleran, W.M., Elias, P.M. and Feingold, K.R. Permeability barrier disruption coordinately regulates mRNA levels for key enzymes of cholesterol, fatty acid, and ceramide synthesis in the epidermis. *J. Invest. Dermatol.* 109:783–787, 1997.
26. Feingold, K.R., Brown, B.E., Lear, S.R., Moser, A.H. and Elias, P.M. Localization of *de novo* sterologenesis in mammalian skin. *J. Invest. Dermatol.* 81:365–369, 1983.
27. Proksch, E., Elias, P.M. and Feingold, K.R. Localization and regulation of epidermal 3-hydroxy-3-methylglutaryl coenzyme A reductase activity by barrier requirements. *Biochim. Biophys. Acta* 1083:71–79, 1991.
28. Grubauer, G., Feingold, K.R. and Elias, P.M. The relationship of epidermal lipogenesis to cutaneous barrier function. *J. Lipid Res.* 28:746–752, 1987.
29. Ottey, K.A., Wood, L.C., Grunfeld, C., Elias, P.M. and Feingold, K.R. Cutaneous permeability barrier disruption increases fatty acid synthetic enzyme activity in the epidermis of hairless mice. *J. Invest. Dermatol.* 104:401–405, 1995.
30. Monger, D.J., Williams, M.L., Feingold, K.R., Brown, B.E. and Elias, P.M. Localization of sites of lipid biosynthesis in mammalian epidermis. *J. Lipid Res.* 29:603–612, 1988.
31. Holleran, W.M., Feingold, K.R., Man, M.Q., Gao, W.N., Lee, J.M. and Elias, P.M. Regulation of epidermal sphingolipid synthesis by permeability barrier function. *J. Lipid Res.* 32:1151–1158, 1991.
32. Holleran, W.M., Gao, W.N., Feingold, K.R. and Elias, P.M. Localization of epidermal sphingolipid synthesis and serine palmitoyl transferase activity: alterations imposed by permeability barrier requirements. *Arch. Dermatol. Res.* 287:254–258, 1995.
33. Chujor, C.S.N., Feingold, K.R., Elias, P.M. and Holleran, W.M. Glucosylceramide synthase activity in murine epidermis: quantitation, localization, regulation and requirement for barrier homeostasis. *J. Lipid Res.* 39:277–285, 1998.
34. Brown, M.S. and Goldstein, J.L. A receptor mediated pathway for cholesterol homeostasis. *Science* 232:34–47, 1986.
35. Ashby, M.N. and Edwards, P.A. Identification and regulation of a rat liver cDNA encoding farnesyl pyrophosphate synthetase. *J. Biol. Chem.* 264:635–640, 1989.
36. Rosser, D.S., Ashby, M.N., Ellis, J.L. and Edwards, P.A. Coordinate regulation of 3-hydroxy-3-methylglutaryl-coenzyme A synthase, 3-hydroxy-3-methylglutaryl-coenzyme A reductase and prenyltransferase synthase but not degradation in HepG2 cells. *J. Biol. Chem.* 264:12653–12656, 1989.
37. Molowa, D.T. and Cimis, G.M. Coordinate regulation of low density lipoprotein receptor and 3-hydroxy-3-methylglutaryl CoA reductase and synthase gene expression in HepG2 cells. *Biochem. J.* 260:731–736, 1989.
38. Guan, G., Jiang, G., Koch, R.L. and Shecter, I. Molecular cloning and functional analysis of the promoter of the human squalene synthase gene. *J. Biol. Chem.* 270:21958–21965, 1995.
39. Brown, M.S. and Goldstein, J.L. The SREBP pathway: Regulation of cholesterol metaoblism by proteolysis of a membrane bound transcription factor. *Cell* 89:331–340, 1997.
40. Feingold, K.R., Pollock, A., Moser, A.H., Shigenaga, J.K. and Grunfeld, C. Discordant regulation of proteins of cholesterol metabolism during the acute phase response. *J. Lipid Res.* 36:1474–1482, 1995.
41. Yokoyama, C., Wang, X., Briggs, M.R., Admon, A., Wu, J., Hua, X., Goldstein, J.L. and Brown, M.S. SREBP-1, a basic-helix-loop-helix-leucine zipper protein that controls transcription of the low density lipoprotein receptor gene. *Cell* 75:187–197, 1993.
42. Hua X., Yokoyama, C., Wu, J., Briggs, M.R., Brown, M.S., Goldstein, J.L. and Wang, X. SREBP-2, a second basic-helix-loop-helix-leucine zipper protein that stimulates transcription by binding to a sterol regulatory element. Proc. Natl. Acad. Sci. 90:11603–11607, 1993.
43. Wang, X., Sato, R., Brown, M.S., Hua, X. and Goldstein, J.L. SREBP-1, a membrane-bound transcription factor released by sterol regulated proteolysis. *Cell* 77:53–62, 1994.
44. Baeverle, P.H. and Henkel, T. Function and activation of NF-Kappa B in the immune system. *Annu. Rev. Immunol.* 12:141–179, 1994.
45. Yang, J., Sato, R., Goldstein, J.L. and Brown, M.S. Sterol-resistant transcription in CHO cells caused by gene rearrangement that truncates SREBP-2. *Genes Dev.* 8:1910–1919, 1994.
46. Sheng, Z., Otani, H., Brown, M.S. and Goldstein, J.L. Independent regulation of sterol regulatory element binding proteins 1 and 2 in hamster liver. *Proc. Natl. Acad. Sci.* 92:935–938, 1995.
47. Havel, R.J. Lipoproteins and lipid disorders. In: *Metabolic Control and Disease,* 8th ed., Bondy, P.K. and Rosenberg, L.E. (eds.), W.B. Saunders, Philadelphia, pp. 394–494, 1980.

48. Feingold, K.R., Man, M.Q., Proksch, E., Menon, G.K., Brown, B.E. and Elias, P.M. The lovastatin-treated rodent: A new model of barrier disruption and epidermal hyperplasia. *J. Invest. Dermatol.* 96:201–209, 1991.
49. Tontonoz, P., Kim, J.B., Graves, R.A. and Spiegelman, B.M. ADD1: a novel helix loop helix transcription factor associated with adipocyte determination and differentiation. *Mol. Cell. Biol.* 13:4753–4759, 1993
50. Kim, J.B., Spotts, G.D., Halvorsen, Y.D., Shih, H.M., Ellenberger, T., Towle, H.C. and Spiegelman, B.M. Dual DNA binding specificity of ADD1/SREBP-1 controlled by a single amino acid in the basic helix-loop-helix domain. *Mol. Cell. Biol.* 15:2582–2588, 1995.
51. Bennett, M.K., Lopez, J.M., Sanchez, H.B. and Osborne, T.F. Sterol regulation of fatty acid synthase promoter. Coordinate feedback regulation of two major lipid pathways. *J. Biol. Chem.* 270:25578–25583, 1995.
52. Lopez, J.M., Bennett, M.K., Sanchez, H.B., Rosenfeld, J.M. and Osborne, T.F. Sterol regulation of acetyl CoA carboxylase: a mechanism for coordinate regulation of cellular lipid. *Proc. Natl. Acad. Sci.* 93:1049–1053, 1996.
53. Harris, I.R., Farrell, A.M., Holleran, W.M., Jackson, S., Grunfeld, C., Elias, P.M. and Feingold, K.R. Parallel regulation of sterol regulatory element binding protein-2 and the enzymes of cholesterol and fatty acid synthesis but not ceramide synthesis in cultured human keratinocytes and murine epidermis. *J. Lipid Res.* 39:412–422, 1998.
54. Feingold, K.R., Man, M.Q., Menon, G.K., Cho, S.S., Brown, B.E. and Elias, P. Cholesterol synthesis is required for cutaneous barrier function in mice. *J. Clin. Invest.* 86:696–702, 1990.
55. Man, M.Q., Elias, P.M. and Feingold, K.R. Fatty acids are required for epidermal barrier function. *J. Clin. Invest.* 92:791–798, 1993.
56. Holleran, W.M., Man, M.Q., Gao, W.N., Menon, G.K., Elias, P.M. and Feingold, K.R. Sphingolipids are required for mammalian barrier function: inhibition of sphingolipid synthesis delays barrier recovery after acute perturbation. *J. Clin. Invest.* 88:1338–1345, 1991.
57. Ziboh, V.A. and Chapkin, R.S. Metabolism and function of skin lipids. *Prog. Lipid Res.* 27:81–105, 1988.
58. Dykes, P.J., Marks, R., Davies, M.G. and Reynolds, D.J. Epidermal metabolism in heredopathia atactica polyneuritoformis (Refsum's disease). *J. Invest. Dermatol.* 70:126–129, 1978.
59. Steinberg, D.J., Herndon, Jr., J.H., Uhlendorf, B.W., Mine, C.E., Avigan, J. and Milne, G.W. Refsum's disease: nature of the enzyme defect. *Science* 156:1740–1742, 1967.
60. Holleran, W.M., Takagi, Y., Menon, G.K., Jackson, S.M., Lee, J.M., Feingold, K.R. and Elias, P.M. Permeability barrier requirements regulate epidermal B-glucocerebrosidase. *J. Lipid Res.* 35:905–911, 1994.
61. Holleran, W.M., Takagi, Y., Menon, G.K., Legler, G., Feingold, K.R. and Elias, P.M. Processing of epidermal glucosylceramides is required for optimal mammalian cutaneous permeability barrier function. *J. Clin. Invest.* 91:1656–1664, 1993.
62. Holleran, W.M., Ginns, E.I., Menon, G.K., Groundmann, J.U., Fartasch, M., McKinney, C.E., Elias, P.M. and Sidransky, E. Consequences of beta-glucocerebrosidase deficiency in epidermis. Ultrastructure and permeability barrier alterations in Gauder disease. *J. Clin. Invest.* 93:1756–1764, 1994.
63. Sidransky, E., Fartasch, M., Lee, R.E., Metlay, L.A., Abella, S., Zimran, A., Fao, W., Elias, P.M., Ginns, E.I. and Holleran, W.M. Epidermal abnormalities may distinguish type 2 from type 1 and type 3 of Gauder disease. *Pediatr. Res.* 39:134–141, 1996.
64. Man, M.Q., Feingold, K.R., Jain, M. and Elias, P.M. Extracellular processing of phospholipids is required for permeability barrier homeostasis. *J. Lipid Res.* 36:1925–1935, 1995.
65. Mauro, T., Holleran, W.M., Grayson, S., Gao, W.N., Kriehuber, E., Man, M.Q., Feingold, K.R. and Elias, P.M. Barrier recovery is impeded at neutral pH, independent of ionic effects. *Arch. Dermatol. Res.* 290:215–222, 1998.
66. Lee, S.H., Elias, P.M., Proksch, E., Menon, G.K., Man, M.Q. and Feingold, K.R. Calcium and potassium are important regulators of barrier homeostasis in murine epidermis. *J. Clin. Invest.* 89:530–538, 1992.
67. Menon, G.K., Elias, P.M., Lee, S.H. and Feingold, K.R. Localization of calcium in murine epidermis following disruption and repair of the permeability barrier. *Cell Tissue Res.* 270:503–512, 1992.

68. Menon, G.K., Price, L.F., Bommannan, B., Elias, P.M. and Feingold, K.R. Selective obliteration of the epidermal calcium gradient leads to enhanced lamellar body secretion. *J. Invest. Dermatol.* 102:789–795, 1994.
69. Menon, G.K., Elias, P.M. and Feingold, K.R. Integrity of the permeability barrier is crucial for maintenance of the epidermal calcium gradient. *Br. J. Dermatol.* 130:139–147, 1994.
70. Lee, S.H., Elias, P.M., Feingold, K.R. and Mauro, T. A role for ions in barrier recovery after acute perturbation. *J. Invest. Dermatol.* 102:976–979, 1994.
71. Menon, G.K., Grayson, S. and Elias, P.M. Ionic calcium reservoirs in mammalian epidermis: ultrastructural localization by ion-capture cytochemistry. *J. Invest. Dermatol.* 84:508–512, 1985.
72. Malmquut, K.G., Carlson, L.E., Forslind, B. and Roomans, G.M. Proton and electron microprobe analysis of human skin. *Nucl. Instr. Methods Phys. Res.* 3:611–617, 1984.
73. Forslind, B. Quantitative X-ray microanalysis of skin. *Acta Derm. Venereol.* (*Stockholm*) (Suppl.) 134:1–8, 1987.
74. Mauro, T., Bench, G., Sidderas-Haddad, E., Feingold, K.R., Elias, P. and Cullander, C. Acute barrier perturbation abolishes the CA^{++} and K^{+} gradients in murine epidermis: quantitative measurement using PIXE. *J. Invest. Dermatol.* 111:1198–1201, 1998.
75. Man, M.Q., Mauro, T., Bench, G., Warren, R., Elias, P.M. and Feingold, K.R. Calcium and potassium inhibit barrier recovery after disruption, independent of the type of insult in hairless mice. *Exp. Dermatol.* 6:36–40, 1997.
76. Lee, S.H., Choi, E.H., Feingold, K.R., Jiang, S. and Ahn, S.K. Effect of iontophoresis on stratum corneum structure and the epidermal calcium gradient. *J. Invest. Dermatol.* 111:39–43, 1998.
77. Brown, E.M. Extracellular Ca^{2+} and other ions as extracellular (first) messengers. *Physiol. Rev.* 17:371–411, 1991.
78. Lo, J.S., Oriba, H.A., Maibach, H.I. and Bailin, P.L. Transepidermal potassium ion, chloride ion, and water flux across delipidized and cellophane tape stripped skin. *Dermatologica* (*Basal*) 180:66–68, 1990.

6 Permeability Barrier Homeostasis: The Role of Lipid Processing

Peter M. Elias, Walter M. Holleran, Cornelia J. Calhoun, Danielle Quiec, Barbara E. Brown, Martin Behne, and Kenneth R. Feingold

CONTENTS

6.1 BACKGROUND

Until the mid-1970s, the stratum corneum (SC) was considered a metabolically inert, homogeneous tissue, analogous to a plastic film.[70,71] Then, through a variety of techniques, the SC was shown to be structurally and biochemically heterogeneous, with all of its constituent lipids sequestered in expanded extracellular domains.[11,13] With tracer perfusion and freeze-fracture replication, the permeability barrier was shown to form coincident with the secretion of lamellar body (LB) contents at the stratum granulosum (SG)–SC interface.[13] Most importantly, the delivery of LB contents to the SC interstices is associated with the formation of broad membrane bilayers, with the freeze-fracture characteristics of hydrophobic lipids.[13] In this chapter, we will consider recent evidence that the SC is not dead or inert, but instead it possesses certain types of metabolic activity that regulate barrier formation, together called *extracellular processing* (ECP).

This two-compartment concept of the SC provides new insights into the pathogenesis of both disorders of cornification (DOC) and diseases associated with important barrier abnormalities.[81,82] Moreover, variations in intercellular lipid content and membrane structure also provide a structural basis for the wide variations in permeability of different human skin sites (e.g., palms/soles vs. leg vs. abdomen vs. face).[9,40] Finally, the delivery of LB contents to the SC interstices causes an increase in the volume fraction of the SC intercellular compartment, and the SC produces both the "reservoir function" of the SC, as well as the SC interstices as the putative intercellular transport route.[63]

0-8493-7520-7/00/$0.00+$.50

We and others have described the changes in lipid composition that accompany epidermal differentiation (reviewed in Reference 72). Briefly, these studies demonstrated the loss of phospholipids (PL) and the emergence of the neutral lipids cholesterol (Chol) and ceramides (Cer) in the SC. The Cer in mammalian SC comprise a surprisingly well-conserved family of seven different species, which demonstrate important species-to-species variations in sphingoid base structure, N-acyl chain length, and α/ω hydroxylation.[72] Moreover, the two ω-hydroxylated species, Cer-1 and Cer-4, contain an ω-esterified linoleate moiety (= acylceramide).[3,4,24,69,79] The last two species have two putative functions: (1) the "molecular rivets" are proposed to link adjacent membrane bilayers; and (2) the de-esterified ω-hydroxy group is proposed to bind covalently to the cornified envelope, forming the lipid-bound envelope. The other major species comprise a mixture of Cer with or without α-hydroxylated N-acyl groups, which are presumed to form the bulk of the intercellular bilayers. Finally, the free fatty acids (FFA) in SC comprise both essential and nonessential species, with the latter comprising the bulk of the FFA in the membrane bilayers. The essential FA, linoleic acid, comprises only a small proportion of the FFA; instead, it is largely present as an ω-esterified moiety on Cer-1 and Cer-4.[69,79] Finally, a further gradient in lipid transformation occurs during the final stages of terminal differentiation and barrier formation, i.e., small amounts of GlcCer and PL persist in the lower SC, but disappear from the outer SC (i.e., the stratum disjunctum).[12] In addition, the cholesterol sulfate (CS) content is maximal in the SG and stratum compactum, decreasing in the stratum disjunctum.[12,43] These biochemical alterations, coupled with evidence for extensive membrane remodeling within the SC (see the following), provide presumptive evidence of the tissue's metabolic activity.

LB-containing subcellular fractions are enriched in both polar lipids (GlcCer, PL, and Chol), as well as a selected family of hydrolytic enzymes (phospholipases [PLases], triacylglycerol lipase [TAGase], sphingomyelinase [SMase], acid phosphatase, and certain glycosidases and proteases).[19,20] Curiously, both CS and steroid sulfatase (SS) are not concentrated in LB, though they ultimately reach the SC interstices. Subsequent cytochemical and biochemical studies showed that several of these lipases are concentrated in the SC interstices.[12,58,68] This process of hydrolase delivery correlates with a series of membrane structural transformations within the SC interstices that lead to barrier formation.[12,16]

Recent studies have shown that LB originate from a trans-Golgi-like (TGN) reticulum, which is widely dispersed in the apical cytosol of the outermost granular cell.[15] This widely disbursed TGN is one of several structural and metabolic specializations that allow this cell (the secretory granulocyte) to deliver LB contents rapidly following acute barrier disruption. The signal for accelerated LB secretion is a decline in extracellular calcium, associated with loss of the calcium gradient following barrier disruption.[49,59,60] Following exocytosis, the secreted disk-like contents begin to change their structural organization immediately.[55] The so-called disk contents of the LB actually are compressed pleated sheets, which unfurl, followed initially by end-to-end elongation and then by compaction/transformation into lamellar unit structures (reviewed in Reference 13).

Whereas freeze-fracture replication and osmium vapor fixation reveal a multilamellar system of broad membrane bilayers in the SC interstices, application of ruthenium tetroxide (RuO_4) postfixation revealed further details of membrane structure.[16,34,44] RuO_4 postfixation reveals the intercellular lamellae to be organized into pairs of continuous lamellae, alternating with a fenestrated lamellae, forming the lamellar basic unit structure.[16,34,44] These intercellular lamellae lie external to a lipid-bound envelope, which resists solvent extraction and is covalently bound to the cornified envelope.[76]

6.2 MAINTENANCE OF BARRIER FUNCTION BY EPIDERMAL METABOLISM

A basic tenant of this work holds that the SC is not dead, but actually possesses a limited form of metabolic activity. Equally important, the SC is a biosensor that signals the underlying epidermis to respond to external stresses. The principle metabolic response to such stresses is a temporary increase in lipid synthesis, localized to the underlying epidermis.[10,17] This synthesis response is relatively autonomous from circulating influences because (1) barrier homeostasis is not altered in animals with either very high or very low serum lipids,[85] and (2) only very small amounts of infused lipids are incorporated into the epidermis, even when the barrier is disrupted.[22,54] Despite its autonomy from the influences of circulating lipids, epidermal lipid synthesis is regulated by barrier requirements (reviewed in References 10 and 17). Thus, acute insults such as organic solvent treatment, cellophane tape stripping, and surfactant treatment induce a localized increase in Chol, Cer, and FA synthesis.[22,27,65] Furthermore, the increase in lipid synthesis is attributable to an antecedent increase in mRNA expression, enzyme content, and enzyme activity, as well as alterations in the phosphorylation state of some of the key enzymes of lipid synthesis.[25,36,67] Barrier requirements not only regulate epidermal lipid synthesis, but, in addition, the barrier regulates mRNA for certain proteins involved in lipid transport, such as apoprotein E and the LDL receptor,[4,36] suggesting that not only lipid synthesis, but also lipid transport systems are regulated by barrier requirements. Furthermore, while all of the nucleated cell layers retain the capacity to synthesize lipid with various types of acute and chronic barrier disruption, distinctive changes in lipid synthesis and enzyme activity occur within specific epidermal cell layers.[10,17] Finally, the burst in lipid synthesis results in a return of SC lipids, previously removed during barrier disruption, to the SC in parallel with barrier restoration.[21]

Finally, using specific pharmacologic inhibitors of the rate-limiting enzymes of these lipids, i.e., HMG CoA reductase,[18] serine palmitoyl transferase,[28] and acetyl CoA carboxylase,[46] we showed that each of these lipids is required both specifically and individually.

6.3 EXTRACELLULAR PROCESSING

As noted previously, the unique two-component organization of the SC is attributable to the secretion of LB-derived lipids and co-localized hydrolases at the SG–SC interface. Under basal conditions, the rate of LB secretion appears to be slow, but sufficient to provide for barrier integrity in the absence of stress.[55] LB secretion requires active metabolism, since neither new organelle formation nor secretion occurs at 4°C.[23] Moreover, calcium is an important regulator of LB secretion with the epidermal calcium gradient restricting LB secretion to low, maintenance levels under basal conditions.[15,42,59,60] With acute barrier disruption, the preformed pool of LB in the outermost SG cell is largely and quickly secreted,[15,55] in response to a decline in the epidermal calcium gradient.[57,59,60]

6.3.1 Terminal Differentiation

During the final stages of epidermal differentiation, a sequence of membrane transitions occurs within the SC extracellular domains (Figure 1). Extrusion of LB contents at the SG–SC interface is followed sequentially by unfurling, elongation, and processing into mature lamellar bilayer unit structures (reviewed in References 13, 41, 16, and 50). Concurrently, marked alterations in lipid composition occur, including the elimination of GlcCer and PL, with the accumulation of Cer and FFA in the SC[72] (Table 1). As noted earlier, LB deliver not only GlcCer, PL, and Chol, but also a family of hydrolytic enzymes to the SC interstices. These observations lead to early suggestions that the LB is a type of lysosome and to speculation that the enzymatic contents of LB might regulate SC desquamation.[64] Whereas it has been shown that LB-derived hydrolases, particularly certain types of proteases, mediate desquamation,[8] strong circumstantial evidence links LB-derived hydrolases to barrier homeostasis. For example, several of these hydrolases are localized within the outer epidermis, within LB, and specifically within SC membrane domains (reviewed in Reference 13). Three of these enzymes, β-glucocerebrosidase (β-GlcCer'ase), secretory phospholipase A_2 (sPLA), and steroid sulfatase (SSase), have been extensively studied and shown to be critical for processory. (Additional circumstantial evidence for the occurrence of regulated extracellular processing in barrier homeostasis has come from studies in a dominant-negative, transgenic mouse model, which overexpresses an abnormal RARα transcript.[35]) Through further heterodimerization with nuclear receptors for T_3, 1,25 $(OH)_2$ vitamin D_3, and PPAR ligands, the abnormal RAR-ligand complexes could compromise the regulation of epidermal differentiation and/or barrier homeostasis. Moreover, the abnormal,

TABLE 1
Precursors and Products of Stratum Corneum Extracellular Processing Enzymes

Lamellar Body Lipids	Extracellular Hydrolase	Mature SC Membranes
Phospholipids	Phospholipases (several)	Free fatty acids, glycerolipids, lysolecithin
Sphingomyelin	Sphingomyelinase	Ceramides
Cholesterol sulfate	Steroid sulfatase	Cholesterol[a]
Glucosylceramides	β-Glucocerebrosidase	Ceramides[b]
Acylglucosylceramides[b]	Acidic/neutral lipases	Ceramides[b]

Note: Metabolic intermediates in degradative pathways have putative signaling functions.

[a] Most cholesterol derives unchanged from lamellar body contents.

[b] These can be further metabolized to sphingoid base plus free fatty acids by ceramidase.

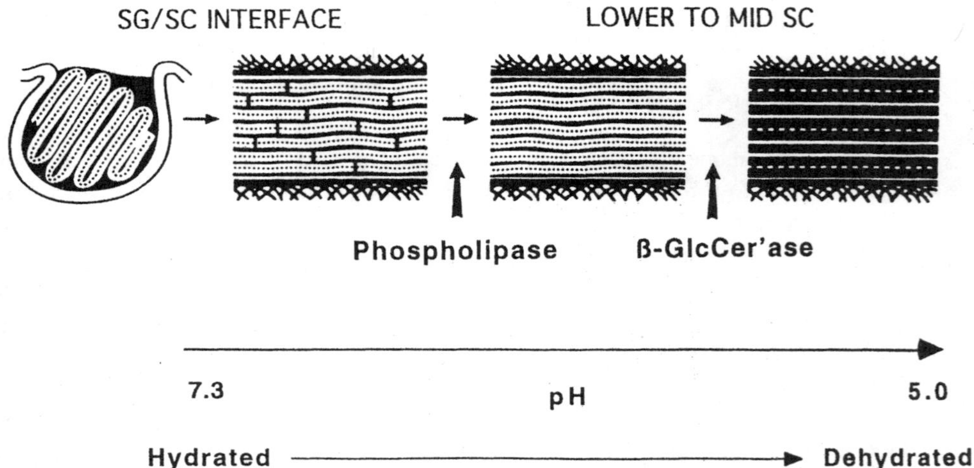

FIGURE 1 Sequence of membrane transitions occurring within the SC extracellular domains during the final stages of epidermal differentiation.

truncated RARα, by heterodimerization with RXR, creates a deficiency of this nuclear regulatory protein. It is the sequence homology of the DNA binding domain of these receptors that apparently explains both the profound effects of these diverse agents on growth/differentiation and their shared ability to up-regulate so many functionally diverse processes. In this model, LB formation and secretion are normal, but a major defect in barrier function occurs in association with a failure to form normal intercellular membrane structures.

6.3.2 GlucCer-to-Cer Metabolism by β-Glucocerebrosidase

The most compelling direct evidence for the central role of extracellular processing in barrier formation comes from studies in GlucCer-to-Cer processing. Just as with the other lipid hydrolases described earlier, β-glucocerebrosidase (β-GlcCer'ase) is concentrated in the outer epidermis with the highest levels in SC,[30] and, more specifically, in membrane domains.[77] In contrast, endogenous-β-glycosidase activity is low in the SC of mucosal epithelia,[4] which display a less stingent barrier requirement than epidermis. Moreover, in mucosal epithelia, glycosylCer (type(s) unspecified) predominates over Cer; untransformed LB contents persist into the outer SC; and mature membrane structures do not form.[78,80] GlycosylCer also predominates over Cer, and immature LB-derived membranes persist within the SC interstices of marine cetaceans, which again have lesser barrier requirements than their terrestrial counterparts.[56] Recently, these correlative observations have been supported by direct evidence for the role of β-GlcCer'ase in the extracellular processing of GlcCer-to-Cer. (1) Applications of specific conduritol-type inhibitors of β-GlcCer'ase both delay barrier recovery after acute perturbations,[32] and produce a progressive abnormality in barrier function when applied to intact skin.[31] Moreover, the barrier dysfunction produced by the various conduritol inhibitors correlates with the extent of β-GlcCer'ase inhibition in the treated epidermis. (2) In a transgenic murine model of Gaucher disease (GD), produced by targeted disruption of β-GlcCer'ase, homozygous animals are born with an ichthyosiform dermatosis and a severe barrier abnormality, attributable to absent epidermal enzyme activity.[29,75] (3) Likewise, in the severe type 2 neuronopathic form of GD, infants present with a similar clinical phenotype, including an ichthyosiform erythroderma.[29,75]

In all three situations (inhibitor treated, transgenic murine knockout, and type 2 GD), the functional barrrier deficit is accompanied by accumulation of GlcCer in the SC and persistence of immature LB-derived membrane structures within the SC interstices.[29,31,75] Moreover, the barrier deficit appears to be attributable to accumulation of GlcCer rather than to depletion of Cer, because application of Cer with the conduritol inhibitors reverses neither the structural nor the functional abnormalities. Finally, levels of β-GlcCer'ase enzyme activity and mRNA are regulated by barrier requirements.[32] Together, these studies point to a critical role for GlcCer-to-Cer processing in barrier homeostasis.

6.3.3 PL-to-FFA Catabolism by Phospholipases

Phospholipids, which are integral components of cell membranes, harbor within their structures bioactive moieties, such as arachidonic acid at the sn-2 position, whose generation is rate limiting for the production of eicosanoids and other lipid mediators. Both the 85-kD cytosolic PLA ($cPLA_2$), which is calcium dependent and regulated by phosphorylation, and the type 2 $sPLA_2$ (14 kD), which is less calcium sensitive and regulated transcriptionally and posttranscriptionally by cytokines and other agonists, play crucial roles in the stimulus-coupled release of arachidonic acid (reviewed in References 51 and 62). The fatty acids and lysophospholipids, resulting from $cPLA_2$ and type 2 $sPLA_2$ action, can themselves act as second messengers, or they can be metabolized further into proinflammatory lipid mediators. In contrast, the type 1 $sPLA_2$ also is a 14-kD secretory isoenzyme, with separate functions in membrane remodeling and PL degradation.[51,62] Whereas type 1 $sPLA_2$ has been studied most extensively in pancreatic juices, it also has been localized to several nonpancreatic tissues.[51] While the types of PLA_2 present in mammalian epidermis have not been extensively studied, recent studies have shown that both the $cPLA_2$ and type 2 $sPLA_2$ are constitutively expressed in epidermis under basal conditions and that the type 2 $sPLA_2$, but not the $cPLA_2$, is up-regulated severalfold in psoriasis.[1] Pertinently, the enzyme is localized preferentially to the outer epidermis under basal conditions and is expressed further in the lower epidermis in psoriasis. We showed recently that both bromphenacyl bromide (BPB) and MJ-33, a selective type 1 inhibitor (Figure 2), but not MJ-45 (a type 2 $sPLA_2$ inhibitor), modulate barrier function both in intact skin and after acute disruption.[47,48] Our results suggest, but do not prove, a role for the type 1 rather than the type 2 isoenzyme in barrrier function. Although epidermal barrier function appears to require an $sPLA_2$ with characteristics of the type 1 (degradative) form, we have been unable to detect this enzyme in Northern blots either before or after barrier disruption. Hence, epidermis may contain a unique type of PLA_2 activity. In contrast, the prior work on the type 2 $sPLA_2$ in epidermis is consistent with a putative role for this isoenzyme in the pathogenesis of inflammation, rather than barrier homeostasis.[1] These characteristics fit our models of extracellular processing well; i.e., that $sPLA_2$ would be most active as an early participant, becoming less active as the SC interstices become progressively more acidified and dehydrated (Figure 1).

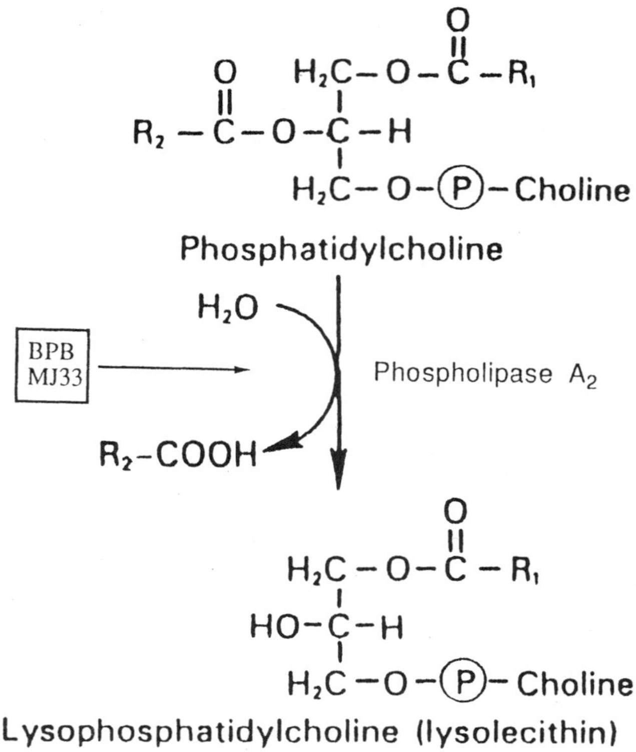

Phosphatidylcholine

H_2O

BPB
MJ33

Phospholipase A_2

R_2-COOH

Lysophosphatidylcholine (lysolecithin)

FIGURE 2 BPB and MJ-33 modulate barrier function in both intact skin and after acute disruption.

6.3.4 CS-to-Chol Catabolism by Steroid Sulfatase

Just as with GlucCer, CS content increases with epidermal differentiation and then decreases quantitatively between the inner and outer SC.[12,43] Since both CS and SSase are concentrated in the SC within membrane domains, but not in LB, it is likely that alternate pathway(s) account for their delivery to the SC intertices. That CS plays a critical role in desquamation is demonstrated definitively by the accumulation of CS in SC membranes in recessive X-linked ichthyosis,[14,86] and by the ability of topical CS to induce hyperkeratosis, while topical Chol reverses the scaling phenotype both in RXLI and in association with topical CS applications.[45,86] CS presumably influences desquamation by its capacity as a protease inhibitor in epidermis, e.g., CS regulates the acrosome reaction, a proteolytically triggered process, in spermatozoa.[26]

In addition to its role in desquamation, CS expression is linked to keratinization in retinoid-induced differentiation models, where it regulates the expression of certain protein kinase C isoenzymes and keratin 1, proteins linked to epidermal differentiation.[7,38,74] Recent studies have shown that CS, in addition to its apparent roles in desquamation and differentiation, is also an important participant in barrier homeostasis. The fact that CS content increases to 10 to 12%, while Chol content decreases by 50% in RXLI,[83] raised the possibility that CS could provide an important precursor pool for Chol in the SC. Moreover, patients with RXLI display abnormal barrier formation under basal conditions,[37,86] and a dramatic delay in recovery occurs after acute disruption.[86] However, an abundant and sufficient pool of Chol is available from LB secretion directly without further modifications.[20] Moreover, topical applications of CS to intact skin induces a barrier abnormality.[45] These studies suggest that excess CS not only induces excess scale, but also induces a barrier abnormality. The latter can be attributed, however, to substrate accumulation, rather than to product depletion, consistent with the barrier abnormality in RXLI.[102] CS also could function in the barrier by additional or unrelated mechanisms, e.g., as an activator of $sPLA_2$.[39]

TABLE 2
Stratum Corneum Intercellular Acidification: Possible Mechanisms

1. Surface microbial metabolism
2. Sebum-derived fatty acids
3. Outward proton flux
4. Insertion of proton pumps
5. Hydrolysis of phospholipids to FFA
6. Bulk hydrolysis in outer epidermis
7. Hydrolysis of specific proteins, e.g., filaggrin → urocanic acid

Activity of SS, a close relative of arylsulfatase C, is absent in RXLI (reviewed in Reference 81). This microsomal enzyme, which is expressed in high levels in the outer epidermis of mammals,[14] hydrolyzes sulfate from the 3-β-hydroxy group on a variety of steroids.[73] The gene that encodes this 62-kD polypeptide has been cloned, characterized, and localized to the distal short arm of the X-chromosome.[73] Major mutations of this region produce ichthyosis and more complex phenotypes.[81]

6.3.5 Acid Sphingomyelinase

Recent studies have shown that acidic sphingomyelinase (aSMase) is required for normal permeability barrier homeostasis.[33] Patients with severe Tay Sachs disease and aSMase trangenic knockout mice display an ichthyotic phenotype, consistant with a barrier abnormality. Moreover, applications of two different classes of aSMase inhibitors after acute barrier disruption provoke a delay in barrier recovery, associated with biochemical and morphological evidence for abnormal extracellular processing. Whether sphingomyelin is a source of one specific fraction(s) of the seven known Cer species in SC is unknown at present. But it is important to note that the SM precursor could originate in either LB or the plasma membrane, both of which are rich, potential sources of this lipid.

6.3.6 pH and Ions

That the SC displays an acidic external pH ("acid mantle") is well documented, and such acid conditions are considered crucial for the resistance to microbial invasion. However, the origin of the acid mantle is not known — passive mechanisms, including net catabolic processes, sebaceous gland-derived fatty acids, and microbial metabolism and apical proton flux due to the high electrical resistance of the SC, have been implicated (Table 2). Alternatively, protons could also be generated actively, e.g., by ion pumps inserted in the plasma membrane, analogous to the urinary bladder where such a process contributes to the acidification of urine. If the limiting membrane of the LB contained such pumps, as suggested by recent inhibitor studies,[2,5] then acidification of the ECS could begin with insertion of such pumps coincident with LB secretion. Ongoing proton secretion at the SG–SC interface, perhaps coupled with one or more of the passive mechanisms described previously, could explain the pH gradient, which we and others have described across the SC interstices. Such a pH gradient could explain the different pH optima of those hydrolases already known to reside in the interstices (Figure 1). Furthermore, the acidic pH of the SC is required for normal barrier homeostasis. Damaged skin that is exposed to a neutral pH buffer recovers more slowly than when exposed to an acidic pH.[50] This pH effect is independent of buffer type and of concurrent changes in ion concentrations. Finally, there is direct evidence for the requirement for an acidic pH for β-Glc-Cer'ase activation in the SC.[50] Together, these studies provide a potential mechanism whereby ECP could occur in a sequential and orchestrated fashion (Figure 1).

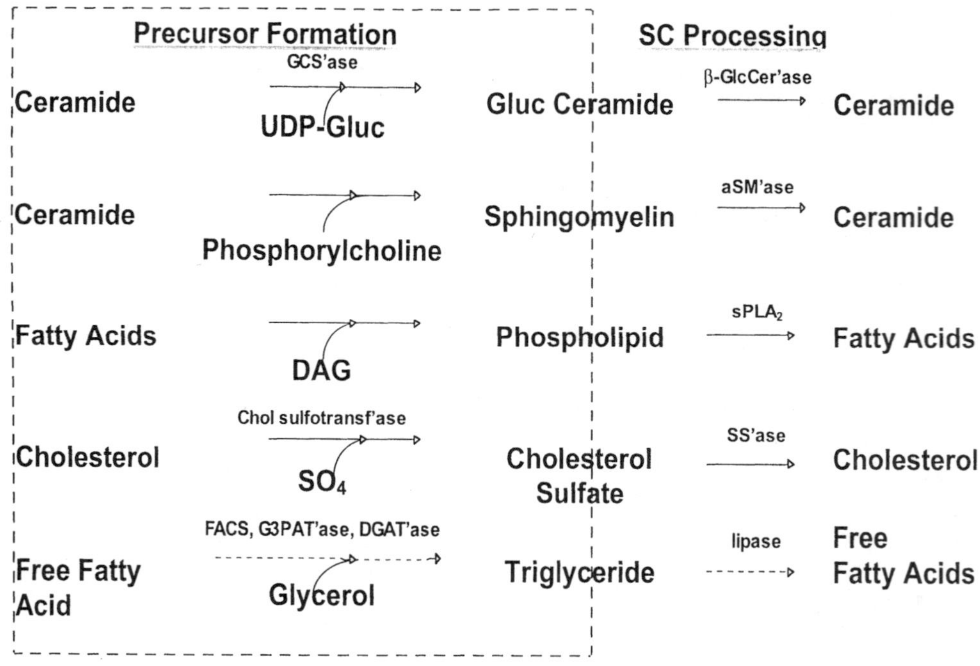

FIGURE 3 Enzymes that synthesize those lipids that are the immediate precursors of the SC lipids.

Attention has focused recently on the enzymes that synthesize those lipids that are the immediate precursors of the SC lipids (Figure 3). One of these enzyme, glucosylCer synthase (GC synthase), catalyzes the formation of glucosylCer from Cer. Utilizing specific inhibitors, we showed that this step is required both for barrier homeostasis and for the formation of normal LB.[6] In contrast, GC synthase is not regulated by acute changes in barrrier requirements. This lack of regulation also appears to extend to enzymes of triglyceride, PL, and CS synthesis. Moreover, transgenic mice with a knockout of the diacylglycerol acyl transferase (DGAT), an enzyme required for triglyceride synthesis, display a normal or even supernormal barrier (B.E. Brown, P.M. Elias, K.R. Feingold, unpublished observations). Finally, cholesterol sulfotransferase, the enzyme that generates CS from Chol, is not regulated by barrier requirements. Whether this enzyme is required for normal desquamation is not known. Studies to date show that none of the late synthetic enzymes are regulated by barrier requirements, and only glucosylCer synthase is required.

6.4 ACKNOWLEDGMENTS

This work was supported by NIH grants AR19098, AR46019, and AR39448 (PP), as well as the Medical Research Service at the Veterans Affairs Medical Center. Sue Allen and Sonia West capably prepared the manuscript.

REFERENCES

1. Andersen S, Sjursen W, Laegrid A, Volden G, Johansen B: Elevated expression of human nonpancreatic phospholipase A_2 in psoriatic tissue. *Inflammation* 18:1–12, 1994.
2. Behne M, Yuko O, Holleran, WM, Mauro T: The sodium/hydrogen antiporters (NHE) in epidermal pH regulation. *J Invest Dermatol* 112: 620A, 1999.

3. Bowser PA, Nguteren DH, White RJ, Houtsmuller UMT, Prottey C: Identification, isolation, and characterization of epidemal lipids containing linoleic acid. *Biochim Biophys Acta* 834:419–428, 1985.
4. Chang F, Wertz PW, Squier CA: Comparison of glycosidase activities in epidermis, palatal epithelium, and buccal epithelium. *Comp Biochem Physiol* [*B*] 100:137–139, 1991.
5. Chapman SJ, Walsh A: Membrane-coating granules are acidic organelles which possess proton pumps. *J Invest Dermatol* 93:466–470, 1989.
6. Chujor CSN, Holleran WM, Feingold KR, Elias PM: Glucosylceramide synthase activity in murine epidermis: quantitation, localization, regulation, and requirement for barrier homeostasis. *J Lipid Res* 39:277–288, 1998.
7. Denning MF, Kazanietz MG, Blumberg PM, Yuspa SA: Cholesterol sulfate activates multiple protein kinase C isoenzymes and induces granular cell differentiation in cultured murine keratinocytes. *Cell Growth Differ* 6:1619–1626, 1995.
8. Egelrud T, Hofer PA, Lundström A: Proteolytic degradation of desmosomes in plantar stratum corneum leads to cell dissociation *in vitro*. *Acta Derm Venereol* 68:93–97, 1988.
9. Elias PM, Cooper ER, Korc A, Brown BE: Percutaneous transport in relation to stratum corneum structure and lipid composition. *J Invest Dermatol* 76:297–301, 1981.
10. Elias PM, Feingold KR: Lipids and the epidermal water barrier: metabolism, regulation, and pathophysiology. *Semin Dermatol* 11:176–182, 1992.
11. Elias PM, Friend DS: The permeability barrier in mammalian epidermis. *J Cell Biol* 65:180–191, 1975.
12. Elias PM, Menon GK, Grayson S, Brown BE: Membrane structural alterations in murine stratum corneum: relationship to the localization of polar lipids and phospholipids. *J Invest Dermatol* 91:3–10, 1988.
13. Elias PM, Menon GK: Structural and lipid biochemical correlates of the epidermal permeability barrier. *Adv Lipid Res* 24:1–26, 1991.
14. Elias PM, Williams ML, Maloney ME, Bonifas JA, Brown BE, Grayson S, Epstein EH Jr: Stratum corneum lipids in disorders of cornification: steroid sulfatase and cholesterol sulfate in normal desquamation and the pathogenesis of recessive X-linked ichthyosis. *J Clin Invest* 74:1414–1421, 1984.
15. Elias PM, Cullander C, Mauro T, Rassner U, Kömüves LG, Brown BE, Menon GK: The secretory granular cell: the outermost granular cell as a specialized secretory cell. *J Invest Dermatol Symp Proc* 3:87–100, 1998.
16. Fartasch M, Bassukas ID, Diepgen TL: Structural relationship between epidermal lipid lamellae, lamellar bodies and desmosomes in human epidermis: an ultrastructural study. *Br J Dermatol* 128:1–9, 1993.
17. Feingold KR: The regulation and role of epidermal lipid synthesis. *Adv Lipid Res* 24:57–79, 1991.
18. Feingold KR, Mao-Qiang M, Menon GK, Cho SS, Brown BE, Elias PM: Cholesterol synthesis is required for cutaneous barrier function in mice. *J Clin Invest* 86:1738–1745, 1990.
19. Freinkel RK, Traczyk TN: Acid hydrolases of the epidermis: subcellular localization and relationship to cornification. *J Invest Dermatol* 80:441–446, 1983.
20. Grayson S, Johnson-Winegar AG, Wintroub BU, Isseroff RR, Epstein EH Jr, Elias PM: Lamellar body-enriched fractions from neonatal mice: preparative techniques and partial characterization. *J Invest Dermatol* 85:289–295, 1985.
21. Grubauer G, Elias PM, Feingold KR: Transepidermal water loss: the signal for recovery of barrier structure and function. *J Lipid Res* 30:323–333, 1989.
22. Grubauer G, Feingold KR, Elias PM: Relationship of epidermal lipogenesis to cutaneous barrier function. *J Lipid Res* 28:746–752, 1987.
23. Halkier-Sorensen L, Elias PM, Menon GK, Thestrup-Pederse K, Feingold KR: Cutaneous barrier function after cold exposure in hairless mice. A model to demonstrate how cold interferes with homeostasis among workers in the fish-processing industry. *Br J Dermatol* 132:391–401, 1995.
24. Hamanaka S, Asagami C, Sukzuki M, Inagaki F, Suzuki A: Structure detemination of glucosy1β1-N-(ω-o-linoleoyl)-acylsphingosines of human epidermis. *J Biochem* (*Tokyo*) 105:68–590, 1989.
25. Harris IR, Farrell AM, Grunfeld C, Holleran WM, Elias PM, Feingold KR: Permeability barrier disruption coordinately regulates mRNA levels for key enzymes of cholesterol, fatty acid, and ceramide synthesis in the epidermis. *J Invest Dermatol* 109:783–787, 1997.
26. Hobkirk R: Steroid sulfotransferases and steroid sulfate sulfatases: characteristics and biological role. *Can J Cell Biol* 63:1127–1144, 1985.

27. Holleran WM, Feingold KR, Mao-Qiang M, Gao WN, Lee JM, Elias PM: Regulation of epidermal sphingolipid synthesis by barrier requirements. *J Lipid Res* 32:1151–1158, 1991.
28. Holleran WM, Mao-Qiang M, Gao WN, Menon GK, Elias PM, Feingold KR: Sphingolipids are required for mammalian barrier function: II. Inhibition of sphingolipid synthesis delays barrier recovery after acute perturbation. *J Clin Invest* 88:1338–1345, 1991.
29. Holleran WM, Sidransky E, Menon GK, Fartasch M, Grundmann J-U, Ginns EI, Elias PM: Consequences of β-glucocerebrosidase deficiency in epidermis: ultrastructure and permeability barrier alterations in Gaucher disease. *J Clin Invest* 93: 1756–1764, 1994.
30. Holleran WM, Takagi Y, Imokawa G, Jackson S, Lee JM, Elias PM: β-Glucocerebrosidase activity in murine epidermis: characterization and localization in relationship to differentiation. *J Lipid Res* 33:1201–1209, 1992.
31. Holleran WM, Takagi Y, Jackson SM, Tran HT, Feingold KR, Elias PM: Processing of epidermal glucosylceramides is required for optimal mammalian cutaneous permeability barrier function. *J Clin Invest* 91:1656–1664, 1993.
32. Holleran WM, Takagi Y, Menon GK, Jackson SM, Feingold KR, Elias PM: Permeability barrier requirements regulate epidermal β-glucocerebrosidase. *J Lipid Res* 35:905–912, 1994.
33. Holleran WM, Mao-Qiang M, Gao WN, Feingold KR, Elias PM: Extracellular processing of sphingomyelin by acid sphingomyelinase is required for normal permeability barrier homeostasis. *J Clin Invest* Submitted.
34. Hou SYE, Mitra AK, White SH, Menon GK, Ghadially R, Elias PM: Membrane structures in normal and essential fatty acid deficient stratum corneum: characterization by ruthenium tetroxide staining and X-ray diffraction. *J Invest Dermatol* 96:215–223, 1991.
35. Imakado S, Bickenbach JR, Brundman DS, Rothnagel JA, Attar PS, Wang X-J, Walczak VR, Wisniewski S, Pote J, Gordon JS, Heyman RA, Evans RM, Roop DR: Targeting expression of a dominant-negative retinoic acid receptor mutant in the epidermal of transgenic mice reults in loss of barrier function. *Genes Dev* 9:317–329, 1995.
36. Jackson SM, Wood LC, Lauer S, Taylor JM, Cooper AD, Elias PM, Feingold KR: Effect of cutaneous permeability barrier disruption on HMG CoA reductase, LDL receptor and apoprotein E mRNA levels inthe epidermis of hairless mice. *J Lipid Res* 33:1307–1314, 1992.
37. Johansen JD, Ramsing D, Vejlsgaard G, Agner T: Skin barrier properties in patients with recessive x-linked ichthyosis. *Acta Derm Venereol* 75:202–204, 1995.
38. Kawabe S, Ikuta T, Ohba M, Kazuhiro C, Ueda E, Yamanishi K, Kuroki T: Cholesterol sulfate activates transcription of transglutaminase 1 gene in normal human keratinocytes. *J Invest Dermatol* 111:1098–1102, 1998
39. Kinkaid AR, Wilton DC: Enhanced hydrolysis of physphatidylcholine by human Group II non-pancreatic secreted phospholipase A_2 as a result of interfacial activation by specific anions. *Biochem J* 308:507–512, 1995.
40. Lampe MA, Burlingame AI, Whitney J, Williams ML, Brown BE, Roitman E, Elias PM: Human stratum corneum lipids: characterization and regional variations. *J Lipid Res* 24:120–150, 1983.
41. Landmann L: The epidermal permeability barrier. *Anat Embryol* 178:1–10, 1988.
42. Lee SH, Elias PM, Proksch E, Menon GK, Mao-Qiang M, Feingold KR: Calcium and potasssium are important are important regulators of barrier homeostasis in murine epidermis. *J Clin Invest* 89:530–538, 1992.
43. Long SA, Wertz PW, Strauss JS, Downing DT: Human statum corneum polar lipids and desquamation. *Arch Dermatol Res* 277:284–287, 1985.
44. Madison KC, Swartzendruber DC, Wertz PW, Downing DT: Presence of intact intercellular lamellae in the upper layers of the stratum corneum. *J Invest Dermatol* 88:714–718, 1987.
45. Maloney ME, Williams ML, Epstein EH Jr., Law MYL, Fritsch PO, Elias PM: Lipids in the pathogenesis of ichthyosis: topical cholesterol sulfate-induced scaling I hairless mice. *J Invest Dermatol* 83:253–256, 1984.
46. Mao-Qiang M, Elias PM, Feingold KR: Fatty acids are required for epidermal permeability barrier function. *J Clin Invest* 92:791–798, 1993.
47. Mao-Qiang M, Feingold KR, Jain M, Elias PM: Secretory phospholipase A_2 activity is required for permeability barrier homeostasis. *J Lipid Res* 106:57–63, 1996.

48. Mao-Qiang M, Jain M, Feingold KR, Elias PM: Secretory phospholipase A_2 activity is required for permeability barrier homeostasis. *J Invest Dermatol* 106:57–63, 1996.
49. Mauro T, Bench G, Sidderas-Haddad E, Feingold K, Elias PM, Cullander C: Acute barrier perturbation abolishes the Ca^{2+} and K^+ gradients in the epidermis: quantitative measurement using PIXE. *J Invest Dermatol* 111:1198–1201, 1998.
50. Mauro T, Holleran WM, Grayson S, Gao WN, Mao-Qiang M, Kriehuber E, Behne M, Feingold KR, Elias PM: Barrier recovery is impeded at neutral pH, independent of ionic effects: implications for extracellular lipid processing. *Arch Dermatol Res* 290:215–222, 1998.
51. Mayer RJ, Marshall LA: New insights on mammalian phospholipase A_2 (s): comparison of arachidonoyl — selective and non-selective enzymes. *FASEB J* 7:339–348, 1993.
52. Menon GK, Elias PM, Feingold KR: Integrity of the permeabilty barrier is crucial for maintenance of the epidermal calcium gradient. *Br J Dermatol* 130:139–147, 1994.
53. Menon GK, Elias PM: Ultrastructural localization of calcium in psoriatic and normal human epidermis. *Arch Dermatol* 127:57–63, 1991.
54. Menon GK, Feingold KR, Moser AH, Brown BE, Elias PM: De novo sterologenesis in the skin. II. Regulation by cutaneous barrier requirements. *J Lipid Res* 26:418–427, 1985.
55. Menon GK, Feingold KR, Elias PM: The lamellar body secretory response to barrier disruption. *J Invest Dematol* 98:279–289, 1992.
56. Menon GK, Grayson S, Brown BE, Elias PM: Lipokeratinocytes of the epidemis of a cetacean, (*Phocena phocena*): histochemistry, ultrastructure, and lipid composition. *Cell Tissue Res* 244:385–394, 1986.
57. Menon GK, Grayson S, Elias PM: Ionic calcium reservoirs in mammalian epidermis: ultrastructural localization with ion capture cytochemistry. *J Invest Dermatol* 84:508–512, 1985.
58. Menon GK, Grayson S, Elias PM: Cytochemical and biochemical localization of lipase and sphingomyelinase activity in mammalian epidermis. *J Invest Dermatol* 86:591–597, 1986.
59. Menon GK, Lee S, Elias PM, Feingold KR: Localization of calcium in murine epidermis following disruption and repair of the permeability barrier. *Cell Tissue Res* 270:503–512, 1992.
60. Menon GK, Price LF, Bommannan B, Elias PM, Feingold KR: Selective obliteration of the epidermal calcium gradient leads to enhanced lamellar body secretion. *J Invest Dermatol* 102:789–795, 1994.
61. Mommaas-Kienhuis A-M, Grayson S, Wijsman MC, Vermeer BJ, Elias PM: LDL receptor expression on keratinocytes in normal and psoriatic epidermis. *J Invest Dermatol* 89:513–517, 1987.
62. Mukherjee AB, Miele L, Pattabiraman N: Phospholipase A_2 enzymes: regulation and physiological role. *Biochem Pharmacol* 48:1–10, 1994.
63. Nemanic MK, Elias PM: *In situ* precipitation: a novel cytochemical technique for visualization of permeability pathways in mammalian stratum corneum. *J Histochem Cytochem* 28:573–578, 1980.
64. Odland GP, Holbrook K: The lamellar granules of the epidermis. *Curr Probl Dermatol* 9:29–49, 1987.
65. Ottey K, Wood LC, Elias PM, Feingold KR: Cutaneous permeability barrier disruption increases fatty acid synthetic enzyme activity in the epidermis of hairless mice. *J Invest Dermatol* 104:401–405, 1995.
66. Ponec M, Havekes L, Kempenaar J, Vermeer BJ: Cultured human skin fibroblasts and keratinocytes: differences in the regulation of cholesterol synthesis. *J Invest Dermatol* 81:125–130, 1983.
67. Proksch E, Elias PM, Feingold KR: Regulation of 3-hydroxy-3-methyl-glutaryl-coenzyme A reductase activity in murine epidermis: modulation of enzyme content and activation state by barrier requirements. *J Clin Invest* 85:874–882, 1990.
68. Rassner UA, Crumrine DA, Nau P, Elias PM: Microwave incubation improves lipolytic enzyme preservation for ultrastructural cytochemistry. *Histochem J* 29:387–392, 1997.
69. Robson KJ, Stewart ME, Michelsen S, Lago ND, Downing DT: 6-Hydroxy-4-sphingenine in human epidermal ceramides. *J Lipid Res* 35:2060–2068, 1994.
70. Rushmer RF, Beuttner KJK, Short JM, Odland GF: The skin. *Science* 154:343–348, 1966.
71. Scheuplein RJ, Blank IH: Permeability of the skin. *Physiol Rev* 51:702–747, 1971.
72. Schurer NY, Elias PM: The biochemistry and function of stratum corneum lipids. *Adv Lipid Res* 24:27–56, 1991.
73. Shapiro LJ, Yen P, Pomerantz D, Martin E, Rolemic L, Mohandas T: Molecular studies of deletions at the human steriod sulfatase locus. *Proc Natl Acad Sci USA* 86:8427–8481, 1989.

74. Sidransky E, Fartasch M, Lee RE, Metlay LA, Abella S, Zimran A, Gao W, Elias PM, Ginns EI, Holleran WM: Epidermal abnormalities may distinguish type 2 from type 1 and type 3 of Gaucher disease. *Pediatr Res* 39:134–141, 1996.
75. Swartzendruber DC, Wertz PW, Kitko DJ, Madison KC, Downing DT: Evidence that the corneocyte has a chemically-bound lipid envelope. *J Invest Dermatol* 88:709–713, 1987.
76. Takagi Y, Kriehuber E, Imokawa G, Elias PM, Holleran WM: β-Glucocerebrosidase activity in mammalian stratum corneum. *J Lipid Res* 40:861–869, 1999.
77. Wertz PW, Cox PS, Squier CA, Downing DT: Lipids of epidermis and keratinized and non-keratinized oral epithelia. *Comp Biochem Physiol* [*B*] 83:529–531, 1986.
78. Wertz PW, Downing DT: Ceramides of pig epidermis: structure determination. *J Lipid Res* 24:759–765, 1983.
79. Wertz PW, Kremer M, Squier SM: Comparison of lipids from epidermal and palatal stratum corneum. *J Invest Dermatol* 98:375–378, 1992.
80. Williams ML: Lipids in normal and pathological desquamation. *Adv Lipid Res* 24:211–252, 1991.
81. Williams ML, Elias PM: From basketweave to barrier: unifying concepts for the pathogenesis of the disorders of cornification. *Arch Dermatol* 129:626–629, 1993.
82. Williams ML, Elias PM: Stratum corneum lipids in disorders of cornification: I. Increased cholesterol sulfate content of stratum corneum in recessive X-linked ichthyosis. *J Clin Invest* 68:1404–1410, 1981.
83. Williams ML, Rutherford SL, Mommaas-Kienhuis A-M, Grayson S, Vermeer BJ, Elias PM: Free sterol metabolism and low density lipoprotein receptor expression as differentiation markers in cultured human keratinocytes. *J Cell Physiol* 1332:428–440, 1987.
84. Wu-Pong S, Elias PM, Feingold KR: Influence of altered serum cholesterol levels and fasting on cutaneous cholesterol synthesis. *J Invest Dermatol* 102:799–802, 1994.
85. Zettersten E, Mao-Qiang M, Sato J, Denda M, Farrell A, Ghadially R, Williams ML, Feingold KR, Elias PM: Recessive x-linked ichthyosis: role of cholesterol-sulfate accumulation in the barrier abnormality. *J Invest Dermatol* 111:784–790, 1998.

7 Particle Probes and Skin Physiology

Bo Forslind and Jan Pallon

CONTENTS

7.1 INTRODUCTION

The condition of the skin, whether it is normal, dry, eczematous, etc., reflects its physiology/pathophysiology. Only during the past two and a half decades has it been possible to probe the physiology of human skin, and this has been achieved through the means of particle probes. The electron (see Chapter 8 by Warner) and the proton probe both rely on the production of secondary X-ray quanta

0-8493-7520-7/00/$0.00+$.50

emission, which allows identification of elements as well as quantification of them. Since it has become clear during the past two decades that there exists no actual substitute for human skin in experimental approaches to clinically normal and pathological skin conditions, this chapter is devoted to the study of element and particularly trace element distributions in normal and pathological human skin.

It is interesting to note that the development of modern medicine from the moment of the discovery of X-rays has been closely linked to the development of physics. Almost immediately after his discovery of X-rays in December 1895, Konrad Röntgen made an image of his left hand carrying a finger ring. From a historical point of view, this can truly be regarded as the first clinical X-ray image. It is a fact that this image had a tremendous impact on the contemporary medical body, and the clinical applications of the method were greeted with great enthusiasm among medical doctors. It became obvious that the density of the material was related to the degree of X-ray absorption, i.e., the bones were seen easily against the background of soft tissue. In clinical practice this resulted in the invention of contrast media which allowed, for example, the intestinal system to be imaged with a fair amount of detail.

Early on, X-rays were used for structure determination, and Bragg, father and son, are justly regarded as portal figures in this basic research application of the "mysterious rays." The development of this and other analytical methods based on X-ray techniques has had a pronounced impact on modern biology and is expected to be even more important in the future, a fact that can be gained from recent overviews in the literature. This chapter will briefly outline the history of X-ray absorption in biological research and then concentrate on the application of proton probes in experimental dermatology. References to results from other techniques will, however, be included.

7.2 THE BEGINNING — QUANTITATIVE MICRORADIOGRAPHY

The UV-absorption method, which today is one of the quickest and most reliable ways to assess cancers through quantitative determination of DNA in tissue sections, provided the inspiration for the development of X-ray spectrographic methods at the end of the 1940s. The quantitative X-ray analysis methods were developed to provide quantitative elementary analysis on a histochemical and cytochemical scale, i.e., quantitative elemental analysis of tissues *in situ* and at a subcellular level. Engström[1] formulated how the problem could be attacked in the following way:

- *Alternative 1* — Quantitative analysis of the element in question in a very small piece of tissue, microdrop, or something similar; the localization of the element in question in the tissue being obtained in the *preparation** of the analysis object
- *Alternative 2* — Quantitative determinations of the element in question, which has a relatively low atomic number, within a cell or a very small area in a microscopic section of a tissue, but retaining the structure; resulting in the analysis being *directly* correlated to the cytological structure

The second alternative was developed in Engström's thesis, "Quantitative micro- and histochemical elementary analysis by roentgen absorption spectrography," which he published in 1946, and his method became known as *quantitative microradiography*.[1] A satisfactory resolution was granted by fine-grain Lippmann emulsions, available in the 1930s, and this film material allowed a resolution in the 10-μm range.

This spectrographic method which allowed chemical elementary analysis of single mammalian cells was based on the selective absorption of monochromatic X-rays measured directly in the

* Microdissection without previous histological staining or any other sort of chemical interference.

spectrometer or by photometry of the X-ray photographic image of the cell/tissue. By exposing the same object for X-rays on each side of the absorption edge for the element to be determined, quantitative data were obtained, e.g., concentrations when the mass of the exposed area/volume was determined by a "white" radiation exposure. In early studies, ^{15}P and ^{20}Ca were determined in 10-μm bone sections within an area of 10 × 10 μm, and the amounts determined were of the order of 10^{-9} to 10^{-12} g. The error of the analysis was estimated to be 5 to 10%. The photographic recording provided a precise localization of the area measured, and grain density can be determined by photometry, out of which quantitative data can be calculated.

Engström's method was further developed and refined by the work of Lindström[2] (Figure 1). He expanded the theoretical basis for X-ray absorption spectrophotometry and constructed an X-ray spectrophotometer with a bent crystal that produced high intensity monochromatic X-rays of varying wavelengths.[14] The basis provided by the work of Engström and Lindström is presently put to good use in fully automatic microradiographic systems and standard tools in, for example, dental research.

7.3 INERT PREPARATION — CRYO-METHODS FOR ELEMENTAL ANALYSIS OF TISSUE SAMPLES

The content of a cell can be regarded as a gel in which ions are free to move at appreciable speed with minor restrictions. The study of the physiology of a cell in a particular phase of its activity must be done on a sample where all ionic movements have been instantaneously arrested. Chemical fixation relies on the diffusion of the fixing agent into the cell and its contents and will obviously perturb the particular conditions sought. If the tissue temperature can be instantaneously lowered to produce vitreous ice this would be an ideal preparative choice.[3,4] However, the heat conductive properties of organic material are far from excellent, and, therefore, we expect a gradient of temperature to move down into a tissue block exposed to a freezing medium. It has been shown that the depth to which a complete momentary freezing will reach is only about 50 to 100 μm. Further down in the tissue a temperature gradient will cause ice crystals to form, and these ice crystals not only disrupt the morphology of the cell, but also create redistribution of movable ions in a freezing-out process. Therefore, only a surface portion of a cryo-fixed tissue block is suitable.

After the subsequent sectioning of only the outer part of the frozen tissue block, we should ideally have a tissue section with a vitrified cellular gel containing all ions in their "natural" morphological positions. But cryo-sectioning is actually a process of shearing. The shearing process may actually cause a rise in the temperature of the section surface unless precautions against this are taken. Samples aimed for high resolution analysis require that sectioning be performed preferably in a temperature-controlled chamber at an ambient temperature of lower than –100°C. Also, the knife temperature must be controlled and kept very close to this temperature if very thin sections (<200 nm) are desired.[4] This is especially the case for X-ray microanalysis (EMP) in the scanning transmission electron microscope (STEM).

7.4 ENERGY DISPERSIVE X-RAY MICROANALYSIS IN THE ELECTRON MICROSCOPE

The original electron probes were *wavelength dispersive,* utilizing a crystal spectrometer for analyzing the particular characteristic X-ray emission from an element sought for. It was realized in the 1960s that the scanning electron microscope (SEM) actually represented an analysis system, i.e., had a potential of being a versatile analysis instrument. In addition to the secondary electrons used for imaging, the electron beam of an SEM produces a number of signals, e.g., back-scattered electrons, X-rays, cadluminiscent light, Auger electrons, electric current, etc.

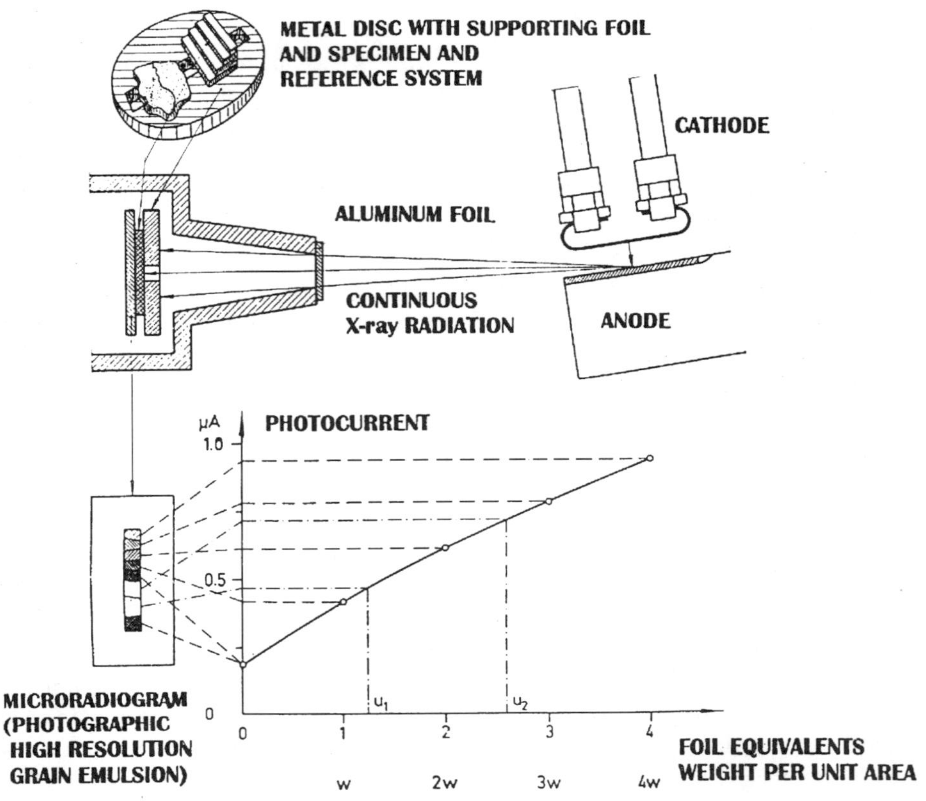

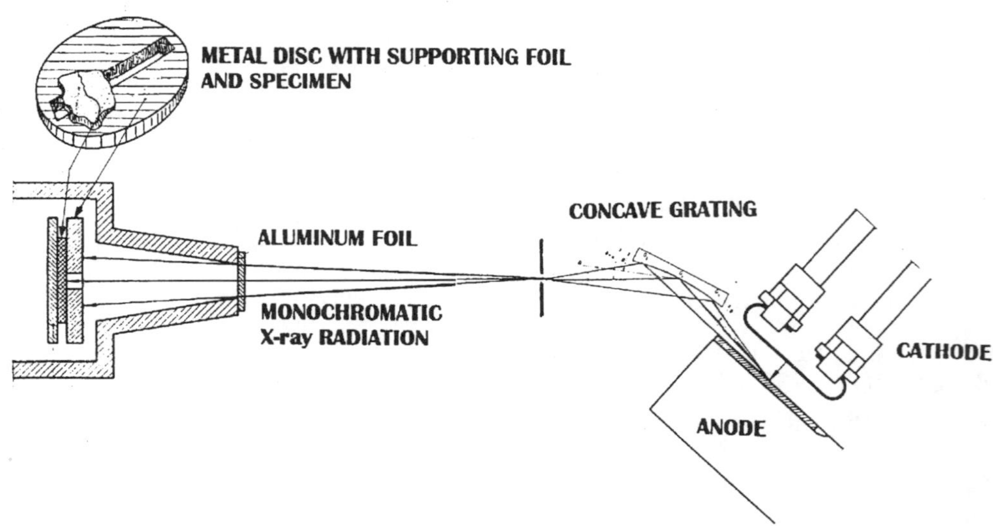

FIGURE 1 Top: The principle of microradiography — an X-ray absorption technique for quantitative assessment of dry weight (mass). Bottom: In addition to the mass information, a specified element can be quantitatively assessed by using two monochromatic radiation wavelengths on each side of an absorption edge for the element. (Adapted from Lindström. B., *Acta Radiologica Suppl* 125, p. 206, 1955.)

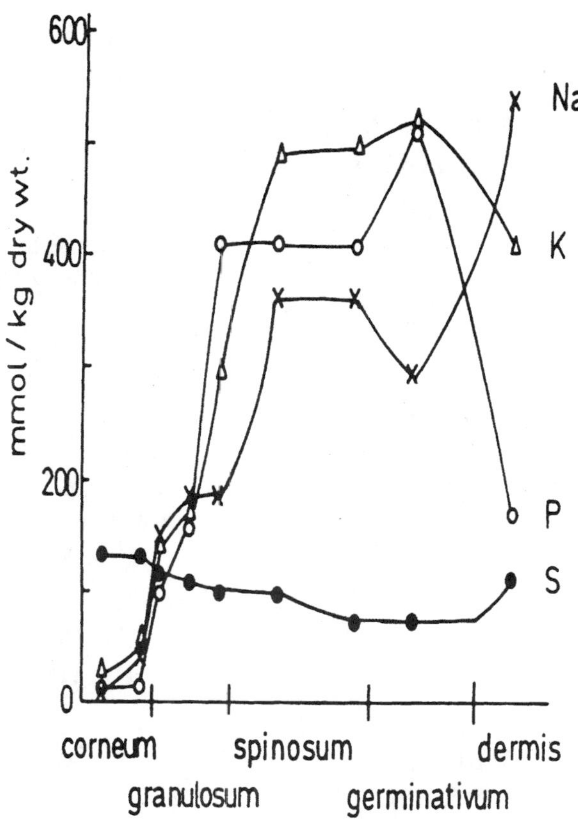

FIGURE 2 STEM X-ray spectrum from a skin sample.[36] Note that there is a conspicuous shift in the Na/K ratio moving from the dermis into the basal cell layer. Again, moving into the stratum spinosum, Na increases and K is lowered, a ratio shift which suggests that the spinosum cells are incapable of entering the mitosis cycle.

In the early 1970s when the *energy dispersive detectors* of semiconductor origin were commercially introduced, they actually revolutionized elemental analysis in the electron microscope. X-ray microanalysis (XRMA)* almost immediately found numerous applications in medical and biological sciences. The energy-dispersive detectors allowed a simultaneous recording of "all" elements in the irradiated volume. Cytochemical methods are hampered by the obvious drawback of not allowing multi-element analysis in the same section. The particle probes present a great advantage because virtually all elements of physiological interest can be measured *simultaneously* within one and the same volume. Consequently, comparisons of the relative contents and formation of elemental ratios, e.g., Na/K, that provide sensitive markers for cellular function[5] (Figure 2), are often more sensitive indicators of a physiological change than the absolute amounts of an ion (i.e., an element). The additional fact that the electron beam could scan a surface area of the object meant that elemental mapping now in principle was possible. However, it is clear for what was hinted previously that the XRMA technique requires inert preparation in order to minimize ion flux during the preparation and analysis. In the past three decades, cryo-fixation and cryo-sectioning methods, as well as freeze-drying techniques, have consequently been the focus for preparation technique development.[3,6]

* X-ray microanalysis (XRMA) in the scanning electron microscope (SEM) or scanning tranmission electron microscope (STEM) is often denoted EDX (energy-dispersive X-ray) analysis or just XRMA.

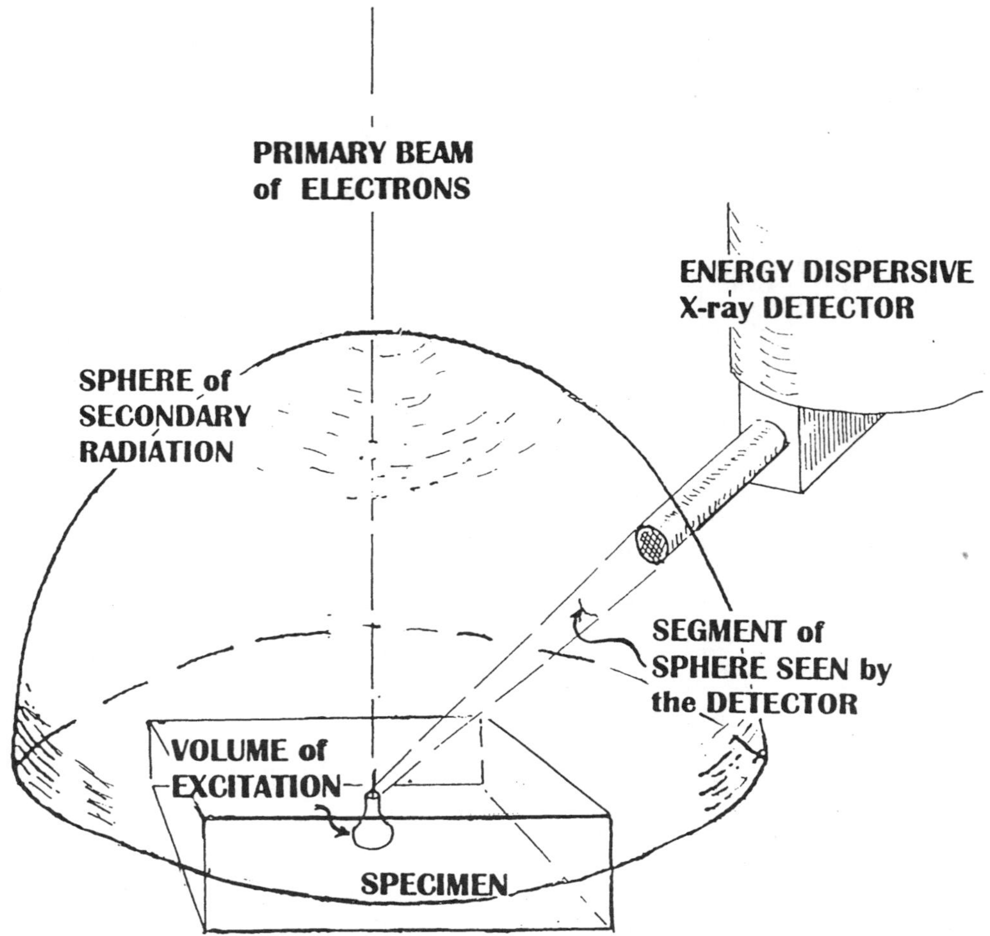

FIGURE 3 Sphere of secondary radiation. The detector "sees" only a fraction of the total number of emitted X-ray quanta. (Adapted from Lindström, B., *Acta Radiologica Suppl 125,* p. 206, 1955.)

7.5 DETECTION OF THE X-RAY SIGNAL

In the particle probe analysis systems, X-rays are generated from the elements due to an excitation caused by the impinging particles, whether they are electrons or protons, and these secondary X-rays are emitted in all directions. However, the detector can only cover a small part of the sphere of secondary radiation (Figure 3), even if the geometry of the experimental setup allows the detector to come very close to the object which will increase the spatial angle from which the detector "sees" the volume of analysis. Already, here we see a factor which influences markedly the sensitivity of the analysis method.

The X-rays generated represent quanta of energy. Since characteristic X-ray quanta represent "fingerprints" of the atom they are originating from, a detector which can sort quanta according to their energy will allow identification of elements present in the excited specimen volume. The number of quanta recorded will be proportional to the amount of that particular element present (Figure 4). The energy-dispersive system is a fast detector system that uses a signal processor which transforms the incoming X-ray quanta into electric pulses, subsequently fed into a multichannel analyzer which recognizes the different energies. The energy resolution of the system depends on the channel width that is usually set to 10 to 20 eV (Figure 4). The information collected in such a multichannel analyzer can be presented as an energy spectrum, which presents the relative

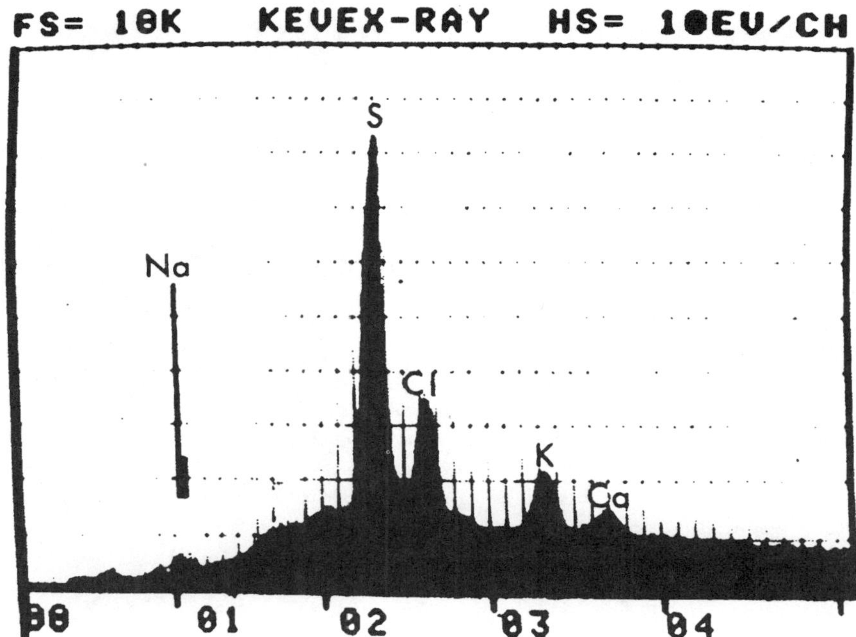

FIGURE 4 An X-ray spectrum from a skin sample. Note that the Na peak is very weak (due to absorption in the detector window), almost buried in the continuous background (Bremsstrahlung) radiation.

intensities of the X-ray signals from the object. As is generally the rule for spectrographic techniques, calibration of the system is done for absolute quantitation.

7.6 PROTON PROBE ANALYSIS

The use of particles heavier that electrons, and especially proton-induced X-ray emission analysis, was developed under the supervison of Professor Sven Johansson at Lund University, Sweden, during the 1970s. Generally referred to as PIXE (particle- or proton-induced X-ray emission) analysis, it has proven to be a sensitive trace element technique. The initial response among medical researchers was a cautious one, most likely due to the fact that the problems of specimen preparation initially were not fully appreciated by the physicists or even among biologists. Hence, the interpretation of results obtained from ill-prepared specimens were difficult, if not impossible, to make.

From what was given earlier, it is clear that PIXE analysis of tissue physiology requires cryomethods for tissue preparation. But are the data obtained with PIXE compatible with those given by the EMP (XRMA)?

7.7 COMPARISONS BETWEEN ELECTRON AND PROTON PROBES

Using standards for biological quantitation as specimens, we have compared XRMA and PIXE and obtained identical results — a correlation coefficient of 0.996 between the methods was obtained for elements such as ^{16}S and ^{28}Ni.[7] Hence, as analysis techniques these methods are fully complementary.

But how well do the XRMA and PIXE compare in practice? The advantages and disadvantages of the two techniques are summarized in Table 1. It can be recognized that even if EMP and PIXE are fully compatible concerning sensitivity for a number of physiologically important elements, there are some notable differences in two important aspects: their sensitivity to trace elements and their spatial resolution.

TABLE 1
The Advantages and Disadvantages of XRMA and PIXE

XRMA		PIXE	
Advantages	**Disadvantages**	**Advantages**	**Disadvantages**
High spatial resolution, 0.2 μm (200 nm)	Need for very thin *cryo-sections* (<200 nm), *cumbersome preparation*	*High sensitivity, < 1 ppm* Allows trace element analysis, e.g., Ca, Fe, Zn	Comparatively *low spatial resolution* ≤ *5 μm* which can be improved with loss of sensitivity
Sensitivity ~200 ppm *Simultaneous recording* of elements within a specified volume which allows formation of elemental ratios which can be used as sensitive monitors of physiological balance and unbalance in cells and tissues, e.g., Na/K	Absolute quantitation is not a straightforward procedure, appropriate *standards* and some approximations of *correction factors* are always involved in the practical application	Sensitivity 1 ppm *Simultaneous recording* of elements within a specified volume which allows formation of elemental ratios which can be used as sensitive monitors of physiological balance and unbalance in cells and tissues, e.g., Ca/K, Ca/Zn, Fe/Zn	Need for rather cumbersome *cryo-preparation*
Mass determination by background absorption	Rapid *burnout of the organic scaffold* causes registration of higher than normal contents of elements	*Mass determination* by back scattered protons or STIM, light element detection by nuclear complementary techniques, e.g., back scattering (C,N,O), photon tagged nuclear reaction analysis, pNRA for detection of B, Li, Na	Thick samples require *correction factors* Quantitation of thin samples is straightforward
Elemental mapping to depict distributions of elements over the *mass distribution image* or a *secondary electron image*	Mapping, even of small areas, requires very long analysis time on the order of hours	*Elemental mapping* to depict distributions of elements over tissue section is a routine *Low thermic load* on specimen due to scanning data acquisition	*Very long acquisition* times may result in *burnout of the organic scaffold*, causing a virtual higher than normal contents of elements

7.7.1 Sensitivity

PIXE analysis has a sensitivity which allows analysis of most of the physiologically important elements down to 1 ppm level with the notable exception of Na. The characteristic X-ray quanta from Na have a low energy and are therefore, to a great extent, suffering self-absorption within the specimen, but also attenuation by the detector window. However, Na can be quantified concomitantly with energy detection via γ-detectors by utilizing the nuclear reaction occurring as a result of proton capture by the Na nucleus.[8]

The heavy particles used in PIXE analysis are not as easily retarded as electrons by biological materials, and this results in a negligible background production allowing even weak secondary X-rays to be detected, hence the high sensitivity of 1 ppm.

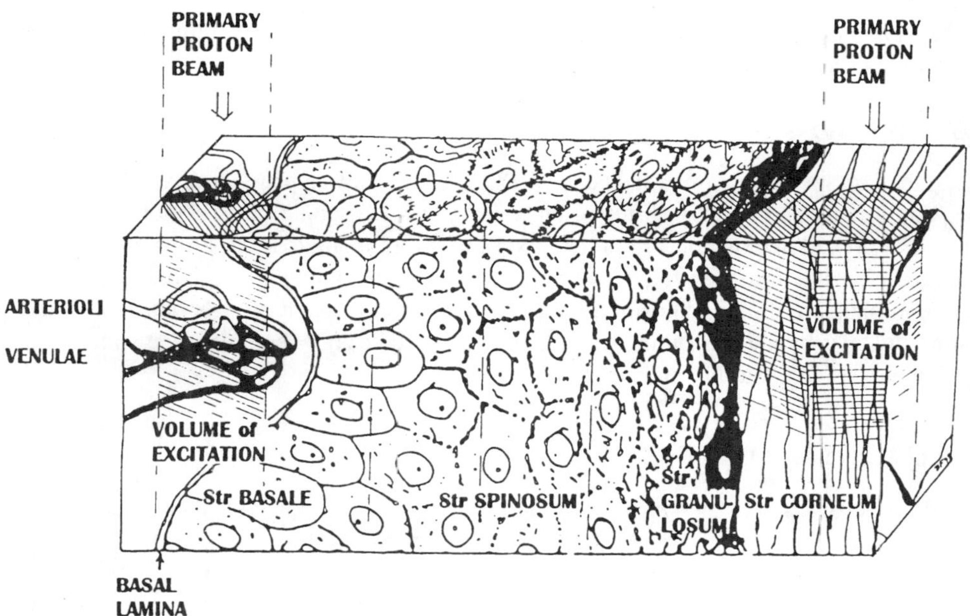

FIGURE 5 The secondary X-ray information will emerge from cellular structures in the depth of the section within volume of the proton beam (shadowed areas). In addition, a probe diameter of 5 μm will result in lateral overlap of cellular compartments. Hence, the spatial resolution of the proton probe is restricted to strata rather than single cells. The resolution can be improved by diminishing the probe diameter (<2 μm) and the section thickness (<6 μm) at the cost of a substantial increase in acquisition time.

The XRMA can generally be said to analyze elements down to contents of 200 ppm and is therefore essentially insensitive to trace elements such as Ca, Fe, and Zn, which are denoted trace elements in biological tissues. The reason for this insensitivity is the fact that the light electrons impinging on the section are subject to multiple scattering and retardation, effects that produce a significant background of continuous radiation in which the weak trace element signals are buried (Figure 4).

7.7.2 Spatial Resolution

The cross section of the electron probe is often of the order of 2 nm, and with a section thickness approximately 100 nm a subcellular resolution is allowed. Considering the fact that physiologically interesting elements generally are freely dispersed in the cytosol, it is clear that local variations in concentration in biological tissues are to be expected. Therefore, analysis data are retrieved from sets of spots in regions of the tissue deemed to be representative of the structure under investigation.

In order to get reasonable acquisition times for data, the sections used for PIXE generally are 15 μm thick. This thickness causes an overlap of the secondary X-ray emission information from cellular structures in the depth of the section precluding a subcellular resolution at analysis (Figure 5). Furthermore, when the width of the PIXE probe is ≤5 μm, this represents another factor that diminishes the spatial resolution of PIXE. Thus, PIXE analysis superposes the intra- and extracellular compartment data during analysis depending both on the comparatively low spatial resolution of the measuring system and on the thickness of the sections (~15 μm), which of necessity must contain both compartments in a cross section. These facts relate to the considerable smoothing of curves describing the elemental and mass distribution over the cellular layers of a differentiated epidermis (Figure 6, bottom panel). The effect is perhaps most conspicuous in the very narrow stratum corneum region (a total width in a section of approximately 10 μm) where the mass curve is rather wide in these experiments. In general terms, this means that generally analysis *within* a defined cell compartment is not possible, and data are generally referred to as originating from a defined morphological entity, e.g., a stratum of an epithelium, a special structure in the brain, etc.

7.7.3 Limitations of PIXE Analysis

The number of specimens investigated in a PIXE study may appear small in comparison with corresponding numbers used in different types of light microscopic investigations or biochemical studies. The typical acquisition time for a pixel map from a single section is generally about 2 h when trace elements are analyzed. Costs/benefit aspects of running an experiment will obviously require optimization of data acquisition for evaluation. To assess a number of data that would allow statistical analysis by the algorithm used, the time allowed has not been sufficient so far to quantify such elements as Mg, Cu, Ni, and Se.

7.8 ELEMENTAL MAPPING

In PIXE applications spot analysis was initially the dominating analysis method, but during the 1980s scanning procedures were developed which allowed pixel mapping of the specimen. With a probe size of 5 μm, a tissue surface of 200 × 200 μm can be covered by the pixel map in an acquisition time of approximately 2 h, i.e., within this time period a representative area of the tissue section can be analyzed for all elements and mass (Figure 6, middle panel). A further important advantage in PIXE mapping is the markedly diminished thermal load on the volumes of analysis that results in more reliable data when the influence of burnout of the organic matrix material was minimized.

From pixel maps obtained by the scanning proton probe, cross-section profiles of elemental distributions can be extracted (Figure 6, bottom panel). For elements present in trace amounts, long acquisition times are needed as mentioned. A corresponding map obtained with the EMP would require at least a five times longer acquisition time, which is the reason why elemental mapping for elements present in low concentrations has not been favored in XRMA.

7.8.1 Pixel Maps Provide Information on the Dynamics of Tissue Activity

Analysis of PIXE pixel maps reveals as one conspicuous feature the variation in the distribution of elements and trace elements seen in the sequel as well as in different sections. This is a finding which occurs both in the normal skin and in the clinically normal psoriatic skin. Such variations in the distribution of elements, and especially trace elements, indicate that there are obvious differences in the detailed cellular physiology of the differentiating keratinocytes. Such findings harmonize with our previous experience from electron microscopic studies of contact irritative reactions. These studies show that the correlation between the morphological image and the quantitative elemental data is not a direct one.[9-11] Although morphologically similar, certain stratum cells reveal their different stage of differentiation in the patterns of elemental distributions as suggested by the elemental maps. The combination of immunological techniques to tag different markers of differentiation in parallel with elemental analysis should provide an additional detailed insight into the keratinization process programmed to develop a complete stratum corneum with a functional barrier.

7.8.2 Multivariate Analysis Identifies Co-Variations of Elements and Strata

A recent development of proton probe analysis involves multidimensional statistical analysis of all data extracted from mass and elemental maps. The SIMCA™ program, which essentially analyzes co-variations of factors, allows not only comparisons of elemental levels within strata of an epidermal cross section, but it also allows comparisons between strata, elements, individuals, etc.[12]

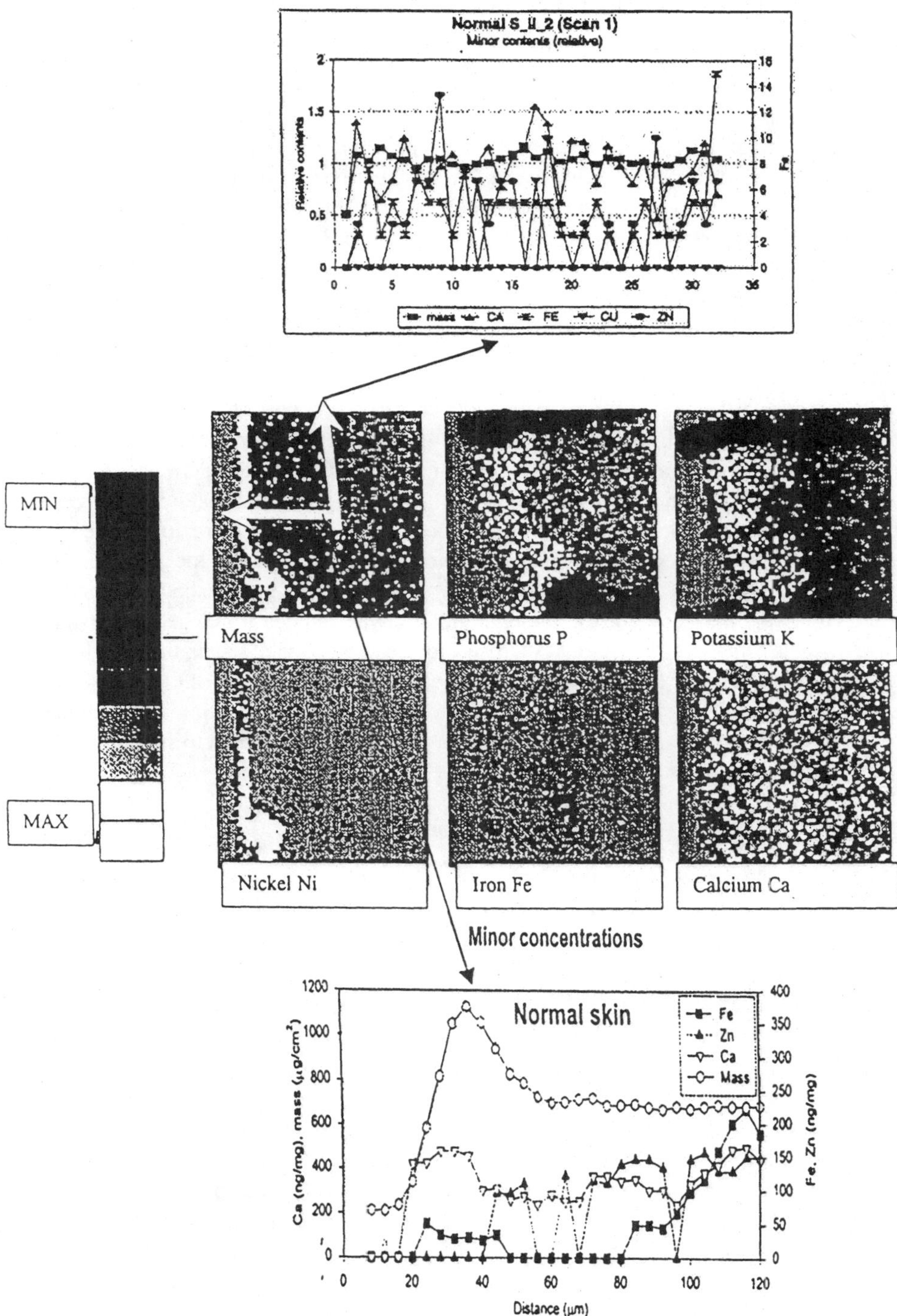

FIGURE 6 Proton probe analysis of a normal skin sample. The middle panel demonstrates mass, P, K, Ca, Fe, Ni, and Zn distributions. Note that Ni is solely confined to the stratum corneum (Ni pixel map lower row, left). The top panel represents a "horizontal" scan parallel to the basal cell layer (vertical arrow in mass pixel map). The bottom panel represents a cross section (white horizontal arrow in mass pixel map) demonstrating distributions of mass, Ca, Fe, and Zn.

7.9 TRACE ELEMENT ANALYSIS IS POSSIBLE WITH THE PROTON PROBES

In the initial studies of trace elements of human skin cross sections, a Ca profile evolved which was increasing from the basal, germinative level of the epidermis toward the horny layer. The drastic concentration drop of Ca concentration down to threshold values at the border of the stratum germinativum and the stratum corneum was a particularly interesting feature.[12-14] Only a few years later this finding could be correlated to the fact that a Ca concentration >0.1 mmol was essential if a fully cornified stratum corneum was to be obtained in cell culture. This relationship between Ca and terminal differentiation of the epidermal cells was recently verified in a PIXE study of epidermal cell cultures.[15]

7.9.1 THE CA^{2+} SIGNAL

The influence of trace elements on the normal and abnormal physiology of the skin has not yet reached a full understanding. The role of calcium for epidermal differentiation has been demonstrated in a series of elegant studies using ion capture cytochemistry at transmission electron microscopic resolution by Elias and co-workers.[16] In the normal murine skin the most prominent localization of Ca^{2+} was noted in the upper stratum granulosum and the dermis, whereas the basal region was virtually free from Ca^{2+} precipitates. When the barrier was broken by acetone treatment, a redistribution of Ca^{2+} took place with a conspicuous accumulation of precipitates in the extracellular space of the stratum corneum and loss of the stratum granulosum localization. Treating the barrier-disrupted skin with isoosmolar sucrose containing Ca^{2+} replenished the epidermal Ca^{2+} reservoir. However, the secretion of lamellar bodies was impeded and hence barrier recovery. Conversely, treatment with isoosmolar sucrose only lead to barrier repair through lamellar body secretion in the absence of the normal Ca^{2+} gradient. The conclusion of the authors was that loss of the Ca^{2+} reservoir is an important signal for restoration of barrier function after damage. In spite of these investigations there is obviously a need for fully quantitative data to support these findings, and such quantitative data can be obtained using PIXE analysis.

7.9.2 CA^{2+} AND PROGRAMMED CELL DEATH OR APOPTOSIS

The importance of Ca^{2+} as a signal for various cell functions is now established. A further aspect of the Ca^{2+} function is its property to promote "programmed cell death" (or apoptosis). Zn^{2+} has been shown to inhibit this effect.[17] As of yet, it is not clear what role such a phenomenon plays in the sequel of cellular differentiation of the epidermis. This process can be regarded as a kind of programmed cell death which involves the complete dissolution of nucleic acid material in the stratum granulosum. One indication on the importance of increased Ca levels in this cellular stratum is related to the finding that a full differentiation of the epidermis does not occur in tissue culture unless the Ca content equals at least 0.1 m*M*.[18] One may speculate that these findings suggest an explanation to the sporadic occurrence of parakeratotic cells in the stratum corneum in the paralesional psoriatic epidermis where unusually high zinc levels are recorded in the stratum granulosum zone. Whether this effect is directly coupled to an increased cellular activity in the germinative pool may be a matter of speculation, but the actual high levels of iron compared to normal skin suggest such an increased activity. Further detailed analyses, including particle probe studies, are required before this question can be settled.

The skin dependence on appropriate availability of Zn^{2+} for normal function is a subject that has not been completely resolved.[19,20] However, it is conceivable that these problems can at least partially be solved using particle probe analysis.

7.9.3 IRON AND ZINC

Iron (Fe) has a high peak value in the basal cell region, drops to values less than half the peak value in the uppermost epidermal layers, and is not detectable in the stratum corneum region.[13]

Zinc (Zn), which is represented in the dermis by concentrations below or just at the detection level of the system, shows a comparatively stable level over the Malpighian epidermis and disappears coincidentally with Fe in the stratum corneum region.[12,13] So far, the PIXE data obtained from normal skin suggest an approximate ratio of Zn content in epidermis/dermis of 3:1 to be compared with a 6:1 ratio given by neutron activation analysis.[21] Copper (Cu) is just barely detectable in the Malpighian layers, and generally no quantitation is possible within the acquisition times used in most of our experiments.

7.9.4 Mass and Elemental Distributions of the Epidermis

The mass distribution curves reach a peak in the stratum corneum region, flatten out in the basal cell region, and then rise again in the dermis in full agreement with the previous XRMA data. The S distribution curves follow the mass curves in concert.

Around 50 μm below the maximum mass peak, at a region corresponding to the stratum spinosum, we find the P distribution peak. Chlorine (Cl) has a weak minimum approximately where the P distribution has its peak. In the vicinity of stratum corneum, which is virtually free from Cl, there is a conspicuous drop in the Cl content. Conversely, the Cl content rises in the dermis compared to the epidermal content. K reaches its highest levels in the Malpighian layers and drops to nil in the stratum corneum. In the dermis relatively low values are recorded, as is expected for the extracellular compartment.

7.9.5 Recycling of Diffusible Ions

Summing up the data on the distribution of physiologically important elements, it is interesting to note that at the border between the viable epidermis and the stratum corneum their contents are close to or below the detection limit of the particle probes with the particular exception of calcium (see Chapter 8). The disappearance of the diffusible ions can be understood if we consider the fact that the water content is roughly constant over the epidermal cross section, finally dropping to low values within the stratum corneum.[22,23] The mass content of the cells increase continuously on the passage from the cells of the basal layer to the final fully cornified corneocyte. Since keratin binds water, we can see that the amount of *free* water available for the freely diffusible ions decreases with increasing mass. This creates a downhill gradient directed toward the dermis. Therefore, the recycling of freely diffusible ions requires no special energy-consuming mechanism.

7.9.6 Local Variations of Element and Trace Element Distributions

There are slight, but obvious variations in the elemental distribution patterns from one section to another, although a general trend can clearly be discerned. The Fe and Zn distributions have their centers of gravity in the stratum spinosum/stratum granulosum area, but Zn is more clearly confined to the basal layer.

7.9.7 Horizontal Elemental Distributions

The element distribution curves have generally been extracted from pixel "channels" which cover the cross section from stratum corneum down into the papillary dermis. When data are retrieved so as to represent pixel channels which cover a specified stratum horizontally, it can be seen that the mass distribution along the basal lamina of normal skin varies somewhat along the horizontal scan (Figure 6, top panel). However, it remains approximately constant at the upper level (the level of the stratum spinosum/granulosum). This obviously relates to the fact that the basal cells may be in different phases of the cell division cycle, whereas the stratum spinosum cells are more synchronized in their development. K and Cl co-vary with mass in the basal region, but the variation is more independent in the stratum spinosum region as expected from cross-section distribution.[10]

As expected S co-varies to a great extent with the mass distribution. In both regions (stratum spinosum and basal) more conspicuous variations in relation to mass are seen in the P distribution.

There is an extensive variation in the Fe and Zn distributions in the basal region. The Fe content is close to or below the detection limit in the upper region; the Zn content shows some peaks above the detection limit. Single off-limit values in these trace elements were seen.

Ca appears to stay rather constant within each horizontally scanned band, which is consistent with the fact that the increase in Ca toward the stratum corneum is likely to be related to the physiological and regulatory effects of this ion.

7.10 ELECTRON AND PROTON PROBE DATA FROM PATHOLOGICAL SKIN

7.10.1 PSORIASIS

An early XRMA study in which compared skin from healthy, normal persons with uninvolved and involved (a stable plaque) psoriatic skin revealed that Mg, P, and K were increased in the involved skin corresponding to what is recorded in highly proliferative, non-neoplastic cells.[24,25] Previously Burkhart and Burnham had recorded a significant increase in P and Ca content in involved psoriatic skin compared to uninvolved skin from the same patients.[26] Later, Kurtz et al. reported corresponding findings from a PIXE study of psoriatic skin, but found no difference between the Zn content of control skin and uninvolved skin from psoriatic patients.[27] However, in pinpoint lesions they recorded a significant increase of Zn corresponding to neutron activation analysis data given by Molin and Wester (Table IV).[28,29]

Our PIXE data have demonstrated that noninvolved psoriatic skin has a mass distribution with the same general features as that of normal skin, although generally at a lower level (absolute mass content). The P and S distributions are not conspicuously different from those of normal skin.

Some interesting aspects on the elemental distribution were revealed in a recent study of uninvolved psoriatic skin.[30] Ca shows a twofold or even higher increase in the stratum granulosum region compared to normal skin, but in contrast to the Ca distribution in normal skin, that of psoriasis follows the mass distribution more closely. In many sections there is an additional Ca peak in the vicinity of the basal cell layer, but the full significance of this is not clear at the moment.

The trace element distributions of uninvolved psoriatic skin merit special comments. The main Fe peak appears closer to the mass distribution peak than in normal skin. Also, there are obvious variations in the Fe content in different strata (cell layers), and the lowermost values are consistently at least twice as high as those in normal skin. Our PIXE investigation substantiates the previously reported finding that psoriatic patients lose Fe through the shedding of stratum corneum cells in lesional areas by demonstrating that clinically normal skin of psoriatic patients contains higher than normal amounts of Fe.[28,29]

The Zn content of the uninvolved psoriatic skin is increased in the stratum spinosum especially, except in one single section where the Zn follows suit with Fe distribution. Such variations are likely to occur as a function of the cell cycle position of a particular cell.

Since the Cu concentrations as a rule are below the detection threshold, they are therefore not considered in these contexts.

7.10.2 ELEMENTAL DISTRIBUTIONS IN DIFFERENT STRATA OF PSORIATIC NORMAL-LOOKING SKIN — HORIZONTAL SCANS

In comparison to the control skin there are high mean values and prominent variations in the trace elements, notably Fe and Zn, in the upper level of the epidermis. However, the mass distribution pattern essentially follows that of normal control skin with some variations in the upper layer. There were more spots of Cu above the detection limit in the psoriatic skin sections both in the basal and the upper level in comparison to the control skin where Cu is a spurious finding. The issue is still unclear and needs further exploration.

In spite of the fact that the spatial resolution does not allow discrimination between the intra- and extracellular compartments, PIXE data nevertheless reveal some crucial points concerning the physiology of normal-appearing psoriatic skin as opposed to the normal skin. The Ca distribution profile, which in the normal skin remains at an almost constant level over the skin cross section, shows a slight increase in the stratum granulosum region in certain specimens. This differs from data of a previous preliminary study based on selected point measurements in different strata of skin sections.[12] However, with the new information obtained from the elemental maps such a variation is likely to occur as an expression of the continuous changes occurring *in vivo*. Continuous changes like these are represented in similar studies using quench frozen specimens by a "snap-shot" depicting momentarily what are actually transient processes.

In order to elucidate the background to these abnormal elemental distributions further studies including psoriatic plaques will be needed. Recent data from dry skin of atopics also present elemental distributions which vary conspicuously from those found in normal.[12,31] These facts challenge our experimental imagination to produce answers to what faults in the cellular mechanisms are at hand in these skin disorders.

7.10.3 Metal Allergy

In the Western Hemisphere Ni allergy has very rapidly grown to be a major dermatological problem. The penetration profile of this metal ion through the skin remained largely unknown, in spite of previous studies on Ni penetration through human skin using XRMA, due to the insensitivity of the method.[10,32,33] In a recent PIXE study of skin samples from individuals tested for Ni allergy, it was demonstrated that the Ni accumulated in the stratum corneum and that only trace levels passed through the skin barrier.[34] These findings suggest that extremely minute amounts of Ni are needed to elicit an allergic reaction in an Ni-sensitized individual. It corresponds to the observation that just a single, very brief contact with a dry nickel-plated object may elicit an allergic reaction.

7.10.4 Multidimensional Statistical Analysis Using SIMCA

Primary data are not always easy to interpret to give a functional picture of the tissue physiology. Ratios of elements such as Ca/Zn can provide interesting information when one realizes that Zn may be antagonistic to effects elicited by Ca. But comparisons and correlations of data from different strata, individuals, and disorders are still problematic. From a physiological/biological point of view correlations may provide more pertinent information than straightforward statistics which just provide statistical significances. The recent introduction of multidimensional statistical analysis (SIMCA) conspicuously broadens the possibility of meaningful interpretations of primary data. Using SIMCA to study the dry skin of atopic individuals, it turns out that when we look for correlations between strata of the epidermis and elements, the dry atopic skin proves to be very immature compared to the unafflicted skin of normal (control) individuals. A SIMCA scatter plot shows that the stratum basale and spinosum co-variate in the atopic skin, but are well separated in the control skin.[35] Such information suggests that the stratum spinosum of the atopic skin is immature. Multidimensional statistical analysis allows us to understand data in physiological terms and will undoubtedly have an impact on the analysis of skin disorder obtained by biochemical and immunological means.

In a recent study of clinically normal skin from patients with psoriasis, a high Fe content of the horny layer was demonstrated, whereas there was no detectable Fe in the horny layer of normal healthy control individuals.[30] Obviously, this finding in psoriasis demonstrates that the entire differentiating epidermis of these patients is involved in the disorder, whether clinically expressed or not.

7.11 SUMMARY AND CONCLUSIONS

In this chapter, as well as in Chapter 8, the feasibility of skin physiology studies using particle probe analysis has been demonstrated. The EMP or XRMA analysis of biological tissues has allowed the study of physiological processes which cannot be attacked using common physiological techniques, e.g., microelectrode registrations. An example of "impossible physiology" that was subsequently allowed by the XRMA is the study of the physiology of the differentiating epidermis (Figure 2).[36] Thus, we were able to show that the cells on the basal lamina separating the fibrous tissue of the dermis from the cellular tissue of the epidermis are the only cells upholding a normal Na/K ratio. Already the next cellular level has suffered an increase in the Na and a decrease in K, meaning that these cells either leak ion or that their membrane pumps are deficient. A consequence of this is that only the basal cells with a normal Na/K ratio can go through the mitosis cycle producing a progeny. The biological meaning of this is obviously one of cell division control, resulting in a smooth skin surface.

Further, the EMP has allowed studies of the water profile over the skin cross section,[22,23] the physiological changes at irritative reactions,[9-11] and psoriasis.[24] A comprehensive overview of the EMP application is given in a recent overview paper.[37]

The application of X-ray analysis methods to biological problems has proven to be of great, sometimes unsurpassed, value. Recent developments of computer software, statistical programs, etc. have tremendously broadened the possibility of data retrieval and handling. The reason why we do not find more biologically oriented work in the literature is obviously due to an information gap, i.e., an educational problem — biologists/medical researchers know too little about X-ray physics, and physicists know to little about biological systems and the effects of biological tissue preparation.

Particle probe analysis and, in particular, proton probe analysis which is sensitive to trace element levels in tissue sections have been demonstrated to reveal important details about cellular physiology in the differentiating epidermis of normal and pathological skin. Such a physiological approach will serve to complement data from histochemistry, immunology, and other morphological techniques. A future collective approach of this kind will make it possible to understand how a dry and/or eczematous skin develops and also what the mechanisms of subsequent healing are.

REFERENCES

1. Engström, A., Quantitative micro- and histochemical elementary analysis by roentgen absorption spectrography. Thesis. *Acta Radiologica Suppl* 63, pp 1–106, 1946.
2. Lindström, B., Roentgen absorption spectrophotometry in quantitative cytochemistry. Thesis. *Acta Radiologica Suppl 125,* pp 1–206, 1955.
3. Roomans, G.M., Shelburne, J.D., (Eds), *Basic Methods in Biological X-Ray Microanalysis.* Scanning Electron Microscopy Inc., Chicago (AMF O'Hare), 1983.
4. Roomans, G.M., Gupta, B.L., Leapman, R.D., von Zglinicki, T., (Eds), *The Science of Biological Microanalysis.* Suppl. 8., Scanning Electron Microscopy Inc., Chicago (AMF O'Hare), 1994.
5. Von Zglinicki, T., Ziervogel, H., Bimmler, M., Binding of ions to nuclear chromatin. *Scanning Microsc* 3:1231–1239, 1989.
6. Ingram, P., Shelburne, J.D., Roggli, V.L., *Microprobe Analysis in Medicine.* Hemishpere Publ. Corp., New York, 1989.
7. Forslind, B., Kunst, L., Malmqvist, K.G., Carlsson, L.-E., Roomans, G.M., Quantitative correlative proton and electron microprobe analysis of biological specimens. *Histochemistry* 82:425–427, 1985.
8. Kristiansson, P., Al-Suhaili, S., Elfman, M., Malmqvist, K.G., Pallon, J., Sjöland, K.A., Photon-tagged nuclear reaction analysis — evaluation of the technique for a nuclear microprobe. *Nucl. Instr. Methods* B 136–138: 362–367, 1998.
9. Lindberg, M., Roomans, G.E., Elemental redistribution and ultrastructural changes in guinea-pig epidermis after dinitrochlorobenzene (DNCB) exposure. *J Invest Dermatol* 81:303–308, 1983.

10. Lindberg, M., Sagström, S., Roomans, G.M., Forslind, B., Sodium lauryl sulfate enhances nickel penetration through guinea-pig skin. Studies with energy dispersive X-ray microanalysis. *Scanning Microsc* 3:221–224, 1989.
11. Lindberg, M., Forslind, B., Sagström, S., Roomans, G.M., Elemental changes in guinea-pig epidermis at repeated exposure to sodium lauryl sulfate. *Acta Derm Venereol (Stockholm)* 72:428–431, 1992
12. Pallon, J., Knox, J., Forslind, B., Werner-Linde, Y., Pinheiro, T., Applications in medicine using the new Lund microprobe. *Nucl Instr Methods Phys Res B* 77:287–293, 1992.
13. Malmquist, K.G., Carlsson, L.-E., Akselsson, K.R., Forslind, B., Proton-induced X-ray emission analysis — a new tool in quantitative dermatology. *Scanning Electron Microscopy* 4:1815–1825, 1983.
14. Forslind, B., Roomans, G.M., Carlsson, L.-E., Malmqvist, K.G., Akselsson, K.R., Elemental analysis on freeze dried sections of human skin: studies by electron microprobe and particle induced X-ray emission analysis. *Scanning Electron Microscopy* 2:755–759, 1984.
15. Vicanova, J., Mommaas, A.M., Kempenaar, J., Forslind, B., Pallon, J., Egelrud. T., Koerten, H.K., Ponec, M., Normalization of epidermal calcium distribution profile in reconstructed human epidermis is related to improvement of terminal differentiation and stratum corneum formation. *J Invest Dermatol* 111:97–106, 1998.
16. Menon, G., Elias, P.M., Seung, H.L., Feingold, K.R., Localization of calcium in murine epidermis following disruption and repair of the permeability barrier. *Cell Tissue Res* 270:504–512, 1992.
17. Barr, P.J., Tomei, L.D., Apoptosis and its role in human disease. *Biotechnology* 12:487–493, 1994.
18. Ponec, M., Kempenaar, J., Calcium induced modulation of lipid synthesis in cultured human epidermal keratinocytes. *J Invest Dermatol* 84:452, 1985.
19. Goolamali, S.K., Comaish, J.S., Zinc and the skin. *Int J Dermatol* 14:182–187, 1973.
20. Nelder, K.H., The biochemistry and physiology of zinc metabolism. In L. Goldsmith (Ed.) *Physiology, Biochemistry and Molecular Biology of the Skin,* 2nd ed., Oxford University Press, New York, pp 1329–1350, 1991.
21. Molokia, M., Portnoy, B., Neutron activation analysis of trace elements in the skin. III. Zinc in normal skin. *Br J Dermatol* 81:759–763, 1969.
22. von Zglinicki, T., Lindberg, M., Roomans, G.M., Forslind, B., Water and ion distribution profiles in human skin. *Acta Derm Venereol (Stockholm)* 73:340–343, 1993.
23. Warner, R.R., Myers, M.C., Taylor, D.A., Electron probe analysis of human skin. Determination of the water concentration profiles. *J Invest Dermatol* 90:218–224, 1988.
24. Grundin, T., Roomans, G.M., Forslind, B., Lindberg, M., Werner, Y., X-ray microanalysis of psoriatic skin. *J Invest Dermatol* 85:378–380, 1986.
25. Smith, N.R., Sparks, R.L., Pool, T.B., Cameron, I.L., Differences in the intracellular concentrations of elements in normal and cancerous liver cells determined by X-ray microanalysis. *Cancer Res* 38:1952–1959, 1978.
26. Burkhart, C.G., Burnham, J.C.V., Elevated phosphorus in psoriatic skin determined energy dispersive X-ray microanalysis. *J Cutan Pathol* 10:171–177, 1983.
27. Kurtz, K., Steuigleder, G.K., Bischof, W., Gonsior, B., PIXE analysis in different stages of psoriatic skin. *J Invest Dermatol* 88:223–226, 1987.
28. Molin, L., Wester, P.-O., Iron content in normal and psoriatic epidermis. *Acta Derm Venereol (Stockholm)* 53:473–476, 1973.
29. Molin, L., Wester, P.-O., Cobalt, copper and zinc in normal and psoriatic epidermis. *Acta Derm Venereol (Stockholm)* 53:477–480, 1973.
30. Werner-Linde, Y., Pallon, J., Forslind, B., Physiologically important trace elements of paralesional psoriatic skin. Quantitative analysis of distributions using scanning proton probe technique. Vol. 4. *Scanning Microscopy,* Accepted for publication. 1997.
31. Werner-Linde, Y., Pallon, J., Forslind, B., Physiological aspects on atopic skin. Elemental analysis using PIXE. Manuscript submitted 1999.
32. Forslind, B., Lindberg, M., Emilson, A., Sagström, S., Roomans, G.M., Malmqvist, K.G., Themner, K., Nickel penetration through skin. In S. Jasienska, L.J. Maksymowicz (Eds.), *Particle Probe Analysis,* Proceeding of 12th ICXOM, Cracow, Academy of Mining and Metallurgy, Cracow, Poland, pp 587–591, 1989.
33. Lindberg, M., Forslind, B., Roomans, G.M., Elemental changes at irritant reactions due to chromate and nickel in guinea-pig epidermis. *Scanning Electron Microscopy* 3:1243–1247, 1983.

34. Forslind, B., Lindberg, M., Pallon, J., Epidermal physiology at epicutaneous patch testing for Ni-allergy assessed by PIXE. *Scanning Microscopy*, Accepted for publication, 1998.
35. Forslind, B., Pallon, J., Werner-Linde, Y., Elemental analysis mirrors epidermal differentiation. *Acta Derm-Venereol* 79:12–17, 1999.
36. Wei, X., Roomans, G.M., Forslind, B., Elemental distribution in guinea-pig skin as revealed by X-ray microanalysis in the scanning transmission electron microscope. *J Invest Dermatol* 79:167–169, 1982.
37. Forslind, B., Lindberg, M., Roomans, G.M., Pallon, J., Werner-Linde, Y., Aspects on the physiology of human skin. Studies using particle probe analysis. (Invited and accepted paper to special issue of MRT on the molecular histology of the skin). *Microsc Res Technique* 38:373–386, 1998.

8 The Distribution and Function of Physiological Elements in Skin

Ronald R. Warner

CONTENTS

8.1 INTRODUCTION

All epithelia of the body have a barrier function by which they divide compartments and control the transfer of water, solutes, and electrolytes across their borders. Usually this barrier function is studied by measuring fluxes, electrical parameters, and intracellular solute/electrolyte concentrations. These investigations owe much to fundamental studies of frog skin.[1] As a result of 50 years of research, there is an enormous wealth of data on water and electrolyte fluxes and concentrations for all epithelia of the body **but** mammalian skin, and as evidenced by the prominent inclusion of such data in reference texts, this knowledge is pivotal in the understanding of organ function in nonskin tissues. Electrolytes in nonskin tissues play functional roles, and changes in cellular concentrations reflect altered function or pathology. The paucity of similar data for mammalian skin has undoubtedly contributed to the current poor understanding of proliferation/differentiation disorders and barrier function, and this paucity is all the more ironic given the historical importance, the wealth of data, and the ongoing investigations on electrolytes in frog skin.

This brief review of what is known about element concentrations in mammalian skin will deal exclusively with the major physiological elements Na, P, S, Cl, K, and Ca. Due to the known importance of Ca in skin, and the greater attention it has received, this element will be discussed separately in the latter portion of this chapter. Of course, element concentrations are not independent of the water content; given that water levels change across the skin[2,3] and given a near

0-8493-7520-7/00/$0.00+$.50

absolute lack of quantitative data on this water distribution,[4] any discussion of element concentrations must be, at best, semiquantitative in nature. Nearly all data on elements in skin suffer from this uncertainty.

A major aim of this chapter is not only to provide perspective and to highlight what is known about elements in skin, but also to point out deficiencies in our knowledge in this area. The importance of understanding element concentrations in skin must not be underestimated. The questions left unanswered are fundamental, with important ramifications. For instance, what ionic strength is appropriate for the study of stratum corneum (SC) enzymes *in vitro*? Is barrier repair[5,6] mediated via osmotic effects on cellular electrolytes or by element gradients? Which elements? Are keratinocytes in the granular layer metabolically (energetically) healthy? Are the element concentrations of the keratinocytes altered in disease? As occurs in other tissues, it is quite possible that therapies addressing keratinocyte electrolyte imbalances may one day improve skin health; currently, however, that discovery process has hardly started.

8.2 CONVENTIONAL STUDIES OF PHYSIOLOGICAL ELEMENTS IN SKIN

There are few conventional studies on the handling of physiological elements by mammalian skin. It is known that electrolytes have a very low permeability across skin,[7-10] the epidermal transudate has an extremely low electrolyte content,[11,12] and the Na^+ and Cl^- activities measured at the surface of dry skin range from 10 to 120 and 10 to 70 m*M*, respectively.[13] Amazingly little wet chemistry appears to have been done on the electrolyte content of skin. Rothman reviews studies on the electrolyte content of both whole skin, which would be dominated by the dermis, and heat-separated epidermis, which would contain significant amounts of extracellular space.[14] The Na and K values obtained for the epidermis were 50 and 80 mmol/kg wet weight, respectively; the resulting K/Na ratio is substantially different from other organs.[14] This author is aware of only one study that quantitatively measured an intracellular electrolyte in mammalian skin, that being Na in fetal sheep skin.[15] In that study, intracellular Na levels were 29 m*M*, which increased to 43 m*M* in the presence of an antidiuretic hormone.[15] Even in the classic calcium-jump studies of keratinocyte cultures[16,17] as well as in *in vivo* studies,[18] changes in keratinocyte electrolyte concentrations were not measured (excluding calcium, discussed subsequently) or, if measured, were reported not as absolute values, but as percent change from control.[19-21] It would appear that accurate quantitative values for the average concentrations of electrolytes in mammalian keratinocytes, determined by conventional wet chemical techniques, are simply not available.

8.3 PARTICLE-BEAM STUDIES OF PHYSIOLOGICAL ELEMENTS IN SKIN

Unlike all other epithelia, most determinations of cellular elemental content in mammalian skin have been based on X-ray microanalysis using particle beams of either electrons (electron microprobe analysis, analytical electron microscopy [AEM]) or proton-induced X-ray emission (PIXE). These techniques are difficult, tedious, and measure cellular concentrations one cell at a time. Sample preparation is critical. The accuracy and sensitivity of results, and the spatial resolution that can be obtained, strongly depend on the approach taken. One of the earliest investigations of skin using X-ray microanalysis compared the fidelity of different sample preparation procedures.[22] Similar to results obtained by others,[23,24] preparation techniques other than the analysis of fast-frozen, freeze-dried tissue (cryosections) resulted in the elimination of physiological elements and a reduction in the amount of insoluble sulfur-containing protein.[22] The earliest study of diffusible elemental distributions in skin cryosections was that by Forslind et al.[25] Subsequent work in this area has been done primarily by this Swedish group (B. Forslind, G.M. Roomans, and M. Lindberg),[3,26-37] with contributions from others,[38-40] including our own laboratory.[2,41,42]

There are important differences between the methodology we have used and that of all other laboratories that have measured element profiles in skin using particle-beam analysis. These differences have led to some disagreements, and perspective in this area is useful. Compared to others, our methodology involves sectioning samples at lower temperatures (<–100°C), analyzing sections that are more than an order of magnitude thinner (0.5 to 1.0 μm), and analyzing at a higher (electron beam) accelerating voltage (100 kV). As a consequence, we have a smaller analytical volume and a superior analytical spatial resolution (<0.2 μm) in which intracellular and extracellular spaces are easily distinguished. These advantages come at the cost of difficulty and slowness. An alternative approach using much thicker cryostat sections has an analytical spatial resolution of ~10 μm,[26] and as a consequence it is possible that underlying or adjacent intercellular spaces (with much different electrolyte concentrations) could inadvertently be included in the analyses of intracellular cytoplasm.[3,26,27]

Finally, PIXE analysis (a technique we have not used) has enormously enhanced sensitivity allowing for trace element analysis. However, PIXE also suffers from an analytical spatial resolution that is only slightly better than 10 μm. For all PIXE skin analyses, cryostat sections were analyzed with similar dangers of mixing intra- and intercellular concentrations. Although there is a world of skin biology to explore at a 10-μm level of resolution, particularly for trace elements, understanding the role of elements in cell function (and in the stratum corneum) will be aided by submicron (organelle-level) resolution.

8.3.1 Element Profiles across Skin

The distribution of physiological elements across the human skin epithelium[41] is shown in Figure 1. All measurements were obtained from intracellular cytoplasm. For each panel, the skin surface is at the left, the basal layer at the right. Note that element profiles appear to be relatively constant across the viable tissue, although concentrations appear slightly elevated in the basal layers. In contrast, at the SC/granulosum interface, almost nothing is constant. Sulfur and Cl increase, P falls, K initially falls, and Na initially remains constant. In the outer SC, all elements but P increase to high levels. The element profiles across the skin epithelium can be visualized directly in X-ray maps of human skin cryosections,[42] as illustrated in Figure 2. In this figure, the upper left morphological (STEM) image shows a (torn) granular layer at the bottom, with the skin surface at the top. Element concentration is depicted in grayscale in the X-ray maps, with white being the highest value. Although the element gradients across the SC are not as large as those of Figure 1, gradients are nevertheless apparent.

The element profiles of Figure 1 appear very different from those of the Swedish group[3,25,30,36] (and others[39]), which typically show marked drops in concentration from the basal layer to the SC and very low values in the SC. In part these differences are due to the different units for expressing concentration. The other groups report element concentrations per unit dry mass. Such units are useful when tissue dry mass is reasonably constant, and the mass normalization corrects for differences in the amount of sample. However, in skin where the dry mass distribution is known to increase (and water content decrease) across the epithelium, particularly for the stratum corneum,[2,4] division by a variable mass may be inappropriate. If an element were to exist at a uniform concentration per unit volume of tissue across the skin, then expressing its concentration per unit mass would produce a large drop of the apparent concentration across the SC; in contrast, expressing concentrations per liter of water would produce a large increase in apparent concentration across the SC. In one study of human skin,[3] measurement of both local element concentration and water content permitted element concentrations to be expressed in the appropriate form of moles per liter of water. In this instance, the element profiles were relatively constant across the skin, as shown in Figure 3, similar to our observations per unit volume in Figure 1.

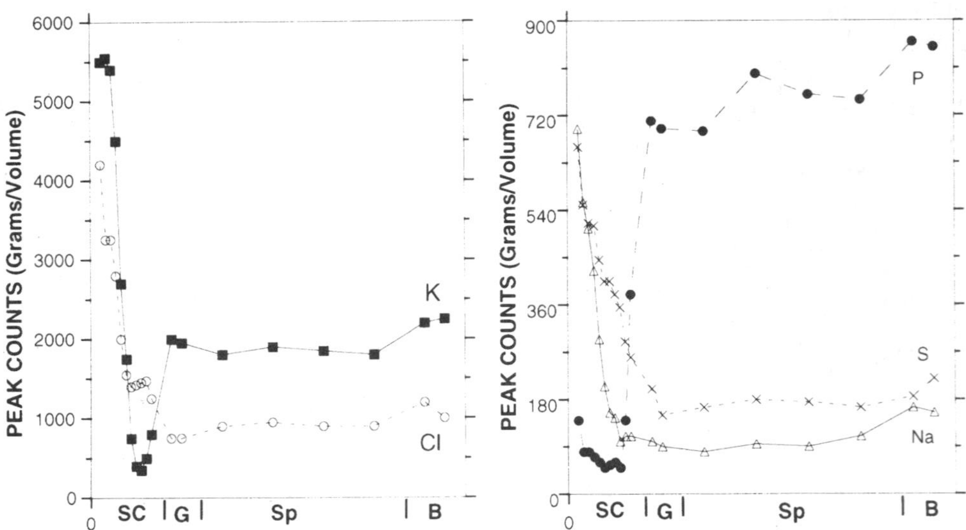

FIGURE 1 Element profiles across human skin. The vertical axis is in arbitrary units proportional to grams (or moles) per unit volume. The horizontal axis indicates position within the tissue measured from the outer SC cell. SC = stratum corneum, G = stratum granulosum, Sp = stratum spinosum, and B = basal layer. The widths of these morphological regions are not drawn to scale. ■ = K, ○ = Cl, ● = P, × = S, Δ = Na. (From Warner, R. R., Myers, M. C., Taylor, D. A., Electron probe analysis of human skin: element concentration profiles, *J. Invest. Dermatol.*, 90, 78–85, 1988. Reprinted by permission of Blackwell Science, Inc.)

8.3.2 Element Profiles across the Stratum Corneum

As indicated in Figures 1 and 2, steep element gradients exist across the SC. In the outer SC, concentrations are high at the surface and decrease toward the SC interior. In our experience, the magnitude of these gradients is quite variable from person to person, but a gradient is always present. Since the high concentrations are at the skin surface, the most likely source of these elements is sweat salts or residues from personal skin products. There may be a functional role for high element concentrations at the skin surface, such as the control of enzyme activity involved in desquamation.[41]

Element profiles in the inner SC, shown in Figures 1 and 2, are more consistent in magnitude from person to person than those of the outer SC. There is a systematic progression in element concentration as keratinocytes "mature" into corneocytes.[42] These position-dependent alterations in corneocyte element composition, shown in more detail in Figure 4, likely relate to the reclamation of intracellular solutes back into the viable tissue. From mass-balance considerations, the loss of the major intracellular solutes K and P from the inner SC strongly suggests that they are recycled to the underlying tissue. Since the granular layer is entrusted with the formation of the skin's lipid barrier,[43,44] yet is 100 μm away from a capillary bed, a release of nutrients at the SC interface may be important to the metabolic activity of this layer. Because the K gradient across the cell membrane is typically the primary determinant of the cellular membrane potential,[45] a sudden surge of extracellular K would have profound effects on the membrane potential of the granular cell and could readily account for altered cellular function such as the lamellar body secretory response known to occur after acute barrier disruption.[46] Indeed, K is known to affect barrier repair[47] and to be decreased in the outer epidermis following barrier perturbation.[39] It is very possible that the profound release of intracellular solutes at the SC interface has very important ramifications for proper skin function. Many of these ideas were included in a model for inorganic element cycles within human skin,[41] reproduced in Figure 5.

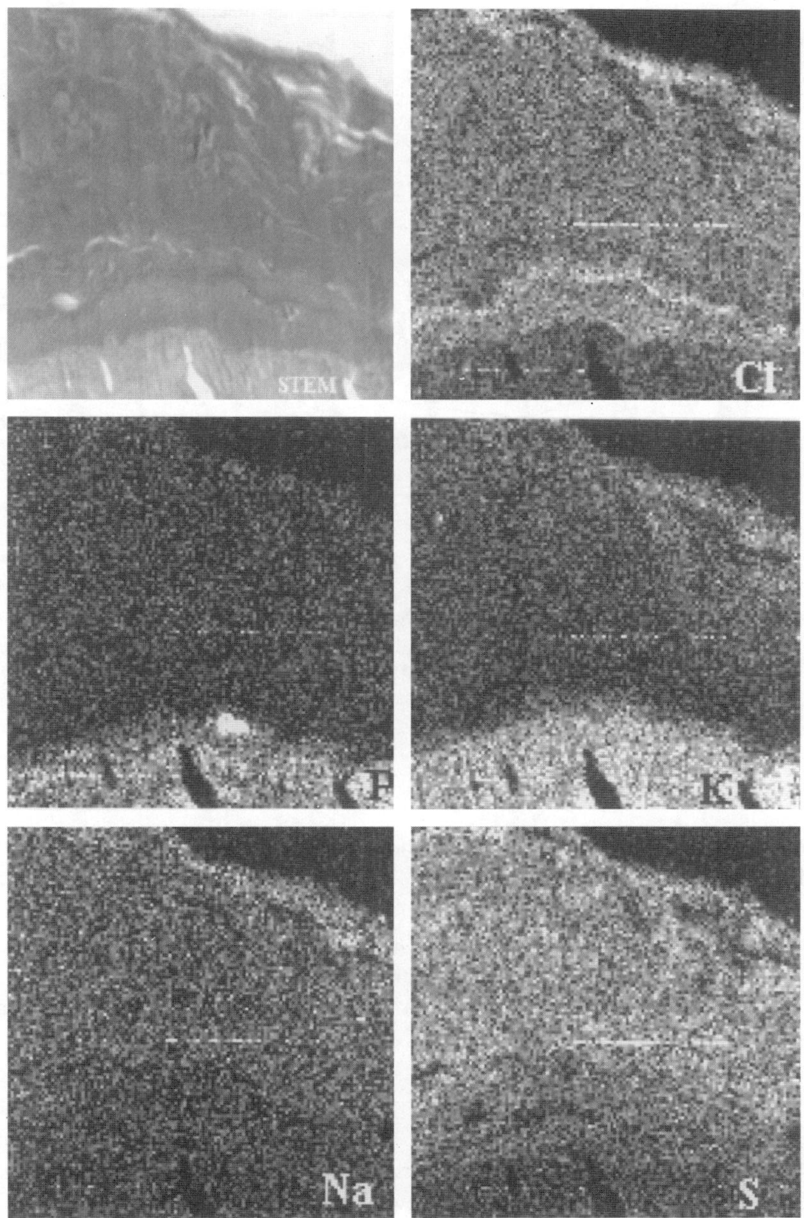

FIGURE 2 Upper left image is a STEM (scanning transmission electron microscope) micrograph from a human skin cryosection showing a portion of the viable tissue at the bottom and the skin surface at the top. Separations between corneocytes are likely artifacts of cryosectioning. The grayscale of the corresponding element maps for Cl, P, K, Na, and S is related to grams of element per unit volume of tissue, where black denotes the absence of the element, white the highest value.

Figure 4 shows that each element has a novel distribution within the inner SC. Note that in the innermost two corneocytes the Cl concentration is increasing, the K concentration is falling, and the Na concentration is unchanging. These opposing Cl and K movements within the corneocyte, unbalanced by other inorganic electrolytes, would suggest that an electrical charge imbalance is created. Such an imbalance must be offset by the generation or movement of organic ions not detected by AEM. We have proposed that generation of intracellular acidity due to filaggrin breakdown could account for the K and Cl movements.[42]

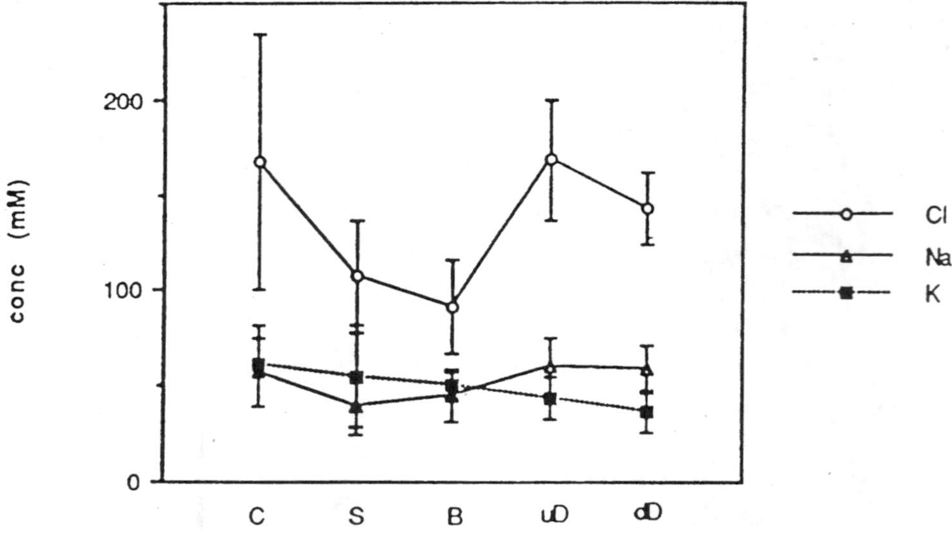

FIGURE 3 Electrolyte concentration profiles across human skin; data from Reference 3, Figure 4. The horizontal axis indicates position within the tissue; C = stratum corneum, S = stratum spinosum, B = basal layer, uD = upper dermis, dD = deep dermis. The widths of these morphological regions are not drawn to scale. ■ = K, ○ = Cl, Δ = Na. (From Von Zglinicki, T., Lindberg, M., Roomans, G. M., Forslind, B., Water and ion distribution profiles in human skin, *Acta Derm. Venereol. (Stockh.)*, 73, 340, 1993. Reprinted by permission of Scandinavian University Press.)

8.3.3 Intracellular Electrolyte Concentrations in Skin

All quantitative particle probe analyses involve demanding techniques where insidious errors can occur with little notice. In skin this technology has a particularly difficult problem: given the deplorable absence of knowledge concerning intracellular concentrations within keratinocytes by alternative techniques, there is no direct way to assess the presence of systematic errors in measurements done by particle probe analysis. This inability to objectively determine the accuracy of an analysis of skin, to know when a measurement is substantially incorrect, is an enormous disadvantage. It is likely for this reason that precision in the determination of keratinocyte concentrations appears to be lacking, as suggested by the large variations in keratinocyte concentrations reported in the literature. For control, untreated guinea pig skin, values for the Na concentration in keratinocytes in the spinosum layer have varied from 95 to 374 mmol/kg dry weight, and for K from 118 to 560 mmol/kg dry weight[25,34] (expressing concentrations per kilogram dry weight is awkward; since the epidermis is approximately two thirds water,[48] dividing the concentrations by three would convert the units to a more user-friendly kilogram wet weight). Values for the K/Na ratio within keratinocytes in the spinosum have varied from 0.6 to 1.1.[29,34] In control, untreated human skin, values for the intracellular K/Na ratio in the spinosum varied from 0.8 to 1.7,[3,37] and in the basal layer a K/Na value of 0.7 was reported.[37] These K/Na ratios are much lower than typical cellular values in other tissues.[7]

Claims with considerable significance to skin physiology are based on such uncertain measurements. For instance, it has been claimed that in passage from the basal layer to the SC, keratinocytes are unable to maintain a constant intracellular K/Na ratio.[25,36] Is this due to energy limitations of the differentiated keratinocyte? It has been proposed that there is nearly ionic equilibrium for Na, K, and Cl across the entire skin, SC to dermis, and that high levels of K must be bound within the epithelium and dermis.[3] Could there be only small concentration differences between extracellular and intracellular compartments in skin? Guinea pigs killed and kept at room temperature for 24 h had spinosum and basal layer keratinocyte concentrations that were not different from freshly killed

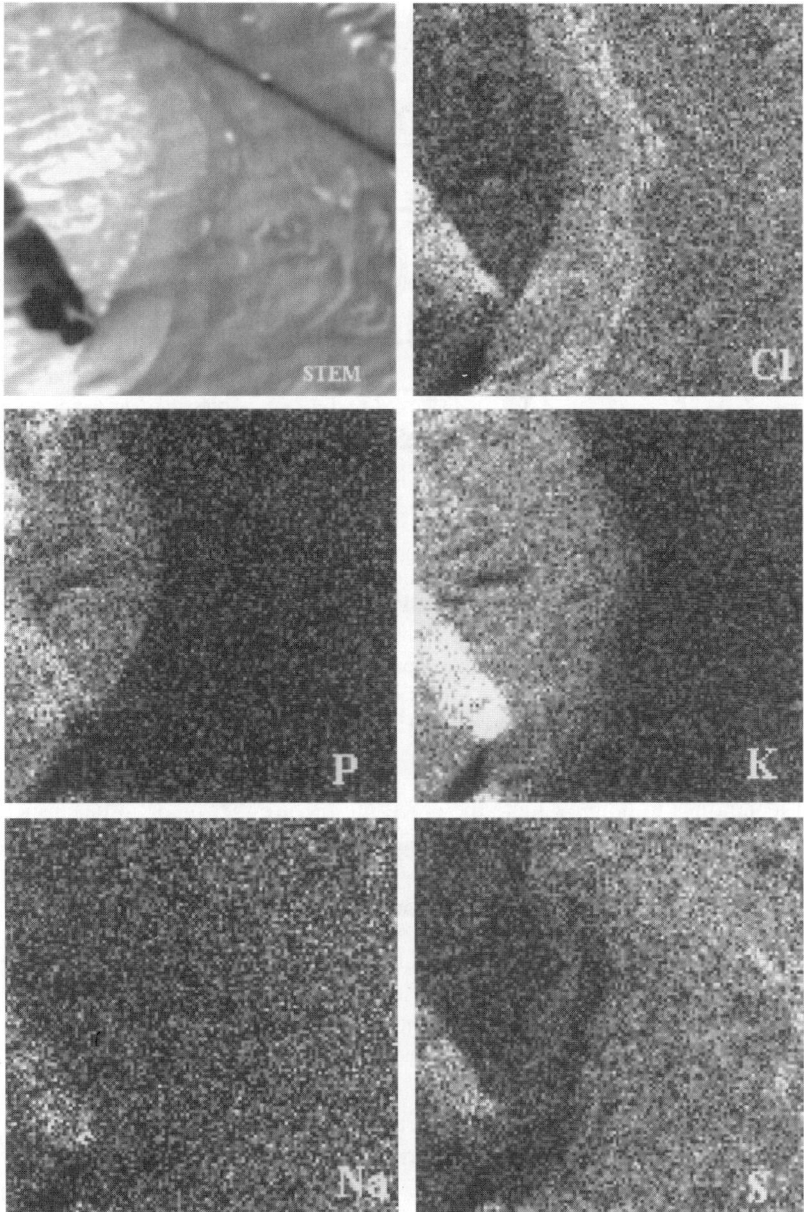

FIGURE 4 Top left image is a STEM micrograph from a human skin cryosection showing granular layers at the far left of the image followed by six to seven inner SC corneocyte layers. The dark cylindrical shape at the left edge of this cryosection is tissue debris from cryosectioning, and it serves as a useful marker pointing to the innermost corneocyte in the corresponding elemental maps. The dark line at the top right corner of this image is a contamination track formed by the electron beam during a prior extended (2 h) linescan; the width of the contamination track indicates the analytical resolution.

controls.[26] Is it possible that the skin can derive sufficient oxygen from diffusion across the SC that it is all but isolated from dependence on the circulation? In untreated human skin, many keratinocyte intracellular K/Na ratios were less than 1.[3,37] Such electrolyte distributions would make skin a very unique tissue in the body. Conventional measurement of electrolyte concentrations do exist for the dermis,[49,50] and they are very different from the microprobe results;[3] hence, the proposal for high binding of extracellular K[3]. The point is that there is little or no published data on skin using more

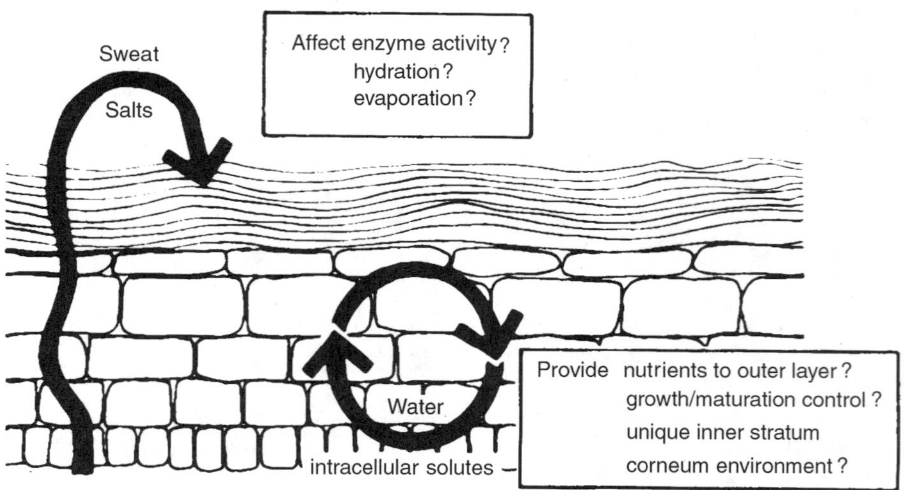

FIGURE 5 Proposed model of inorganic element cycles in human skin. Salts from sweat are delivered to the skin surface; carrier evaporation leaves high salt concentrations that diffuse into the outer SC and potentially affect enzyme activity and skin hydration. Within the viable tissue, K, P, and likely other intracellular solutes potentially support metabolism in cell layers far removed from a nutrient source, participate in maturation or barrier control, or by their simple exclusion from upper layers, provide a unique environment necessary for barrier formation. (From Warner, R. R., Myers, M. C., Taylor, D. A., Electron probe analysis of human skin: element concentration profiles, *J. Invest. Dermatol.*, 90 (1), 78–85, 1988. Reprinted by permission of Blackwell Science, Inc.)

conventional techniques to help evaluate the emerging picture that the skin has a metabolism and elemental makeup considerably different from any other organ system.

8.3.4 Intracellular Electrolytes in Pathological Conditions

It is well known that ions influence cellular functions, and many therapeutic drugs act by directly modifying the ionic traffic across cell membranes. Elements are known to play a role in the pathogenesis of some diseases. Knowledge of ionic alterations in skin disease may provide needed insight for future therapies. Although particle probe analysis of skin may have had difficulties in determining absolute values for cellular electrolytes, it should have less trouble in detecting relative changes in electrolyte levels. A number of particle probe studies have addressed element levels and pathology, particularly concerning the action of irritants and control of hyperplasia. The intradermal injection of 1% nickel sulfate in guinea pig increased Na and Cl and decreased K in the viable tissue of skin, indicating cell injury (and possibly a stimulation of mitotic activity).[27] A similar injection of 0.05% potassium chromate had less effect, and only increased Cl (and decreased P) achieved statistical significance.[27] Application of the irritant dinitrochlorobenzene (10%) led to a loss of K and P with a gain of Ca, also indicating cellular injury.[26] Application of *n*-hexadecane resulted in a decrease in Na and increase in K and Mg, with increased K/Na ratio; the tissue hyperplastic response to the irritant appeared to precede the elemental changes.[33] In contrast, treatment of skin with 5% sodium lauryl sulfate (SLS) produced an increase in intracellular Na, K, and Cl that preceded a hyperplastic response,[32,34] followed by a normalization of Na and a higher K/Na ratio at later times.[34] Contrasting responses were elicited in a direct comparison of two different irritants, 80% nonanoic acid (NAA) and 4% SLS; at 6 h K increased with SLS and decreased with NAA.[37] Although irritants produce a common hyperplastic response, it would seem that different irritants do not have a common effect on intracellular concentrations. In other investigations, K, P, and Mg were increased in psoriasis, interpreted as typical for highly proliferative, nonneoplastic cells.[29,38] In the skin of the elderly, K was lower and Ca higher than the skin of a younger group.[40]

8.4 CALCIUM AND KERATINOCYTE DIFFERENTIATION

Calcium is unique among physiological elements in that its intracellular ionic concentration has been measured in keratinocytes. Intracellular Ca^{+2} was determined in cultured cells using fluorescent dyes; values ranged from 20 to 200 n*M*, depending on external Ca and other culture conditions.[51-56] This focus on calcium in skin occurred following the demonstration that extracellular calcium could regulate growth and differentiation in cultured keratinocytes. When extracellular Ca^{+2} was increased ("switched") to 0.1 m*M* or higher, keratinocytes ceased proliferation and terminally differentiated.[16,21] The calcium-induced terminal differentiation was associated with a sustained increase in both intracellular Ca^{+2} and endoplasmic reticulum (ER) Ca^{+2} stores.[51,53] An increase in ER Ca^{+2} stores was associated with an increased expression of the spinous cell markers K1 and K10, a redistribution of E-cadherin to the cell membrane, and suppression of DNA synthesis.[53,54] It was suggested that the "fullness" status of the ER Ca^{+2} stores and/or levels of intracellular Ca^{+2} regulate proliferation.[53] In contrast to the regulation of K1 and K10, expression of granular cell differentiation markers loricrin and profilaggrin were closely linked simply to an increase in intracellular ionic calcium.[53,54] A Ca^{+2}-sensitive regulatory element has been identified in the profilaggrin gene.[57] Increased extracellular calcium also produces changes in distribution and activity of isozymes of protein kinase C.[58] It should be noted that Ca^{+2} levels in the dermis have been measured and are in excess of 1 m*M*;[49,50] it would seem that in tissue the "calcium switch" would always be in the "on" position.

Potassium has been shown to modulate Ca^{+2}-induced keratinocyte differentiation. Extracellular-calcium-induced terminal differentiation elevates Na and K; by inhibiting the increase in intracellular K with ouabain or very low extracellular K, the calcium-induced terminal differentiation is blocked.[19-21] Similarly, K^+ channel blockers inhibited Ca^{+2}-induced keratinocyte differentiation, suggesting these K^+ channels are required for differentiation; these K^+ channels were shown to be present *in vivo* in human and mouse skin.[56] In other studies, amiloride, which blocks here a non-specific cation channel, inhibited both the long-term rise of intracellular Ca^{+2} and aspects of terminal differentiation induced by raised extracellular calcium.[59] Additional Ca^{+2}-activated channels identified in keratinocytes include a large-conductance cation channel[60] and a Cl channel.[61]

Calcium appears to be involved in a number of disease states. For instance, 1,25-dihydroxyvitamin D3, an effective treatment for psoriasis,[62] is known to increase keratinocyte intracellular Ca^{+2} and to promote Ca^{+2}-induced differentiation at the level of both gene expression and mRNA stability.[63-65] Calcium is also known to be a factor in surfactant-induced irritant contact dermatitis, contact hypersensitivity, and atopic eczema.[66-69]

Calcium may be involved in the formation of lipid lamellar bilayers of the SC. In *in vitro* studies, unilamellar liposomes (formed from lipids matching the composition of the SC) slowly transformed into broad lamellar sheets after the addition of calcium.[70]

Calcium directly affects desquamation, the final act of terminal differentiation. In addition to being involved in desmosome formation,[71,72] calcium appears to protect corneodesmosomes from degradation.[72] In particular, calcium chelators accelerate SC disaggregation,[73,74] which can be blocked by the addition of exogenous calcium.[75] Calcium may afford this protection by inhibiting SC proteolytic enzymes involved in desquamation.[76]

8.5 THE CALCIUM GRADIENT IN SKIN

Calcium levels are considerably higher in the epidermis than in other nonbone organs of the body, including the brain, kidney, heart, and liver.[77] Where is this calcium? One of the more intriguing aspects of calcium in skin was the demonstration of a Ca^{+2} gradient in murine epidermis using "ion capture cytochemistry." With this calcium localization technique, the highest density of calcium was observed in the upper stratum granulosum,[78] as reproduced in Figure 6. Both extracellular and intracellular Ca^{+2} exhibited this gradient,[78] although the gradient was most apparent in the extracellular space.[79] This calcium gradient was also observed in humans, although the extracellular calcium gradient was not as pronounced.[80] The presence of this Ca^{+2} gradient suggests that calcium could play a role in regulating epidermal growth and differentiation *in vivo*, analogous to its role in cultured keratinocytes discussed previously. Implicit in this argument is the acceptance that the composition of the extracellular space in the granular layer is abnormally high for calcium, as also suggested for potassium.[3]

It must be mentioned that ion capture cytochemistry is a precipitation approach for element localization that has often been criticized in the literature[23,24,81-83] and has largely been avoided in nonskin fields. In studies of the intracellular distribution of calcium in smooth muscle cells, very different results were obtained between the rigorous cryological sample preparation and that of oxalate and pyroantimonate precipitation.[84] Nevertheless, a wealth of studies on the Ca^{+2} gradient using ion capture cytochemistry has built a convincing body of evidence not only in support of this gradient, but in support of its critical role in barrier repair and normal keratinocyte differentiation (described later).

Independent confirmation of a Ca^{+2} gradient in skin was provided by PIXE in studies of thick cryosections[30,39,40,85,86] (although not always observed[40,86]). However, localization by PIXE is limited by its resolution of 5 to 10 μm — the image of Figure 4 would be seen as a single pixel by PIXE! Understanding events at the cellular level is very limited with such resolution. It is likely that AEM with optimized instrumentation could provide both the detection sensitivity and the resolution needed to answer the very important questions concerning calcium handling in this tissue, but these studies have not been done. Our own exploration of alternative instrumentation suggests that dynamic secondary ionization mass spectroscopy (SIMS)[87] offers considerable advantages over that of PIXE. With dynamic SIMS, the sample surface is gradually eroded by the primary ion beam (sputtering); the ejected secondary ions represent the sample composition and are detected using mass spectrometry. Element sensitivity is high, and the ability to distinguish isotopes opens up the possibility for distinguishing between intrinsic element pools and externally applied elements in transit.[88,89] Data can be obtained as element maps, as shown in the Na, K, Ca, and Mg maps of human skin in Figure 7. The spatial resolution can be 0.5 μm with the instrument used (Cameca IMS-3f ion microscope). Although this is not as good as that of AEM, it is a substantial improvement over PIXE. In Figure 7 the tissue is oriented with the SC at the top of the image; the frozen-hydrated 1-μm-thick cryosection was pressed into indium metal prior to freeze drying[90] in order to keep the section electrically conductive and flat, but the right-hand side of the section has slightly curled out of the image plane, distorting the upper-right SC. The level of brightness within an individual SIMS image is directly proportional to the concentration of the element (isotope). In Figure 7, high Na levels are present in the SC. In contrast, K is present at high concentrations throughout the viable tissue, with much lower levels in the SC. Especially noticeable are high concentrations of K in the nuclei of the viable tissue (long arrows). The K/Na ratios were approximately 12 in the viable cells, representing physiologically relevant concentrations of these elements and reflecting the quality of cryopreservation throughout the sample preparation steps. There appears to be a relatively constant level of K and Mg in the keratinocyte cytoplasm from the mid-spinous layer at the bottom of the image up to the abrupt drop at the SC/granulosum border.

The calcium distribution of Figure 7 shows remarkable diversity. There appear to be several, almost stepwise increases in calcium in the cytoplasm of the viable tissue and then an abrupt drop at the SC interface (the central crack in the tissue is a good reference marker between images). There is then a reappearance of calcium in the upper SC (arrowheads), somewhat similar to the K distribution we observed by AEM (Figure 1). Very high levels of calcium are in the upper SC, a region where high calcium levels might be expected to be found due to personal cleansing products,[66]

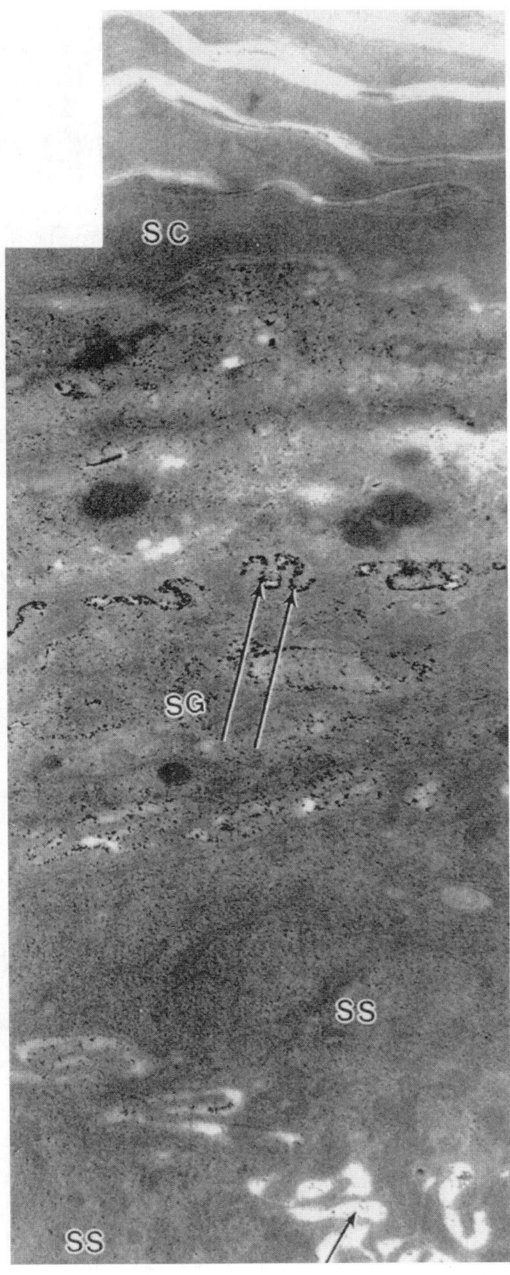

FIGURE 6 Demonstration of a calcium gradient across murine epidermis using ion capture cytochemistry. The intercellular domains at lower cell levels contain little calcium-containing precipitates, but the precipitates progressively increase toward the outer epidermis, reaching the highest density within the intercellular spaces of the upper stratum granulosum. The intracellular calcium content displays a similar enrichment with position. The SC was free of precipitates. (From Menon, G. K., Elias, P. M., Lee, S. H., Feingold, K. R., Localization of calcium in murine epidermis following disruption and repair of the permeability barrier, *Cell Tissue Res.*, 270, 503, 1992. Reprinted with permission from Springer-Verlag, New York.)

but a region where ion capture cytochemistry typically did not detect calcium.[78] However, there is a consensus by a variety of techniques that a calcium gradient is present across the viable tissue, with a maximum at the granular layer.

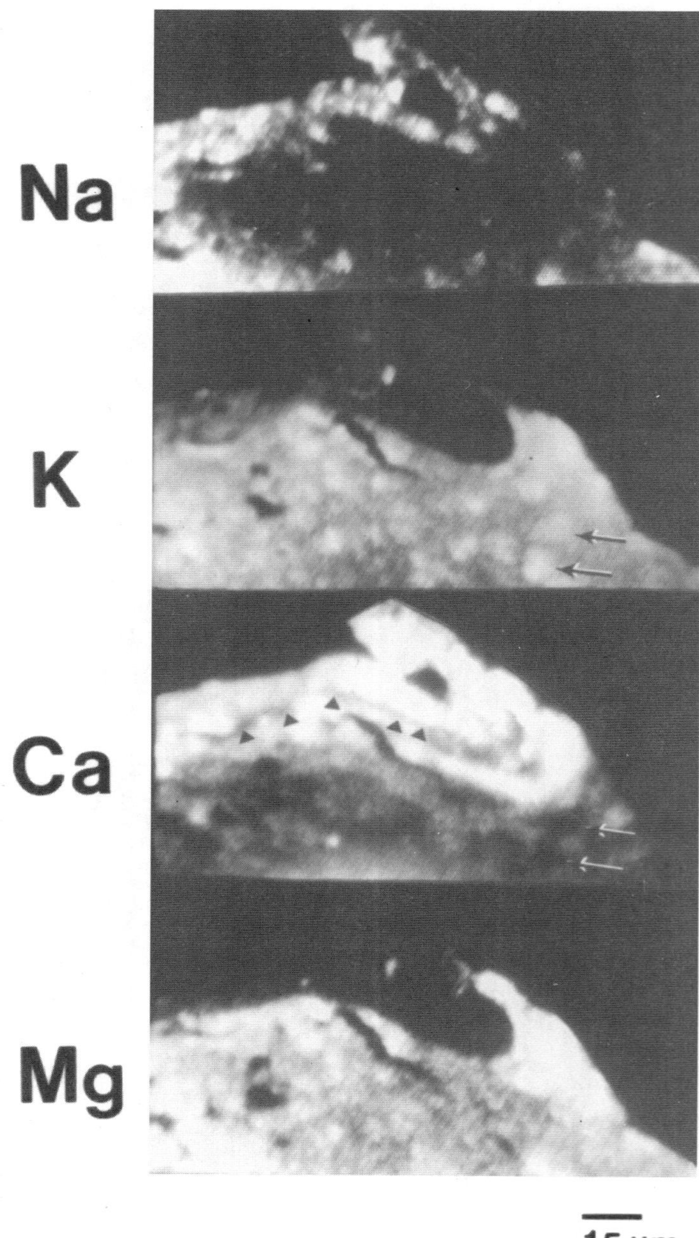

FIGURE 7 Dynamic SIMS images for Na, K, Ca, and Mg in a human skin cryosection. The SC is at the top of the image and spinosum is at the bottom. The long arrows highlight the high K, low Ca concentration within nuclei. The calcium image shows two apparent stepwise increases in concentration as the stratum corneum is approached, followed by a drop in concentration at the SC/granulosum border. Arrowheads highlight a subsequent abrupt increase in calcium within the SC. Across the viable tissue, concentrations for K and Mg appear relatively constant in the keratinocyte cytosol. (S. Chandra and R. Warner, unpublished data.)

8.6 THE CALCIUM GRADIENT AND LIPID BARRIER REPAIR

Calcium is involved in the repair of the lipid bilayers of the SC. Following SC barrier disruption by either topical acetone treatment, surfactant treatment, or tape stripping, recovery of normal transepidermal water loss (TEWL) in mice was inhibited by topical solutions containing calcium or potassium; calcium plus potassium produced a synergistic inhibition.[47,85] Both phosphate and magnesium produced a modest inhibition.[47] This inhibition by calcium and potassium could be overcome by the addition of calcium channel blockers, suggesting cellular uptake of calcium played a crucial role in regulating barrier homeostasis.[47] Potassium channels also appear to be involved in this barrier repair, and appropriate extracellular and intracellular potassium concentrations appear to be required for calcium to affect barrier homeostasis.[91]

The effect of external calcium on barrier repair suggested the Ca^{+2} gradient might have a role in this repair, and this was demonstrated in a variety of ion capture studies. Disruption of the lipid barrier with acetone application, surfactant, or tape stripping resulted in an immediate, marked decrease in Ca^{+2} in the stratum granulosum,[85,92] along with the massive secretion of lamellar bodies known to occur following barrier disruption.[46] Barrier disruption caused the calcium of the granular layer to move into the SC, where it accumulated within corneocytes and in the intercellular spaces of the lower SC.[85,92,93] Restoration of the Ca^{+2} gradient in the granular layer occurred in parallel with barrier recovery.[92] After barrier disruption followed by exposure to isoosmolar sucrose or a vapor-impermeable wrap, the Ca^{+2} gradient did not return, and both lamellar body secretion and barrier recovery occurred. In contrast, after exposure to an external calcium-containing solution following barrier disruption, the extracellular calcium gradient was restored (but not intracellular gradient), barrier repair was impeded, and the enhanced lamellar body secretion did not occur. It was suggested that loss of the elevated Ca^{+2} in the granular layer was the signal that initiates lamellar body secretion leading to barrier repair.[92] In support of this concept, high frequency sonophoresis was used to alter the calcium distribution without altering barrier function. Using sonophoresis with a Ca^{+2}-free solution, extracellular calcium was displaced downward toward the basal layer and dermis and resulted in accelerated lamellar body secretion as predicted. Sonophoresis with a Ca^{+2} solution resulted in excess intracellular Ca^{+2} at all levels of the epidermis and resulted in basal rates of lamellar body secretion as predicted, strongly supporting the hypothesis that changes in the Ca^{+2} gradient, not barrier disruption, controls lamellar body secretion.[79] Similarly, iontophoresis had no effect on SC barrier function as measured by TEWL, but both positive and negative iontophoresis caused a disappearance of the calcium gradient with marked decrease in Ca^{+2} content in the granular layer. Positive iontophoresis increased Ca^{+2} in the basal layer and dermis, and negative iontophoresis increased Ca^{+2} in the SC, but both caused an increase in lamellar body secretion as predicted from the decrease in granular layer Ca^{+2} content.[94]

In a recent study, PIXE demonstrated a calcium gradient across the epithelium that disappeared after barrier disruption and partially reformed as the barrier recovered, confirming results from ion capture cytochemistry. This study also observed a similar epithelial gradient for potassium, which also partially reformed with barrier recovery. In contrast, chloride and phosphorous gradients were unaffected by barrier disruption.[39] Calcium and potassium have been mentioned together throughout this chapter. Increasingly, evidence supports a central role for both of these elements in barrier repair and keratinocyte differentiation.

8.7 THE CALCIUM GRADIENT AND SKIN DISEASE

The role of Ca^{+2} in keratinocyte differentiation of cultured cells was discussed earlier. Does the Ca^{+2} gradient play a role in differentiation within the intact epithelium? In psoriasis, a disease characterized by defects in both proliferation and differentiation, the Ca^{+2} gradient is altered. Although uninvolved psoriatic lesions had a calcium gradient similar to that of normal human tissue, involved psoriatic lesions were characterized by less Ca^{+2} in both intracellular and extracellular regions of the basal layer, very high levels in all suprabasal viable cells (indicating loss of the normal Ca^{+2} gradient), and increased levels of Ca^{+2} in the intercellular regions of the lower SC.[80] It was felt that these calcium abnormalities might underlie the abnormal desquamation and permeability barrier in psoriasis.[80] In two other chronic models of barrier dysfunction, the essential-fatty-acid-deficient mouse (EFADM) and the chronic topical-lovastatin-treated mouse, the Ca^{+2} distributions were similar to that of psoriasis, with enhanced extracellular Ca^{+2} throughout the epidermis, including the basal layer, and variable but relatively high levels of intracellular Ca^{+2} in suprabasal keratinocytes. In addition, large clusters of Ca^{+2} occurred frequently in the intercellular regions of the SC.[93] Artificial barrier restoration with a water-vapor-impermeable wrap in the EFADM caused the Ca^{+2} distribution to revert toward normal.[93] In an acne model using topical applications of oleic acid to induce comedones, the calcium gradient was lost within the follicular epidermis, with increased calcium levels throughout the tissue with the exception of decreased levels in the stratum granulosum.[95] In a model for incomplete differentiation, that of the *in vitro* reconstructed human epidermis generated in serum-containing medium, the tissue was characterized by a Ca^{+2} gradient similar to that of viable tissue in normal human skin, but with large quantities of intracellular and some extracellular Ca^{+2} throughout the entire SC.[96] Use of a serum-free medium containing vitamin and lipid supplements led to a marked improvement in SC ultrastructure and in parallel a normalization of the Ca^{+2} distribution with the highest levels in the stratum granulosum and low levels in the inner SC. Addition of retinoic acid resulted in an altered keratinocyte differentiation and reappearance of large quantities of Ca^{+2} in the SC.[96]

It has been suggested that the modulation of keratinocyte intracellular Ca^{+2} may be an important pathway for further development of cutaneous pharmaceuticals.[53]

8.8 PROPOSED MODEL: ELEMENT RECYCLING FORMS THE CALCIUM GRADIENT AND PARTICIPATES IN TERMINAL DIFFERENTIATION — THERAPEUTIC IMPLICATIONS

Given the strong evidence that a Ca^{+2} gradient exists across the viable epithelium and plays a major role in differentiation, lipid barrier repair, and possibly lipid barrier formation, questions arise on how this gradient is formed and maintained, how it goes awry in disease, and how it might be manipulated to treat skin pathology or improve general skin health. For instance, the incidence of skin xerosis increases with winter and with age and may be related to a decrease in SC lipids in winter and age.[97] A therapy that would reduce Ca^{+2} in the granular layer, thus enhancing lipid synthesis, could have potential benefits in treating the decreased lipid synthesis which occurs in the elderly[98] and in restoring the depleted SC lipids which occur in winter.[97]

Previous investigations concluded that the Ca^{+2} gradient was formed from the movement of Ca^{+2}-containing fluid across the basement membrane and viable tissue; at the SC, water flux would continue, but the co-migrating Ca^{+2} would remain trapped beneath the SC. Disruption of the barrier or occlusion with impermeable membranes changed the water flux and hence calcium delivery.[93] Although this hypothesis accounted for much of the data on the Ca^{+2} gradient, the fate of the other elements in the migrating fluid, some at concentrations two orders of magnitude higher than Ca^{+2}, was not accounted for.

Figure 8 presents an alternative model for the creation of the Ca^{+2} gradient, based on the concepts of Figure 5 and a synthesis of existing literature. Although speculative, there are testable elements of this model. At the bottom of Figure 8 is a keratinocyte from the first granular layer (G1). In the extracellular space there is a Ca^{+2} gradient, indicated by the large right-hand arrow, and perhaps a gradient for K and P. The enhanced extracellular Ca^{+2} results in an enhanced Ca^{+2} influx and an increase in cytoplasmic Ca^{+2}. The increase in intracellular Ca^{+2} leads to the expression of profilaggrin,[53,54] likely due to a Ca^{+2}-sensitive regulatory element in the gene.[57] High levels of intracellular Ca^{+2} are toxic to cells, so a continued increase in Ca^{+2} influx presents problems as the keratinocyte advances into the upper granular layer (G2, Figure 8) with yet higher extracellular Ca^{+2}. However, because profilaggrin is a calcium-binding protein,[99] its continued production serves as a sink for an increased calcium influx. In addition to the calcium-binding domains of profilaggrin, additional calcium may be bound to this protein within the developing keratohyalin granules due

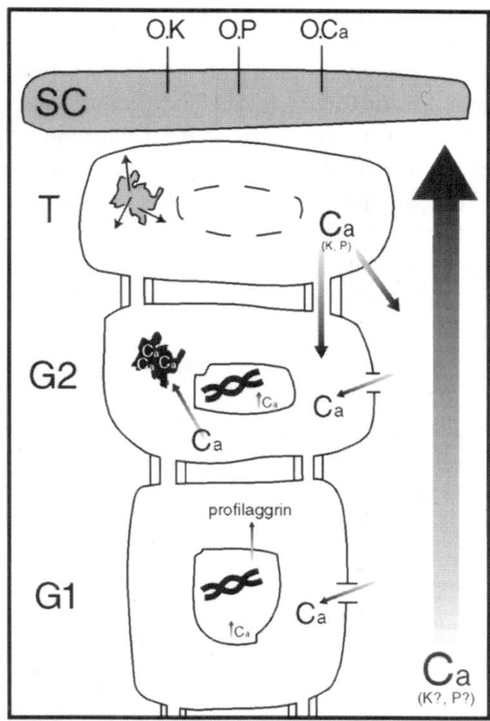

FIGURE 8 Proposed model for generation of calcium gradient across the viable tissue. In the lower granular cell (G1), Ca^{+2} influx increases due to the high extracellular Ca^{+2}, increasing cytosol and nuclear levels and increasing production of profilaggrin. Since profilaggrin is a calcium-binding protein, enhanced Ca^{+2} influx is buffered by profilaggrin within keratohyalin granules in the upper cell (G2). In the transitional cell (T), profilaggrin breakdown into filaggrin releases large amounts of Ca^{+2} (and P), which leaves the cell either into the extracellular space, creating the Ca^{+2} gradient, or into the lower viable tissue via communicating gap junctions.

to the many phosphoserine residues known to be present in each filaggrin repeat.[100] Finally, in the transitional stage (T, Figure 8), the breakdown of profilaggrin would release this large amount of stored calcium (along with considerable phosphate). As shown by ion capture cytochemistry (Figure 6) and SIMS (Figure 7), calcium is normally not found in the inner SC. Consequently, the entire intracellular calcium content (and K and P [Figures 2, 4, and 5], and Mg [Figure 7]) of the transitional cell either must leave the cell into the extracellular space or leave the cell through gap junctions[101,102] into the underlying granular cell. It is unlikely that the underlying granular cell could tolerate a huge influx of Ca^{+2}, and high Ca^{+2} is known to uncouple gap junctions,[103] so it is likely that the high calcium content of the transitional cell would enter the extracellular space, creating the calcium gradient.

One of the common observations of ion capture cytochemistry was the appearance of Ca^{+2} in the SC following barrier disruption or altered differentiation,[85,92,93] which was attributed to alterations in water flux across the tissue.[79,93] This author believes a more likely explanation is an altered differentiation in which the calcium content of the transitional cell is not entirely lost to the extracellular space, and the newly formed corneocyte carries calcium (and likely other intracellular elements) with it into the SC.

Evidence for an involvement of K^+ in epidermal differentiation, skin pathology, and response to barrier abrogation and repair was presented earlier. In particular, the involvement of Ca^{+2} in switching on differentiation in cultured keratinocytes could be blocked by K^+ modulation,[19-21,56] the involvement of calcium in inhibiting barrier repair was strongly impacted by potassium,[47,85,91] and the calcium gradient appears to be linked with a potassium gradient.[39] In the model of Figure 8, K^+, P, and Mg must also be recycled, since they too are absent from the inner SC (Figures 4 and 7). This presents interesting consequences, particularly for K^+. The potassium ion is usually the primary determinant of the cell membrane potential. Elevated extracellular K^+ would likely depolarize the keratinocyte cell membrane, which would decrease the electromotive force for calcium influx, perhaps offsetting the effect of elevated extracellular Ca. Phosphorus recycling also has potential consequences. If P moves through gap junctions, it could be reutilized in the formation of profilaggrin. Many scenarios are possible; it is likely that the last hours of the transitional cell are highly choreographed, as suggested by the two proteolytic stages of profilaggrin.[104] Measuring changes in element pools during this process would likely be informative.

8.9 CONCLUSIONS

There is essentially no knowledge of electrolyte concentrations in mammalian skin based on conventional wet chemistry techniques, and there is considerable confusion concerning electrolyte concentrations measured by particle probe technologies. Electrolytes and their channels have been largely ignored in dermatology, but they are likely critical players in skin function. Available evidence suggests extraordinarily unique concentrations exist within keratinocytes or extracellular space in the skin epithelium. This uniqueness, if true, likely has a unique function in both skin health and pathology. For instance, if element recycling occurs through the granular layer, hyperproliferative responses may deplete the pool of these elements by loss into the SC, resulting essentially in nutrient deprivation limiting proper keratinocyte maturation. Knowledge of the granular cell extracellular milieu, of the ion channels present in the granular cell, and of the control of these channels will likely be critical to understanding the terminal differentiation of keratinocytes and to the design of potential new therapies for treating disorders of proliferation, differentiation, barrier repair, and skin moisturization.

REFERENCES

1. Ussing, H. H., Zerahn, K., Active transport of sodium as the source of electric current in the short-circuited isolated frog skin, *Acta Physiol. Scand.*, 23, 110, 1951.
2. Warner, R. R., Myers, M. C., Taylor, D. A., Electron probe analysis of human skin: determination of the water concentration profile, *J. Invest. Dermatol.*, 90, 218, 1988.
3. von Zglinicki, T., Lindberg, M., Roomans, G. M., Forslind, B., Water and ion distribution profiles in human skin, *Acta Derm. Venereol.* (*Stockh.*), 73, 340, 1993.
4. Warner, R. R., Lilly, N. A., Correlation of water content with ultrastructure in the stratum corneum, in *Bioengineering of the Skin: Water and the Stratum Corneum*, Elsner, P., Berardesca, E., Maibach, H. I., Eds., CRC Press, Boca Raton, FL, 1994, 3.
5. Grubauer, G., Elias, P. M., Feingold, K. R., Transepidermal water loss: the signal for recovery of barrier structure and function, *J. Lipid Res.*, 30, 323, 1989.
6. Denda, M., Sato, J., Masuda, Y., Tsuchiya, T., Koyama, J., Kuramoto, M., Elias, P. M., Feingold, K. R., Exposure to a dry environment enhances epidermal permeability barrier function, *J. Invest. Dermatol.*, 111, 858, 1998.
7. Rothman, S., *Physiology and Biochemistry of the Skin*, University of Chicago Press, 1954, 36.
8. Tregear, R. T., The permeability of mammalian skin to ions, *J. Invest. Dermatol.*, 46, 16, 1966.
9. Wahlberg, J. E., Some attempts to influence the percutaneous absorption rate of sodium and mercuric chlorides in the guinea pig, *Acta Derm. Venereol.*, 45, 335, 1965.
10. Scheuplein, R. J., Blank, I. H., Permeability of the skin, *Physiol. Rev.*, 51, 702, 1971.
11. Grice, K., Sattar, H., Baker, H., The cutaneous barrier to salts and water in psoriasis and in normal skin, *Br. J. Dermatol.*, 88, 459, 1973.

12. Grice, K., Sattar, H., Casey, T., Baker, H., An evaluation of Na^+, Cl^-, and pH ion-specific electrodes in the study of the electrolyte contents of epidermal transudate and sweat, *Br. J. Dermatol.*, 92, 511, 1975.
13. Green, M., Berendt, H., Libien, G., Successive determination of Na^+, Cl^-, and H^+ activities on the skin surface with ion-selective electrodes, *Clin. Chem.*, 18, 427, 1972.
14. Rothman, S., *Physiology and Biochemistry of the Skin*, University of Chicago Press, Chicago, IL, 1954, 500.
15. France, V. M., Active sodium uptake by the skin of foetal sheep and pigs, *J. Physiol. (London)*, 258, 377, 1976.
16. Hennings, H., Michael, D., Cheng, C., Steinert, P., Holbrook, K., Yspa, S. H., Calcium regulation of growth and differentiation of mouse epidermal cells in culture, *Cell*, 19, 245, 1980.
17. Hennings, H., Steinert, P., Buxman, M. M., Calcium induction of transglutaminase and the formation of (γ-glutamyl)lysine cross-links in cultured mouse epidermal cells, *Biochem. Biophys. Res. Commun.*, 102, 739, 1981.
18. Dykes, P. J., Marks, R., The effect of serum calcium levels on the rate of epidermal renewal in the rat, *Br. J. Dermatol.*, 111, 191, 1984.
19. Hennings, H., Holbrook, K., Extracellular calcium regulates growth and terminal differentiation of cultured mouse epidermal cells, in *Ions, Cell Proliferation, and Cancer*, McKeehan, W. L., Boynton, A., Whitfield, J. F., Eds., Academic Press, New York, 1982, 499.
20. Hennings, H., Holbrook, K., Yuspa, S. H., Potassium mediation of calcium-induced terminal differentiation of epidermal cells in culture, *J. Invest. Dermatol.*, 81, 50s, 1983.
21. Hennings, H., Holbrook, K., Yuspa, S. H., Factors influencing calcium-induced terminal differentiation in cultured mouse epidermal cells, *J. Cell. Physiol.*, 116, 265, 1983.
22. Holbrook, K. A., Holbrook, J. R., Odland, G. F., A comparison of the effects of sample preparation on the X-ray microanalysis and ultrastructure of the thin sectioned specimens of human skin, *Scanning Electron Microscopy/1976/*IITRI, SEM Inc., Chicago, 1976, 265.
23. Lechene, C. P., Warner, R. R., Ultramicroanalysis: X-ray spectrometry by electron probe excitation, *Annu. Rev. Biophys. Bioeng.*, 6, 57, 1977.
24. Chandler, J. A., The application of X-ray microanalysis in TEM to the study of ultrathin biological specimens — a review, in *Electron Probe Microanalysis in Biology*, Erasmus, D. A., Ed., Chapman and Hall, London, 1978, 37.
25. Forslind, B., Wei, X., Roomans, G. M., Elemental distribution in cross sections of guinea-pig epidermis: X-ray microanalysis in the electron microscope, in *Stratum Corneum,* Marks, R., Plewig, G., Eds., Springer-Verlag, Heidelberg, 1983, 217.
26. Lindberg, M., Roomans, G. M., Elemental distribution and ultrastructural changes in guinea pig epidermis after dinitrochlorobenzene (DNCB) exposure, *J. Invest. Dermatol.*, 81, 303, 1983.
27. Lindberg, M., Forslind, B., Roomans, G. M., Elemental changes at irritant reactions due to chromate and nickel in guinea-pig epidermis, *Scanning Electron Microscopy/1983/III*, SEM Inc., Chicago, 1983, 1243.
28. Forslind, B., Roomans, G. M., Carlsson, L.-E., Malmqvist, K. G., Akselsson, K. R., Elemental analysis on freeze-dried sections of human skin: studies by electron microprobe and particle induced X-ray emission analysis, *Scanning Electron Microscopy/1984/II*, SEM Inc., Chicago, 1984, 755.
29. Grundin, T. G., Roomans, G. M., Forslind, B., Lindberg, M., Werner, Y., X-ray microanalysis of psoriatic skin, *J. Invest. Dermatol.*, 85, 378, 1985.
30. Forslind, B., Grundin, T. G., Lindberg, M., Roomans, G. M., Werner, Y., Recent advances in X-ray microanalysis in dermatology, *Scanning Electron Microscopy/1985/II*, SEM Inc., Chicago, 1985, 687.
31. Forslind, B., Particle probe analysis in the study of skin physiology, *Scanning Electron Microscopy/1986/III*, SEM Inc., Chicago, 1986, 1007.
32. Lindberg, M., Grundin, T. G., Elemental changes in guinea-pig epidermis in the hyperplastic response to irritant stimuli, *Br. J. Dermatol.*, 116, 477, 1987.
33. Lindberg, M., Sagström, S., Changes in sodium-potassium ratio in guinea-pig epidermis in n-hexadecane-induced hyperplasia, *Acta Derm. Venerol. (Stockh.)*, 69, 369, 1989.
34. Lindberg M., Forslind, B., Sagström, S., Roomans, G. M., Elemental changes in guinea pig epidermis at repeated exposure to sodium lauryl sulfate, *Acta Derm. Venerol. (Stockh.)*, 72, 428, 1992.

35. Emilson, A., Lindberg, M., Forslind, B., The temperature effect on *in vitro* penetration of sodium lauryl sulfate and nickel chloride through human skin, *Acta Derm. Venereol. (Stockh.)*, 73, 203, 1993.
36. Forslind, B., Lindberg, M., Malmqvist, K. G., Pallon, J., Roomans, G. M., Werner-Linde, Y., Human skin physiology studied by particle probe microanalysis, *Scanning Microsc.*, 9, 1011, 1995.
37. Grängsjö, A., Leijon-Kuligowski, A., Törmä, H., Roomans, G. M., Lindberg, M., Different pathways in irritant contact exzema?, *Contact Dermatitis*, 35, 355, 1996.
38. Kurz, K., Steigleder, G. K., Bischof, W., Gonsior, B., PIXE analysis in different stages of psoriatic skin, *J. Invest. Dermatol.*, 88, 223, 1987.
39. Mauro, T., Bench, G., Sidderas-Haddad, E., Feingold, K., Elias, P., Cullander, C., Acute barrier perturbation abolishes the Ca^{2+} and K^+ gradients in murine epidermis: quantitative measurement using PIXE, *J. Invest. Dermatol.*, 111, 1198, 1998.
40. Bunse, T., Steigleder, G. K., Höfert, M., Gonsior, B., PIXE analysis in uninvolved skin of atopic patients and in aged skin, *Acta Derm. Venereol. (Stockh.)*, 71, 287, 1991.
41. Warner, R. R., Myers, M. C., Taylor, D. A., Electron probe analysis of human skin: element concentration profiles, *J. Invest. Dermatol.*, 90, 78, 1988.
42. Warner, R. R., Bush, R. D., Ruebusch, N. A., Corneocytes undergo systematic changes in element concentrations across the human inner stratum corneum, *J. Invest. Dermatol.*, 104, 530, 1995.
43. Elias, P. M., Friend, D. S., The permeability barrier in mammalian epidermis, *J. Cell Biol.*, 65, 180, 1975.
44. Elias, P. M., Cooper, E. R., Korc, A., Brown, B. E., Percutaneous transport in relation to stratum corneum structure and lipid composition, *J. Invest. Dermatol.*, 76, 297, 1981.
45. Goldman, D. E., Potential, impedance, and rectification in membranes, *J. Gen. Physiol.*, 27, 37, 1943.
46. Menon, G. K., Feingold, K. R., Elias, P. M., Lamellar body secretory response to barrier disruption, *J. Invest. Dermatol.*, 98, 279, 1992.
47. Lee, S. H., Elias, P. M., Proksch, E., Menon, G. K., Mao-Quiang, M., Feingold, K. R., Calcium and potassium are important regulators of barrier homeostasis in murine epidermis, *J. Clin. Invest.*, 89, 530, 1992.
48. Zheutlin, H. E. C., Fox, C. L., Sodium and potassium content of human epidermis, *Arch. Dermatol. Syphilol.*, 61, 397, 1950.
49. Gilányi, M., Ikrényi, C., Fetete, J., Ikrényi, K., Kovách, A. G. B., Ion concentrations in subcutaneous interstitial fluid: measured vs. expected values, *Am. J. Physiol.*, 255, F513, 1988.
50. Linhares, M. C., Kissinger, P. T., Determination of endogenous ions in intercellular fluid using capillary ultrafiltration and microdialysis probes, *J. Pharm. Biomed. Anal.*, 11, 1121, 1993.
51. Kruszewski, F. H., Hennings, H., Tucker, R. W., Yuspa, S. H., Differences in the regulation of intracellular calcium in normal and neoplastic keratinocytes are not caused by *ras* gene mutations, *Cancer Res.*, 51, 4206, 1991.
52. Pillai, S., Bilke, D. D., Role of intracellular-free calcium in the cornified envelope formation of keratinocytes: differences in the mode of action of extracellular calcium and 1,25 dihydroxyvitamin D_3, *J. Cell. Physiol.*, 146, 94, 1991.
53. Li, L., Tucker, R. W., Hennings, H., Yuspa, S. H., Inhibitors of the intracellular Ca^{2+}-ATPase in cultured mouse keratinocytes reveal components of terminal differentiation that are regulated by distinct intracellular Ca^{2+} compartments, *Cell Growth Differ.*, 6, 1171, 1995.
54. Li, L., Tucker, R. W., Hennings, H., Yuspa, S. H., Chelation of intracellular Ca^{2+} inhibits murine keratinocyte differentiation *in vitro*, *J. Cell. Physiol.*, 163, 105, 1995.
55. Xiong, Y., Harmon, C. S., Evidence that diazoxide promotes calcium influx in mouse keratinocyte cultures by membrane hyperpolarization, *Skin Pharmacol.*, 8, 309, 1995.
56. Mauro, T., Dixon, D. B., Komuves, L., Hanley, K., Pappone, P. A., Keratinocyte K^+ channels mediate Ca^{2+}-induced differentiation, *J. Invest. Dermatol.*, 108, 864, 1997.
57. Jang, S., Markova, N. G., Steinert, P. M., Positive and negative elements involved in the transcription of the human profilaggrin gene, *J. Invest. Dermatol.*, 100, 501, 1993.
58. Denning, M. F., Dlugosz, A. A., Williams, E. K., Szallasi, Z., Blumberg, P. M., Yuspa, S. H., Specific protein kinase C isozymes mediate the induction of keratinocyte differentiation markers by calcium, *Cell Growth Differ.*, 6, 149, 1995.
59. Mauro, T., Dixon, D. B., Hanley, K., Isseroff, R. R., Pappone, P. A., Amiloride blocks a keratinocyte nonspecific cation channel and inhibits Ca^{2+}-induced keratinocyte differentiation, *J. Invest. Dermatol.*, 105, 203, 1995.

60. Galietta, L. J. V., Barone, V., De Luca, M., Romeo, G., Characterization of chloride and cation channels in cultured human keratinocytes, *Pfluegers Arch.,* 418, 18, 1991.
61. Mauro, T. M., Pappone, P. A., Isseroff, R. R., Extracellular calcium affects the membrane currents of cultured human keratinocytes, *J. Cell. Physiol.*, 143, 13, 1990.
62. Berth-Jones, J., Hutchinson, P. E., Vitamin D analogues and psoriasis, *Br. J. Dermatol.*, 127, 71, 1992.
63. MacLaughlin, J. A., Cantley, L. C., Hollick, M. F., 1,25$(OH)_2D_3$ increases calcium and phosphatidylinositol metabolism in differentiating cultured human keratinocytes, *J. Nutr. Biochem.*, 1, 81, 1990.
64. Bittiner, B., Bleehen, S. S., MacNeil, S., 1α,25$(OH)_2$ vitamin D_3 increases intracellular calcium in human keratinocytes, *Br. J. Dermatol.*, 124, 230, 1991.
65. Su, M.-J., Bikle, D. D., Mancianti, M.-L., Pillai, S., 1,25-dihydroxyvitamin D_3 potentiates the keratinocyte response to calcium, *J. Biol. Chem.*, 269, 14723, 1994.
66. Warren, R., Ertel, K. D., Bartolo, R. G., Levine, M. J., Bryant, P. B., Wong, L. F., The influence of hard water (calcium) and surfactants on irritant contact dermatitis, *Contact Dermatitis*, 35, 337, 1996.
67. Diezel, W., Gruner, S., Diaz, L. A., Anhalt, G. J., Inhibition of cutaneous hypersensitivity by calcium transport inhibitors lanthanum and diltiazem, *J. Invest. Dermatol.*, 93, 322, 1989.
68. Stern, R., Khalsa, J. H., Cutaneous adverse reactions associated with calcium channel blockers, *Arch. Intern. Med.,* 149, 829, 1989.
69. Devlin, J., David, T. J., Intolerance to oral and intravenous calcium supplements in atopic eczema, *J. R. Soc. Med.*, 893, 497, 1990.
70. Abraham, W., Wertz, P. W., Landmann, L., Downing, D. T., Stratum corneum lipid liposomes: calcium-induced transformation into lamellar sheets, *J. Invest Dermatol.,* 88, 212, 1987.
71. Watt, F. M., Mattey, D. L., Garrod, D. R., Calcium induced reorganization of desmosomal components in cultured human keratinocytes, *J. Cell Biol.*, 99, 2211, 1984.
72. Takeichi, M., Cadherins: a molecular family important in selective cell–cell adhesion, *Annu. Rev. Biochem.*, 59, 237, 1990.
73. Bissett, D. L., McBride, J. F., Patrick, L. F., Role of protein and calcium in stratum corneum cell cohesion, *Arch. Dermatol. Res.,* 279, 184, 1987.
74. Lundström, A., Egelrud, T., Cell shedding from human plantar skin *in vitro*: evidence of its dependence on endogenous proteolysis, *J. Invest. Dermatol.*, 91, 340, 1988.
75. Brysk, M. M., Santshi, C., Bell, T., Rajaraman, S., Predesquamin inhibits desquamation, *Exp. Cell Res.*, 209, 301, 1993.
76. Lundström, A., Egelrud, T., Cell shedding from human plantar skin *in vitro*: evidence that two different types of protein structures are degraded by a chymotrypsin-like enzyme, *Arch. Dermatol. Res.,* 282, 234, 1990.
77. Hoath, S. B., Pickens, W. L., Tanaka, R., Ross, R., Ontogeny of integumental calcium in relation to surface area and water content in the perinatal rat, *J. Appl. Physiol.*, 73, 458, 1992.
78. Menon, G. K., Grayson, S., Elias, P. M., Ionic calcium reservoirs in mammalian epidermis: ultrastructural localization by ion-capture cytochemistry, *J. Invest. Dermatol.*, 84, 508, 1985.
79. Menon, G. K., Price, L. F., Bommannan, B., Elias, P. M., Feingold, K. R., Selective obliteration of the epidermal calcium gradient leads to enhanced lamellar body secretion, *J. Invest. Dermatol.*, 102, 789, 1994.
80. Menon, G. K., Elias, P. M., Ultrastructural localization of calcium in psoriatic and normal human epidermis, *Arch. Dermatol.*, 127, 57, 1991.
81. Simson, J. A. V., Spicer, S. S., Selective subcellular localization of cations with variants of the potassium (pyro)antimonate technique, *J. Histochem. Cytochem.*, 23, 575, 1975.
82. Chandler, J. A., *X-ray Microanalysis in the Electron Microscope*, Glauert, A. M., Ed., North-Holland Publishing, Amsterdam, 1977, 400.
83. Morgan, A. J., Davies, T. W., Erasmus, D. A., Specimen preparation, in *Electron Probe Microanalysis in Biology*, Erasmus, D. A., Ed., Chapman and Hall, London, 1978, 94.
84. Popescu, L. M., De Bruijn, W. C., Zelck, U., Ionescu, N., Intracellular distribution of calcium in smooth muscle: facts and artifacts, *Rev. Roum. Morphol. Embryol. Physiol. Morphol. Embryol.*, 3, 251, 1980.
85. Mao-Qiang, M., Mauro, T., Bench, G., Warren, R., Elias, P. M., Feingold, K. R., Calcium and potassium inhibit barrier recovery after disruption, independent of the type of insult in hairless mice, *Exp. Dermatol.,* 6, 36, 1997.

86. Pallon, J., Malmqvist, K. G., Werner-Linde, Y., Forslind, B., PIXE analysis of pathological skin with special reference to psoriasis and atopic dry skin, *Cell. Mol. Biol.*, 42, 111, 1996.
87. Chandra, S., Morrison, G. H., Ion microscopy in biology and medicine, *Methods Enzymol.,* 158, 157, 1988.
88. Chandra, S., Fullmer, C. S., Smith, C. A., Wasserman, R. H., Morrison, G. H., Ion microscopic imaging of calcium transport in the intestinal tissue of vitamin D-deficient and vitamin D-replete chickens: a ^{44}Ca stable isotope study, *Proc. Natl. Acad. Sci. U.S.A.,* 87, 5715, 1990.
89. Chandra, S., Fewtrell, C., Millard, P. J., Sandison, D. R., Webb, W. W., Morrison, G. H., Imaging of total intracellular calcium and calcium influx and efflux in individual resting and stimulated tumor mast cells using ion microscopy, *J. Biol. Chem.,* 269, 15186, 1994.
90. Sod, E. W., Crooker, A. R., Morrison, G. H., Biological cryosection preparation and practical ion yield evaluation for ion microscopic analysis, *J. Microsc.,* 160, 55, 1990.
91. Lee, S. H., Elias, P. M., Feingold, K. R., Mauro, T., A role for ions in barrier recovery after acute perturbation, *J. Invest Dermatol.,* 102, 976, 1994.
92. Menon, G. K., Elias, P. M., Lee, S. H., Feingold, K. R., Localization of calcium in murine epidermis following disruption and repair of the permeability barrier, *Cell Tissue Res.*, 270, 503, 1992.
93. Menon, G. K., Elias, P. M., Feingold, K. R., Integrity of the permeability barrier is crucial for maintenance of the epidermal calcium gradient, *Br. J. Dermatol.*, 130, 139, 1994.
94. Lee, S. H., Choi, E. H., Feingold, K. R., Jiang, S., Ahn, S. K., Iontophoresis itself on hairless mouse skin induces the loss of the epidermal calcium gradient without skin barrier impairment, *J. Invest. Dermatol.*, 111, 39, 1998.
95. Choi, E. H., Ahn, S. K., Lee, S. H., The changes of stratum corneum interstices and calcium distribution of follicular epithelium of experimentally induced comedones (EIC) by oleic acid, *Exp. Dermatol.*, 6, 29, 1997.
96. Vicanová, J., Boelsma, E., Mommaas, A. M., Kempenaar, J. A., Forslind, B., Pallon, J., Egelrud, T., Koerten, H. K., Ponec, M., Normalization of epidermal calcium distribution profile in reconstructed human epidermis is related to improvement of terminal differentiation and stratum corneum barrier formation, *J. Invest. Dermatol.*, 111, 97, 1998.
97. Ghadially, R., Brown, B. E., Sequeira-Martin, S. M., Feingold, K. R., Elias, P. M., The aged epidermal permeability barrier. Structural, functional, and lipid biochemical abnormalities in humans and a senescent murine model, *J. Clin. Invest.*, 95, 2281, 1995.
98. Rogers, J., Harding, C., Mayo, A., Banks, J., Rawlings, A., Stratum corneum lipids: the effect of ageing and the seasons, *Arch. Dermatol. Res.*, 288, 765, 1996.
99. Markova, N. G., Marekov, L. N., Chipev, C. C., Gan, S.-Q., Idler, W. W., Steinert, P. M., Profilaggrin is a major epidermal calcium-binding protein, *Mol. Cell. Biol.*, 13, 613, 1993.
100. Presland, R. B., Bassuk, J. A., Kimball, J. R., Dale, B. A., Characterization of two distinct calcium-binding sites in the amino-terminus of human profilaggrin, *J. Invest. Dermatol.*, 104, 218, 1995.
101. Kạm, E., Melville, L., Pitts, J. D., Patterns of junctional communication in skin, *J. Invest. Dermatol.*, 87, 748, 1986.
102. Salomon, D., Saurat, J.-H., Meda, P., Cell-to-cell communication within intact human skin, *J. Clin. Invest.*, 82, 248, 1988.
103. Loewenstein, W. R., The cell-to-cell channel of gap junctions, *Cell*, 48, 725, 1987.
104. Resing, K. A., Al-Alawi, N., Blomquist, C., Fleckman, P., Dale, B. A., Independent regulation of two cytoplasmic processing stages of the intermediate filament-associated protein filaggrin and role of in the second stage, *J. Biol. Chem.*, 268, 25139, 1993.

9 Desquamation

Torbjörn Egelrud

CONTENTS

9.1 INTRODUCTION

The stratum corneum is a cellular tissue. Its building blocks, the corneocytes, are highly resistant to physical and chemical trauma. The mechanical strength of an individual corneocyte, emanating from its tightly packed keratin bundles and the cross-linked proteins of the cornified envelope, is outstanding. The mechanical resistance of individual corneocytes is mirrored by the pronounced mechanical strength of the entire stratum corneum, implying a strong cell cohesion within the tissue. The corneocytes and their intercellular cohesive structures are prerequisites for the function of the stratum corneum as the physical-chemical barrier between body interior and exterior, serving as an important part of the barrier as well as a backbone for the intercellular barrier lipids.

The stratum corneum is continuously being formed in the process of terminal keratinocyte differentiation. The rate of stratum corneum renewal is determined by the rate of cell proliferation in the basal layer of the epidermis. The fact that the thickness of the stratum corneum is fairly constant at a given body site implies that a fraction of the most superficial parts of the stratum corneum must be continuously shed at a rate which balances *de novo* production of corneocytes. This process, desquamation, normally occurs invisibly with shedding of individual cells or small aggregates of cells, resulting in the smooth appearance of the skin surface associated with a "normal" skin condition. Disturbances in this process, due to either increased production of corneocytes or a decreased rate of cell shedding, results in the accumulation on the skin surface of only partially detached cells with or without a concomitant thickening of the stratum corneum. The severity of the disturbance may vary from modest to very pronounced, from a barely visible scaling combined with a feeling of roughness and dryness of the skin surface to the accumulation of thick brittle scales such as in psoriasis or in the various forms of ichthyosis.

Thus, it can be concluded that there must be mechanisms within the stratum corneum which are responsible for a well regulated desquamation. A closer look at criteria which must be fulfilled by these mechanisms suggests that they are likely to be of significant complexity. As stated previously, the barrier function of the stratum corneum depends on a strong cohesion between individual corneocytes. The elimination of cell cohesion, a prerequisite for desquamation, would be deleterious if it took place in the barrier-forming parts of the stratum corneum. Under normal

0-8493-7520-7/00/$0.00+$.50

conditions the turnover time of the stratum corneum is two to four weeks. Moreover, corneocytes are "dead" in the sense that they have no protein synthesis, they have no active turnover of cell surface structures, and they are unresponsive to cellular signaling. Thus, chemical reactions leading to structural and functional changes within the stratum corneum may be considered as the final steps of a series of events inititated in viable parts of the epidermis. The process, which occur spontaneously without further input of regulatory signals, but yet in a well-regulated manner, depends on enzymes and other components produced by still living keratinocytes. In other words, at the time when a viable keratinocyte of the stratum granulosum is transformed to a corneocyte of the stratum corneum, the cell and the tissue it becomes part of must be "programmed" in a way that allows the cell to be strongly linked to contiguous cells for a certain period of time, after which its cohesion to its neighbors should decrease to an extent which will eventually allow it to be shed from the skin surface.

It seems reasonable to believe that a better understanding of desquamation and the mechanisms involved would give us possibilities to design better treatments for skin disorders associated with disturbances in stratum corneum turnover, be they common "dry skin problems" or results of more or less handicapping skin diseases. One strategy to understand desquamation would be to first identify mechanisms of cell cohesion in the stratum corneum, the structures involved, and the changes these structures undergo as cell cohesion decreases. The next step would be the identification of chemical reactions taking place, which would immediately give clues as to the nature of enzymes likely to be involved. Another fruitful strategy would be to elucidate the molecular basis and pathophysiology of diseases such as ichthyoses (see Chapter 10). The elucidation of ichthyosis-like conditions induced by certain drugs may also be expected to be productive in this context.[1,2]

The most likely site at which the events which eventually lead to desquamation take place is the stratum corneum intercellular space. As described in other chapters of this book, the chemical composition, organization, and interactions of this part of the stratum corneum are extremely complex. The stratum corneum intercellular space may be considered as a multiphase system consisting of a complex mixture of lipids in which structural proteins, enzymes, and other non-structural proteins; a range of low molecular weight substances with different degrees of hydrophilicity; and water in low but significant concentrations are dispersed and interact with each other. A full understanding of stratum corneum cell cohesion and desquamation will rely on our understanding of the complex interactions of the many constituents of the intercorneocyte space. Although important steps forward have been taken in recent years, much has still to be learned. It should therefore be stated that our present knowledge about desquamation is quite rudimentary. Some clues have emerged, however, and will be summarized below.

9.2 SKIN DISEASES WITH DESQUAMATION DISTURBANCES

An accumulation of scales on the skin surface may be due to either an increased production of corneocytes, such as in psoriasis, or to a delayed desquamation. It may be predicted that conditions with delayed desquamation, once their pathophysiology on the molecular level is understood, will be highly informative with regards to the understanding of desquamation. Two such conditions are recessive X-linked ichthyosis (RXI) and lamellar ichthyosis.

The elucidation of the molecular genetics RXI has had a major impact on our understanding of stratum corneum turnover. Individuals with RXI lack an enzyme, cholesterol sulfatase,[3,4] which catalyzes the transformation of cholesterol sulfate to cholesterol and free sulfate. As a result there is an accumulation of cholesterol sulfate in the stratum corneum intercellular space. Possible mechanisms by which this change in intercellular lipid composition of the stratum corneum can cause disturbances in desquamation, leading to ichthyosis, will be discussed later.

A group of individuals with severe ichthyosis (recessive autosomal lamellar ichthyosis) has been found to have mutations in the gene for epidermal transglutaminase.[5-7] By means of catalyzing cross-linking of constituent proteins, this enzyme plays a crucial role in the formation of the cornified envelope of the corneocyte. How this type of molecular defect can cause ichthyosis is totally unknown. It may be expected that further studies on this condition will give important contributions to our understanding of desquamation. Similarly, we can expect that the soon-to-come elucidation of the molecular genetics of inherited lamellar ichthyoses with similar phenotypes, but without transglutaminase mutations,[8] will be informative.

9.3 STRATUM CORNEUM CELL DISSOCIATION INVOLVES PROTEOLYSIS

Experimental evidence that protein structures are involved in stratum corneum cell cohesion was presented by Bisset et al.[9] They induced cell dissociation in pig and human nonpalmo-plantar stratum corneum by means of incubation of the tissue in the presence of the zwitterionic surfactant 6-octadecyldimethyl ammoniohexanoate. Cell dissociation could not be induced when the tissue had been pretreated with the serine protease inhibitor phenylmethylsulfonyl fluoride (PMSF). The fact that cell dissociation was found only in the presence of EDTA suggested a role also for calcium in stratum corneum cell cohesion.

Lundström and Egelrud[10] found a unipolar spontaneous cell dissociation in pieces of hypertrophic human plantar stratum corneum incubated in a simple buffer. The cell dissociation occurred only at the surface which had faced outward *in vivo*. The rate of cell dissociation was increased in the presence of EDTA. It was inhibited by inhibitors of serine proteases, but not by inhibitors of other groups of proteases. Since the tissue had not been treated with exogenous proteases before the experiments, it was concluded that the observed cell dissociation was mediated by an endogenous serine protease. This experimental system has been used as an *in vitro* model of desquamation. In addition to information about the enzyme(s) involved in the cell dissociation, it has provided information about the nature of the cohesive structures in the stratum corneum (see later).

There is evidence that protein structures are also responsible for cell cohesion in nonpalmo-plantar stratum corneum. When punch biopsies of normal human gluteal skin were incubated in a buffer containing a mixture of the zwitterionic surfactant *N,N,*-dimethyldodecylamine and the anionic surfactant sodium dodecyl sulfate,[11] there was dissociation of cells in the stratum corneum but not in the rest of the epidermis. The cell dissociation took place only in the presence of EDTA and was inhibited by the serine protease inhibitor aprotinin.[12] Suzuki et al.[13,14] presented evidence that spontaneous cell dissociation in nonpalmo-plantar stratum corneum could be inhibited by a combination of inhibitors of trypsin-like and chymotrypsin-like enzymes. Thus, nonpalmo-plantar stratum corneum contains endogenous proteases that mediate cell dissociation.

9.4 DESMOSOMES AND CORNEODESMOSOMES

Desmosomes mediate mechanical contacts between viable eptihelial cells such as keratinocytes.[15-18] A desmosome is a round or oval, button-like structure with a diameter of 0.2 to 1 mm. It consists of two symmetrical halves, each one belonging to one of two contiguous cells and consisting of an intracellular, a transmembranal, and an extracellular part. Inside the cell, just below the plasma membrane, is the desmosomal plaque. To this structure are linked intracellular keratin filaments as well as glycoproteins belonging to the cadherin family named desmogleins and desmocollins. (For a review of desmosomal cadherins, see Reference 19.) These glycoproteins cross the plasma membrane, and their glycosylated parts occupy the extracellular space where they interact with their counterparts from the contiguous cell, thus forming a cohesive structure between the cells. In the electron microscope the desmosomal plaque is visible as an electron dense structure, approximately 15 nm in width, on the inner aspect of the plasma membrane. The extracellular parts of desmosomes between uncornified keratinocytes has a moderately electron dense, plate-like appearance, approximately 30 nm in width, and has a zigzag formed electron dense central line. Desmosomes and keratin filaments form functional units, the desmosome-intermediate filament complexes.[17] These complexes link the keratin filament cytoskeleton of individual cells into a network comprising the whole epithelium.

The corneodesmosomes, i.e., desmosomes in the stratum corneum, have a somewhat different appearance in the electron microscope.[20-22] Due to the densely packed and electron dense intracellular keratin filaments, it is not possible to identify the intracellular desmosomal plaque. The extracellular plate-like parts of corneodesmosomes have a homogenous and high electron density with no visible central line. Analyses of total number of desmosomes, measured as percentage of the cell periphery occupied by extracellular parts of desmosomes, showed a difference between the stratum corneum in palms and soles and stratum corneum at other body sites. In nonpalmo-plantar stratum corneum the number of desmosomes in deeper layers was comparable to the number of desmosomes in the stratum granulosum, whereas it was only around 20% of this number in the superficial layers close to the skin surface. This was true, however, only if the whole corneocyte periphery was considered. Whereas there were few desmosomes in the central parts of superficial corneocytes, the number of desmosomes per unit length of cell periphery at the overlapping edges of corneocytes was essentially the same as in deeper layers of the tissue. Thus, extracellular parts of desmosomes in the central parts of corneocytes disappear as the cells move upward in the stratum corneum, whereas desmosomes at the edges remain as long as the cells have not been shed. In palmo-plantar stratum corneum the number of desmosomes per unit length of corneocyte periphery is constant and high throughout the tissue until the cells are shed.[23]

The ultrastructural appearance of corneodesmosomes suggest that they are modified during the transition between viable and cornified epidermal layers. Part of this modification may be due to the incorporation of a recently discovered protein, corneodesmosin.[24-26] This is a 52-kD protein which is specifically expressed in keratinizing epithelia. In the stratum granulosum it is found intracellularly in association with lamellar bodies. In the transition zone between the stratum granulosum and the stratum corneum, coinciding with the change in the ultrastructural appearance of the desmosomes, corneodesmosin is translocated to the extracellular parts of desmosomes.[27] Immunoblot analyses have suggested that corneodesmosin is continuously degraded to smaller components in the stratum corneum.[26] It is not yet known to what extent this protein contributes to the cohesive capacity of corneodesmosomes. The possible role of corneodesmosin degradation in desquamation will be discussed later.

9.5 DESQUAMATION INVOLVES DEGRADATION OF CORNEODESMOSOMES

Evidence that degradation of corneodesmosomes is a prerequisite for desquamation comes from ultrastructural and immunochemical studies. In the so-called retention ichthyoses, in which it is believed that a delayed desquamation causes the thickening of the stratum corneum and the accumulation of squames, there is an increased number of corneodesmosomes in the superficial layers of the stratum corneum.[28,29] In plantar stratum corneum undergoing spontaneous cell dissociation (see earlier), electron microscopy of dissociating cells suggested that degradation of the intercellular parts of desmosomes preceded the widening of the intercellular space.[30] Chapman and Walsh[31] showed by means of electron microscopy that desquamation in pig skin was associated with morphological signs of desmosomal degradation.

Immunoblot analyses with antibodies specific for the transmembranal desmosomal glycoprotein desmoglein I (DG I) of plantar stratum corneum undergoing spontaneous cell dissociation[30] showed that whereas the still cohesive tissue contained only intact DG I, dissociated cells contained no intact DG I, but instead they contained degradation products of this protein. Analyses of surface cells that had been shed from plantar skin *in vivo* gave similar results.[32] In xerotic skin superficial stratum corneum contained more extractable intact DG I than in normal skin,[33] suggesting that delayed desmosomal degradation may contribute to the accumulation of squames. Increased amounts of intact DG I in superficial stratum corneum was found also in a mouse model with experimentally induced scaling.[34] Taken together, these ultrastructural and immunochemical results strongly suggest that corneodesmosomes are responsible for cell cohesion in the stratum corneum and that proteolytic degradation of their extracellular parts is a prerequisite for desquamation.

9.6 ENZYMES INVOLVED IN DESQUAMATION

The best-characterized enzyme so far with a proposed function in desquamation is stratum corneum chymotryptic enzyme (SCCE). The discovery of SCCE was a result of the search for the enzyme responsible for the degradation of cohesive structures in the *in vitro* model of desquamation in hypertrophic plantar stratum corneum. SCCE has several properties compatible with a role in desquamation also *in vivo*.[35,36] SCCE has been purified from plantar stratum corneum.[37] It has been cloned and expressed in mammalian cells.[38] In reduced form SCCE has a molecular mass of around 28 kD, it is partially glycosylated, and it has a basic isoelectric point. Although having a neutral to alkaline pH-optimum it is active also at pH 5.5, i.e., it is active at the pH of the stratum corneum.[39] SCCE is produced as an inactive precursor with a pro-peptide seven amino acid residues long. Removal of the pro-peptide by means of trypsin treatment of recombinant pro-SCCE yields a proteolytically active enzyme.[38] The mechanisms of SCCE activation *in vivo* remain to be elucidated. The deduced amino acid sequence contains the conserved regions typical of serine proteases, but is otherwise, at most, only around 40% homologous with other known enzymes. SCCE shows similarities, but also significant differences regarding the activity on peptide substrates and the sensitivity to various protease inhibitors when compared to other chymotryptic enzymes such as bovine chymotrypsin and human cathepsin G.[37] This may be explained, at least partially, by the fact that in SCCE there is an asparagine residue in the bottom of the deduced primary substrate binding pouch, whereas this site is occupied by serine and alanine residues in chymotrypsin and cathepsin G, respectively.[38]

Analyses of mRNA from a large number of various human tissues has shown high expression of SCCE only in the skin.[38] Immunohistochemical studies have shown that SCCE is expressed in high suprabasal keratinocytes in the epidermis. In hair follicles and sebaceous glands it is expressed at a site where there is formation of cornified keratinocytes and hence a need for desquamation-like processes. In the oral cavity SCCE staining is found in the cornified epithelium of the hard palate, but not in the buccal mucosa or at other sites with noncornified epithelium. Thus, these findings suggest that SCCE expression is related to a differentiation process, leading to the formation of a cornified squamous epithelium.[40-43]

Results from enzymologic studies have suggested that SCCE has an extracellular localization in the stratum corneum.[44] This has been corroborated by means of immunoelectron microscopy. With this method SCCE was found intracellularly in association with lamellar bodies in the stratum granulosum. In the transition between the stratum granulosum and the stratum corneum, SCCE is extruded to the extracellular space together with the lamellar bodies. In the stratum corneum specific labelling is found only in the extracellular space, often in association with corneodesmosomes.[45]

Results from *in vitro* experiments, catalytic properties, and tissue localization are all compatible with the role of SCCE in the degradation of intercellular cohesive structures in the stratum corneum as part of the events leading to remodeling of the tissue and eventually to desquamation. Firm proof that this is the physiological function of SCCE is still lacking. There are also other proteases present in the stratum corneum, some of which may be involved in desquamation.[13,14,36,37,46-48] Of these proteases, a 30-kD serine protease which may have a trypsin-like primary substrate specificity may be of special interest. This enzyme appears on zymography gels together with SCCE and has been postulated to have a complementary role to that of SCCE in degradation structures involved in stratum corneum cell cohesion during desquamation.[13] In addition it is a candidate for being responsible for the activation of the SCCE precursor. Additional information in this respect will be crucial for the understanding of the role of SCCE and related enzymes in the formation and turnover of the stratum corneum.

TABLE 1
Mechanisms Which May Be Involved in Regulation of Desquamation

Enzyme activation
- Activation of SCCE

Enzyme inhibition
- Cholesterol sulfate
- Antileukoprotease
- Other protease inhibitors in the stratum corneum

Substrate modification
- Glycosylation
- pH? Water? Ions? Lipids?

Note: See text for references.

9.7 REGULATION OF DESQUAMATION

We are very far from an understanding of how and by which mechanisms desquamation is regulated. If we assume, however, that proteolytic degradation of corneodesmosomes plays a major role in desquamation, a number of possible mechanisms can be postulated on the basis of the present knowledge. These are summarized in Table 1.

The activation of enzyme precursors is likely to be of central importance. A significant fraction of the total SCCE present in the stratum corneum is in the form of inactive pro-enzyme (Lundström, A. and Egelrud, T., unpublished observations and Reference 49). A change in the ratio of precursor to active enzyme may be expected to cause marked changes in the rate of corneodesmosomal degradation. *In vitro* pro-SCCE can be activated by pancreatic trypsin.[38] The physiological SCCE activator remains to be identified. As mentioned earlier, stratum corneum extracts contain a trypsin-like enzyme[13,36] which may possibly have this function. This enzyme still awaits characterization. It is possible that SCCE is just one of a number of enzymes constituting a "proteolytic cascade" in the stratum corneum, in which one enzyme serves as activator of another enzyme.

The stratum corneum is likely to contain a number of inhibitors of the various proteases present. Cholesterol sulfate (CS) may be of special interest. Accumulation of CS in the stratum corneum in XRI may be causative of this disease (see earlier), in which there is evidence of a delayed degradation of desmosomes.[28] CS has been shown to inhibit pancreatic serine proteases *in vitro*, and application of CS on mouse skin *in vivo* causes a scaling condition.[34] In addition to direct effects on enzymes, CS could cause delayed desquamation by acting as a substrate modifier or by changing the physical-chemical conditions in the stratum corneum extracellular space.

A number of protein protease inhibitors are present in the stratum corneum. Of these antileukoprotease has been shown to be an efficient inhibitor of SCCE at physiological concentrations.[50] Extracts of plantar stratum corneum contains covalent complexes between SCCE and α1-antitrypsin (Egelrud. T., unpublished observation).

Also, in autosomal recessive ichthyosis there are findings indicative of an impaired desmosome degradation in the stratum corneum.[29] The mechanisms involved have not been elucidated.

As mentioned previously for CS, substrate modifications could be of significant importance as regulating factors in proteolytic degradation of cohesive structures. Walsh and Chapman showed that pretreatment with glycosidases made preparations of stratum corneum more susceptible to cell dissociation induced by exogenous proteases, suggesting that proteins involved in cell cohesion may be protected by carbohydrates against proteolytic degradation.[51]

There are a vast number of other factors which may be expected to influence the rate of desquamation, for instance, by affecting the rate of proteolytic reactions. pH, water, and ion concentrations, and lipid composition may all be expected to be of importance. Experimental data in this area are very scarce, but some speculations can be made. For instance, the pH dependency of SCCE activity could be of importance. SCCE has optimal activity at pH 7 to 8, but close to half its maximal activity at pH 5.5.[35,36] This implies that rather small variations in either direction of the pH of the extracellular space should have effects on the rate of SCCE-mediated protein degradation. In support of this, the rate of spontaneous cell dissociation observed in plantar stratum corneum *in vitro* showed a marked pH dependency, being highest at neutral to weakly alkaline pH and decreasing at lower pH values.[10]

The effects of chelating agents in *in vitro* models for desquamation suggest that divalent ions such as calcium may play a role in the regulation of desquamation.[12,26,52]

The composition of the stratum corneum intercellular lipids may have profound effects on desquamation. In addition to modifying effects on, e.g., proteolytic enzymes and their substrates,[34] lipids may also be directly involved in corneocyte cohesion. The effects of cholesterol sulfate have already been mentioned. In addition to RXI, there are a number of other hereditary diseases with disorders of desquamation associated with disturbances in lipid metabolism. Furthermore, scaling as a result of treatment with lipid-lowering drugs has been observed (for review, see References 1 and 2).

9.8 CONCLUSION

A normal desquamation is of crucial importance for the maintenance of the function of the stratum corneum and for a normal skin appearance. In recent years some basic knowledge about stratum corneum cell cohesion and the role of proteolysis in desquamation has evolved. Much still has to be learned, however. In the near future we may expect to obtain information about further enzymes involved in desquamation, and the ongoing elucidation of hereditary skin diseases will give new clues with regards to regulation of mechanisms involved in desquamation. Similarly, further studies on the physical chemistry and the chemical composition, including identification of hitherto unknown proteins, of the stratum corneum intercellular space may be expected to give important contributions to this central area of skin biology.

REFERENCES

1. Williams, M. L., Feingold, K. R., Grubauer, G., Elias, P. M., Ichthyosis induced by cholesterol-lowering drugs, *Arch. Dermatol.*, 123, 1535, 1987.
2. Williams, M. L., Lipids in normal and pathological desquamation, *Adv. Lipid Res.*, 24, 211, 1991.
3. Shapiro, L. J., Weiss, R., Webster, D., France, J. T., X-linked ichthyosis due to steroid suphatase deficiency, *Lancet*, 1, 70, 1978.
4. Koppe, G., Marinkovic-Ilsen, A., Rijken, Y., De-Groot, W. P., X-linked ichthyosis. A sulfatase deficiency, *Arch. Dis. Child.,* 53, 803, 1978.
5. Huber, M., Rettler, I., Bernasconi, K., Frenk, E., Lavrisjen, S. P., Ponec M., Bon, A., Lautenschlager, S., Schorderet, D. F., Hohls, D., Mutations of transglutaminase in lamellar ichthysois, *Science*, 267, 525, 1995.
6. Russel, L. J., DiGiovanna, J. J., Rogers, G. R., Hashem, N., Compton, J. G., Bale, S. J., Mutations in the gene for transglutaminase 1 in autosomal recessive lamellar ichthyosis, *Nat. Genet.*, 9, 279, 1995.
7. Parmentier, L., Blanchet-Bardon, C., Nguyen, S., Prud'homme, J.-F., Dubertret, L., Weissenbach, J., Autosomal recessive lamellar ichthyosis: identification of a new mutation in transglutaminase 1 and evidence for genetic heterogeneity, *Hum. Mol. Genet.*, 4, 1391, 1995.
8. Huber, M., Rettler, I., Bernasconi, K., Wyss, M., Hohl, D., Lamellar ichthyosis is genetically heterogenous — cases with normal keratinocyte transglutaminase, *J. Invest. Dermatol.*, 105, 653, 1995.
9. Bisset, D. L., McBride, J. F., Patrick, L. F., Role of protein and calcium in stratum corneum cell cohesion, *Arch. Dermatol. Res.,* 279, 184, 1987.

10. Lundström, A., Egelrud, T., Cell shedding from human plantar skin *in vitro*: evidence of its dependence on endogenous hydrolysis, *J. Invest. Dermatol.,* 91, 340, 1988.
11. Takahashi, M., Aizawa, M., Miyazawa, K., Machida, Y., Effects of surface active agents on stratum corneum cell cohesion, *J. Soc. Cosmet. Chem.,* 38, 21, 1987.
12. Egelrud, T., Lundström, A., The dependence of detergent-induced cell dissociation in non-palmo-plantar stratum corneum on endogenous proteolysis, *J. Invest. Dermatol*., 95, 456, 1990.
13. Suzuki, Y., Nomura, J., Koyama, J., Takahashi, M., Horii, I., Detection and characterization of endogenous protease associated with desquamation of stratum corneum, *Arch. Dermatol. Res.,* 285, 372, 1993.
14. Suzuki, Y., Nomura, J., Koyama, J., Horii, I., The role of proteases in stratum corneum: involvement in stratum corneum desquamation, *Arch. Dermatol. Res.,* 286, 249, 1994.
15. Staehelin, L. A., Intercellular junctions, *Int. Rev. Cytol*., 39, 191, 1974.
16. Arnn, J., Staehelin, L. A., The structure and function of spot desmosomes, *Int. J. Dermatol*., 20, 330, 1981.
17. Cowin, P., Franke, W. W., Grund, C., Kapprell, H.-P., Kartenbeck, J., The desmosome-intermediate filament complex. In: Edelman, G.M. and Thiery, J.-P. (eds.) *The Cell in Contact. Adehsions and Junctions as Morphogenetic Determinants.* John Wiley & Sons, New York, 1985, 427.
18. Skerrow, C. J., Desmosomal proteins. In: Bereiter-Hahn, J., Matoltsy, A. G., and Richards, K. S. (eds.) *Biology of the Integument 2. Vertebrates.* Springer-Verlag, Berlin, Heidelberg, 1986, 762.
19. Buxton, R. S., Cowin, P., Franke, W. W., Garrod, D. R., Green, K. J., King, I.A., Koch, P. J., Magee, A. I., Rees, D. A., Stanley, J. R., Steinberg M. S., Nomenclature of the desmosomal cadherins, *J. Cell Biol.* 121, 481, 1993.
20. Brody, I., An electron-microscopic study of the junctional and regular desmosomes in normal human epidermis, *Acta Derm. Venereol.* (*Stockh.*)., 48, 290, 1968.
21. Raknerud, N., The ultrastructure of the interfollicular epidermis of the hairless (hr/h) mouse III. Desmosomal transformation during keratinization, *J. Ultrastruct. Res.,* 52, 32, 1974.
22. White, F. H., Gohari, K., Some aspects of desmosomal morphology during differentiation of hamster cheek pouch*, J. Submicrosc. Cytol.*, 16, 407, 1984.
23. Skerrow, C. J., Clelland, D. G., Skerow, D., Changes to desmosomal antigens and lectin-binding sites during differentiation in normal human epidermis: a quantitative ultrastructural study, *J. Cell Sci.*, 92, 667, 1989.
24. Serre, G., Mils, V., Haftek, M., Vincent, C., Croute, F., Réano, A., Ouhayoun, J.-P., Bettinger, S., Soleilhavoup, J.P., Identification of late differentiation antigens of human cornified epithelia, expressed in re-organized desmosomes and bound to cross-linked envelopes, *J. Invest. Dermatol.,* 97, 1061, 1991.
25. Guerrin, M., Simon, M., Montezin, M. Haftek, M. Vincent, C., Serre, G., Expression cloning of human corneodesmosin proves its identity with the product of the S gene and allows improved characterization of its processing during keratinocyte differentiation, *J. Biol. Chem.*, 273, 22640, 1998.
26. Lundström, A., Serre, G., Haftek, M., Egelrud, T., Evidence for a role of corneodesmosin, a protein which may serve to modify desmosomes during cornification, in stratum corneum cell cohesion and desquamation, *Arch. Dermatol. Res.,* 286, 369, 1994.
27. Haftek, M., Serre, G., Thivolet, J., Immunochemical evidence for a possible role of cross-linked keratinocyte envelopes in stratum corneum cohesion, *J. Histochem. Cytochem.,* 39, 1531, 1991.
28. Elsayed, A. H., Barton, S., Marks, R., Stereological studies of desmosomes in ichthyosis vulgaris, *Br. J. Dermatol*., 126, 24, 1992.
29. Ghadially, R., Williams, M. L., Hou, S. Y., Elias, P. M., Membrane structural abnormalities in the stratum corneum of the autosomal recessive ichthyoses, *J. Invest. Dermatol.*, 99, 755, 1992.
30. Lundström, A., Egelrud, T., Evidence that cell shedding form plantar skin *in vitro* involves endogenous proteolysis of the desmosomal protein desmoglein I, *J. Invest. Dermatol.,* 94, 216, 1989.
31. Chapman, S. J., Walsh, A., Desmosomes, corneosomes and desquamation. An ultrastructural study of adult pig epidermis, *Arch. Dermatol. Res.,* 282, 304, 1990.
32. Egelrud, T., Lundström, A., Immunochemical analyses of the distribution of the desmosomal protein desmoglein I in different layers of plantar epidermis, *Acta Derm. Venereol.* (*Stockh.*), 69, 470, 1989.
33. Bartolone, J., Doughty, D., Egelrud, T., A non-invasive approach for assessing corneocyte cohesion: Immunochemical detection of desmoglein I, *J. Invest. Dermatol.*, 96, 596 (abstr.), 1991.

34. Sato, J., Denda, M., Nakanishi, J., Nomura, J., Koyama, J., Cholesterol sulfate inhibits proteases that are involved in desquamation of stratum corneum, *J. Invest. Dermatol.*, 111, 189, 1998.
35. Egelrud, T., Lunström, A., A chymotrypsin-like proteinase that may be involved in desquamation in plantar stratum corneum, *Arch. Dermatol. Res.*, 283, 108, 1991.
36. Lundström, A., Egelrud, T., Stratum corneum chymotryptic enzyme: a proteinase which may be generally present in the stratum corneum and with a possible involvement in desquamation, *Acta Derm. Venereol. (Stockh.),* 71, 471, 1991.
37. Egelrud, T., Purification and preliminary characterization of stratum corneum chymotryptic enzyme: a proteinase that may be involved in desquamation, *J. Invest. Dermatol.*, 101, 200, 1993.
38. Hansson, L., Strömqvist, M., Bäckman, A., Wallbrandt, P., Carlstein, A., Egelrud, T., Cloning, expression, and characterization of stratum corneum chymotryptic enzyme, a skin-specific human serine proteinase, *J. Biol. Chem.,* 269, 19420, 1994.
39. Öhman, H., Vahlquist, A., *In vivo* studies concerning a pH gradient in human stratum corneum and upper epidermis, *Acta Derm. Venereol. (Stockh.),* 74, 375, 1994.
40. Sondell, B., Thornell, L.-E., Stigbrand, T., Egelrud, T., Immunolcoalization of stratum corneum chymotryptic enzyme in human skin and oral epithelium with monoclonal antibodies: evidence of a proteinase specifically expressed in keratinizing squamous epithelia, *J. Histochem. Cytochem.*, 42, 459, 1994.
41. Sondell, B., Dyberg, P., Anneroth, G. K. B., Östman, P.-O., Egelrud, T., Association between expression of stratum corneum chymotryptic enzyme and pathological keratinization in human oral mucosa, *Acta Derm.Venereol. (Stockh.)*, 76, 177, 1996.
42. Ekholm, E., Sondell, B., Dyberg, P., Jonsson M., Egelrud, T., Expression of stratum corneum chymotryptic enzyme in normal human sebaceous follicles, *Acta Derm. Venereol. (Stockh.)*, 78, 343, 1998.
43. Ekholm, E., Egelrud, T., The expression of stratum corneum chymotryptic enzyme in human anagen hair follicles. Further evidenc for its involvement in desquamation-like processes, Br. J. Dermatol., 139, 585, 1998.
44. Egelrud, T., Stratum corneum chymotryptic enzyme: evidence of its location to the stratum corneum extracellular space, *Eur. J. Dermatol.,* 2, 50, 1992.
45. Sondell B., Thornell L.-E., Egelrud, T., Evidence that stratum corneum chymotryptic enzyme is transported to the stratum corneum extracellular space via lamellar bodies, *J. Invest. Dermatol.,* 104, 819, 1995.
46. Brysk, M. M., Bell, T., Brysk, H., Selvanayagam, P., Rajaraman, S., Enzymatic activity of desquamin, *Exp. Cell Res.,* 214, 22, 1994.
47. Horikoshi, T., Chen, S.-H., Rajaraman, S., Brysk, H., Brysk, M. M., Involvement of cathepsin D in the desquamation of human stratum corneum, *J. Invest. Dermatol.*, 110, 547 (abstr.), 1998.
48. Watkinson, A., Stratum corneum gelatainase: a novel late differentiation, epidermal cystein protease, *J. Invest. Dermatol.*, 110, 539 (abstr.), 1998.
49. Vicanova, J., Mommaas, M., Forslind, B., Pallon, J., Egelrud, T., Koerten, H. K., Ponec, M., Normalization of epidermal calcium distribution profile in reconstructed human epidermis is related to improvement of terminal differentiation and stratum corneum barrier formation, *J. Invest. Dermatol.*, 111, 97, 1998.
50. Franzke, C. W., Baici, A., Bartels, J., Christophers, E., Wiedow, O., Antileukoprotease inhibits stratum corneum chymotryptic enzyme. Evidence for a regulative function in desquamation, *J. Biol. Chem.*, 271, 21886, 1996.
51. Walsh, A., Chapman, S. J., Sugars protect desmosome and corneosome glycoproteins from proteolysis, *Arch. Dermatol. Res.,* 283, 174, 1991.
52. Lundström, A., Egelrud, T., Cell shedding from plantar skin *in vitro*: evidence that two different types of protein structures are degraded by a chymotrypsin-like enzyme, *Arch. Dermatol. Res.,* 282, 234, 1990.

Part 3

Dry Skin and Hyperkeratotic Conditions

10 Ichthyosis — An Inborn Dryness of the Skin

Anders Vahlquist

CONTENTS

10.1 INTRODUCTION

Patients with ichthyosis often experience severe skin dryness combined with hyperkeratosis that requires life-long application of emollients all over the body several times a day. Thus, it is no wonder that many of these patients become experts in their own right on topical treatment of the skin. However, before discussing therapy of ichthyosis, one should recall that the term encompasses a wide range of keratinizing disorders with completely different pathophysiology, each requiring tailored advice about how to best treat the skin. In some patients, for example, erosions rather than hyperkeratosis and dryness of the skin are the biggest problem. These patients may have a type of ichthyosis that is pathogenetically related to other blistering diseases, such as epidermolysis bullosa simplex, pachonychia congenita, and Dariers's disease.

Interestingly, the etiologies of many of these diseases have recently been elucidated (Figure 1), making it easier in the future to correctly diagnose and to develop new therapies specific for each type of ichthyosis. Whereas today the therapy is mainly symptomatic and based on topical emollients and keratolytic agents, this new knowledge will probably lead to more long-lasting remedies, e.g., gene therapy for the most severe types of keratinizing disorders. With these prospects at hand, a more detailed description of the pathophysiology, clinical presentation, and current treatment of the various ichthyoses are given here (see Table 1 for overview).

10.2 COMMON ICHTHYOSES

The two most common forms of ichthyosis, autosomal dominant ichthyosis vulgaris (IV) and X-linked recessive ichthyosis (XRI), in most populations occur at frequencies of about 1/300 and 1/2,500, respectively.[1] In fact, the two diseases are so relatively common that they sometimes

0-8493-7520-7/00/$0.00+$.50

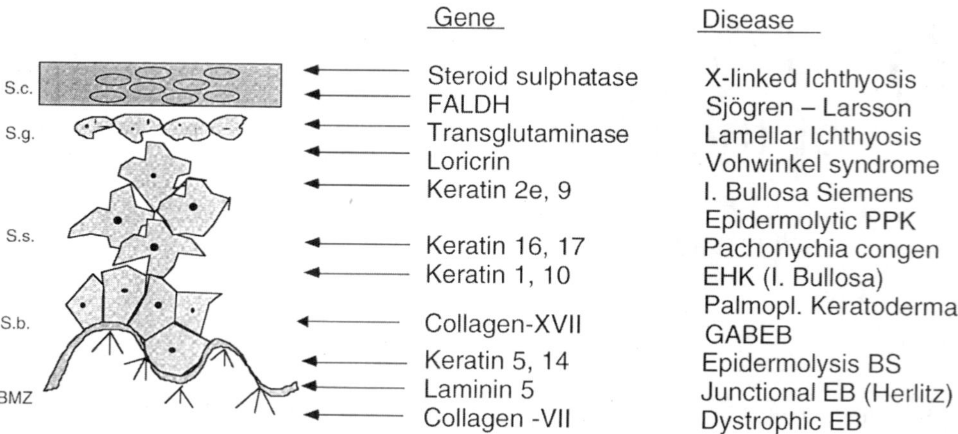

FIGURE 1 Examples of gene mutations causing keratinizing disorders in human skin. Data compiled from the literature in 1998. Abbreviations: S.c. — stratum corneum, S.g. — stratum granulosum, S.s. — stratum spinosum, S.b. — stratum basale, BMZ — basal membrane zone, FALDH — fatty aldehyde dehydrogenase, PPK — palmo-plantar keratoderma, EHK — epidermoltyic hyperkeratosis, GABEB — generalized atrophic benign epidermolysis bullosa, EB — epidermolysis bullosa.

TABLE 1
Common and Rare Forms of Ichthyosis

	Ichthyosis vulgaris	**X-Linked ichthyosis**	**Lamellar Ichthyosis (Non-Bullous ichthyosiform Erythroderma)**	**Epidermolytic Hyperkeratosis (Bullous ichthyosis)**
Incidence:	1/300	1/3000 (boys)	1/100,000	1/300,000
Etiology:	Defective keratohyaline	Steroid sulfatase deficiency	Transglutaminase deficiency (and other)	Keratin mutations
Inheritance:	Autosomal dominant	Recessive X-linked	Autosomal recessive	Autosomal dominant
Appearance:	Early in childhood	Early in childhood	Congenital	Congenital
Symptoms:	Retention hyperkeratosis on extremities; better in summer	Brown scales all over the body; associated features; maternal pregnancy abn.	"Collodion baby"; generalized scaling; large, thick scales; ektropion; hypohidrosis	Intense blistering at birth; later verrucous hyperkeratosis, esp. in body folds; keratoderma ±

co-exist in one and the same family.[2] The incidence and severity of the diseases vary in different countries, depending on both genetic and environmental factors. In a humid climate, these types of ichthyoses need not be a big problem to an affected individual, whereas in a cold and dry climate xerosis and hyperkeratosis may become severe.

Scaling is usually most apparent on the extensor surface of the extremities, but it may also appear on the trunk, especially in XRI (Figure 2). Xerosis of the skin is a prominent feature in most patients, but there is no skin inflammation unless ichthyosis is complicated by atopic eczema (common in IV) or by microbial infections. Histologically, IV and XRI are both characterized by orthohyperkeratosis due to an abnormal retention of corneocytes.

Although there is considerable overlap between symptoms of IV and XRI, the two diseases were first deliniated by Wells and Kerr in the 1960s.[3] Thus, XRI usually starts earlier in life and is more

a

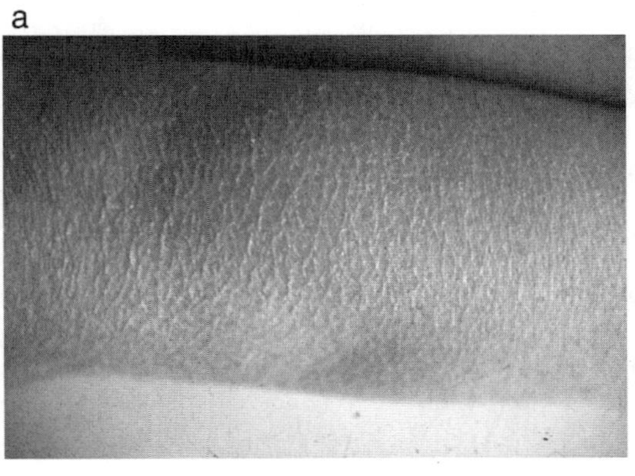

b

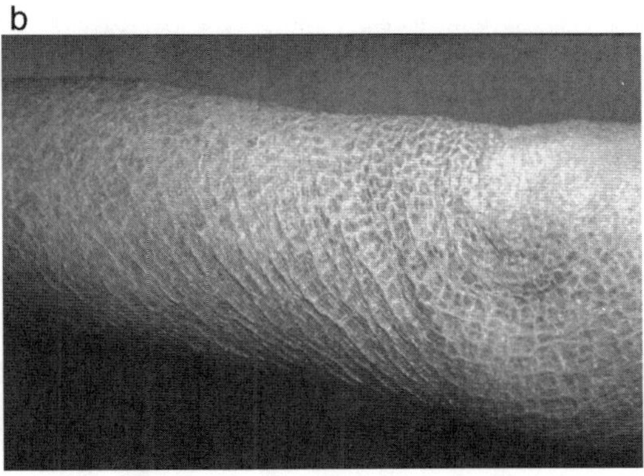

FIGURE 2 Extremities showing (a) ichthyosis vulgaris in a 40-year-old woman and (b) x-linked ichthyosis in a 20-year-old man (from the author's files).

severe than IV. When laboratory diagnosing of XRI became possible in the late 1970s, based on the discovery of steroid sulfatase deficiency in these patients,[4,5] several new features distinguishing XRI from IV emerged[6,7] (Table 2). Diagnosing is facilitated by the fact that a routine lipoprotein electrophoresis will show an abnormal mobility of the ß-band in XRI patients, but not in IV patients.[8] Additionally, a punch biopsy from lesional skin will show that stratum granulosum is normal in XRI, but thin or missing in IV, which is due to a defect in the processing of profilaggrin.[9,10] On electron microscopy, this defect in IV epidermis will appear as tiny and crumbly keratohyalin granules.[11]

10.3 BIOCHEMICAL DIFFERENCES OF THE HORNY LAYER IN IV AND XRI

The lack of fillagrin and keratohyaline in IV results *inter alia* in a deficiency of the natural moisturizing factor (NMF) composed of hygroscopic, amino acid-derived breakdown products.[12] In XRI, on the other hand, due to the steroid sulfatase deficiency, there is an accumulation of cholesterol sulfate (CS) and a decrease in cholesterol in the stratum corneum.[13] This finding, together with recent observations about the many interesting effects of CS in epidermis (Table 3), makes it possible to speculate about why the normal shedding of corneocytes is delayed in XRI. The intercellular lipids are important for corneocyte cohesion and barrier function. Careful monitoring of TEWL in XRI patients has shown a slightly impaired barrier function, despite the hyperkeratosis,[14,15] and this impairment can be reproduced in experimental animals by topical application of CS.[15] The hyperkeratosis can be compensatory, but may also reflect an inhibition of the desquamation process by CS.[16]

TABLE 2
Clinical and Biological Features Distinguishing Ichthyosis Vulgaris (IV) from X-Linked Recessive Ichthyosis (XRI)

Features	IV	XRI
Symptoms appearing <6 months	Rare	Frequent
Brownish scales on the trunk	Rare	Frequent
Flexural involvement	Rare	Frequent
Testicular non-descendence	Rare	Frequent
Corneal opacity	Rare	Frequent
Accentuation of palmar creases	Frequent	Rare
Associated atopic eczema	Frequent	Rare
Associated keratosis follicularis	Frequent	Rare
Scanty or absent stratum granulosum	+	–
High CS/low free cholesterol in stratum corneum	–	+
Abnormal mobility of β-lipoprotein	–	+

TABLE 3
Cholesterol Sulfate and the Skin

CS: Is normally present in stratum granulosum and stratum corneum[46]
Is probably important for the pH gradient in stratum corneum[17]
Accumulates in stratum corneum of patients with X-linked ichthyosis[13]
Accumulates in epidermis during chemical carcinogenesis[47]
Is growth inhibitory to human keratinocytes[48]
Activates PKC (which phosphorylates TGM1)[49]
Induces transcription of the TGM gene[50]
Inhibits certain proteases (SCCE etc.) in stratum corneum[16]
Is reduced in epidermis during retinoid therapy[51]

It is also noteworthy that CS is a weak acid, presumably participating in the formation of a pH gradient over stratum corneum. Thus, in a recent study[17] we found that this gradient, which normally spans from pH 7 in stratum granulosum to pH 4.5 to 5.0 on the surface, is shifted to more acidic values in XRI patients, whereas in IV patients it is shifted to more basic values (Figure 3). These findings are consistent with the accumulation of CS in XRI, and the lack of filaggrin breakdown products (urocanic acid and pyrrolidone carboyxlic acid) in IV skin. Speculatively, changes in the pH gradient may not just reflect the altered chemical compostion of the horny layer, but could also influence the activity of the many pH-dependent enzymes operating in the intercorneocyte space (for review see Reference 18). Whether pH variations also influence the transcorneal diffusion of topically applied acids and bases (e.g., salicylic acid, alpha-hydroxy acids, and certain drugs) is presently unclear.

10.4 TREATMENT OF COMMON ICHTHYOSIS

Several factors have to be taken into consideration when prescribing a topical treatment for ichthyosis, viz: the age of the patients (children generally have thinner skin and a greater skin

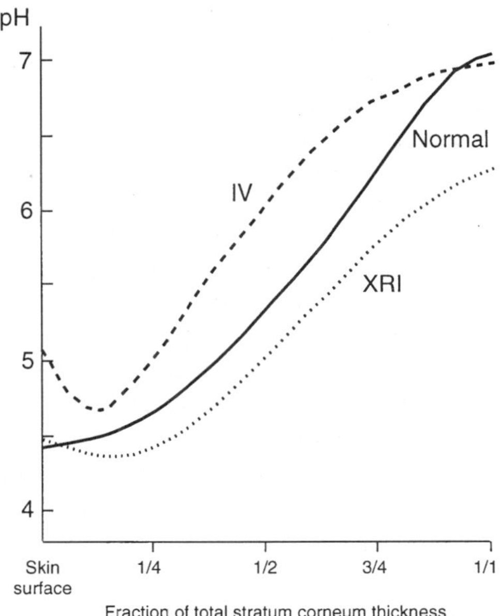

FIGURE 3 Schematic representation of the pH gradients over stratum corneum in normal skin, ichthyosis vulgaris (IV) skin, and x-linked recessive ichthyosis (XRI) skin, respectively. (Reproduced from Öhman, H. and Vahlquist, A., *J Invest Dermatol,* 111, 674, 1998. With permission.)

surface area/body weight ratio than adults), (2) the extent of the skin lesions (whole body application increases the risk for systemic toxicity), (3) regional variations in the degree of symptoms (flexural sites and the face usually need less potent therapy), and (4) presence of fissures and erosions (prevents use of certain types of irritating creams). Also, it is important to recognize that cosmetic acceptability of a cream is a sine qua non for good compliance and that there are probably as many opinions about "the best cream formulation" as there are patients.

The most logical way of treating IV and XRI would be to try and substitute stratum corneum (SC) with the missing components NMF and cholesterol, respectively. In fact, some success with topical cream has been reported in XRI patients,[19] but the overall results are meager and substitution therapy is not a routine in any types of ichthyosis. Instead, standard treatment of mild to moderate IV and XRI is daily application of emollients containing 2 to 10% urea,[20] 5 to 15% lactic acid,[21] or 10 to 25% propylene glycol.[22] In a recent study from Germany, urea in a new lotion base was found to be highly effective and well tolerated by children.[23] Other treatment options include regular baths (salt and oil), UV-irradiation, and climate therapy in the winter. Oral retinoid therapy is rarely indicated except in the most severe cases of XRI. Topical corticosteroids and vitamin D derivatives (calcipotriol) are usually contraindicated in common ichthyosis because (1) they do not alleviate the disease processes and (2) they are associated with a significant risk for systemic absorption when used extensively.

10.5 RARE FORMS OF ICHTHYOSIS

The two most severe types of ichthyosis, lamellar ichthyosis (LI) and epidermolytic hyperkeratosis (EHK), are distinct families of diseases with completely different etiologies (see Figure 1 and Table 1). However, LI and EHK have a few things in common: they are rare, congenital diseases (prevalence <1/100,000) which are characterized by more or less generalized hyperkeratosis and a defective skin barrier.

LI and its closely related variants, nonbullous ichthyosiform congenital erythroderma or erythrodermic lamellar ichthyosis (ELI) (Figure 4), seem to be the results of either failures in the formation of cornified cell envelope or in defective deposition of intercorneocyte lipids. In the former case, mutations in the gene encoding for keratinocyte transglutaminase (TGM1) frequently underlie a recessive disorder characterized by deficient TGM activity in the upper epidermis.[24,25] This causes a defective cross-linking of envelope proteins, such as involucrin and loricrin, which can be visualized on electron microscopy (EM) as an absent or only faint marginal band in the corneocytes.[11] However, there are also several unexplained EM features in LI and ELI, such as numerous lipid droplets and cholesterol clefts in SC and a bizarre accumulation of membrane-like structures in cells from both the granular and the horny layers.[11] This points to a multifactorial pathogenesis in LI and ELI,[26] supported also by genetic analysis of large kindreds of affected families showing coupling to at least two loci other than TGM1 on chromosome 14.[27] In a recent Swedish study, we found about 50% of LI/ELI to be associated with TGM1 mutations that were mostly of the compound heterozygocity type (Pigg et al., to be published). Finding the remaining causes of nonbullous congenital ichthyosis will probably be instrumental in elucidating some of the still unknown mechanisms during normal cornification and also raise the hope for future gene therapy in this disorder.

10.6 TREATMENT OF LAMELLAR ICHTHYOSIS

Although the introduction of systemic retinoids in the late 1970s meant a great deal to many LI patients, the mainstay of therapy remains external and will probably do so until gene therapy eventually finds its way into the therapeutic repertoire. The pros and cons of oral retinoid therapy will not be discussed further in this chapter (for review, see Reference 28).

For years topical emollients and various keratolytic agents have been the most commonly prescribed remedies. The treatment traditions differ from one country to another and even from one hospital center to another. For example, whereas urea-containing lipophilic creams are popular in many European countries, including Sweden, mixtures containing propylene glycol or alpha-hydroxy acids seem to be the first choice in the U.S. and many other countries. Salicylic acid, however, is best avoided when treating large skin areas and children, due to the risk of systemic toxicity. This is very important in collodion babies, especially when urea has been found to penetrate the skin.[29]

The selection of cream base (hydrophilic or lipophilic, non-occlusive or semi-occlusive) is important not only for the pharmacologic effect, but also for compliance reasons (see earlier). By combining two or more keratolytic agents and moisturizers in the same cream base it is usually possible to achieve additative or even synergistic effects without having to use irritating concentrations of either ingredients.[30] Thus, in a recent double-blind trial of 4 different cream mixtures in 20 patients with LI, a mixture of 5% lactic acid and 20% propylene glycol in a semi-occlusive cream for 4 weeks twice daily was significantly more effective than 20% propylene glycol or 5% urea alone in the same vehicle.[31] However, although hyperkeratosis was almost abolished in some patients (Figure 5) and the treatment went well for many months, it was clear from our measurements of TEWL that the skin barrier deteriorated further as a result of therapy. This points to a problematic dualism when effectively reducing a symptom (hyperproliferative hyperkeratosis) that probably represents a compensatory mechanism for the corneocyte defect in LI.

Apart from using emollients and keratolytic agents, LI has also been treated topically with more specific drugs, such as retinoids,[32,33] liarozole,[34] and calcipotriol.[35] Some of these drugs probably act through reducing the epidermal hyperproliferation associated with certain forms of LI. However, the risk of side effects is obvious when using these drugs extensively on a skin suffering from a defect barrier function, and they are not marketed for treatment of LI.

Unfortunately, neither topical nor oral treatment has any profound effect on the failure of normal sweating that many LI patients suffer from in a hot climate or during excercise.[36]

a

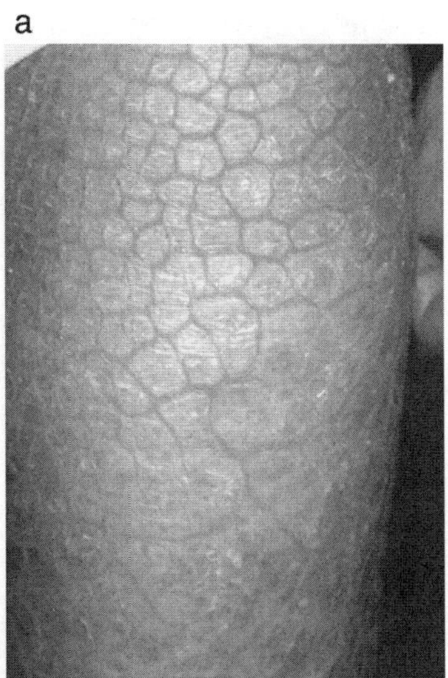

b

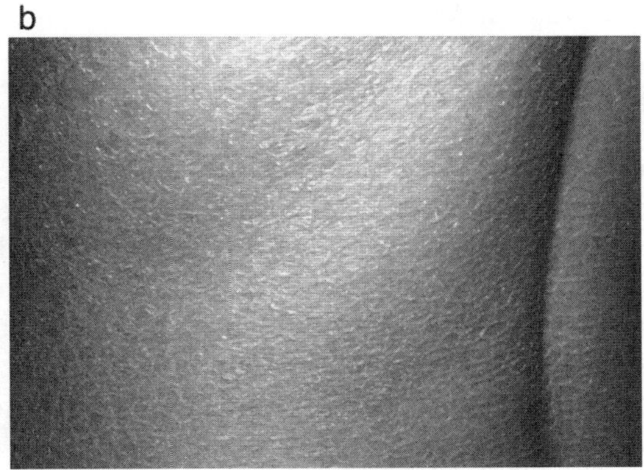

c

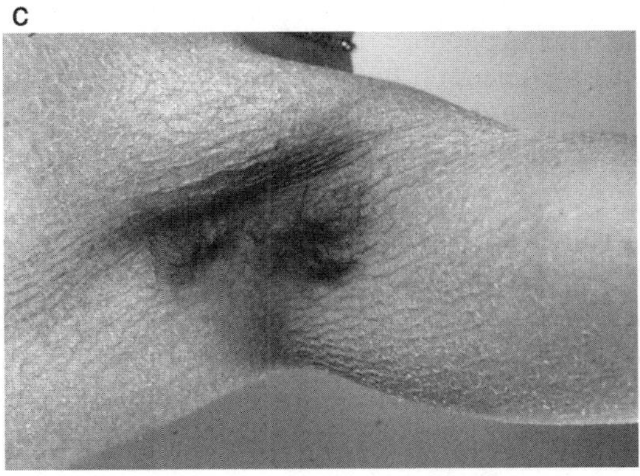

FIGURE 4 Examples of clinical variants of lamellar ichthyosis (LI) and nonbullous congenital ichthyosiform erythroderma (NBCIE). (a) Large scales on the thigh of a man with LI due to transglutaminase mutation, (b) generalized scaling on the trunk of a woman without transglutaminase mutation, and (c) scaling and mild erythroderma in the axillae of a woman also without transglutaminase mutation (c). (From the author's files).

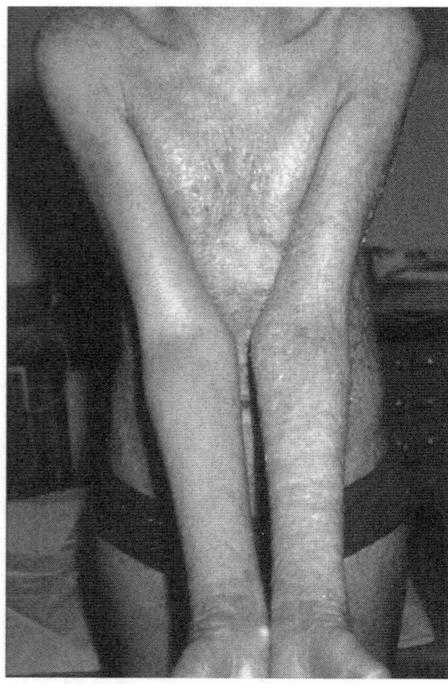

FIGURE 5 Effect of 4 weeks of treatment b.i.d. with a cream base containg 5% lactic acid and 20% propylene glycol on the right arm vs. 5% urea on the left arm. The trunk was treated with indifferent emollients. (Reproduced from Gånemo, A., Virtanen, M., and Vahlquist, A., *Br J Dermatol,* in press. With permission.)

10.7 BULLOUS ICHTHYOSIS, A KERATIN DISORDER

Epidermolytic hyperkeratosis (EHK) and the closely related diseases ichthyosis bulluosa of Siemens, epidermolytic palmo-plantar hyperkeratosis, and pachonychia congenita are all due to dominant negative keratin mutations expressed in the suprabasal layers of epidermis.[37-39] Depending on which keratin pair is affected (K1/10, K2e/9, or K6/16,17), keratinocytes in different parts of the epidermis will collapse, resulting in blisters that easily rupture. Concurrently, however, other parts of the epidermis will remain hyperkeratotic, leading to a mixture of oozing and dry skin lesions that easily become infected.[1] The flexural areas are usually severely affected, but some patients also have a more widespread verrucous type of ichthyosis (Figure 6).

The treatment of EHK is complex. On the one hand, hyperkeratosis should be reduced to minimize the disfiguring and foul-smelling scales. On the other hand, blisters and erosions must be protected and allowed to heal. Thus, a too potent keratolytic treatment will often aggravate the condition by disrupting the epidermal barrier and increasing the risk for painful and easily infected wounds. More than ever the treatment of different body areas has to be individualized.

The problem is the same with topical or systemic retinoids.[40] Although some patients are improved by oral acitretin, the dose must be kept low in order to avoid the epidermolytic side effect of the drug. Other patients actually get worse during retinoid therapy. However, correctly used, even topical tretinoin may be clearly effective in some patients with EHK (Figure 7). It is possible that the response to retinoids is determined by which type of keratin mutation (K1 or K10) underlies the condition (Virtanen and Vahlquist, unpublished observation). As of yet, the topical treatment of EHK mostly relies on the use of bland emollients and a liberal prescription of antiseptics and antibiotics to prevent bacterial infection of the skin.

10.8 EXAMPLES OF OTHER RARE TYPES OF ICHTHYOSIS-LIKE CONDITIONS

Netherton's syndrome (ichthyosis circumflexa and atopic dermatitis) is a congenital disease of unknown etiology. Neonatally, the barrier defect associated with generalized erythroderma may be

a

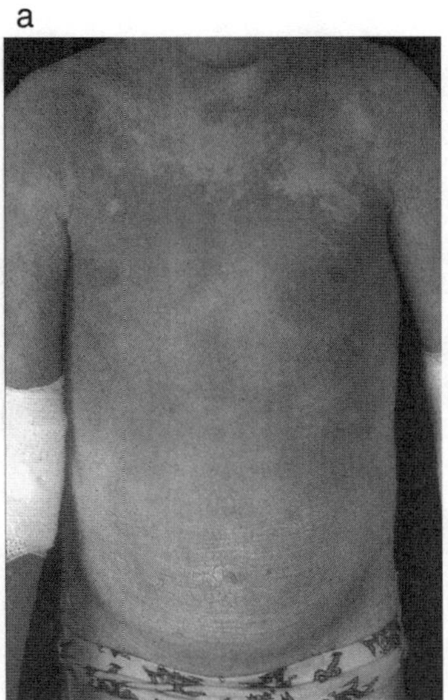

b

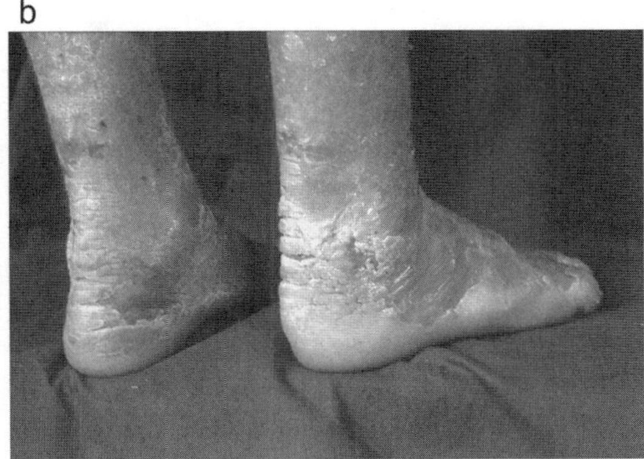

c

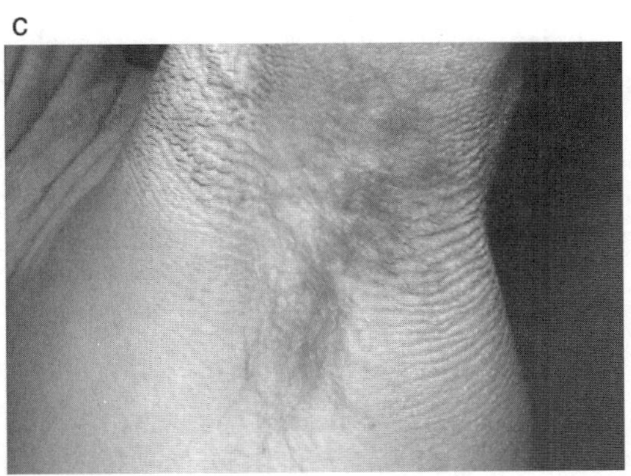

FIGURE 6 Epidermolytic hyperkeratosis in a 10-year-old boy showing (a) extensive hyperkeratosis on the trunk and (b) erosions and scaling around the ankle; and (c) verrucous hyperkeratosis in the axilla of a 25-year-old man carrying a spontaneous deletion in one of his K1 alleles (Vahlquist et al., unpublished observations).

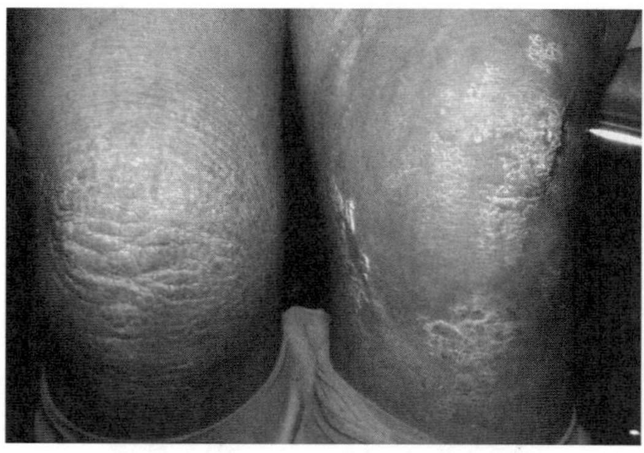

FIGURE 7 Successful topical treatment of EHK with a tretinoin-containing cream on the left knee of a woman with inherited K10 mutation (Vahlquist et al., unpublished observations).

life threatening and can cause severe hyponatrinemia.[1] When children grow older, the ichthyosis become less severe and usually responsive to ordinary topical treatment.

Darier disease (keratosis follicularis) is an autosomal dominant disorder of keratinization which usually starts at puberty. The skin problems have some resemblence to EHK in that hyperkeratosis and acantholysis coexist. However, the cause of the disease is completely different, in this case involving an endoplasmatic ATPase called SERCA2.[41]

There are many types of neuroectodermal syndromes that show ichthyosis as a presenting symptom. Perhaps the most well-known examples are Sjögren-Larsson syndrome and Refsum disease, both of which represent inborn errors of the lipid metabolism.[42,43] Although treatment aiming at rectifying the abnormal accumulation of lipid metabolites in skin and nervous tissue has improved ichthyosis in some cases of Refsum disease, most patients require additional therapy of the same type as in common ichthyosis.

Identification of various other syndromes associated with a vulgaris-like type of ichthyosis is also feasible, as exemplified in recent reports of the so-called KLICK syndrome.[44] Finally, it is important to know that aquired ichthyosis resembling IV and XRI has been noted in association with certain malignancies and as a side effect of hyperlipidemic drugs.[45]

10.9 CONCLUSIONS AND PROSPECTS FOR THE FUTURE

Ichthyosis can be a disabling condition requiring laborious treatments several times a day, but may also be a relatively mild disorder which only occasionally needs application of emollients. From a diagnostic as well as therapeutic point of view, the many different subtypes of ichthyosis represent a problem for the caring physician. For example, a paradoxic combination of barrier failure and massive hyperkeratosis in some types of ichthyosis demands special attention. Choosing the right treatment will be even more important in the future when new therapeutic regimes based on more-detailed knowledge about the pathogenesis of ichthyosis will emerge.

REFERENCES

1. Traupe, H., *The Ichthyoses: A Guide to Clinical Diagnosis, Genetic Counselling and Therapy,* Springer-Verlag, New York, 1989.
2. Mevorah, B., Frenk, E., and Pescia, G., Ichthyosis vulgaris showing features of the autosomal dominant and the x-linked recessive variants in the same family, *Clin Genet,* 13, 462, 1978.
3. Wells, R. and Kerr, C., Clinical features of autosomal dominant and sex-linked ichthyosis in an English population, *Br Med J,* 54, 947, 1966.

4. Jobsis, A., van Duuren, C., de Vries, G., et al., Trophoblast sulfate deficiency associated with x-linked ichthyosis, *Ned Tijdschr Geneeskd,* 120, 1980, 1976.
5. Shapiro, L. and Weiss, R., X-linked ichthyosis due to steroid sulfatase deficiency, *Lancet,* 14, 70, 1978.
6. Bousema, M., van Diggelen, O., van Joost, T., Stolz, E., and Naafs, F., Ichthyosis: reliability of clinical signs in the differentiation between autosomal dominant and sex-linked forms, *Int J Dermatol,* 28, 240, 1989.
7. Okano, M., Kitano, Y., Yoshikawa, K., Nakamura, T., Matsuzawa, Y., and Yuasa, T., X-linked ichthyosis and ichthyosis vulgaris: comparison of their clinical features based on biochemical analysis, *Br J Dermatol,* 119, 777, 1988.
8. Ibsen, H., Brandrup, F., Blaabjerg, I., and Lykkesfeldt, G., Lipoprotein electrophoresis in recessive x-linked ichthyosis, *Acta Derm Venereol,* 66, 59, 1986.
9. Sybert, V., Dale, B., and Holbrook, K., Ichthyosis vulgaris: identification of a defect in synthesis of filaggrin correlated with an absence of keratohyaline granules, *J Invest Dermatol,* 84, 191, 1985.
10. Nirunsuksiri, W., Presland, R. B., Brumbaugh, S. G., Dale, B. A., and Fleckman, P., Decreased profilaggrin expression in ichthyosis vulgaris is a result of selectively impaired posttranscriptional control, *J Biol Chem,* 270, 871, 1995.
11. Anton-Lamprecht, I., Ultrastructural identification of basic abnormalities as clues to genetic disorders of the epidermis, *J Invest Dermatol,* 103, 6S, 1994.
12. Scott, I., Harding, C., and Barrett, J., Histidine-rich protein of the keratohyalin granules. Source of the free amino acids, urocanic acid and pyrrolidone carboxylic acid in the stratum corneum, *Biochim Biophys Acta,* 719, 110, 1982.
13. Williams, M. and Elias, P., Increased cholesterol sulfate content of stratum corneum in recessive x-linked ichthyosis, *J Clin Invest,* 68, 1404, 1981.
14. Lavrijsen, A., Oestmann, E., Hermans, J., Bodde, H., Vermeer, B., and Ponec, M., Barrier function parameters in various keratinzation disorders: transepidermal water loss and vascular response to hexyl nicotinate, *Br J Dermatol,* 129, 547, 1993.
15. Zettersten, E., Man, M.-Q., Sato, J., Denda, M., Farrell, A., Ghadially, R., Williams, M., Feingold, K., and Elias, P., Recessive x-linked ichthyosis: role of cholesterol sulfate accumualtion in the barrier abnormality, *J Invest Dermatol,* 111, 784, 1998.
16. Sato, J., Denda, M., Nakanishi, J., Nomura, J., and Koyama, J., Cholesterol sulfate inhibits proteases that are involved in desquamation of stratum corneum, *J Invest Dermatol,* 111, 189, 1998.
17. Öhman, H. and Vahlquist, A., The pH gradient over the stratum corneum differs in x-linked recessive and autosomal dominant ichthyosis: a clue to the molecular origin of the acid skin mantle?, *J. Invest Dermatol,* 111, 674, 1998.
18. Vahlquist, A., Variations in skin pH during normal and pathologic keratinisation, *Retinoids Lipid-soluble Vitamins Clinical Practice,* 15, 50, 1999.
19. Lykkesfeldt, G. and Hoyer, H., Topical cholesterol treatment of recessive x-linked ichthyosis, *Lancet,* 2, 1337, 1983.
20. Swanbeck, G., A new treatment of ichthyosis and other hyperkeratotic conditions, *Acta Derm Venereol,* 48, 123, 1968.
21. van Scott, E. and Yu, R., Control of keratinization with alpha-hydroxy acids and related compounds, *Arch Dermatol,* 110, 586, 1974.
22. Traupe, H. and Happle, R., Etretinate therapy in children with severe keratinization defects, *Eur J Pediatr,* 143, 166, 1985.
23. Küster, W., Bohnsack, K., Rippke, F., Upmeyer, H., Groll, S., and Traupe, H., Efficacy of urea therapy in children with ichthyosis, *Dermatology,* 196, 217, 1998.
24. Huber, M., Rettle, I., Berbasconi, K., Frenk, E., Lavrijsen, S., Ponec, M., Bon, A., Lautenschlager, S., Schorderet, D., and Hohl, D., Mutations of keratinocyte transglutaminase in lamellar ichthyosis, *Science,* 267, 525, 1995.
25. Choate, K. A., Williams, M. L., and Khavari, P. A., Abnormal transglutaminase 1 expression pattern in a subset of patients with erythrodermic autosomal recessive ichthyosis, *J Invest Dermatol,* 110, 8, 1998.
26. Hennies, H. C., Kuster, W., Wiebe, V., Krebsova, A., and Reis, A., Genotype/phenotype correlation in autosomal recessive lamellar ichthyosis, *Am J Hum Genet,* 62, 1052, 1998.

27. Parmentier, L., Lakhdar, H., Blanchet-Bardon, C., Marchand, S., Dubertret, L., and Weissenbach, J., Mapping of a second locus for lamellar ichthyosis to chromosome 2q33-35, *Hum Mol Genet,* 5, 555, 1996.
28. Vahlquist, A., Role of retinoids in normal and diseased skin, in *Vitamin A in Health and Disease*, ed. R. Blomhoff, Marcel Dekker, Inc., New York, 1994, 365.
29. Beverley, D. and Wheller, D., High plasma urea concentrations in collodion babies, *Arch Dis Child,* 61, 696, 1986.
30. Gånemo, A. and Vahlquist, A., Lamellar ichthyosis is markedly improved by a novel combination of emollients, *Br J Dermatol,* 137, 1011, 1997.
31. Gånemo, A., Virtanen, M., and Vahlquist, A., Improved topical treatment of lamellar ichthyosis: a double-blind study of four different cream mixtures, *Br J Dermatol,* in press.
32. Stege, H., Hofmann, B., Ruzicka, T., and Lehmann, P., Topical application of tazarotene in the treatment of nonerythrodermic lamellar ichthyosis, *Arch Dermatol,* 134, 640, 1998.
33. Steijlen, P. M., Reifenschweiler, D. O. H., Ramaekers, F. C. S., Vanmuijen, G. N. P., Happle, R., Link, M., Ruiter, D. J., and van de Kerkhof, P. C. M., Topical treatment of ichthyoses and Darier's disease with 13-cis-retinoic acid — a clinical and immunohistochemical study, *Arch Dermatol Res,* 285, 221, 1993.
34. van Wauwe, J., Vannyen, G., Coene, M. C., Stoppie, P., Cools, W., Goossens, J., Borghgraef, P., and Janssen, P. A. J., Liarozole, an inhibitor of retinoic acid metabolism, exerts retinoid-mimetic effects in vivo, *J Pharmacol Exp Ther,* 261, 773, 1992.
35. Vandekerkhof, P. C. M., Biological activity of vitamin D analogues in the skin, with special reference to antipsoriatic mechanisms, *Br J Dermatol,* 132, 675, 1995.
36. Kiistala, R., Lauharanta, J., and Kanerva, L., Transepidermal water loss and sweat gland response in lamellar ichthyosis before and during treatment with etretinate: report of three cases, *Acta Derm Venereol,* 62, 268, 1982.
37. Leigh, I. and Lane, E., Mutations in the genes for epidermal keratins in epidermolysis bullosa and epidermolytic hyperkeratosis, *Arch Dermatol,* 129, 1571, 1993.
38. Bowden, P. E., Haley, J. L., Kansky, A., Rothnagel, J. A., Jones, D. O., and Turner, R. J., Mutation of a type II keratin gene (K6a) in pachyonychia congenita, *Nat Genet,* 10, 363, 1995.
39. Fuchs, E. and Cleveland, D. W., A structural scaffolding of intermediate filaments in health and disease, *Science,* 279, 514, 1998.
40. Steijlen, P. M., Vandoorengreebe, R. J., Happle, R., and Vandekerkhof, P. C. M., Ichthyosis bullosa of Siemens responds well to low-dosage oral retinoids, *Br J Dermatol,* 125, 469, 1991.
41. Sakuntabhai, A., Ruiz-Perez, V., Carter, S., Jacobsen, N., Burge, S., Monk, S., Smith, M., Munro, C. S., O'Donovan, M., Craddock, N., Kucherlapati, R., Rees, J. L., Owen, M., Lathrop, M., Monaco, A. P., Strachan, T., and Hovnanian, A., Mutations in ATP2A2, encoding a pump, cause Darier disease, *Nat. Genet.,* 21, 271, 1999.
42. DeLaurenzi, V., Rogers, G., Hamrock, D., et al. Sjögren-Larsson syndrome is caused by mutations in the fatty aldehyde dehydrognease gene, *Nat Genet,* 12, 52, 1996.
43. Herndon, J., Steinberg, D., and Uhlendorf, B., Refsum's disease: defective oxidation of phytanic acid in tissue cultures derived from homozygotes and heterozygotes, *N Engl J Med,* 281, 1034, 1969.
44. Vahlquist, A., Ponten, F., and Pettersson, A., Keratosis linearis with ichthyosis congenita and sclerosing keratoderma (KLICK-syndrome): a rare, autosomal recessive disorder of keratohyaline formation?, *Acta Derm Venereol*, 77, 225, 1997.
45. Williams, M., Feingold, K., Grubauer, G., and Elias, P., Ichthyosis induced by cholesterol-lowering drugs, *Arch Dermatol,* 123, 1535, 1987.
46. Elias, P., Epidermal lipids, barrier function, and desquamation, *J Invest Dermatol,* 80, 44s, 1983.
47. Kiguchi, K., Kagehara, M., Higo, R., Iwamori, M., and DiGiovanni, J., Alterations in cholesterol sulfate and its biosynthetic enzyme during multistage carcinogenesis in mouse skin, *J Invest Dermatol,* 111, 973, 1999.
48. Chida, K., Murakami, A., Tagawa, T., Ikuta, T., and Kuroki, T., Cholesterol sulfate, a second messenger for the n isoform of protein kinase C, inhibits promotional phase in mouse skin carcinogenesis, *Cancer Res,* 55, 4865, 1995.

49. Denning, M., Kazanietz, M., Blumber, P., and Yuspa, S., Cholesterol sulfate activates multiple protein kinase C isoenzymes and induces granular cell differenation in culture murine keratinoyctes, *Cell Growth Differ,* 6, 1619, 1995.
50. Kawabe, S., Ikuta, T., Ohba, M., Chida, K., Ueda, E., Yamanishi, K., and Kuroki, T., Cholesterol sulfate activates transcription of transglutaminase 1 gene in normal human keratinocytes, *J Invest Dermatol,* 111, 1098, 1998.
51. Jetten, A., George, M., and Rearick, J., Down-regulation of squamous cell-specific markers by retinoids: transglutaminase 1 and cholesterol sulfotransferase, *Methods Enzymol,* 190, 42, 1990.

11 Dry Skin in Atopic Dermatitis and Patients on Hemodialysis

Motoji Takahashi and Zenro Ikezawa

CONTENTS

11.1 SUMMARY

We investigated the characteristics of the dry skin in patients with atopic dermatitis (AD) and those on hemodialysis (HD) using noninvasive methods. Transepidermal water loss (TEWL), water content, parakeratotic cells, free amino acid and ceramide in stratum corneum (SC), and skin surface pH were examined on lesional and nonlesional skin in the dorsolumbar part of AD patients, HD patients, and healthy normal controls. The water content in SC on lesional and nonlesional skin was markedly lower in the AD patients than in the normal controls. The water content in SC was also lower in HD patients. The level of free amino acids, which represents the natural moisturizing factor (NMF) in SC, was decreased in both patient groups, which corresponded with the decrease of their water content in SC. TEWL was high in AD patients, but that in HD patients was almost similar to that in the controls. The level of the ceramides, which are closely related to the barrier function of SC, was lower in AD patients than in HD patients or in the controls, which was in agreement with the results of TEWL. In the composition of ceramides, the HD patients showed a

0-8493-7520-7/00/$0.00+$.50

higher percentage of ceramides 2 and 3 and a lower ratio of 1, 4/5, and 6 in comparison with the controls. No parakeratotic corneocytes were found in the controls or HD patients, while they were found in not only the lesional but also nonlesional skin of AD patients, indicating the presence of mild inflammation even in nonlesional skin. The conversion ratio of ornithine, which is a free amino acid component in SC, to citrulline was lower in AD patients than in HD patients or the controls. This suggested increased epidermal proliferation in AD patients. The skin surface pH value was high in both AD and HD patients, and the latter showed a higher value than the former. Except for pH, the results of all of the measurements in the nonlesional skin of AD patients were found to be intermediate between those of the lesional skin and the normal controls, showing that the lesional skin is physiologically different from the nonlesional skin.

These findings suggested that the decrease in free amino acids (= NMF) and inferior barrier function of SC caused the dry skin of AD patients, but the decrease of NMF mainly caused the dry skin in HD patients.

Keywords: atopic dermatitis, hemodialysis, dry skin, skin surface conductance, TEWL, free amino acid, ceramide

11.2 INTRODUCTION

Many important allergic aspects of AD have been reported. For example, most patients show high serum IgE levels due to high response of IgE antibody to various allergens such as foods, dust, mites, and fungi. Also, they show an increase of eosinophils and eosinophil-derived mediators such as eosinophilic cationic protein and major basic proteins in blood during exacerbation of AD. Among the nonallergic aspects of AD, the skin is also known to tend to overreact to irritation and become dry, particularly in winter. Many researchers have analyzed the characteristics of the dryness in skin lesions of AD from the viewpoint of the functions of the SC. Decreased water content in SC,[1,2] enhanced TEWL,[3,4] shortening of the turnover time of SC,[3] reduction of ceramide levels,[5-7] decrease of free amino acid level,[3] and increase of skin surface pH[8] have been reported. However, few investigators have analyzed, compared, and discussed these properties in lesional and nonlesional skin.

On the other hand, although dry skin or skin itchiness has frequently been recognized together with pigmentation in the patients with chronic kidney failure and receiving HD,[9] only a few reports have been made on the characteristics of dry skin (e.g., high pH,[10] decrease of water content in SC, and low TEWL[11]).

Here, we will report the characteristics of dry skin observed in lesional and nonlesional skin of AD patients and patients with chronic kidney failure and undergoing HD from the viewpoints of various functions of SC.

11.3 SUBJECTS AND METHODS

11.3.1 Subjects

The study subjects included 48 patients with AD (27 male and 21 female), 22 patients undergoing HD (7 male and 15 female), and 30 healthy volunteers (15 male and 15 female) who served as controls (Table 1).

11.3.2 Skin Regions and Timing for Measurements

Skin measurements were always made on the dorsolumbar region in HD patients and healthy subjects and whenever possible for lesional and nonlesional skin in AD patients. In some cases, meaurements on the nonlesional skin could not be made because a sufficient area could not be obtained.

TABLE 1
Age Distribution of Subjects

Age Distribution (Years)	Atopic Dermatitis		Hemodialysis		Normal Controls	
	Male	Female	Male	Female	Male	Female
3~9	1	5				
10~19	11	8				1
20~29	7	5			8	11
30~39	6	1			6	3
40~49	1			2	1	
50~59		1			6	
60~69		1	4	4		
70~79	1		3	3		
Total	27	21	7	15	15	15
Mean ± SD	23.3 ± 14.4		64.0 ± 10.1		27.8 ± 4.9	

The targeted skin regions were cleaned with ethanol and distilled water 30 min before the start of measurement. Measurements were made at an ambient temperature of 21 to 23°C and relative humidity of 35 to 50% from December to February when the skin was apt to become dry.

11.4 MEASUREMENTS

11.4.1 Water Content in Stratum Corneum

Skin surface conductance (μS) was determined with Skicon-100 (IBS Company, Hamamatsu, Japan) by measurement of water content in SC. Nine measurements were repeated at a single point, and the mean was taken after excluding the highest and lowest values.

11.4.2 Transepidermal Water Loss (TEWL)

Transepidermal water loss ($g/m^2/h$) was determined with Evaporimeter EP-1 (Servo Med Company, Sweden). Measurements were repeated twice, and the mean was calculated.

11.4.3 Skin Surface pH

Distilled water was dropped on the surface of the skin, and pH was determined with a pH meter (Model D-12, Horiba Manufacturing Co., Ltd., Tokyo, Japan).

11.4.4 Parakeratotic Index of Stratum Corneum

The method of Koyama et al.[12] was used to determine the parakeratotic index of SC. A glass plate was attached to the skin with Scotch tape (Sumitomo 3M, Tokyo, Japan) measuring 25 × 19 mm to remove corneocytes. The adherent horny material was stained with hematoxylin-eosin solution for microscopic inspection of nuclei. The results were scored depending on the number of the nucleated cells in the visual field (0 = none, 1 = small, 2 = relatively large, 3 = very large).

11.4.5 Free Amino Acid in Stratum Corneum

The method proposed by Horii et al.[13] was used for the measurement of free amino acid. The SC was stripped with adhesive cellophane tape (Cello-tape, Nichiban Co. Ltd., Tokyo, Japan). The tape was immersed in toluene to remove the SC, which was then washed with toluene several times and dried in a vacuum desiccator. One milligram of dried sample of SC was precisely weighed and homogenized with 0.1% of sulfosalicylic acid. After centrifugation the supernatant was analyzed with a high-speed amino acid analyzer (Model 835, Hitachi, Tokyo, Japan) to determine the level of total amino acid, ornithine, and citrulline. The conversion ratio of ornithine to citrulline {Cit/(Orn + Cit)} was calculated as an index of amino acid metabolism in the epidermis.

11.4.6 Ceramides in Stratum Corneum

The method of Denda et al.[14] was used to measure ceramides. After SC was stripped with adhesive cellophane tape, it was removed from the tape and washed several times with hexane, followed by drying in a vacuum desiccator. Lipids were extracted from the SC sample in a mixture of chloroform/methanol (2:1). Ceramides were separated with a silica gel column (Bond Elut Sl, Analytichem International, U.S.) and purified for measurement by gas chromatography (GC-14A, Shimazu Manufacturing Co., Ltd., Japan). The composition of ceramides was obtained by high-performance thin layer chromatography and scanned on a recording photodensitometer (TLC Scanner CS930, Shimazu, Japan).

11.5 RESULTS

11.5.1 Water Content in Stratum Corneum

The water content at both lesional and nonlesional sites was markedly lower in the AD patients than in the normal controls (Figure 1). Furthermore, the water content in the lesional skin was lower than that in nonlesional skin, but no significant difference could be recognized between them. The skin surface conductance was also lower in HD patients than in the controls (under one tenth), and the skin of HD patients was dry to the same extent as in AD patients. As the mean age of patients undergoing HD was higher than that in the controls, it is difficult to make a precise comparison without matching the age of the two groups. However, considering the finding that aging did not affect the skin surface conductance on the face,[15] and Kumasaka's[16] report that skin conductance on the crus in the young was about three times as large as that in the elderly, the extent of the dryness in HD patients was larger than the aging effect.

11.5.2 Transepidermal Water Loss

TEWL in both regions was three to four times higher in AD patients than in the control (Figure 2), and the lesional skin gave higher values than the nonlesional skin ($p < 0.05$). On the other hand, the TEWL was only slightly higher in HD patients than in the control (mean value: HD patients, 7.0 $g/m^2/h$, the control, 5.0 $g/m^2/h$). The barrier function of SC in HD patients was similar to that in the control.

11.5.3 Skin Surface pH

AD patients showed a higher pH at lesional and nonlesional sites than the controls ($p < 0.01$). However, the difference between the two sites was not significant. The pH was significantly higher ($p < 0.01$) in HD patients than in the controls (Figure 3).

11.5.4 Parakeratotic Cells in Stratum Corneum

Figure 4 shows the appearence of typical parakeratotic cells in SC obtained by skin surface biopsy with tape stripping. As Figure 5 shows, no nucleated cells were found in either the controls or HD patients, but they were observed frequently on the lesional skin of AD patients. In some AD patients (16 of 31), they were also found on the nonlesional skin.

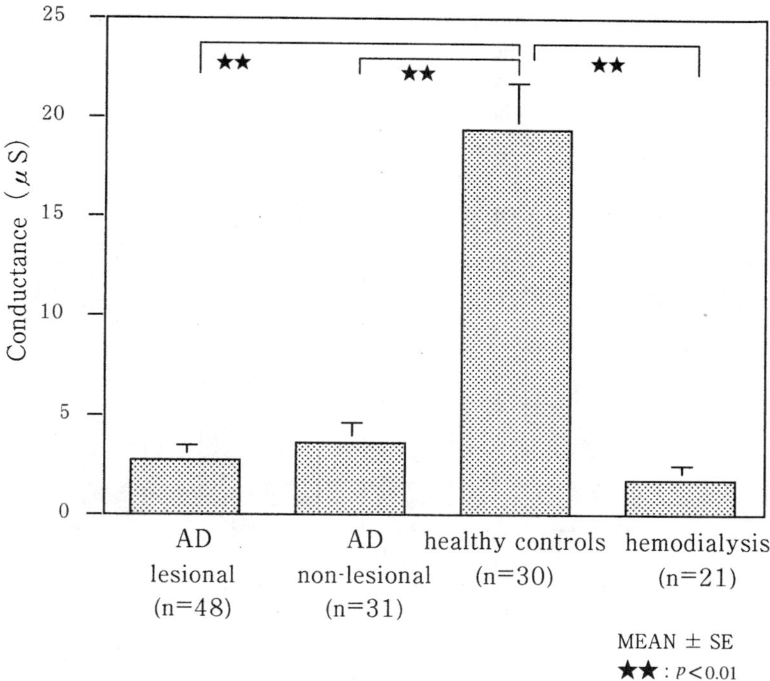

FIGURE 1 Water content in the SC of patients with AD and those on HD.

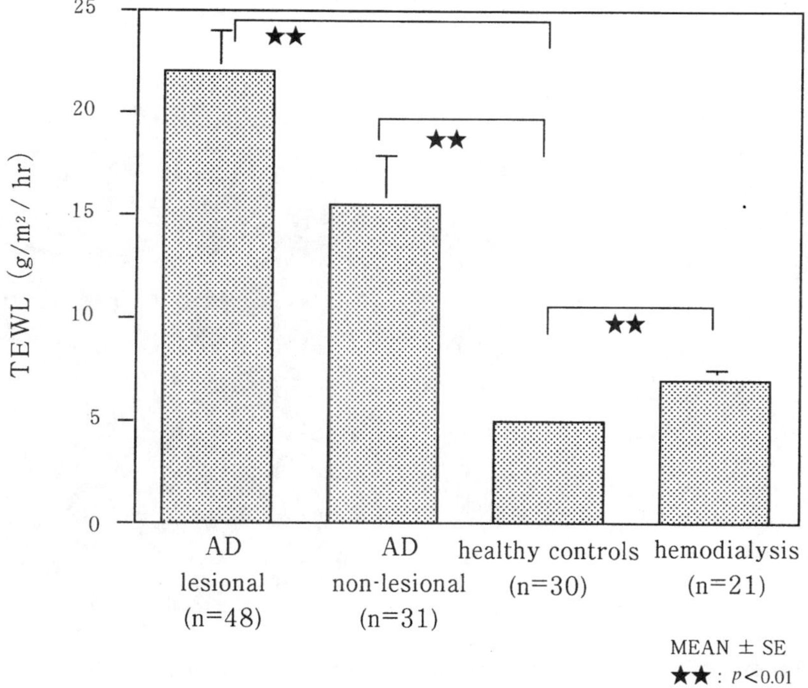

FIGURE 2 TEWL in patients with AD and those on HD.

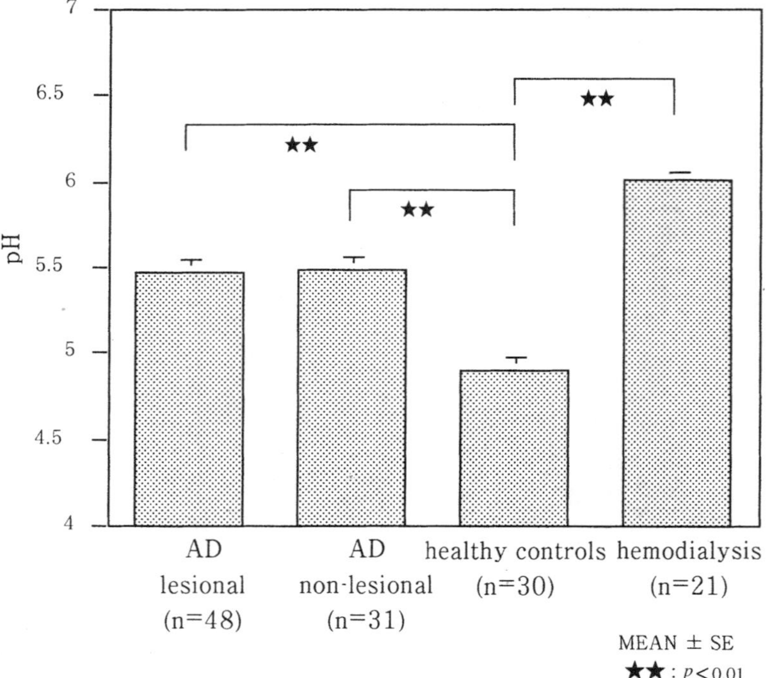

FIGURE 3 Skin surface pH in patients with AD and those on HD.

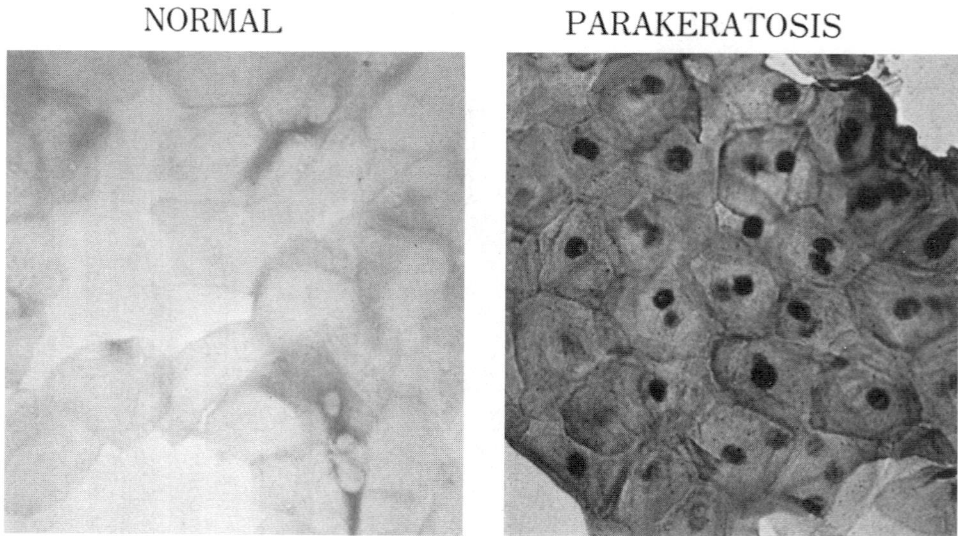

FIGURE 4 Parakeratotic cells detected in the SC obtained by tape stripping. Cells were stained with a hematoxylin-eosin solution.

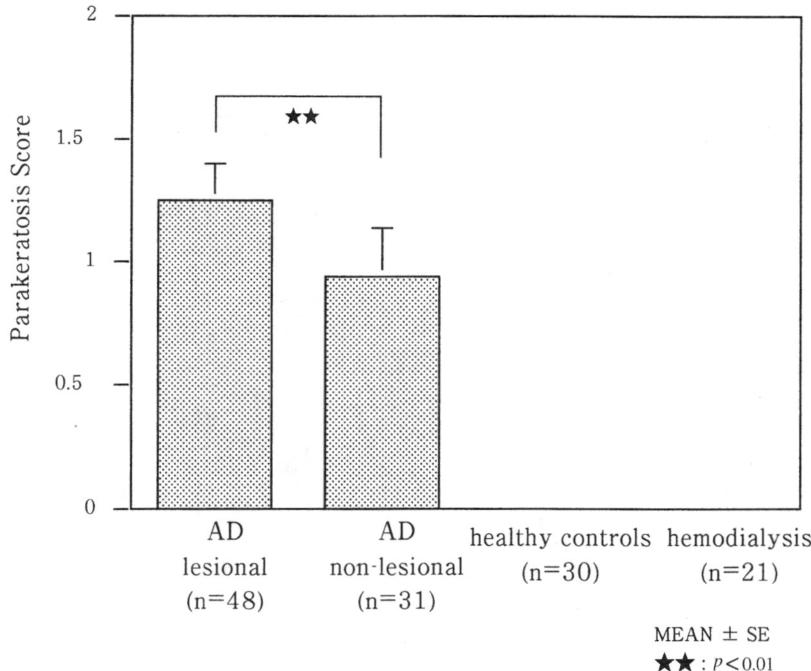

FIGURE 5 Parakeratotic cells in the superficial SC of patients with AD and those on HD.

11.5.5 Free Amino Acid Content in Stratum Corneum

As Figure 6 shows, the levels of free amino acids contained in 1 mg of dry SC were in decreasing order of the controls, HD patients, nonlesional skin of AD patients, and lesional skin of AD patients. Free amino acids act as a moisture holding factor in SC,[17] and their contents are correlated with skin surface conductance.[13] The amino acid levels in both AD and HD patients who had low skin surface conductance were less than half of the control levels. The conversion ratio of ornithine to citrulline {Cit/(Orn+Cit)} is related to the degree of cornification disorder and is negatively correlated with the epidermal proliferation rate.[12] As Table 2 shows, conversion ratios were similar in HD patients and the controls, but showed a significant difference ($p < 0.05$). On the other hand, the conversion ratio of ornithine to citrulline was markedly lower in AD patients, which indicated that the epidermal proliferation was increased in AD patients.

11.5.6 Ceramide Levels in Stratum Corneum

In both lesional and nonlesional sites the ceramide levels were lower in the AD patients than in the controls (Figure 7). This result was in agreement with previous reports.[6,7] The lesional skin gave lower levels than the nonlesional skin on average, but no significant difference could be found. However, the levels were higher in HD patients than in the controls ($p < 0.05$). The quantity of intercellular lipids (or ceramide) was closely related to TEWL.[18,19] This study revealed that ceramide levels were high in the control and HD patients whose TEWLs were low, while AD patients with high TEWL showed low ceramide levels.

Ceramides are classfied into five species (ceramide 1, 2, 3, 4/5, 6) according to their polarity. Yamamoto et al.[6] and Imokawa et al.[7] have reported that AD shows a significant decrease in the proportion of ceramide 1, which is a carrier of linoleate and responsible for water-barrier function.

In HD patients, the proportions of ceramides 2 and 3 were high and those of ceramides 1, 4/5, and 6 were low in comparison with the normal controls.

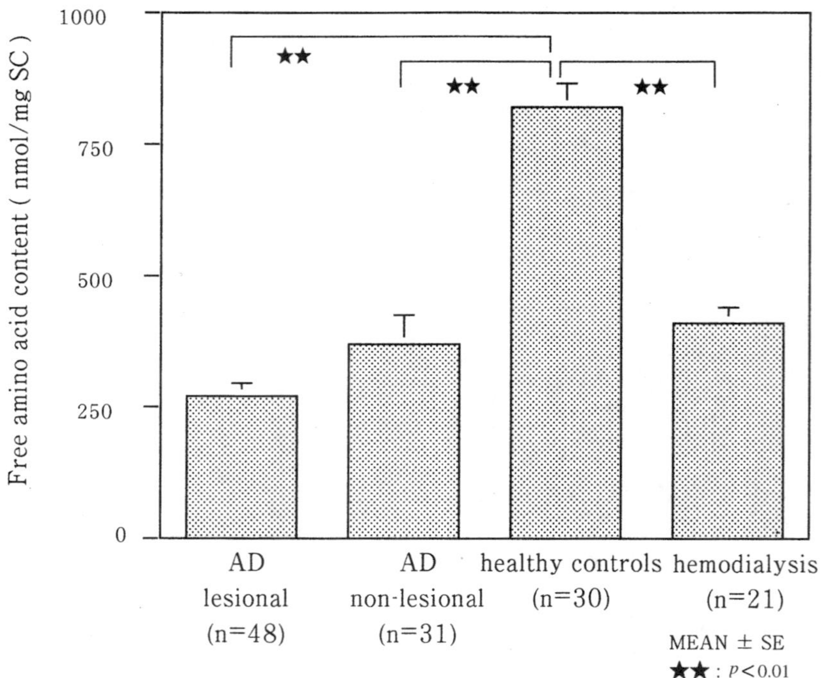

FIGURE 6 Free amino acids in the SC of patients with AD and those on HD.

TABLE 2
Conversion Ratio of Ornithine to Citrulline

	n	Cit/(Orn+Cit) %
AD lesional	48	69.8 ± 2.8[a]
AD nonlesional	31	75.0 ± 2.6[a]
Hemodialysis	21	88.3 ± 1.3[b]
Healthy controls	30	91.8 ± 1.0
		mean ± S.E.

[a] $p < 0.01$ compared with healthy controls.
[b] $p < 0.05$ compared with healthy controls.

11.6 DISCUSSION

The characteristics of the dry skin of AD patients have been widely studied. However, those of HD patients have not been studied in detail, although they also show dry skin with itchiness as in AD patients. In this study, we investigated the functions of SC to characterize the dry skin of AD and HD patients by noninvasive methods.

The water content in SC was low both in AD and HD patients, and their skin was obviously dry. However, there was a great difference between them in TEWL. The TEWL was high in AD patients accompanied with extremely inferior barrier function of SC, while HD patients showed a slightly higher TEWL than the controls and their barrier function proved to be in the mostly normal range. The findings obtained in HD patients resembled the symptoms of senile xerosis[20,21] and

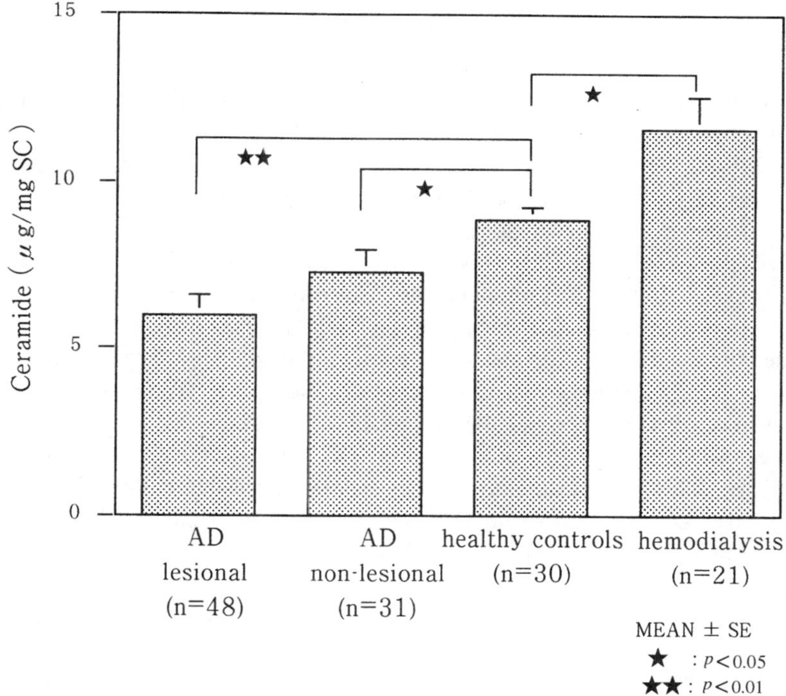

FIGURE 7 Ceramide in the SC of patients with AD and those on HD.

coincided with those reported by Kamiya et al.[11] The difference in TEWL between AD and HD patients and the low water content in SC in both groups were explained by the difference in ceramide levels and low free amino acid levels, respectively.

The extent of parakeratosis was determined by the microscopic inspection of nucleated cells in SC. Parakeratotic cells were detected at a high frequency on the lesional skin of AD patients and were also found on the nonlesional skin in some cases, but at a much lower frequency. This indicates the presence of slight inflammation even at the nonlesional site. On the other hand, the absence of nucleated cells in SC indicated that the skin of HD patients as well as normal controls had no inflammation.

Free amino acids in SC are the metabolites of filaggrin originating from keratohyalin granules.[22] Furthermore, histidine is converted into urocanic acid, ornithine to citrulline, and glutamic acid to pyrrolidone carbonic acid.[12] The conversion ratio of ornithine to citrulline [Cit/(Orn+Cit)] and free amino acid content in SC decreased on the scaly inflammatory skin induced by surface active agents or tape stripping.[12,14] In the dry skin, caused by ichthyosis vulgaris[13] or radiation of UV rays[24] which shows a short turnover time of SC (namely, high proliferation rate in basal cells), the reduced free amino acid levels were recognized.[14,23] The significantly low conversion ratio of amino acids and the observation of some parakeratotic cells even in nonlesional skin suggested that hyperproliferation of keratinocytes induced by slight inflammation caused the decrease in free amino acid levels and the amino acid conversion ratio in AD.

On the other hand, the decrease of free amino acid levels in HD patients could be attributed to the decrease of keratohyalin granules or filaggrin, as found on the crus of the patient with senile xerosis[20,25] or of the elderly,[26] and not to the inflammation nor to the increased epidermal proliferation, because the conversion ratio of amino acid was similar to those in the control and no parakeratotic cells could be observed.

A decrease in ceramide levels and abnormalities in the formation of lamellar bodies and in the extrude process of their components into the corneocytes spaces have been reported in AD patients.[28,29] According to Holleran et al.[30] and Menon et al.,[31] in normal skin ceramides are produced in SC by degradation of glucosylceramides by beta-glucocerebrosidase and by hydrolysis of sphingomyelin by sphingomyelinase. In the epidermis of AD patients an altered metabolic pathway of sphingomyelin was suggested by Murata et al.[32] The activity of sphingomyelin acylase is enhanced, and then large amounts of sphingosylphosphorylcholine and free fatty acids are formed, but the amount of ceramides is decreased. However, no reports on the intercellular lipids in HD patients are available. The ceramide levels were higher than those in the controls. Nevertheless, they had slightly higher TEWL. This might be due to the difference in the composition of ceramides. Though TEWL is correlated with the amount of intercellular lipids, barrier function of the SC also depends on the composition or structure of the intercellular lipids.[33,34] We reported previously[14,23] that on dry skin caused by surface active agents or tape stripping, TEWL was increased with the lack of change in ceramide levels, but the proportion of ceramide 2 was increased while that of ceramide 4/5 decreased. HD patients showed a similar change, and the rise of TEWL was supposed to be caused by the disturbance of the orientation or structure of intercellular lipids. Both AD and HD patients showed a higher skin surface pH than the controls. Ishida et al.[10] have reported that HD patients showed a higher pH on the forehead, forearm, palm, and crus. Anderson[8] also reported that the dry skin in AD or ichthyosis vulgaris showed higher pH. Factors related to skin surface pH are (1) environmental factors, including atmospheric temperature and humidity, and bathing; (2) intracorporeal factors such as menstruation; and 3) factors based on the composition of the skin itself such as SC, sweat, and sebum. However, no established explanations are available yet.

It is quite interesting that the rise in skin surface pH might be related to the drying or itching of the skin in AD or HD patients. The higher pH in HD patients than in AD patients might be partially due to the higher frequency of parhidrosis in the former.

A significant difference was found only in TEWL between the lesional and nonlesional skin of AD patients. However, all the measurements on the nonlesional skin, except for skin surface pH, gave values intermediate between those on the lesional skin and those in the controls. Therefore, lesional and nonlesional skin might have some differences physiologically as well as clinically.

AD patients showed mild inflammation with induction of the parakeratosis, decreased moisture holding ability, and inferior barrier function, while HD patients showed only reduced moisture holding ability with almost normal skin barrier function but without inflammation. Then, it was concluded that the dry skin of AD patients resulted from the lack of moisture holding factor (free amino acids, NMF) and inferior barrier function of SC, while that in HD patients was mainly attributed to the decrease of the moisture holding factors.

REFERENCES

1. Werner Y. The water content of the stratum corneum in patients with atopic dermatitis. *Acta Derm Venereol* (Stockh). 66:281–284(1986).
2. Berardesca E, Fideli D, Borroni G, Maibach H. *In vivo* hydration and water-retention capacity of stratum corneum in clinically uninvolved skin in atopic and psoriatic patients. *Acta Derm Venereol (Stockh)*. 70:400–404(1990).
3. Watanebe M, Tagami H, Horii I, Takahashi M, Kligman AM. Functional analyses of the superficial stratum corneum in atopic xerosis. *Arch Dermatol.* 127:1689–1692(1991).
4. Werner Y, Lindberg M. Transepidermal water loss in dry and clinically normal skin in patients with atopic dermatitis. *Acta Derm Venereol (Stockh)*. 65:102–105(1985).
5. Melnik B, Hollmann J, Hofmann U, Yuh M-S, Plewig G. Lipid composition of outer stratum corneum and nails in atopic and control subjects. *Arch Dermatol Res.* 282:549–551(1990).

6. Yamamoto A, Serizawa S, Ito M, Sato Y. Stratum corneum lipid abnormalities in atopic dermatitis. *Arch Dermatol Res.* 283:219–223(1991).
7. Imokawa G, Abe A, Jin K, Higaki Y, Kawashima M, Hidano A. Decreased levels of ceramides in stratum corneum of atopic dermatitis: an etiologic factor in atopic dry skin. *J Invest Dermatol.* 96:523(1991).
8. Anderson DS. The acid-base balance of the skin. *Br J Dermatol.* 63:283–296(1951).
9. Nielson T, Anderson HKE, Kristansen J. Pruritus and xerosis in patients with chronic renal failure. *Dan Med Bull.* 27:269–271(1980).
10. Ishida K, Kamiya T, Tsuchiya S, Hattori A. Skin surface pH of hemodialysis patients. *Jpn J Dermatol.* 100:1275–1278(1990).
11. Kamiya T, Tsuchiya S, Hara K, Okamoto K, Hattori A, Taguchi N. Study of dry skin in chronic dialysis of skin surface hydration, transepidermal water loss and skin surface structure. *Jpn J Dermatol.* 98:425–430(1988).
12. Koyama J, Horii I, Kawasaki K, Nakayama Y, Morikawa Y, Mitsui T. Free amino acids of stratum corneum as a biochemical marker to evaluate dry skin. *J Soc Cosmet Chem.* 35:183–195(1984).
13. Horii I, Nakayama Y, Obata M, Tagami H. Stratum corneum hydration and amino acid content in xerotic skin. *Br J Dermatol.* 121:587–592(1989).
14 Denda M, Hori J, Koyama J, Yoshida S, Namba R, Takahashi M, Horii I, Yamamoto A, Stratum corneum sphingolipids and free amino acids inexperimentally-induced scaly skin. *Arch Dermatol Res.* 284:363–367(1992).
15. Takahashi M, Watanabe H, Kumagai H, Nakayama Y. Physiological and morphological changes in facial skin with aging. *J Soc Cosmet Chem Jpn.* 23:22–30(1989).
16. Kumasaka K. Functional analysis of the stratum corneum. *J Jpn Cosmet Sci Soc.* 15:254–260(1991).
17. Middleton JD. The mechanism of water binding in stratum corneum. *Br J Dermatol.* 80:437–450(1968).
18. Lampe MA, Burlingame AL, Whitny BJ, Williams ML, Brown BE, Roitman E, Elias PM. Human stratum corneum lipids: characterization and regional variations. *J Lipid Res.* 24:120–130(1983).
19. Grubauer G, Feingold RK, Harris RM, Elias PM. Lipid content and lipid type as determinants of the epidermal permeability barrier. *J Lipid Res.* 30:89–96 (1989).
20. Hara H, Kikuchi K, Watanabe M, Denda M, Koyama J, Nomura J, Horii I, Tagami H. Senile xerosis: functional, morphological, and biological studies. *J. Geriatric Dermatol.* 1,111–120(1993).
21. Sasaki Y, Hashimoto K, Tagami H. The study of the function of the stratum corneum in the aged skin. *J Jpn Cosmet Sci Soc.,* 12:90–94(1991).
22. Scott IR, Harding CR, Barrett JG. Histidine-rich protein of keratohyalin granules: source of the free amino acids, urocaninc acid and pyrrolidone carboxylic acid in the stratum corneum. *Biochim Biophys Acta.* 719:110–117 (1982).
23. Denda M, Koyama J, Takahashi M, Horii I. Changes of sphingolipids and free amino acids in surfactant induced scaly skin. *J Soc Cosmet Chem Jpn.* 27:589–596(1994).
24. Tsuchiya T, Horii I, Nakayama Y. Interrelationship between the change in the water content of the stratum corneum and the amount of natural moisturising factor of the stratum corneum after UVB irradiation. *J Soc Cosmet Chem Jpn.* 22:10–14(1988).
25. Tezuka T. Electron-microscopic changes in xerosis senile epidermis. Its abnormal membrane-coating granule formation. *Dermatologica.* 166:57–61(1983).
26. Tezuka T, Qing J, Saeki M, Kusuda S, Takahashi M. Terminal differentiation of facial epidermis of the aged: immunohistochemical studies. *Dermatology.* 188:21–24(1994).
27. Nooman FP, De Fabo EC, Morrison H. Cis-urocanic acid, a product formed by ultraviolet B irradiation of the skin, initiates an antigen presentation defect in splenic dendritic cells *in vivo. J Invest Dermatol.* 90:92–99(1988).
28. Werner Y, Lindberg M, Forslind B. Membrane-coating granules in 'dry' non-exzematous skin of patients with atopic dermatitis. Acta Derm Venereol (Stockh). 67:385–390(1987).
29. Fartasch M, Bassukas ID, Diepgen TL. Disturbed extruding mechanism of lamellar bodies in dry non-eczematous skin atopics. *Br J Dermatol.* 127:221–227(1992).
30. Holleran WM, Takagi Y, Menon GK, Legier G, Feingolg KR, Elias PM. Processing of epidermal glucocerebrosidase is required for optimal mammalian cutaneous permeability barrier function. *J Clin Invest.* 91:1656–1664(1993).

31. Menon GK, Grayson S, Elias PM. Cytochemical and biochemical localization of lipase and sphingo-myelinase activity in mammalian epidermis. *J Invest Dermatol.* 86:591–597(1986).
32. Murata Y, Ogata J, Higaki Y. Abnormal expression of sphingomyelin acylase in atopic dermatitis: an etiologic factor for ceramide deficiency? *J Invest Dermatol.* 106:1242–1249(1996).
33. Potts RO, Francoeur ML. The influence of stratum corneum morphology on water permeability. J Invest Dermatol.96:495–499(1991).
34. Golden GM, Guzek DB, Kennedy AH, McKie JE, Potts RO. Stratum corneum lipid phase transitions and water barrier properties. *Biochemistry.* 26:2382–2388(1987).

12 Experimentally Induced Dry Skin

Mitsuhiro Denda

CONTENTS

12.1 INTRODUCTION

Dry, scaly skin is characterized by a decrease in the water retention capacity of the stratum corneum (SC),[1] with water content diminished to less than 10%. Barrier function of the SC is usually declined, and transepidermal water loss (TEWL) is increased because of an abnormality on barrier homeostasis.[2] People feel tightness of their skin, and the skin surface becomes rough, scaly, and sensitive. Hyperkeratosis, abnormal scaling, and epidermal hyperplasia are usually observed in the dry skin.[2] Keratinization also shows abnormal features.[2] These phenomena are commonly observed in atopic dermatitis and psoriasis.[3] Dermatitis induced by environmental factors such as exposure to chemicals, low humidity, and UV radiation also show these features. Thus, many researchers have been investigating the cause and treatment of dry skin, and there is currently great interest in adequate model systems for dry skin studies. In this chapter, I will describe several model systems of dry skin for clinical research of dermatitis associated with skin surface dryness.

12.2 DRY, SCALY SKIN INDUCED BY BARRIER DISRUPTION

Barrier disruption is observed in variously induced scaly skin[4] and is known to cause changes in epidermal biochemical processes, including lipid biosynthesis,[5] DNA synthesis,[6] calcium localization,[7] and cytokine production.[8] Up-regulation of specific keratin molecules and adhesion molecules associated with the inflammatory response is also observed.[9] Because a decline of SC barrier function might be related to many types of skin abnormalities, the role of the SC barrier function has recently become the focus of intense research (see Chapters 5 and 6).

In our daily life, the SC barrier is potentially perturbated by chemicals such as surfactants, detergents, and organic solvents. As a good model of this, Gruneward et al. demonstrated[10] damage of the skin by repetitive washing with surfactant solutions. They treated skin following the repeated use of SLS and N-cocoyl protein condensate sodium as a mild wash substance for 1 week. In their report, they suggested that repeated washing with even a mild surfactant damaged skin.

Recent studies suggested that intrinsic factors also affect cutaneous barrier homeostasis. Psychological stress delays barrier recovery after artificial barrier disruption.[11] Also, the SC barrier becomes fragile and the recovery rate is delayed with aging.[12] Thus, a dry skin model induced by barrier disruption might be a good model for clinical research.

0-8493-7520-7/00/$0.00+$.50

TABLE 1
Change of Skin Surface Condition 1 Week After Tape Stripping, Measured at 22°C and 55% RH

	TEWL (g/m^2h)	Conductance (Mean Value/Control)	SC Cell Area (mm^2)
Before treatment	6.3 ± 1.9	1.1 ± 0.3	1047 ± 81
After treatment	8.1 ± 2.5*	0.6 ± 0.3*	956 ± 69***

Note: Each value is the mean ± standard deviation from nine subjects. *$p < 0.05$ and ***$p < 0.001$, significance of difference between normal and scaly skin.

Source: From Denda M. et al. (1992) *Arch Dermatol Res* 363–367. With permission.

Previously,[13] investigators usually used back or forearm skin for the experiment. It was easier to induce scaly skin on back skin than on forearm skin. In the case of back skin, we stripped SC nine times with adhesive cellophane tape. At that time, the transepidermal water loss (TEWL) value was over 10 $mg/cm^2/h$ and most of the SC was removed. In the case of forearm, to induce dry, scaly skin, stripping for 30 to 50 times was needed. One week after treatment, TEWL was higher than the normal level, skin surface conductance decreased, and SC cell area also decreased (Table 1). The skin surface became scaly and flaky. Figure 1 shows skin surface pictures of the forearm skin with and without barrier disruption. Abnormal scaling is observed on the surface of skin which was treated with tape stripping. These phenomena are commonly observed in natural dry skin, such as atopic dermatitis and psoriasis.

Acetone treatment is also used for barrier disruption.[14] Compared to tape stripping, this treatment breaks the SC barrier homogeneously. On the other hand, it takes a longer period of time to break the barrier than by tape stripping.

Treatment with the surfactant is another way to break the barrier, as described earlier.[10] The efficacy depends on each surfactant. Yang et al. suggested[15] that some kinds of anionic surfactant, such as sodium dodecyl sulfate (SDS), affect not only the SC barrier, but also the nucleous layer of the epidermis. Fartasch demonstrated[16] that the topical application of SDS caused cell damage to the nucleated cells of the epidermis and acetone treatment disrupted the lipid structure only in the SC. Thus, if one wants to investigate the effect of the disruption of the SC barrier function, tape stripping or acetone treatment would be better for the study.

UV radiation also causes decline of barrier function, but this method potentially induces various kinds of responses not only in the epidermis, but also in the dermis.[17]

The degree of epidermal hyperplasia correlated with the level and duration of barrier disruption.[14] The effects of repeated barrier disruption have been examined using hairless mice. Not only epidermal hyperplasia, but also cutaneous inflammation, was observed in the case of a longer and higher level of repeated barrier disruption by tape stripping and acetone treatment. Since neither the increase in epidermal cytokine production nor the described changes in cutaneous pathology were prevented by occlusion, the hyperplasia in this model should not be attributed to increased water loss, but rather to epidermal injury resulting in the production and release of epidermal cytokines.

Although repeated barrier disruption induces inflammation, epidermal hyperplasia, and abnormal keratinization, there are several histological differences between this model and psoriasis. Gerritsen et al. reported[19] the absence of some characteristic features of psoriasis in the dry skin induced by repeated tape stripping. They also demonstrated that filaggrin expression in the model system was different from that in psoriasis. The mechanism underlying the clonical skin diseases such as psoriasis remains to be investigated.

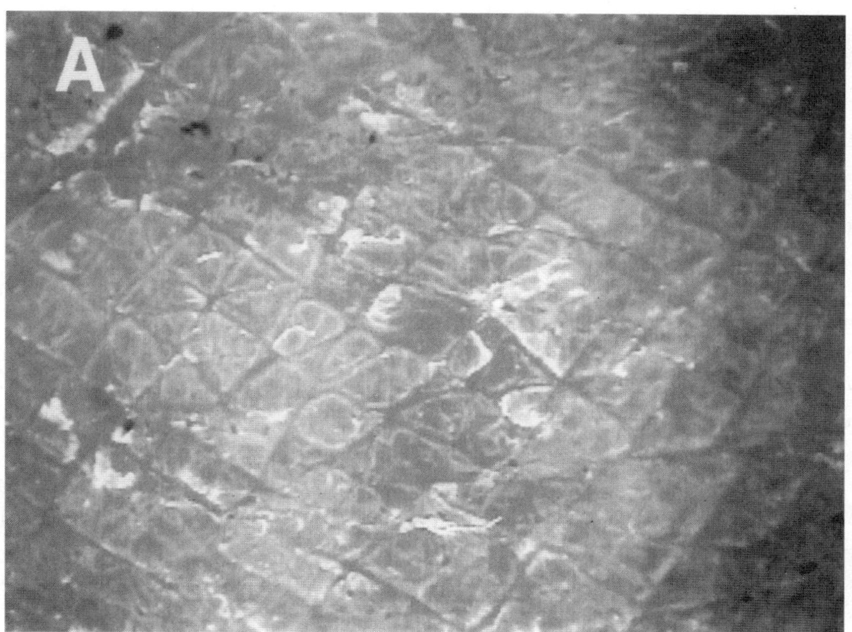

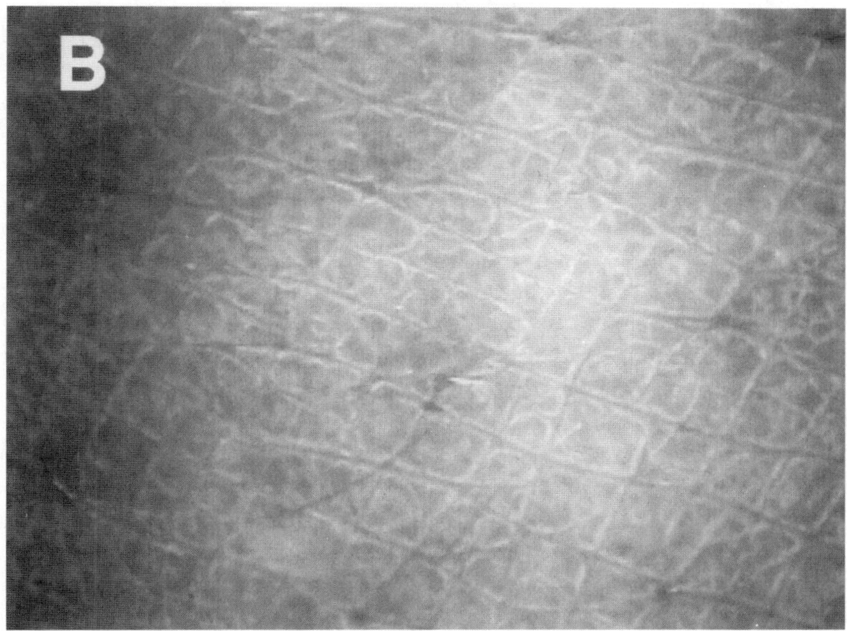

FIGURE 1 Dry, scaly skin induced by tape stripping (A) and untreated control (B). Forearm skin was stripped with adhesive cellophane tape 50 times, and 1 week later, skin surface was observed with a microvision system (Hi-Scope, NH-2000, Panasonic, Japan).

On the other hand, a means to accelerate the barrier recovery rate after barrier disruption induced by environmental insults would be effective in the treatment and prevention of skin trouble induced by barrier damage. We previously demonstrated[20] that t-AMCHA, an antifibrinolytic agent, accelerated barrier recovery and also prevented epidermal hyperplasia induced by repeated barrier disruption. Kitamura et al. already reported[21] the efficacy of this agent for treatment of dry skin.

Thus, one can use the dry skin model, induced by barrier disruption, not only for research of dry skin features, but also for screening of agents effective in the treatment of skin problems.

12.3 DRY, SCALY SKIN INDUCED BY AN OCCLUSIVE SURFACTANT DRESSING

Surfactants have also been used to cause artificial dry skin. Many researchers have reported surfactant-induced dry skin.[22] In our daily life, surfactants, i.e., detergents, are a potential cause of dermatitis. Thus, the dry skin induced by surfactants has been studied not only as a model system of dry skin, but also for clinical study of skin trouble in our daily life.

The effect of a surfactant on skin depends on the type of surfactant as described earlier. Wilhelm et al. demonstrated the irritation potential of anionic surfactants.[23] They evaluated the effects of sodium salts of n-alkyl sulfates with variable carbon chain length on TEWL and found that a C12 analog gave a maximum response. They suggested that the mechanisms responsible for the hydration of SC are related to the irritation properties of the surfactants. Leveque et al. also suggested[24] that the hyperhydration of SC is consecutive to the inflammation process. They demonstrated that the increase of TEWL was induced by SDS without removal of SC lipids. SDS might influence not only SC barrier function, but also the nucleated layer of epidermis and/or dermal system associated with inflammation.[24] Recently, no correlation was found between the level of epidermal hyperplasia and TEWL increase on the SDS-irritated skin.[25] Further work would be needed to determine the effects of surfactants on skin.

In our previous study,[4] we used human forearm skin or back skin for the study. The forearm skin was treated with a 5% aqueous solution of SDS and an occlusive dressing was applied. After treatment, we washed off the surfactant solution with water and then continuously measured TEWL, skin surface conductance, and SC lipid morphology by ATR-IR for 14 days. The lipid morphology in the SC was altered by the treatment, but recovered to normal within 2 days (Figure 2). On the other hand, both TEWL (Figure 3) and skin surface conductance (Figure 4) were abnormal even 2 weeks after the SDS treatment. Single application of the barrier disruption by tape stripping or acetone treatment did not cause such obvious changes. Thus, the occlusive surfactant dressing affects skin not only on the SC, but also on the nucleated layer of the epidermis and dermis as described earlier. Potentially, this method damaged the skin too much. One should pay careful attention to the concentration of the surfactant solution and period of the occlusive dressing. The damage of skin is different in each person. Application of an occlusive dressing substantially increases the irritant response of the skin to repeated short-term treatments with the surfactant.

During the past decade, several reports have demonstrated the decline of sphingolipid metabolism in atopic dermatitis,[26,27] and the cause of dry skin has been shown to be the abnormality of sphingolipid metabolism.[27] However, in experimentally induced dry skin, the total amount of SC ceramide did not change,[13,28] but the amino acid content decreased.[13] Recently, Tanaka et al. reported[29] that amino acid content was reduced in the SC in atopic respiratory disease. They suggested that the free amino acid content is the crucial factor of the dry, scaly features of not only experimentally induced dry skin but also atopic respiratory disease. This is a good example showing that the experimentally induced dry skin model is quite a useful method to investigate dermatitis associated with skin surface dryness.

12.4 DRY, SCALY SKIN INDUCED BY DRY ENVIRONMENT

Seasonal changes affect the condition of normal skin and may trigger various cutaneous disorders.[30,31] In common dermatitis, a decline in barrier function often parallels the increased severity of clinical symptomatology. These conditions all tend to worsen during the winter season when humidity is lower.[30,31] Abundant indirect evidence indicates that decreased humidity precipitates

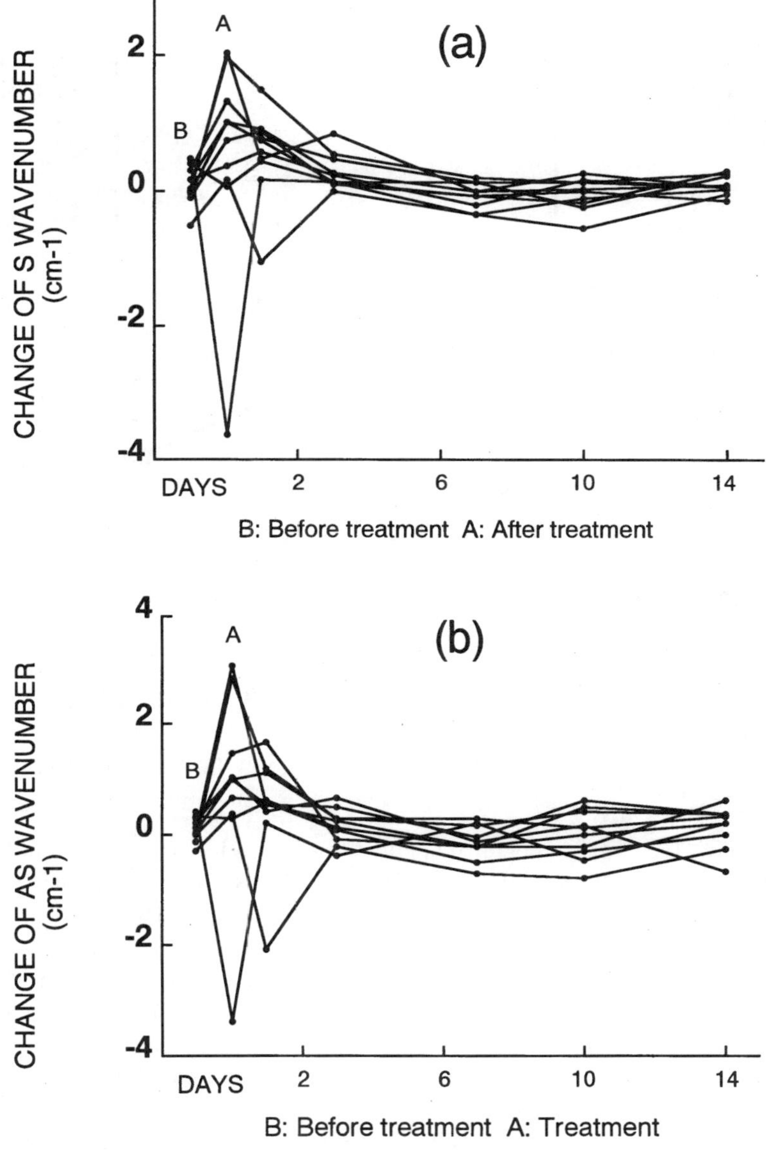

FIGURE 2 Difference from baseline (frequency shift) of symmetric (a) and asymmetric (b) frequency before and after SLS treatment. (From Denda M. et al. (1994) *Arch Dermatol Res* 286:41. With permission.)

these disorders, whereas, in contrast, increased skin hydration appears to ameliorate these conditions. The mechanisms by which alterations in relative humidity might influence cutaneous function and induce cutaneous pathology are poorly understood.

Recently,[32] low humidity has been shown to stimulate epidermal DNA synthesis and to amplify the hyperproliferative response to barrier disruption. SC morphology was also influenced by a dry environment, and abnormal desquamation was observed under low humidity.[33,35] These results suggest that this model system, i.e., dry skin induced by dry environment, is also an important model for clinical research of skin diseases associated with skin surface dryness.

In our study, we used hairless mice.[32,33] Before each experiment, animals were caged separately for at least 4 days. These cages were maintained in a room kept at a temperature of 22 to 26°C and at a relative humidity of 40 to 70%. Animals were kept separately in 7.2-liter cages in which

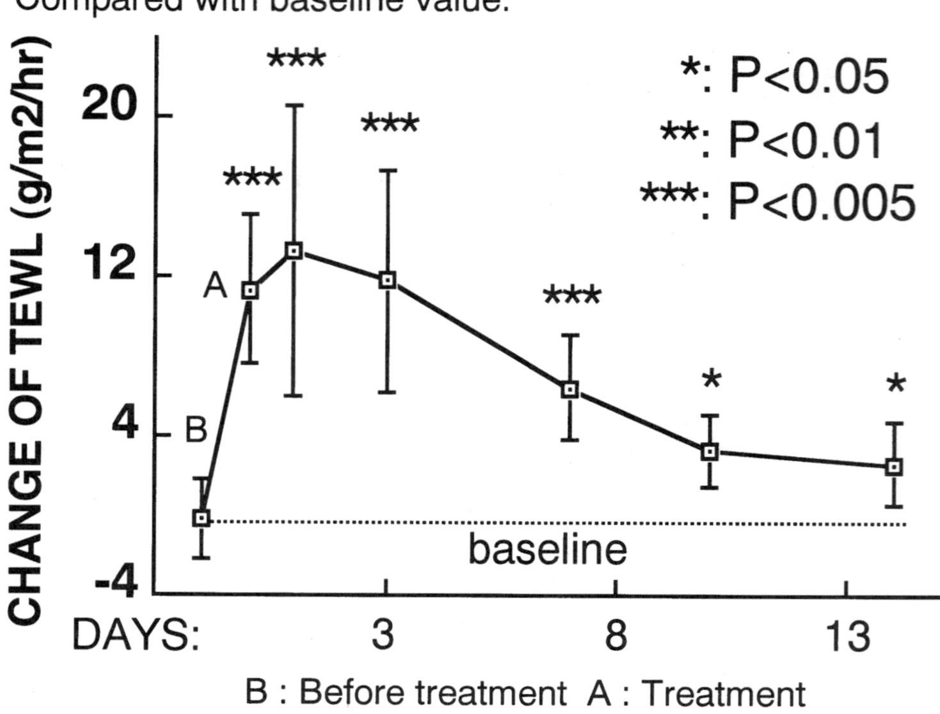

FIGURE 3 Difference of TEWL from baseline value after SLS treatment. (From Denda M. et al. (1994) *Arch Dermatol Res* 286: 41. With permission.)

the relative humidity (RH) was maintained at either 10% with dry air or 80% with humid air. The temperature was the same in all cases (22 to 26°C), and fresh air was circulated 100 times per hour. Animals were kept out of the direct stream of air. The level of NH_3 was always below 1 ppm.

Under a dry condition, epidermal DNA synthesis increased within 12 hours.[34] Abnormal scaling and an increase of SC thickness were also observed within 2 to 3 days.[35] When we treated flank skin of the animals which were kept in a dry condition for 48 hours with acetone, obvious epidermal hyperplasia and mast cell degranulation were observed 48 hours after the acetone treatment.[32] These studies provide evidence that changes in environmental humidity contribute to the seasonal exacerbations/amelioration of cutaneous disorders such as atopic dermatitis and psoriasis, diseases which are characterized by a defective barrier, epidermal hyperplasia, and inflammation. Because these responses were prevented by occlusion with plastic membrane, petrolatum, and humectant,[32] this dry skin model is a good system to evaluate clinical methods to solve skin problems.

12.5 CONCLUSION

As described previously, one can induce dry, scaly skin which shows features very similar to dermatitis such as atopic dermatitis and psoriasis. Use of this experimentally induced dry skin should enable the discovery of a new clinical methodology to cure or care for skin problems. Recently, several excellent *in vitro* skin models have been reported.[36] Although they are also very useful models for the study of cutaneous metabolism, their function and microstructure are still different from those of intact skin. On the other hand, the mechanisms underlying abnormal desquamation, i.e., scaling in the dry skin such as atopic dermatitis, are not completely known. Sato et al. reported[37] that the inhibition of protease in the SC induced scale without affecting epidermal mitosis. This result seems to be no direct relationship between skin surface appearance

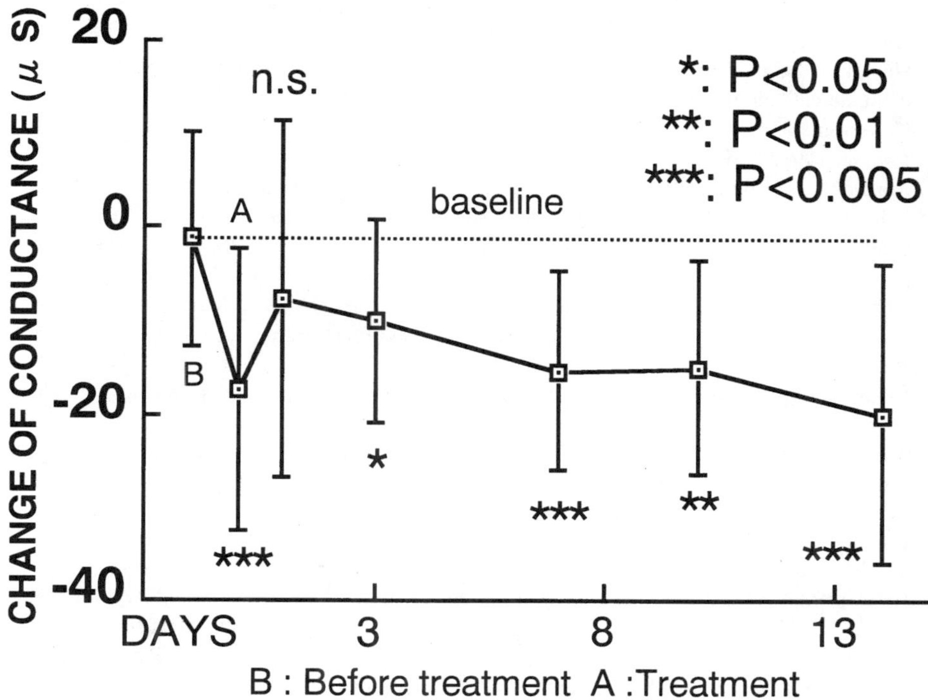

FIGURE 4 Difference of skin surface conductance value from baseline after SLS treatment. (From Denda M. et al. (1994) *Arch Dermatol Res* 286: 41. With permission.)

and epidermal proliferation. However, decline of SC barrier function induced epidermal hyperplasia, as described earlier.[32] The loss of water content from SC also induced epidermal DNA synthesis.[34] Further mechanistic studies on each of the dry skin features are required.

The models described in this section should help clarify the biochemical mechanism of dry skin and lead to improvements in the clinical treatment of various skin problems associated to skin surface dryness.

REFERENCES

1. Tagami H, Yoshikuni K (1985) Interrelationship between water-barrier and reservoir functions of pathologic stratum corneum. *Arch Dermatol* 121:642–645.
2. Black D, Diridollou S, Lagarde JM, Gall Y (1998) Skin care products for normal, dry and greasy skin. In *Textbook of Cosmetic Dermatology,* second edition. Edited by Baran R, Maibach HI. pp 125–150 Martin Dunitz Ltd, London.
3. Sauer GC, Hall JC, Eds. (1996) *Manual of Skin Diseases,* seventh edition. Lippincott-Raven, Philadelphia.
4. Denda M, Koyama J, Namba R, Horii I (1994) Stratum corneum lipid morphology and transepidermal water loss in normal skin and surfactant-induced scaly skin. *Arch Dermatol Res* 286:41–46.
5. Elias PM, Holleran WM, Menon GK, Ghadially R, Williams ML, Feingold KR (1993) Normal mechanisms and pathophysiology of epidermal permeability barrier homeostasis. *Curr Opin Dermatol* 231–237.
6. Proksch E, Feingold KR, Man MQ, Elias PM (1991) Barrier function regulates epidermal DNA synthesis. *J Clin Invest* 87:1668–1673.

7. Menon GK, Elias PM, Lee SH, Feingold KR (1992) Localization of calcium in murine epidermis following disruption and repair of the permeability barrier. *Cell Tissue Res* 270:503–512.
8. Wood LC, Jackson SM, Elias PM, Grunfeld G, Feingold KR (1992) Cutaneous barrier perturbation stimulates cytokine production in the epidermis of mice. *J Clin Invest* 90:482–487.
9. Nickoloff BJ, Naidu Y (1994) Perturbation of epidermal barrier function correlates with initiation of cytokine cascade in human skin. *J Am Acad Dermatol* 30:535–546.
10. Gruneward AM, Gloor M, Gehring W, Kleesz P (1995) Damage to the skin by repetitive washing. *Contact Dermatitis* 32:225–232.
11. Denda M, Tsuchiya T, Hosoi J, Koyama J (1998) Immobilization-induced and crowded environment-induced stress delay barrier recovery in murine skin. *Br. J Dermatol* 138:780–785.
12. Ghadially R, Brown BE, Sequeria-Martin SM, Feingold KR, Elias PM (1995) The aged epidermal permeability barrier. *J Clin Invest* 95:2281–2290.
13. Denda M, Hori J, Koyama J, Yoshida S, Namba R, Takahashi M, Horii I, Yamamoto A (1992) Stratum corneum sphingolipids and free amino acids in experimentally-induced scaly skin. *Arch Dermatol Res* 284:363–367.
14. Denda M, Brown BE, Elias PM, Feingold KR (1997) Epidermal injury stimulates prenylation in the epidermis of hairless mice. *Arch Dermatol Res* 289:104–110.
15. Yang L, Man MQ, Taljebini M, Elias PM, Feingold KR (1995) Topical stratum corneum lipids accelerate barrier repair tape stripping, solvent treatment and some but not all types of detergent treatment. *Br J Dermatol* 133:679–685.
16. Fartasch M (1997) Ultrastructure of the epidermal barrier after irritation. *Microsc Res Tech* 37:193–199.
17. Hawk JLM (1998) Cutaneous photobiology. In *Textbook of Dermatology* Edited by Champion RH, Burton JL, Burns DA, Breathnach SM. pp 973–993 Blackwell Scientific, Oxford.
18. Denda M, Wood LC, Emami S, Calhoun C, Brown BE, Elias PM, Feingold KR (1996) The epidermal hyperplasia associated with repeated barrier disruption by acetone treatment or tape stripping cannot be attributed to increased water loss. *Arch Dermatol Res* 288:230–238.
19. Gerritsen MJP, van Erp PEJ, van Vlijmen-Willems IMJJ, Lenders LTM, van de Kerkhof PCM (1994) Repeated tape stripping of normal skin: a histological assessment and comparison with events seen in psoriasis. *Arch Dermatol Res* 286:455–461.
20. Denda M, Kitamura K, Elias PM, Feingold KR (1997) Trans-4-(aminomethyl) cyclohexane carboxylic acid (T-AMCHA), an anti-fibrinolytic agent, accelerates barrier recovery and prevents the epidermal hyperplasia induced by epidermal injury in hairless mice and humans. J Invest Dermatol 109:84–90.
21. Kitamura K, Yamada K, Ito A, Fukuda M (1995) Research on the mechanism by which dry skin occurs and the development of an effective compound for its treatment. *J Soc Cosmet Chem* 29:133–145.
22. van der Valk PGM, Stam-Westerveld EB, Paye M (1996) A model to study the drying potential of detergent formulations on the skin. In *Dermatologic Research Techniques.* Edited by Maibach HI. pp 195–205 CRC Press, Boca Raton, FL.
23. Wilhelm KP, Cua AB, Wolff HH, Maibach HI (1993) Surfactant-induced stratum corneum hydration in vivo: prediction of the irritation potential of anionic surfactants. *J Invest Dermatol* 101:310–315.
24. Leveque JL, de Rigal J, Saint-Leger D, Billy D (1993) How does sodium lauryl sulfate alter the skin barrier function in man? A multiparametric approach. *Skin Pharmacol* 6:111–115.
25. Welzel J, Metker C, Wolff H, Wilhelm KP (1998) SLS-irritated human skin shows no correlation between degree of proliferation and TEWL increase. *Arch Dermatol Res* 290:615–620.
26. Yamamoto A, Serizawa S, Ito M, Sato Y (1991) Stratum corneum lipid abnormalities in atopic dermatitis. *Arch Dermatol Res* 283:219–223.
27. Imokawa G, Abe A, Jin K, Higaki Y, Kawashima M, Hidano A (1991) Decreased level of ceramides in stratum corneum of atopic dermatitis: an etiological factor in atopic dry skin? *J Invest Dermatol* 96:523–526.
28. Fulmer AW, Kramer GJ (1986) Stratum corneum lipid abnormalities in surfactant-induced dry scaly skin. *J Invest Dermatol* 86:598–602.
29. Tanaka M, Okada M, Zhen YX, Inamura N, Kitano T, Shirai S, Sakamoto K, Inamura T, Tagami H (1998) Decreased hydration state of the stratum corneum and reduced amino acid content of the skin surface in patients with seasonal allergic rhinitis. *Br J Dermatol* 139:618–621.

30. Wilkinson JD, Rycroft RJ (1992) Contact dermatitis. In *Textbook of Dermatology,* fifth edition. Edited by Champion RH, Burton JL, Ebling FJG. pp 614–615 Blackwell Scientific, Oxford.
31. Sauer GC, Hall JC (1996) Seasonal skin diseasses. In *Manual of Skin Diseases,* seventh edition. Edited by Sauer GC, Hall JC. pp 23–28 Lippincott-Raven, Philadelphia.
32. Denda M, Sato J, Tsuchiya T, Elias PM, Feingold KR (1998) Low humidity stimulates epidermal DNA synthesis and amplifies the hyperproliferative response to barrier disruption: implication of seasonal exacerbations of inflammatory dermatoses. *J Invest Dermatol* 111:873–878.
33. Denda M, Sato J, Masuda Y, Tsuchiya T, Koyama J, Kuramoto M, Elias PM, Feingold KR (1998) Exposure to a dry environment enhances epidermal permeability barrier function. *J Invest Dermatol* 111:858–863.
34. Sato J, Denda M, Ashida Y, Koyama J (1998) Loss of water from the stratum corneum induces epidermal DNA synthesis in hairless mice. *Arch Dermatol Res* 290:634–637.
35. Sato J, Denda M, Nakanihi J, Koyama J (1998) Dry conditions affect desquamation of stratum corneum in vivo. *J Dermatol Sci* 18:163–169.
36. Vicanova J, Boelsma E, Mommas AM, Kempenaar JA, Forslind B, Pallon J, Egelrud T, Koerten HK, Ponec M (1998) Normalization of epidermal calcium distribution profile in reconstructed human epidermis is related to improvement of terminal differentiation and stratum corneum barrier function. *J Invest Dermatol* 111:97–106.
37. Sato J, Denda M, Nakanishi J, Nomura J, Koyama J (1998) Cholesterol sulfate inhibits proteases that are involved in desquamation of stratum corneum. *J Invest Dermatol* 111:189–193.

13 Infantile Seborrheic Dermatitis

Donald Rudikoff

CONTENTS

13.1 INTRODUCTION

Seborrheic dermatitis is an inflammatory skin disorder commonly encountered in clinical practice. It occurs in infantile and adolescent/adult forms. The adolescent/adult form presents at or after puberty with dandruff scaling of the scalp and greasy scaling of the nasolabial area, glabella, eyebrows, external ears, and postauricular areas. Infantile seborrheic dermatitis, on the other hand, is controversial in its definition, etiology, clinical manifestations, prognostic significance, and perhaps its very existence as a separate disease entity. One author suggests that infantile seborrheic dermatitis likely reflects the heterogeneous overlapping presentation of several diagnoses such as cradle cap with intertriginous lesions, primary irritant diaper dermatitis with dissemination, intertrigo, infantile psoriasis, atopic dermatitis, and Leiner's disease.[1] Ruiz-Maldonado considers seborrheic dermatitis, in a subset of infants, to be a phase of atopic dermatitis with an oily appearance as a result of increased sebaceous secretion in the first few months of life.[2] Many cases of infantile seborrheic dermatitis diagnosed with assuredness later evolve into garden variety atopic eczema.[3] The relation of seborrheic dermatitis to the adult form is, at best, problematic, and whether the two are the same entity is disputed. This chapter will examine the nosology, etiology, clinical manifestations, differential diagnosis, prognostic implications, and treatment of infantile seborrheic dermatitis.

13.2 DEFINITION AND NOSOLOGY

Infantile seborrheic dermatitis has recently been defined as an "allegedly distinctive eruption" occurring transiently in the weeks following birth, with a predilection for the scalp and proximal flexural areas.[1] There is erythema, vesiculation, and yellow-red greasy scale situated in areas of increased sebaceous gland concentration.[4] Because the relation to sebum production is not known, the condition might, along with the adult form, be better termed dermatitis of the "seborrheic areas." Pruritus, a cardinal feature of atopic dermatitis, is absent or much less prominent in patients with infantile seborrheic dermatitis, although this parameter is not easily measured in infants.[5] Some

0-8493-7520-7/00/$0.00+$.50

authors consider "cradle cap," i.e., seborrhea capitis, to be a separate entity. The situation is further confused by the fact that napkin dermatitis, a characteristic finding in infantile seborrheic dermatitis, occurs on its own, often as a result of irritants, and frequently with a secondary candidal or bacterial infection.[1] It may generalize to produce a clinical picture almost identical to so-called infantile seborrheic dermatitis.

Several authors have subclassified children with infantile seborrheic dermatitis into clinical patterns such as psoriasiform, seborrheic, localized napkin dermatitis, and generalized napkin dermatitis or, another classification system, true seborrheic dermatitis, psoriasiform seborrheic dermatitis, and erythrodermic seborrheic dermatitis.[6,7] A further complication is that studies examining the clinical features and prognosis of infantile seborrheic dermatitis have used different diagnostic criteria For example, Yates et al. in a study of the clinical difference between infantile seborrheic dermatitis and atopic eczema did not distinguish "napkin psoriasis" from seborrheic dermatitis.[8] Some authors consider infantile seborrheic dermatitis to be a variant of atopic dermatitis.[5]

The term seborrhea, often used synonymously with seborrheic dermatitis, should be reserved for excessive oiliness of the skin as a consequence of hyperfunctioning sebaceous glands.[4] The greasy scale that is associated with seborrhea is termed scurf.

Erythrodermic infantile seborrheic dermatitis is customarily referred to as Leiner's disease. True Leiner's disease, a life-threatening disorder, is associated with failure to thrive, protracted diarrhea, and immune abnormalities. One major text recommends referring to severe, erythrodermic infantile seborrheic dermatitis without C5 deficiency and diarrhea as "Leiner's-like seborrheic dermatitis."[4]

Infantile seborrheic dermatitis differs from the adolescent/adult variety in several ways. It is almost always self-limited, more frequently widespread, more likely to involve the groin, and less likely to involve the paranasal area.

13.3 CLINICAL FEATURES

Infantile seborrheic dermatitis starts during the first month of life and if left untreated lasts 3 or 4 months before clearing.[4] This is not a hard and fast rule, and at least one clinical study found a mean age of onset of 4.9 weeks (range 3 to 23 weeks).[8] There is one report of infantile seborrheic dermatitis occurring in the first 2 days of life.[9] The eruption frequently starts in the diaper area, although the face and scalp are also common sites of onset and a bipolar onset is not uncommon.[8] "Cradle cap" is a common finding in many infants. Thickened, greasy scaling, especially over the vertex, may result from the hesitancy of new mothers to wash over the fontanelles.[4] The scaling may occur over mildy erythematous skin and appears white, off-white, brown, or yellowish in color.[10] Hair loss is uncommon, and if present is minimal and transient following removal of scale.[11,12] There may be only fine scaling limited to the scalp, central areas of the face, external ears, and forehead, but the eruption is frequently more widespread even in healthy infants.

Sites of predilection are the parietal region, middle face, neck folds, and central chest. Discrete and coalescent, glazed, greasy, sharply circumscribed erythematous, or salmon-colored plaques often occur in the axillary, inguinal, and intergluteal fold (Figures 1 and 2). In the diaper area, central involvement around the genitalia and anus may spread peripherally to involve the flexures of the groin.[13] There may be microvesicle formation and in some cases truncal lesions reminiscent of guttate psoriasis.[8] Truncal involvement is initially patchy, but may sometimes become confluent.[13]

Infantile seborrheic dermatitis is characteristically nonpruritic. Infants are asymptomatic and comfortable though parents are often disturbed by the cosmetic appearance.[11] It is difficult to assess pruritus in infants who, before the sixth to eighth week of life, lack the capacity to scratch, but the condition is probably much less itchy than atopic dermatitis in the majority of patients. The prognosis of infantile seborrheic dermatitis is quite good, and there is no clear cut progression to adult seborrheic dermatitis. Some infants will go on to develop typical atopic dermatitis and some typical psoriasis, and they may have siblings who develop infantile seborrheic dermatitis as well.

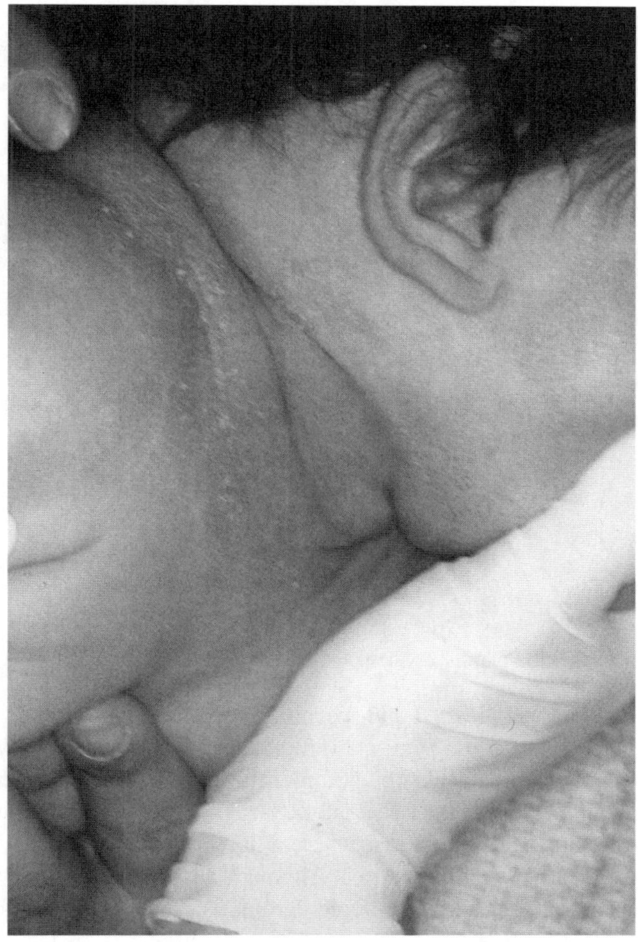

FIGURE 1 Infantile seborrheic dermatitis: proximal flexural involvement with redness and scaling.

In a recent follow-up study of 191 children diagnosed with infantile seborrheic dermatitis, of the 88 who were available for examination, 15% were found to have some kind of skin abnormality.[14] Seven had seborrheic dermatitis, five had atopic dermatitis, and one had psoriasis. Twenty children (23%) had siblings who had also been diagnosed with infantile seborrheic dermatitis. The median follow-up time was 9.6 years (range, 6.3 to 12.8 years).

In another report, 2 of 19 infants with infantile seborrheic dermatitis had affected siblings.[15] In a study of so-called psoriasiform napkin dermatitis with involvement of the diaper area and variable involvement of the face, scalp, trunk, and limbs, 2 of 18 patients subsequently developed atopic dermatitis and 2 of 18 developed psoriasis.[16] Fifty percent of patients grew out *Candida albicans* on culture. There was no association with HLA B13, B17, or Bw37, as is often encountered in psoriasis.

13.4 DIFFERENTIAL DIAGNOSIS

The condition most often confused with infantile seborrheic dermatitis is atopic dermatitis as defined by the criteria of Hanifin and Rajka.[17] Although some authors believe infantile seborrheic dermatitis is a manifestation of atopy, it is important to distinguish the two conditions for prognostic reasons. Infantile seborrheic dermatitis usually clears in a few months on its own, whereas atopic dermatitis may have a protracted course characterized by flares and remissions and be associated with the subsequent development of asthma. Atopic dermatitis usually presents at about 3 months of age

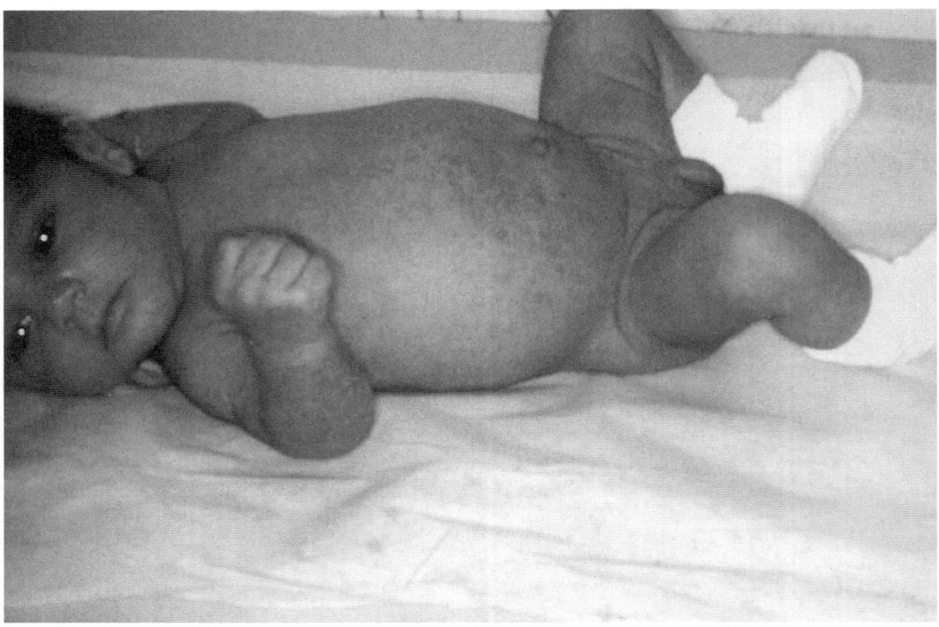

FIGURE 2 Infantile seborrheic dermatitis: erythematous scaly plaques involving the trunk, diaper area, and arms.

with erythematous, eczematous, crusted and weeping patches on the cheeks, and crusted patches on the extensor surfaces of the arms. Yates et al. found scalp involvement, a typical manifestation of infantile seborrheic dermatitis, to also be common in infants with atopic dermatitis and cheek involvement to be equally present in the two conditions.[8] Axillary involvement is not usual in atopic eczema and suggests seborrheic dermatitis, whereas involvement of the extensor aspect of the forearms and shins suggests atopic dermatitis.[8] Although absence of pruritus and lack of oozing and weeping are considered suggestive of atopic dermatitis, Yates et al. did not find the presence or absence of pruritus, family history of atopy, or age of onset of skin lesions helpful in distinguishing the two conditions.[8,10] In that study about one third of seborrheic infants had pruritus, whereas almost 90% of atopic infants itched. The onset of lesions soley in the diaper area favored the diagnosis of infantile seborrheic dermatitis, but this was less helpful if more than one area, e.g., scalp and diaper area, was involved.

Although clinical distinction between infantile seborrheic dermatitis and atopic dermatitis is problematic early on, certain laboratory parameters may be of value.[18] Positive RAST screening tests for egg white or cow's milk and to a lesser extent total IgE levels are helpful in distinguishing the two conditions. Eighty percent of infants with atopic dermatitis displayed positive RAST tests compared with 15% of infants with seborrheic dermatitis. Total eosinophil count and specific IgE levels to house dust mite, pollen, and cat dander are not useful in differentiating infantile seborrheic dermatitis from atopic dermatitis. Podmore et al. found that patients diagnosed with infantile seborrheic dermatitis subsequently had an increased incidence of atopic manifestations and considered infantile seborrheic dermatitis to be part of the spectrum of atopic diseases.[5] In another study, Podmore et al. were unable to differentiate infantile atopic and seborrheic dermatitis on the basis of peripheral blood T-cell subset values.[19] Because it is sometimes so difficult to distinguish the two conditions, a "wait and see attitude" may be indicated in some cases.[8]

Leiner's disease (erythema desquamativum), first described in Vienna in 1908, referred to breast-fed infants who developed failure to thrive; severe, intractable diarrhea; and a generalized erythematous eruption resembling infantile seborrheic dermatitis.[20] The condition is now known not to be confined to breast-fed infants.[21] Affected children may have metabolic disturbances, and death may occur from superimposed bacterial infection, usually pathogenic staphylococci.[21,22]

Leiner's disease probably is the phenotypic expression of a variety of immunodeficiency disorders.[23] Familial cases have been described and were considered to result from a deficiency in the opsonic activity of complement. They were corrected by transfusion of fresh plasma in some patients.[24,25] The plasma of these patients failed to opsonize baker's yeast for phagocytosis by neutrophils. This was thought to be caused by a functional abnormality of C5, but this theory has not been substantiated. Defective yeast opsonization is fairly common in the general population and probably results from impaired deposition of C3b/C3bi consequent to an essential cofactor deficiency.[26,27] Glover et al. described five infants with erythroderma, failure to thrive, and diarrhea with no opsonization defect.[20] Since yeast opsonization defects occur in 5% of the general population and Leiner's syndrome appears without this defect, Glover et al. consider such defects not to be an invariable part of the syndrome as had previously been emphasized in the medical literature.[20,26]

A serious but rare disorder that usually presents with skin manifestations reminiscent of infantile seborrheic dermatitis is Langerhan's cell histiocytosis, sometimes referred to as Histiocytosis X.[28] An erythematous, scaly eruption of the scalp; postauricular areas; and axillae, groin, and perineal areas that on closer inspection reveals reddish-brown and sometimes purpuric papules should suggest that diagnosis. Vesicles and crusted papules may be noted. These infants develop fever, anemia, thrombocytopenia, hepatosplenomegaly, and lymphadenopathy. Once considered invariably fatal, treatment is often beneficial, and spontaneous remissions have been recorded. Wiskott-Aldrich syndrome and other congenital immune deficiencies may present with a generalized eczematous eruption.

Acrodermatitis enteropathica is a rare disorder caused by zinc deficiency that may sometimes mimic severe infantile seborrheic dermatitis. Classically, there is periorificial blistering erythema and erosion and acral erythema with scaling.[12] Involvement of the folds may occur with chronic acrodermatitis enteropathica. The condition may result from a congenital defect in zinc absorption or insufficient zinc in the diet in some breast-fed infants.

13.5 HISTOPATHOLOGY

Infantile seborrheic dermatitis is usually not biopsied unless it fails to respond to topical treatment. Histopathological examination demonstrates scale-crust containing collections of plasma and neutrophils, especially at the margins of the follicular ostia.[12] In the epidermis there is focal spongiosis that may involve the follicular infundibula. The dermis is mildy edematous, with dilated venules and a sparse perivascular lymphohistiocytic infiltrate with few neutrophils. Seborrheic dermatitis may be differentiated histologically from psoriasis by the presence of plasma in mounds of parakeratosis, epidermal and infundibular spongiosis, and a lesser degree of psoriasiform hyperplasia.[12] The presence of neutrophils in the horny layer, thinning of the suprapapillary plates, and tortuous capillaries in elongated dermal papillae favor the diagnosis of psoriasis. Direct immunoflourescence examination of lesional skin of patients with infantile seborrheic dermatitis reveals no significant deposits of IgG, IgM, IgE, IgA, C1q, C3, properdin, or fibrinogen either at the dermo–epidermal junction or in a perivascular location.[29] The inflammatory infiltrate in patients with infantile seborrheic dermatitis consists for the most part of T-helper cells located in a perivascular location with a few scattered T-helper cells in the epidermis.

13.6 ETIOLOGY

Theories as to the etiology of seborrheic dermatitis center around nutritional abnormalities, infection by bacteria or yeasts, hormonal influences, sebum excretion, and lipid abnormalities. There is no apparent relationship between maternal age, birth weight, type of feeding, vitamin usage, or drug administration to mother or infant and subsequent development of infantile seborrheic dermatitis.[15] In early reports, increased prevalence of infantile seborrheic dermatitis associated with wartime food shortages suggested that nutritional deficiencies might be involved in the etiology. Some of these studies, though uncontrolled, suggested that parenteral biotin was an effective treatment of generalized infantile seborrheic dermatitis.[21,30] Later controlled studies do not support this notion.

Essential fatty acid deficiency has been suggested as a cause of infantile seborrheic dermatitis. A similar eruption may develop in infants fed on milk low in fat and linoleic acid. Tollesson et al. have demonstrated abnormal patterns of essential fatty acids in the serum of patients with infantile seborrheic dermatitis.[31] Linoleic acid (LA, 18:2w6) and its metabolic products, gamma linolenic acid (GLA, 18:3w6), and arachidonic acid (AA, 20:4w6) are considered essential for maintenance of a normal epidermal barrier in the skin.[31] Tollesson et al. detected increased levels of FA (20:2w6), an elongation product of LA (18:2w6), and an absence of GLA (18:3w6), the normal product of desaturation of LA. Impaired function of the enzyme delta-6-desaturase (Δ-6-D) which desaturates LA to GLA would explain these abnormalities. An immaturity of the enzyme system is thought to be responsible. At 6 to 11 months of age or earlier, essential fatty acid abnormalities normalize and there is clinical recovery.[31] Levels of arachidonic acid, important for phospholipids and leukotrienes, were found to be normal in infants with seborrheic dermatitis.

These investigators also demonstrated a beneficial effect of topical borage oil, a natural source of gamma linoleic acid, in infantile seborrheic dermatitis when applied to the diaper area.[32] Not only did the eruption clear in the diaper area, but in distant sites as well. In another study, Tolleson et al., using an evaporimeter, demonstrated increased transepidermal water loss (TEWL) in infants with seborrheic dermatitis on noninvolved forearm skin, suggesting a generalized deficit in the barrier function of the skin.[33] TEWL on the forearm returned to normal after borage oil treatment to the diaper area. These investigators concluded that GLA seems to be readily absorbed through the skin and exerts its beneficial effects at locations distant to the site of application.

The role of sebum excretion in infantile seborrheic dermatitis is controversial. In the adult form of seborrheic dermatitis, variation in the pool of residual sebum on the skin is thought to have a permissive effect on the development of the eruption by favoring the growth of *Pityrosporum ovale*.[34] This is thought to occur also in patients with Parkinsonism and other neurological disorders who develop seborrheic dermatitis. Because sebum excretion rates are not increased in seborrheic dermatitis, it had been dismissed by some authors as an etiological factor. The role of increased residual sebum on the skin, rather than its rate of production, may be the critical factor. The proposition that infantile seborrheic dermatitis resolves as a direct result of declining levels of sebum production in late infancy remains to be proven.[1]

Both *C. albicans* and *P. ovale* have been suggested as factors involved in the pathogenesis of infantile seborrheic dermatitis.[35] In a study of 50 infants with seborrheic dermatitis, Ilchyshyn found positive skin cultures for *C. albicans* in only nine patients (18%).[36] In adults, studies have demonstrated little if any difference in the number of *P. ovale* between patients with seborrheic dermatitis and controls or between healthy skin and lesional skin within patient groups.[35] Studies of serum IgG antibodies in adult patients with dandruff and seborrheic dermatitis have had conflicting results. One study showed significant differences in IgG antibody titers to a *P. ovale* cell wall protein extract between adult patients with seborrheic dermatitis and controls. Normal controls had the highest antibody titers, and patients with severe seborrheic dermatitis had the lowest.[35] A majority of young adults demonstrate sensitization to *P. ovale* on lymphocyte transformation tests, though it is a less powerful antigenic stimulant than C. albicans.[37] Other differences have been found in the immune response to *P. ovale* between adult seborrheic dermatitis patients and controls. Peripheral blood lymphocytes from normal donors showed marked proliferative responses to stimulation by a *P. ovale* extract, whereas PBMCs from patients with seborrheic dermatitis were unresponsive.[38] Moreover, IL-2 and IFNγ production from adult seborrheic dermatitis patients was markedly depressed compared to controls, but interestingly IL-10 synthesis was significantly increased.

Ruiz-Maldonado studied infants with infantile seborrheic dermatitis, atopic dermatitis, skin disorders exclusive of these two diagnoses, and healthy infants. Samples were taken from the scalp, face, midchest, and inguinal areas.[2] The number of infants who had positive cultures and/or smears for *P. ovale* was significantly higher ($p < 0.05$) in the infantile seborrheic dermatitis group (73%) than in any of the other groups. *Pityrosporum* was detected in 53% of healthy infants and in 33% of patients with AD or other dermatoses. In addition, positive smears and/or cultures from four body sites were much more commonly seen in infantile seborrheic dermatitis patients. These patients had a good response to ketoconazole cream within 2 weeks. Broberg and Faergemann studied 20 infants with seborrheic dermatitis and found positive cultures for *Mallesezia furfur* (*P. ovale*) in 18 of 20 patients compared to 4 of 20 controls.[39] It is not clear that the healing effect of ketoconazole in infants with seborrheic dermatitis results from its direct antifungal action. This compound has also been shown to have direct anti-inflammatory properties equivalent to 1% hydrocortisone.[40]

Tollesson et al. studied the prevalence of *M. furfur* (*P. ovale*) in patients with infantile seborrheic dermatitis at the time of diagnosis, immediately after complete healing, and after 1 year.[41] With each child serving as his or her own control, no significant change in colonization rates was seen after clearing or after 1 year. These investigators did find aberrant patterns of essential fatty acids in the serum that they considered to be of possible etiological significance.

13.7 TREATMENT

The most important consideration in the management of infants with seborrheic dermatitis is calm reassurance to anxious parents that the condition is benign, that the prognosis is excellent, and that ultimate clearing is the rule.[13] It should also be stressed that complications are rare. Loose-fitting clothing is suggested to avoid excessive perspiration, and no special diet is required. Parents in search of some external etiology or allergy should be advised that restrictive diets may be deleterious.

Seborrheic dermatitis is typically located in oil-gland-bearing skin and is responsive to topical corticosteroid therapy. Steroid applications are more effective if scales are removed with mineral oil or shampoo, but parents should be warned that excessive soaping of the skin or more aggressive attempts to remove sebum may be deleterious.[42,43] Superpotent topical corticosteroid preparations should be avoided as they can cause skin atrophy, telangiectasia, striae distensae, and, if applied to large areas, adrenal suppression. The face and flexural areas are particularly sensitive to these adverse effects.

Irritating substances and alkaline soaps should be avoided, and overaggressive, inappropriate treatments can induce an eczematous "id" reaction with weeping, crusting, and pruritus.[12,44] Addition of peanut oil, bran, or cornstarch to the infant's bath water has been advocated.[44] Schachner recommends bathing with oatmeal baths once or twice a day followed by application of 1% hydrocortisone cream.[11] Some authors have advocated the use of salicylic acid (3%) in olive oil or salicylic acid shampoo to remove scale crust.[11,42] It should be remembered that continued use of salicylic acid preparations may be irritating and can cause systemic toxicity if applied to large areas of damaged skin. Thus, such preparations should be used cautiously.

Gentle use of a soft-bristled toothbrush with a mild shampoo may be helpful to remove scales from the scalp.[23] Ketoconazole shampoo has been determined to be safe for infants.[45] In 13 infants less than 1 year of age, shampooed twice weekly for 1 month, there was no change in liver function tests and no detectable plasma levels of ketoconazole (limit of quantification 2 ng/ml). Taieb et al. found topical ketoconazole 2% cream to be effective within 10 days in 79% of infants treated for seborrheic dermatitis.[46] The cream was well tolerated, and there was no significant accumulation of ketoconazole in the plasma.

A number of early reports suggested that parenteral biotin was helpful in the treatment of generalized seborrheic dermatitis, but this is no longer considered a useful treatment by most authors.[21] Keipert found no advantage of oral biotin 2 mg twice daily over placebo.[15] That study was confounded, however, by the administration of topical betamethasone valerate to both patient groups. This may have masked any potential beneficial event of biotin. As mentioned previously, topical borage oil may be a useful treatment.

Treatment of Leiner's disease includes hospitalization with treatment of infection, infusions of fresh frozen plasma or purified C5 in some cases, and topical hydrocortisone 1% ointment.[15]

Some patients with infantile seborrheic dermatitis will go on to develop atopic dermatitis or psoriasis and will require ongoing management.

13.8 SUMMARY

Infantile seborrheic dermatitis is a skin disorder that is still not well understood. Its relation to the adult form of seborrheic dermatitis has never been substantiated, and it may, in fact, be a reaction pattern particular to this age group that develops in susceptible individuals. The prognosis is excellent, although some patients will go on to develop atopic dermatitis or psoriasis. Future research should focus on the role of barrrier disruption resulting from fatty acid irregularities and the effects of *Candida* and *Pityrosporum* colonization on cutaneous immune responses in these patients.

The author would like to thank Steven R. Cohen, M.D., for contributing the photographs used in this chapter and Victoria White for her valuable editorial comments.

REFERENCES

1. Rook, A., Willkinson, D. S., Champion, R. H., Ebling, F. J. G., *Textbook of Dermatology*, Blackwell Science, Oxford, 1998.
2. Ruiz-Maldonado, R., Lopez-Matinez, R., Perez Chavarria, E. L., Rocio Castanon, L., Tamayo, L., *Pityrosporum ovale* in infantile dermatitis, *Pediatr Dermatol,* 6, 16, 1989.
3. Solomon, L. M., Esterly, N. B., *Neonatal Dermatology. Volume IX; Major Problems in Clinical Pediatrics,* W.B. Saunders, Philadelphia, 1973.
4. Ruiz-Maldonado, R., Parish, L. C., Beare, J. M., *Textbook of Pediatric Dermatology,* Grune & Stratton, Philadelphia, 1989.
5. Podmore, P., Burrows, D., Eedy, D. J., Stanford, C. F., Seborrhoeic eczema — a disease entity or a clinical variant of atopic eczema? *Br J Dermatol*, 115, 341, 1986.
6. Neville, E. A., Finn, O. A., Psoriasiform napkin dermatitis — a follow-up study, *Br J Dermatol*, 92, 279, 1975.
7. Menni, S., Piccinno, R., Baietta, S., Ciuffreda, A., Scotti, L., Infantile seborrheic dermatitis: seven-year follow-up and some prognostic criteria, *Pediatr Dermatol*, 6, 13, 1989.
8. Yates, V. M., Kerr, R. E., MacKie, R. M., Early diagnosis of infantile seborrhoeic dermatitis and atopic dermatitis — clinical features, *Br J Dermatol*, 108, 633, 1983.
9. Leung, A. K. C., Neonatal seborrheic dermatitis [letter], *West J Med*, 142, 558, 1985.
10. Janniger, C. K., Infantile seborrheic dermatitis: an approach to cradle cap, *Cutis*, 51, 233, 1993.
11. Schachner, L. A., Hansen, R. C., Editors. *Pediatric Dermatology*, Churchill Livingstone, New York, 1988.
12. Caputo, R., Gelmetti, C., Annessi, G., *Pediatric Dermatology and Dermatopathology — a Text and Atlas,* Williams & Wilkins, Baltimore, 1997.
13. Keipert, J. A., Rashes commonly starting in the first few months: various form of dermatitis. In Keipert J.A., Ed., *Essential Pediatric Dermatology,* Harwood Academic Publishers, London, 1990.
14. Mimouni, K., Mukamel, M., Zeharia, A., Mimouni, M., Prognosis of infantile seborrheic dermatitis, *J Pediatr,* 127, 744, 1995.
15. Keipert, J. A., Oral use of biotin in seborrheic dermatitis of infancy: a controlled trial, *Med J Aust*, 1, 584, 1976.
16. Rasmussen, H. B., Hagdrup, H., Schmidt, H., Psoriasiform napkin dermatitis, *Acta Dermatol Venereol (Stockh)*, 66, 534, 1986.
17. Hanifin, J. M., Rajka, G., Diagnostic features of atopic dermatitis, *Acta Derm Venereol (Suppl)* 92, 44, 1980.
18. Yates, V. M., Kerr, R. E., Frier, K., Cobb, S. J., MacKie, R. M., Early diagnosis of infantile seborrhoeic dermatitis and atopic dermatitis — total and specific IgE levels, *Br J Dermatol*, 108, 639, 1983.

19. Podmore, P., Burrows, D., Eedy D., T-cell subset assay. A useful differentiating marker of atopic and seborheic eczema in infancy?, *Arch Dermatol*, 124, 1235, 1988.
20. Glover, M. T., Atherton, D. J., Levinsky, R. J., Syndrome of erythroderma, failure to thrive, and diarrhea in infancy: a manifestation of immunodeficiency, *Pediatrics*, 81, 66, 1988.
21. Messaritakis, J., Kattamis, C., Karabula, C., Matsaniotis, N., Generalized seborrhoeic dermatitis. Clinical and therapeutic data of 25 patients, *Arch Dis Child,* 50, 871, 1975.
22. Goodyear, H. M., Harper, J. I., Leiner's disease associated with metabolic acidosis, *Clin Exp Dermatol*, 14, 364, 1989.
23. Mallory, S. B., Neonatal skin disorders, *Pediatr Clin North Am*, 38, 745, 1991.
24. Miller, M., Nilsson, U., A familial deficiency of the phagocytosis-enhancing activity of serum related to a dysfunction of the fifth component of complement (C5), *N Engl J Med,* 282, 354, 1970.
25. Jacobs, J., Miller, M., Fatal familial Leiner's disease: a deficiency of the opsonic activity of serum complement, *Pediatrics*, 49, 225, 1972.
26. Soothill, J. F., Harvey, B.A., Defective opsonization. A common immunity deficiency, *Arch Dis Child*, 51, 91, 1976.
27. Turner, M. W., Seymour, N. D., Kazatchkine, M. D., Mowbray, J. F., Suboptimal C3b/C3bi deposition and defective yeast opsonization. I. Evidence for the absence of essential co-factor activity, *Clin Exp Immunol*, 62, 427, 1985.
28. Hurwitz, S., The reticuloendothelial disorders. In Hurwitz S. Ed., *The Skin and Systemic Disease in Children*, Year Book Medical Publishers, Chicago, 1985.
29. Oranje, A. P., van Joost, T., van Reede, E. C., Vuzevski, V. D., Dzoljic-Danilovic, G., ten Kate, F. J., Stolz, E., Infantile seborrheic dermatitis. Morphological and immunopathological study, *Dermatologica,* 172, 191, 1986.
30. Nisenson, A., Barness, L. A., Treatment of seborrheic dermatitis with biotin and vitamin B complex, *J Pediatr*, 81, 630, 1972.
31. Tollesson, A., Frithz, A., Berg, A., Karlman, G., Essential fatty acids in infantile seborrheic dermatitis, *J Am Acad Dermatol*, 28, 957, 1993.
32. Tollesson, A., Frithz, A., Borage oil, an effective new treatment for infantile seborrhoeic dermatitis, *Br J Dermatol*, 129, 95, 1993.
33. Tollesson, A., Frithz, A., Transepidermal water loss and water content in the stratum corneum in infantile seborrheic dermatitis, *Acta Dermatol Venereol* (*Stockh*), 73, 18, 1993.
34. Cowley, N. C., Farr, P. M., Shuster, S., The permissive effect of sebum in seborrhoeic dermatitis: an explanation of the rash in neurological disorders, *Br J Dermatol*, 122, 71, 1990.
35. Bergbrandt, I. M., Faergemann, J., The role of *Pityrosporum ovale* in seborrheic dermatitis, *Semin Dermatol*, 9, 262, 1990.
36. Ilchyshyn, A., Mendelsohn, S. S., MacFarlane, A., Verbov, J., Candida albicans and infantile seborrheic dermatitis, *Br J Clin Pract*, 41, 557, 1987.
37. Sohnle, P. G., Collins-Lech, C., Relative antigenicity of P. orbiculare and C. albicans, *J Invest Dermatol*, 75, 279, 1980.
38. Neuber, K., Kroger, S., Gruseck, E., Abeck, D., Ring, J., Effects of *Pityrosporum ovale* on proliferation, immunoglobulin (IgA, G, M) synthesis and cytokine (IL-2, IL-10, IFN gamma) production of peripheral blood mononuclear cells from patients with seborrhoeic dermatitis, *Arch Dermatol Res*, 288, 532, 1996.
39. Broberg, A., Faergemann, J., Infantile seborrhoeic dermatitis and *Pityrosporum ovale*, *Br J Dermatol*, 120, 359, 1989.
40. Van Cutsem, J., Van Gerven, F., Cauwenbergh, G., Odds, F., Janssen, P. A., The antiinflammatory effects of ketoconazole, *J Am Acad Dermatol*, 25, 257, 1991.
41. Tollesson, A., Frithz, A., Stenlund, K., Masassezia furfur in infantile seborrheic dermatitis, *Pediatr Dermatol*, 14, 423, 1997.
42. Braun-Falco, O., Wolff, H. H., Plewig, G., Winkelmann, R. K., *Dermatology*, Springer-Verlag, New York, 1991.
43. Weston, W. L., Lane, A. T., Morelli, J. G., *Color Textbook of Pediatric Dermatology*, C. V. Mosby, St. Louis, 1996.
44. Schopf, R., Seborrheic eczema. In Marks R., Ed., *Eczema,* Martin Dunitz, London, 1992.

45. Brodell, R. T., Patel, S., Venglarcik, J. S., Moses, D., Gemmel, D., The safety of ketoconazole shampoo for infantile seborrheic dermatitis, *Pediatr Dermatol*, 15, 406, 1998.
46. Taieb, A., Legrain, V., Palmier, C., Lejean, S., Six, M., Maleville, J., Topical ketoconazole for infantile seborrhoeic dermatitis, *Dermatologica*, 181, 26, 1990.

14 Effects of Moisturizer and Keratolytical Agents in Psoriasis

Joachim W. Fluhr and Enzo Berardesca

CONTENTS

14.1 INTRODUCTION

Psoriasis is a chronic disease with hyperproliferation of the epidermis and inflammation of the dermis and epidermis. Psoriasis is characterized by an elevated turnover rate of keratinocytes. The duration of the cell cycle is shortened. The inflammation in the dermal immune reaction is characterized by the production of cytokines and a predomination of CD4+ cells in psoriasis-affected patients. Scaling marks the clinical feature associated by pruritus, inflammatory signs, and dryness. The different treatment modalities of psoriasis do not offer a cure to the patient. Only disease control or suppressive therapy is possible. The aims of the treatment should be a decrease or remission of scaling, pruritus, inflammation, burning, and dryness. The classical treatments are of a topical nature, including dithranol, coal tar, keratolytical agents, and emollients. Photo-chemotherapy with systemic PUVA, bath PUVA, and recently cream PUVA and photo-therapy with classical UVB-light (wavelength: 300 to 320 nm) have been shown to be effective. Methotrexate, etretinate, systemical corticosteroids, cyclosporin, and fumaric acid have shown their efficacy especially in severe cases.

The aim of this chapter is to analyze the actual knowledge and indications of moisturizing agents in the topical treatment of psoriasis. The most important indications of emollients and moisturizing agents are an adjuvant therapy of classical psoriasis treatment modalities and the supportive treatment in relapse-free phases. Very mild forms of psoriasis should be treated with compounds showing a low side effect rate and low cosmetic problems.

For topical therapy Greaves and Weinstein[1] scored emollients the *lowest,* taking into account the following:

- Relapse rate
- Side effects
- Cosmetic problems
- Efficacy

0-8493-7520-7/00/$0.00+$.50

Emollients were followed by keratolytical agents, coal tar, dithranol, and corticosteroids. For the adjuvant therapy of mild cases there must be a low risk rate (side effects, cosmetic problems) and no necessity for a strong and rapid efficacy. These assumptions can be fulfilled by emollients and moisturizing and keratolytical agents by reducing scaling, subjective discomfort, and a better hydration of dry stratum corneum.

A second indication for keratolytical and some moisturizing agents (e.g., urea) is the penetration enhancement of topically applied antipsoriatic drugs (e.g., salicylic acid in the dithranol and coal tar treatment).

14.2 EFFECTS OF MOISTURIZER AND KERATOLYTICAL AGENTS IN PSORIASIS

14.2.1 Salicylic Acid

Since the beginning of the 20th century salicylic acid has been known to exert a keratoplastic effect. Salicylic acid is widely used as a keratolytic agent in the treatment of hyperkeratotic dermatoses like psoriasis.[2] It can be used in concentrations of 0.5 to 60% in almost any vehicle.

In 1929 Moncorps reported different penetration properties of salicylic acid with different ointments.[3] The concentration depends not only on the concentration within the same ointment, but also on the type of ointment.[3] The resorption rate of salicylic acid on psoriatic lesions is higher with a faster and longer resorption than on the skin of healthy subjects.[4] The resorption rate also depends on the severity of the inflammation.[4] In a recent study the liberation of salicylic acid from different formulations did not correlate with the penetration rate into the skin.[5] An additional study of the same group showed a dose-depending percutaneous absorption of salicylic acid *in vivo*.[6]

In contrast to the keratoplastic properties of salicylic acid on pathological hyperproliferation of the epidermis, a promotion of the epidermopoiesis in normal guinea pig skin has been shown with a 1% salicylic acid–acetone–ethanol solution.[7] The mitotic index was increased by 17%, the epidermis thickness by 40%, and the thickness of the deep epidermis by 19%.[7] These results are not based on data collected from human skin. In contrast, Pullmann et al. did not find a change in the proliferation rate of psoriatic epidermal cells in humans in an autoradiographic study.[8] Roberts et al. showed a reduction of stratum corneum cell layers especially after 3 weeks.[9] The keratolytic effect was shown with the surfometry and the scanning electron microscopy by Davies and Marks.[10] Huber and Christophers showed that for a 50% salicylic acid solution, the corneocytes did not change their morphology, while the intercellular structure was altered.[11] This treatment resulted in a desquamation of the corneocytes. *In vivo*, with the silver nitrate staining technique, Nook could prove a keratolytic effect for the combination of a water-soluble ointment containing 5% salicylic acid and 10% urea in comparison to 5 and 10% salicylic acid alone in petrolatum.[12] The combination therapy was as effective as 10% salicylic acid and significantly more effective than a 5% salicylic acid formulation. The keratolytic effect of salicylic acid 6% in an isopropyl solution has been shown with the cantharidin blister method.[13]

Going et al. reported the successful treatment of scalp psoriasis with salicylic acid gel with a negligible absorption of salicylic acid.[14] The negative interaction of dithranol and zinc oxide in pastes could be partly inhibited by the addition of salicylic acid.[15] The addition of salicylic acid to dithranol formulations improves the clinical efficacy of dithranol due to the antioxidant properties of salicylic acid. [16]

The major problem in the topical treatment of psoriasis with salicylic acid is the possible chronic and acute intoxication with the symptoms of burning of oral mucosa, frontal headache, CNS symptoms, pH deviation (metabolic acidose), tinnitus, nausea, vomiting, and gastric symptoms.[17-19] These symptoms may occur in topical treatment, especially in children.[20-22] Even lethal cases are reported.[23-24] Therefore, a concentration higher than 10% and an application on larger surfaces especially in children are not suitable.

14.2.2 Urea

The moisturizing effect of urea in dry and scaly skin conditions is widely studied and accepted.[25-28] Urea is known to exert a proteolytical, keratolytical, hydrating, hygroscopical, penetration enhancing, epidermis thinning, and antipruritic effect.[29] An increased water-binding capacity was be shown under treatment with water-in-oil (w/o) emulsion containing 10% urea.[30] Recent data could not prove an increased hydration comparing 10% urea to 5% in both o/w and w/o emulsions.[31]

In vitro and *in vivo* data showed a lowered DNA-synthesis index with a thinning of the epidermis and a reduction of the epidermal cells in the cell cycle.[32] The mechanisms of urea on the epidermis result in thinning of the epidermis (~–20%), a reduction of the cells in DNA synthesis in the stratum basale (~–45%), and a prolongation of the generation time of the postmitotic epidermal cells.[33]

A penetration enhancement for glucocorticosteroids by urea is well studied.[34-41] Such a penetration enhancement leads to a steroid sparing effect and an increased clinical effectivity of steroid ointments containing urea. The maximum of the steroid penetration is within psoriatic lesions. But it still remains unclear if penetration enhancers are clinically effective within psoriatic lesions.

Dithranol in combination with urea is widely used in psoriasis to improve the clinical efficacy, to minimize the dithranol concentration, to achieve the desired effect, to shorten the contact in the short-contact treatment, to get a better hydration of the stratum corneum, and to decrease the proliferation of the keratinocytes. Gabard and Bieli showed an increased keratolytical effect of salicylic acid by adding 10% urea.[42]

Some data about the effect of urea in the treatment of psoriasis are available. Hagemann and Proksch[44] showed the following data in ten patients with psoriasis under a 2-week treatment with an ointment containing 10% urea: an increased stratum corneum hydration, a small decrease in TEWL, a reduction in epidermal thickness (–29%), and a decreased epidermal proliferation (–51%). The altered expression of involucrin and cytokeratins as markers for epidermal proliferation was partially reversed.[43] With topically applied 10% urea ointment, Sasaki et al. showed an improvement of the water content, the hygroscopicity, and the TEWL in patients with psoriasis vulgaris.[44]

14.2.3 Alpha Hydroxy Acids

In a recent study, 12 patients affected by psoriasis were treated with a glycolic acid lotion 15%, without occlusion, or with a 0.05% betamethasone valerate cream.[45] TEWL (Evaporimeter EP1, ServoMed, Sweden), Laser Doppler (Perimed-Periflux, Sweden), and skin color (Chroma Meter CR-200, Minolta, Japan) were taken at baseline and on days 5, 10, and 15 on psoriatic lesions. Erythema a* values were used for monitoring. The results of the study showed the following.

1. TEWL values decreased significantly within 15 days in both sites, particularly for the corticosteroid-treated site ($p < 0.01$ glycolic, $p < 0.005$ betamethasone). No significant differences in TEWL between glycolic acid and betamethasone were found during the study.
2. Erythema a* values decreased significantly during the treatment. Significant differences were found between basal and final readings ($p < 0.01$ glycolic, $p < 0.009$ betamethasone). No significant differences were found between glycolic acid and betamethasone.
3. Laser Doppler values decreased significantly during the study (glycolic $p < 0.001$, betamethasone $p < 0.0001$). Significant differences appeared at days 5, 10, and 15 between the two products, with lower values in the corticosteroid-treated site ($p < 0.05$, < 0.01, and < 0.05, respectively).

The results showed significant improvement of TEWL, a* value, and Laser Doppler after treatment with both products. No significant differences appear in TEWL and erythema between glycolic acid and betamethasone; on the other hand, a significantly decreased Laser Doppler is recorded in the sites treated with betamethasone, confirming the higher effect of corticosteroid compounds in terms of vasoconstriction and reduction of inflammation. The results were confirmed clinically with a definite reduction of hyperkeratosis and erythema induced by both treatments. The study shows that alpha hydroxy acids are useful not only in the control of hyperkeratosis, but also in the modulation of keratinocyte proliferation, which occurs in the disorders of keratinization such as psoriasis. Similar effects were reported from topical retinoids.[46] Further research is necessary to confirm these preliminary findings and to compare instrumental data with histological and immunohistochemical parameters in order to better understand these mechanisms. Presently, alpha hydroxy acids could be regarded as an adjuvant therapy in psoriasis.

14.2.4 Omega Fatty Acids and Psoriasis

It has been shown that oral or topical supplements of eicosapentanoic acid (EPA) and/or omega-3 derivatives can decrease not only skin dryness and scaling, but also the severity of skin diseases such as psoriasis.[47-49] Omega-3 derivatives can be incorporated into cell membranes and can be utilized as a substrate for phospholipase activity. This can lead to an increase of free EPA, which can be used as substrate for cyclooxygenase and lipooxygenase activities resulting in an increased production of anti-inflammatory leukotrienes LTB5 and PG3.[49] Abnormal serum fatty acid profiles in Darier's disease, ichthyosis vulgaris, psoriasis, and Sjögren-Larsson syndrome have been reported, suggesting that this may be a nonspecific finding in some epidermal diseases.[50] Hartop et al.[51] monitored TEWL on different psoriatic plaques treated topically with linoleic acid in comparison to clobetasole.

In a recent study with 12 healthy volunteers, barrier damage and skin irritation were induced after a single acute SLS application.[52] The data show that, besides topical corticosteroids, 5% linoleic acid led to an improvement of barrier function. Formulations containing omega-3 and omega-6 fatty acids may help in the restoration of barrier properties. Higher efficacy of these products may be achieved by combining different classes of stratum corneum lipids.[52] For topical fish oil, Escobar et al.[47] showed a clinical improvement of scaling and plaque thickness compared to the base-treated site in a 4-week treatment. In contrast Henneicke-von Zepelin et al. could not confirm these findings.[53]

They could see the same improvement of psoriatic lesions in omega-3-polyunsaturated fatty acid-treated areas as in the ointment-treated psoriatic sites. Further studies are necessary to evaluate the role of omega fatty acids in psoriasis.

14.3 EMOLLIENTS IN PSORIASIS

In the literature it has been reported that in chronic plaque psoriasis water-in-oil emollients could be used as a steroid-sparing agent.[54] The replacement of one of the twice daily applications of bethametasone dipropionate treatment by a water-in-oil emollient showed the same efficacy. Similar data were reported from Singh et al.[55] In an early study it was shown that white soft paraffin inhibited the development of Koebner response in psoriasis.[56] Finlay reported an effective cream therapy adjunct to dithranol for the treatment of chronic plaque psoriasis.[57]

REFERENCES

1. Greaves M. W., Weinstein G. D., Treatment of psoriasis, *N. Engl. J. Med.*, 332, 581, 1995.
2. Lebwohl M., The role of salicylic acid in the treatment of psoriasis, *Int. J. Dermatol.*, 38, 16, 1999.
3. Moncorps C., Untersuchungen über die Pharmakologie und Pharmakodynamik von Salben und salbeninkorporierten Medikamenten. II. Mitteilung: Über die Resorption und Pharmakodynamik der salbeninkorporierten Salizylsäure, *Arch. Exp. Pathol. Pharm.*, 141, 50, 1929.

4. Arnold W., Trinnes F., Schroeder I., Zur Hautresorption von Salicylsäure bei Psoriatikern und Hautgesunden, *Beitr. Gerichtl. Med.*, 37, 325, 1979.
5. Gabard B., Treffel P., Schwarb F., Surber C., Bieli E., Lüdi S., Salicylic acid release from topical formulations does not predict *in vitro* skin absorption, *Dermatology*, 195, 198, 1997.
6. Schwarb F., Gabard B., Jost G., Rufli Th., Surber C., Percutaneous absorption of salicylic acid in man following topical administration of different formulations, *Dermatology*, 195, 198, 1997.
7. Weihrich E. G., Longauer J. K., Kirkwood A. H., Effect of topical salicylic acid on animal epidermopoiesis, *Dermatologica*, 156, 89, 1978.
8. Pullmann H., Lennartz K.-J., Steigleder G. K., Die Wirkung der Salicylsäure auf die Proliferationskinetik psoriatischer Epidermiszellen, *Arch. Dermatol. Forsch.*, 251, 271, 1975.
9. Roberts D. L., Marshall R., Marks R., Detection of action of salicylic acid on the normal stratum corneum, *Br. J. Dermatol.*, 103, 191, 1980.
10. Davies M., Marks R., Studies on the effect of salicylic acid on normal skin, *Br. J. Dermatol.*, 95, 187, 1976.
11. Huber C., Christophers E., Keratolytic effect of salicylic acid, *Arch. Dermatol. Res.*, 257, 293, 1977.
12. Nook T. H., *In vivo* measurement of the keratolytic effect of salicylic acid in three ointment formulations, *Br. J. Dermatol.*, 117, 243, 1987.
13. Gloor M., Beier B., Untersuchungen zum keratoplastischen Effekt von Salicylsäure, Schwefel und einem Tensidgemisch, *Z. Hautkr.*, 59, 1657, 1984.
14. Going S. M., Guyer B. M., Jarvie D. R., Hunter J. A. A., Salicylic acid gel for scalp psoriasis, *Clin. Exp. Dermatol.*, 11, 260, 1986.
15. Hulsebosch H. J., Ponec-Waelsch M., The interaction of anthralin, salicylic acid and zinc oxide in pastes, *Dermatologica,* 144, 287, 1972.
16. Runne U., Zur Anthralin-Salicylsäure-Therapie der Psoriasis, *Hautarzt*, 25, 199, 1974.
17. Diem E., Fritsch P., Salicylatvergiftung durch percutane Resorption, *Hautarzt,* 24, 552, 1973.
18. Zesch A., Short and long-term risks of topical drugs, *Br. J. Dermatol.*, 115, Suppl. 31, 63, 1986.
19. Chapman B. J., Proufoor A. T., Adult salicylate poisoning: deaths and outcome in patients with high plasma salicylate concentrations, *J. Int. Med.* 72, 699, 1989.
20. Péc J., Strmenova M., Palencarova, E., Pullmann R., Funiakova S., Visnovsky P., Buchancec J., Lazarova Z., Salicylate intoxication after use of topical salicylic acid ointment by a patient with psoriasis, *Cutis*, 50, 307, 1992.
21. Luderschmidt C., Plewig G., Die chronische perkutane Salicylsäureintoxikation, *Hautrarzt*, 26, 643, 1975.
22. Germann R., Schindera I., Kuch M., Seitz U., Altmeyer S., Schindera F., Lebensbedrohliche Salicylatintoxikation durch perkutane Resorption bei einer schweren Ichthyosis vulgaris, *Hautarzt*, 47, 624, 1996.
23. Taylor J. R., Halprin K. M., Percutaneous absorption of salicylic acid, *Arch. Dermatol.*, 111, 740, 1975.
24. Weiss J. F., Lever W. F., Percutaneous salicylic acid intoxication in psoriasis, *Arch. Dermatol.*, 90, 614, 1964.
25. Lodén M., Urea-containing moisturizers influence barrier properties of normal skin, *Arch. Dermatol. Res.*, 288, 103, 1996.
26. Lodén M., Barrier recovery and influence of irritant stimuli in skin treated with a moisturizing cream, *Contact Dermatitis*, 36, 256, 1997.
27. Bettinger J., Gloor M., Gehring W., Wolf W., Influence of emulsions with and without urea on water-binding capacity of the stratum corneum, *J. Soc. Cosmet. Chem.*, 46, 247, 1995.
28. Treffel P., Gabard B., Stratum corneum dynamic function measurements after moisturizer or irritant application, *Arch. Dermatol. Res.*, 287, 474, 1995.
29. Müller K. H., Pflugshaupt C., Harnstoff in der Dermatologie, *Hautarzt*, 40, Suppl. 9, 1, 1989.
30. Wohlrab W., Der Einfluß von Harnstoff auf die Wasserbindungskapazität der menschlichen Hornschicht, *Dermatol. Monatsschr.*, 174, 822, 1988.
31. Fluhr J. W., Vrzak G., Gloor M., Hydratisierende und die Steroidpenetration verbessernder Effekt von Harnstoff und Glycerin in Abhängigkeit von der verwendeten Grundlage, *Z. Hautkr.*, 73, 210, 1998.
32. Wohlrab W., Schiemann S., Untersuchungen zum Mechanismus der Harnstoffwirkung auf die Haut, *Arch. Dermatol. Res.*, 255, 23, 1976.

33. Wohlrab W., Harnstoff — ein bewährter Wirkstoff in der Dermatologie und Kosmetik, *Pharm. Ztg.*, 33, 2483, 1992.
34. Wohlrab W., Wiederfindungsrate von extern angewandten Glukokortikosteroiden auf der Hautoberfläche, *Dermatol. Monatsschr.,* 174, 615, 1986.
35. Feldmann R. J., Maibach H. I., Percutaneous penetration of hydrocortisone with urea, *Arch. Dermatol.,* 109, 58, 1974.
36. Wohlrab W., The influence of urea on the penetration kinetics of topically applied corticosteroids, *Acta Dermatol.Venereol. (Stockh.),* 64, 233,1984.
37. Stüttgen G., Promoting penetration of locally applied substances by urea. *Hautarzt,* 40, Suppl. 9, 27, 1989.
38. Müller K. H., Pflugshaupt Ch., Harnstoff in der Dermatologie, *Zbl. Hautkr.,* 142, 157, 1979.
39. Gloor M., Lindemann J., Über die Wirkung von Keratolytika und Moisturizern auf die Bioverfügbarkeit von Triamcinolonacetonid in der Haut bei topischer Anwendung, *Dermatol. Monatsschr.,* 166, 102, 1980.
40. Kalbitz J., Neubert R., Wohlrab W., Modulation der Wirkstoffpenetration in die Haut, *Pharmazie,* 51, 619, 1996.
41. Fluhr J. W., Gloor M., Influence of the ointment on drug liberation of topically applied hydrocortison, triamcionoloneacetonide and betamethasonevalerate (submitted).
42. Gabard B., Bieli E., Salizylsäure und Harnstoff — mögliche Beeinflussung der keratolytischen Wirkung von Salizylsäure durch Harnstoff, *Hautarzt*, 40, Suppl. 9, 71, 1989.
43. Hagemann I., Proksch E., Topical treatment by urea reduces epidermal hyperproliferation and induces differentiation in psoriasis, *Acta Derm. Venereol. (Stockh.),* 76, 353, 1996.
44. Sasaki Y., Tadaki T., Tagami H., The effects of a topical application of urea cream on the function of pathological stratum corneum, *Acta Dermatol. Kyoto,* 84, 581, 1989.
45. Berardesca E., Vignoli G. P., Distante F., Rona C., Effects of glycolic acid on psoriasis, *Clin. Exp. Dermatol.,* 23, 189, 1998.
46. Marks R., Lowe N., Topical retinoids for psoriasis. In: Lowe N, Marks R (Eds): *Retinoids. A Clinician's Guide.* Dunitz, London, 1998.
47. Escobar S. O., Achenbach R., Iannantuono R., Torem V., Topical fish oil in psoriasis — a controlled and blind study, *Clin. Exp. Dermatol.,* 17, 159, 1992.
48. Dewsbury C. E., Graham P., Darley C. R., Topical eicosapentaenoic acid (EPA) in the treatment of psoriasis, *Br. J. Dermatol.,* 120, 581, 1989.
49. Kragballe K., Voorhees J. J., Goetzl E. J., Leukotriene B5 derived from eicosapentaenoic acid does not stimulate DNA synthesis of cultured human keratinocytes but inhibits the stimulation induced by leukotriene B4, *J. Invest. Dermatol.,* 84, 349, 1985.
50. Williams M. L., Lipids in normal and pathological desquamation, *Adv. Lipid Res.,* 24, 211, 1991.
51. Hartop P. J., Allenby C. F., Prottey C., Comparison of barrier function and lipids in psoriasis and essential fatty acid-deficient rats, *Clin. Exp. Dermatol.,* 3, 259, 1978.
52. Berardesca E., Borroni G., Oral and topical supplementation of linoleic acid and skin disease, *Med. Biol. Environ.*, 26, 159, 1998.
53. Henneicke-von Zepelin H.-H., Mrowietz U., Färber L., Bruck-Borchers K., Schober C., Huber J., Lutz G., Kohnen R., Christophers E., Welzel D., Highly purified omega-3-polyunsaturated fatty acids for topical treatment of psoriasis. Results of a double-blind, placebo-controlled multicentre study, *Br. J. Dermatol.,* 129, 713, 1993.
54. Watsky K. L., Frieije L., Lenevue M.-C., Wenck H. A., Leffell D. J., Water-in-oil emulsions as steroid-sparing adjunctive therapy in the treatment of psoriasis, *Cutis*, 50, 383, 1992.
55. Singh S., Gopal J., Mishra R. N., Pandey S. S., Topical 0.05% betamethasone dipropionate: efficacy in psoriasis with once a day vs. twice a day application, *Br. J. Dermatol.,* 133, 497, 1995.
56. Comaish J. S., Greener J. S., The inhibiting effect of soft paraffin on the Koebner response in psoriasis, *Br. J. Dermatol.,* 94, 195, 1976.
57. Finlay A.Y., Emollients as adjuvant therapy for psoriasis, *J. Dermatol. Treatm.*, 8 Suppl. 1, S25, 1997.

Part 4

Formulations and Interactions with the Skin

15 Physico-Chemical Considerations

Eleanor J. Fendler

CONTENTS

15.1 INTRODUCTION

Both the physiological effect on skin condition and the aesthetic characteristics of moisturizers are determined by the physico-chemical interactions between the skin and the moisturizer. Moisturizers can modify the physical and chemical nature of the skin's surface, making it smoother, softer, and more pliable. Moisturizers can also alter the moisture content of the stratum corneum and the skin barrier function. A physico-chemical understanding of the moisturizer as well as of the skin barrier is essential to the development and appropriate use of products. Moisturizers are widely used in dermatologic and cosmetic skin treatments and can improve skin condition by several mechanisms. Several reviews[1-6] and a considerable amount of research[7-26] have been published in this area recently. A fundamental understanding of the physico-chemical effects of moisturizers on the basic functions of the skin barrier will allow the development of physiologically effective products for the prevention and treatment of irritant contact dermatitis and related skin conditions.

15.2 SKIN BARRIER STRUCTURE AND FUNCTION

The primary function of the human skin barrier is to provide an enclosure of the body that controls water loss since water homeostasis is a strict requirement for normal physiological function. Normal skin can be considered to be essentially water tight, and the loss of this barrier function in even a small area of skin can threaten survival. Control of water loss is the main concern for burn victims.

Interest in allergic and irritant contact dermatitis as well as in percutaneous penetration has focused attention on the barrier properties of the stratum corneum. Lipids were identified early as playing a critical role in barrier function; however, the "brick and mortar" model was presented only in 1975 by Michaels et al.[27] In this conceptual model the stratum corneum is viewed as a two-compartment hydrophilic/hydrophobic structure where the corneocytes with their hydrophilic keratin represent the hydrophilic bricks and the lipids represent the hydrophobic mortar. Pioneering

0-8493-7520-7/00/$0.00+$.50

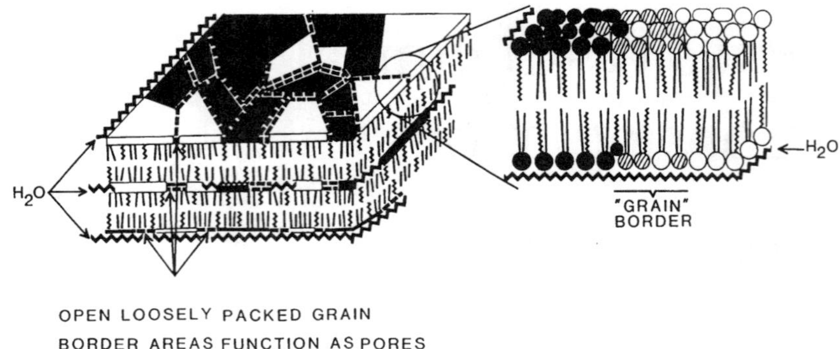

FIGURE 1 The domain mosaic model including grain borders. Lipids with very long chain lengths are aggregated into domains in the crystalline/gel phase separated by grain borders populated by lipids with relatively short chain lengths in the liquid crystalline state. (From Forslind, B., *Acta Dermato Venereologica* (Stockholm), 74, 5, 1994. With permission.)

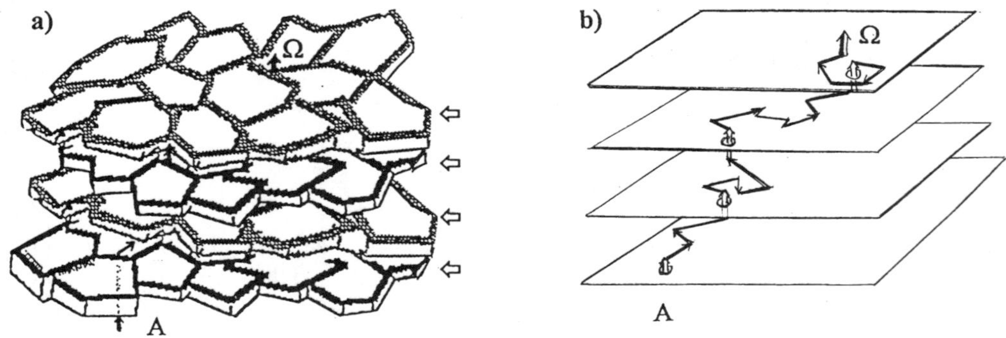

FIGURE 2 The domain mosaic model depicts lipid bilayers stacked on top of each other. (a) In each layer lipid domains form a mosaic where the water-impermeable crystalline domains are separated by "grain" borders essentially made up of lipids and fatty acids in the fluid crystalline state. Through these fluid crystalline phases water molecules can diffuse across a bilayer and then along the water "tablet" separating each double layer. (b) Therefore, a water molecule has a meandering, "random walk" way out of the system through the stacked lipid bilayer structure of the stratum corneum extracellular space. (From Forslind, B. et al., *Journal Dermatology Science*, 14, 119, 1997. With permission.)

work on the skin barrier function by Elias and co-workers in 1979[28-30] suggested that lipids present in the intercellular regions of the stratum corneum would form a bilayer structure. Friberg and Osborne[31] found that a fatty acid salt/fatty acid/water system formed lamellar liquid crystals at physiologic skin pH. This lamellar structure was used as a basis to form the layered structure earlier postulated by Elias and co-workers.[28-30] Subsequently, it has been established that water passes more or less freely through the corneocytes, while the intercorneocyte space is the true pathway for essentially all other substances. In 1994, Forslind published the "domain mosaic model" for the lipid epidermal barrier.[32] Unlike the "brick and mortar model," the domain mosaic model (Figure 1) takes lipid structure and composition into account as a means of explaining the properties of the human skin barrier.[33,34] In this two-compartment model, lipids in the crystalline (gel) state represent the dominant part (Figure 2). These lipids are domains surrounded by lipids in the liquid crystalline state. This structure-function model is an invaluable framework for an understanding of the physico-chemical interactions of "moisturizers" with the stratum corneum and their consequent physiological effects.

15.3 EPIDERMAL BARRIER DAMAGE

Damage to the skin barrier can be caused by numerous external factors, including friction, weather, chemical irritants, water, organic solvents, and soaps and surfactants. Regardless of the cause of the barrier damage and consequent dysfunction, the physical consequences usually include excessive dryness, chapping, cracking, and scaling; redness; roughness; and loss of elasticity and pliability. Damage to the stratum corneum affects the functions which normally control the passage of water through the skin, allowing only a small amount (0.5 $g/m^2/h$) to evaporate. Skin barrier damage is frequently associated with abnormally high transepidermal water loss and decreased water content of the stratum corneum which, in turn, may lead to abnormal desquamation of corneocytes. For normal, healthy skin which is elastic and pliable, the water content of the stratum corneum must be at least 10%. "Dry" or xerotic skin involves more than just low water content. Electron micrographic studies have demonstrated that for dry skin the stratum corneum is thicker, fissured, and disorganized. The scaly appearance and "whitening" of dry skin may be due, in part, to the failure of corneocytes to desquamate normally.

The physico-chemical interactions that result in dry skin depend on the cause of the barrier damage, e.g., the effect of detergents. In Forslind's model, lipids with very long chain lengths are segregated into domains in the crystalline (gel) phase separated by grain borders populated by lipids with relatively short chain lengths in the liquid crystalline state. Detergents and surfactants are postulated to primarily infiltrate the fluid parts of the barrier, i.e., the grain borders in Forslind's model, and dissolve the lipids from the barrier. The transepidermal water loss then increases and the liquid crystallinity of the lipid barrier is lost, resulting in dry, rough, scaly skin.

15.4 EPIDERMAL BARRIER REPAIR: ROLE OF MOISTURIZERS

Once the skin has been damaged and the stratum corneum barrier function impaired, barrier repair can only occur if the loss of moisture is retarded. This is the primary function of moisturizers. Remoisturization of the skin has been found to occur as a four-phase physiological process: (1) initiation of barrier repair by the moisturizer forming a film on the skin, (2) alteration of the cutaneous moisture partition coefficient, (3) diffusion of water from the dermis to the epidermis, and (4) lipid synthesis and reconditioning of the intercellular lipids enabling them to again control water distribution through the epidermis.[35] There are two primary physico-chemical mechanisms for rehydrating the stratum corneum: (1) use of a hydrophobic barrier or "occlusion" and (2) the use of hydrophilic humectants. Moisturizing ingredients used in skin care products can be considered to be the *biomimectic counterparts* of stratum corneum components (Table 1). An increase in stratum corneum moisturization by either of these mechanisms or by a combination is thought to improve skin condition and barrier function.

15.5 FUNCTION OF HYDROPHOBIC LIPIDS

Hydrophobic lipids such as petrolatum, beeswax, lanolin, and oils are generally believed to exert their effect by forming an inert, occlusive, epicutaneous film or membrane which reduces transepidermal water loss by preventing evaporation from the stratum corneum. However, topically applied lipids have been found to penetrate the viable epidermis, be metabolized, and significantly modify endogenous epidermal lipids.[36] It is also probable that topically applied lipids, such as fatty acids, triglycerides, and phospholipids, can penetrate the stratum corneum and be incorporated into the lamellar bilayers.

Petrolatum is usually considered to be the most "occlusive" of the hydrophobic lipids used in skin care products. However, if skin with a damaged barrier is occluded with a vapor-impermeable wrap, the synthesis of intercellular lipids is blocked. "Occlusion" with a vapor-permeable wrap, however, does not prevent barrier recovery. Consequently, transepidermal water loss is necessary

TABLE 1
Moisturizers: Components of Skin and Moisturizers

Stratum Corneum Component	Biomimectic Moisturizer Ingredient
Hydrophobic Lipids	
Sterols/sterol esters	Cholesterol
	Fatty alcohol
	Lanolin
Ceramides	Ceramides
Fatty acids/fatty alcohols	Fatty alcohols (cetyl alcohol)
	Lanolin
	Fatty acid esters
Squalene/waxes	Petrolatum
	Beeswax
Triglycerides	Vegetable, animal, and marine oils
Complex lipids: sphingolipids, glycerophospholipids, glycerol lipids	Phospholipids, sphingolipids
Others	
Hydrophilic Humectants	
Keratinocytes/keratin fibers	
Natural moisturizing factor:	
Amino acids	Amino acids
Inorganic salts	
Pyrrolidone carboxylic acid	Pyrrolidone carboxylic acid and salts
Lactates	α-Hydroxy acids and salts (glycolates, lactates)
Urea	Urea
Others	Polyhydric alcohols: glycerine, propylene glycol, sorbitol

for initiation of the synthesis of lipids that allow barrier repair and skin reconditioning to occur. Petrolatum neither forms nor acts like an epicutaneous, impermeable membrane. Instead, it penetrates the stratum corneum, where it is localized in intercellular domains, and interacts with the bilayer system in some places, while in others it forms separate lamellar domains.

Unlike an occlusive film or wrap, petrolatum was found to accelerate barrier recovery after acetone defatting. Other lipids may perform more like the occlusive plastic film and interfere with the skin's ability to repair the damaged barrier by proper lipid synthesis.

15.6 USE OF HYDROPHOBIC LIPIDS WITH HUMECTANTS IN BARRIER REPAIR PRODUCTS

These investigations of petrolatum provided truly exciting possibilities for skin protection and skin therapy. Based on this research and on the predicted effects of other lipids and humectants, skin care products containing high levels of petrolatum were formulated to promote the repair of the barrier for severely damaged skin. Prototypes both with and without hydrocortisone and silicone oil were evaluated using visual and skin bioengineering techniques on large panels of automotive technicians. The panels were divided into product test groups and a control group that used no product. The products were used in the workplace for a period of at least 2 weeks, with baseline measurements being made before product use and after week one and week two. All of the products significantly improved skin condition as determined by visual grading and measurements of transepidermal water loss and skin hydration. No significant differences were found for the products containing hydrocortisone and/or silicone oil.

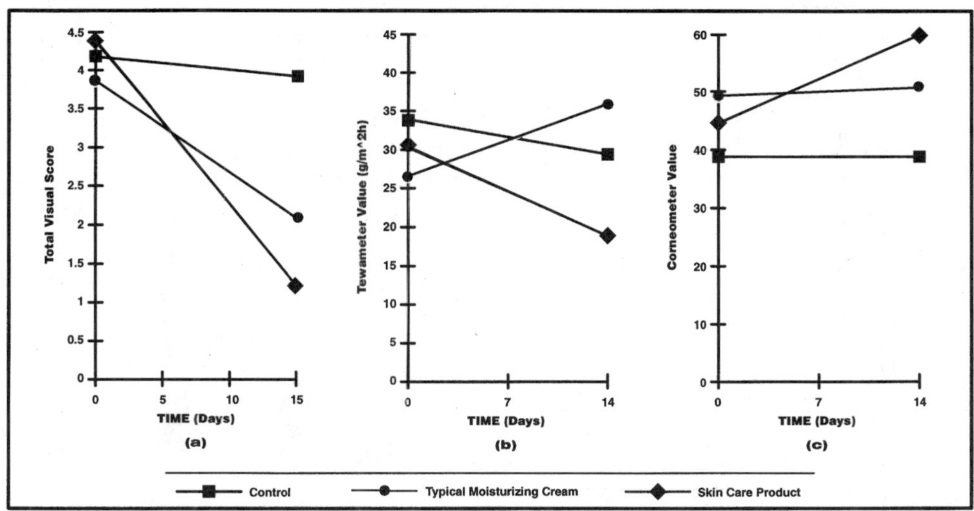

FIGURE 3 Effects of skin care products on damaged skin are evaluated using (a) visual ratings of expert grader, (b) transepidermal water loss measurements on a Tewameter TM210, and (c) skin hydration measurements on a Corneometer CM820PC.

The skin care product without either of these ingredients was then compared to a typical moisturizing cream using the same methodology. Remarkably, the skin care product significantly improved the skin condition, while the typical moisturizer exhibited little effect (Figure 3).

15.7 FUNCTION OF HYDROPHILIC HUMECTANTS

Humectants used as moisturizers are substances which attract water, mimicking the role of the dermal glycosaminoglycans and other hydrophilic components of the stratum corneum (Table 1). They are absorbed into the stratum corneum and there, by attracting water, increase hydration. Humectants draw water largely from the dermis to the epidermis and rarely from the environment, when conditions of relative humidity exceed 70%. Humectants are considered valuable moisturizers since they have the ability to bind moisture over a wide range of humidities. Since the skin's ability to hold moisture varies with relative humidity, humectants enable the skin to maintain a higher than normal equilibrium moisture content. Under low humidity conditions, humectants, such as glycerine, can actually draw moisture from the skin and increase transepidermal water loss. The effect of glycerine was determined on model lipids.[37] Although glycerine did not alter the water loss at 6% relative humidity, it maintained the liquid crystalline state of the lipid at that very low humidity. In the absence of glycerine, the model lipids showed substantial crystallization and exhibited multiple phases. This study suggests that the addition of substances which maintain the liquid crystalline structure under dry environmental conditions may provide an alternate mechanism for moisturization. This approach could be potentially useful for "winter" xerosis and use in dry climates. Froebe and co-workers[37] also found that glycerine acts as a moisturizer, even in a dry atmosphere, by inhibiting the lipid phase transition from liquid to solid crystals.

15.8 PHYSICO-CHEMICAL INTERACTIONS OF INGREDIENTS

Cosmetic and dermatologic products for use in improving "dry" skin problems are formulated using a wide variety of chemical ingredients. These ingredients include the hydrophylic humec-

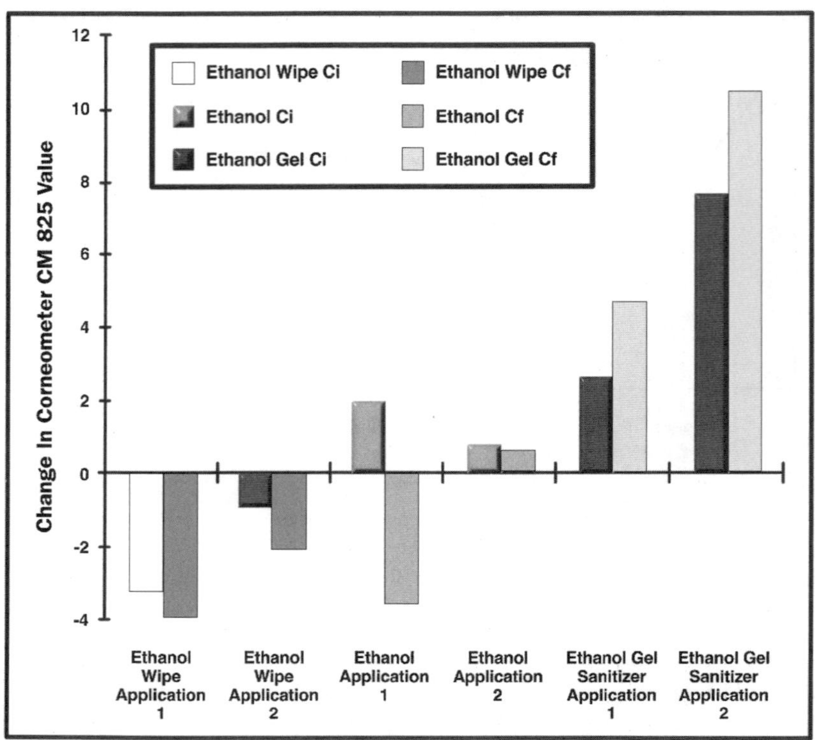

FIGURE 4 Effects of alcohol treatments on skin hydration. Ci = skin hydration: initial Corneometer CM825 reading at time zero. Cf = skin moisture capacity: Corneometer reading after 1.5 min occlusion.

tants discussed earlier, which penetrate the stratum corneum and bind water via hydrogen bonding, and the hydrophobic lipids that may form a barrier that decreases the rate of water loss from the stratum corneum. Other ingredients have no physiological function, but improve the skin's softness, smoothness, and pliability by essentially "lubricating" or filling in the spaces between "dry" partially desquamated skin flakes on the skin surface. These types of ingredients can be considered to be the "active" or functional ingredients in a formulated product. Most products also contain inactive ingredients whose function is to solubilize, emulsify, suspend, and/or disperse the other ingredients or to simply provide aesthetically pleasing attributes to the product. Unfortunately, the interactions, and resulting effects, of the active ingredients on each other as well as the effects of the inactive ingredients on the active ones are too often overlooked. Consideration of these physico-chemical interactions can lead to functionally superior products based on positive synergies between the ingredients.

Use of a combination of physico-chemical interactions and mechanisms in a single product can even overcome the dehydrating effects of other ingredients. An example of this is the alcohol hand sanitizer (Purell® Instant Hand Sanitizer). It is formulated with 62% ethanol, a neutralized film forming carobmer, glycerine (an humectant), propylene glycol, and isopropyl myristate (hydrophobic lipids). Its effect on skin hydration and moisture capacity was compared to that of 62% ethanol and a 62% ethanol wipe (Figure 4). The results clearly indicate that the alcohol wipe dehydrates the skin, and the alcohol itself has an insignificant effect. However, the same alcohol combined with biomimectic moisturizing ingredients in the alcohol hand sanitizer increases both skin hydration and skin moisture capacity, an effect which increases with a repeated application (Figure 4).

REFERENCES

1. Zhai H. and Maibach H. I., Moisturizers in Preventing Irritant Contact Dermatitis: An Overview, *Contact Dermatitis*, 38, 241–244, 1998.
2. Hannuksela M., Moisturizers in the Prevention of Contact Dermatitis, *Curr Probl Dermatol,* 25, 214–220, 1996.
3. Lodén M., Biophysical Properties of Dry Atopic and Normal Skin with Special Reference to Effects of Skin Care Products, *Acta Derm Venereol*, Suppl. 192, 1–48, 1995.
4. Rieger M. M., Skin, Water and Moisturization, *Cosmet Toiletries*, 104, 41–51, 1989.
5. Idson, B., Dry Skin, Moisturizing and Emoliency, *Cosmet Toiletries*, 107, 69–78, 1992.
6. Blichmann C. W., Serup J., and Winther A., Effects of Single Application of a Moisturizer: Evaporation of Emulsion Water, Skin Surface Temperature, Electrical Conductance, Electrical Capacitance, and Skin Surface (Emulsion) Lipids, *Acta Derm Venereol* (Stockh.), 69, 327–330, 1989.
7. Serup J., Winther A., and Blichmann C. W., Effects of Repeated Application of a Moisturizer, *Acta Derm Venereol* (Stockh.), 69, 457–459, 1989.
8. Lodén M. and Lindberg M., The Influence of a Single Application of Different Moisturizers on the Skin Capacitance, *Acta Derm Venereol* (Stockh.), 71, 79–82, 1991.
9. Ghadially R., Halkier-Sørensen L., and Elias P. M., Effects of Petrolatum on Stratum Corneum Structure and Function, *J Am Acad Dermatol*, 26, 387–396, 1992.
10. Hannuksela A. and Kinnunen T., Moisturizers Prevent Irritant Dermatitis, *Acta Derm Venereol* (Stockh.), 72, 42–44, 1992.
11. Swanbeck G., Urea in the Treatment of Dry Skin, *Acta Derm Venereol* (Stockh.), Suppl. 177, 7–8, 1992.
12. Serup J., A Three-Hour Test for Rapid Comparison of Effects of Moisturizers and Active Constituents (Urea), *Acta Derm Venereol* (Stockh.), Suppl. 177, 29–33, 1992.
13. Serup J., A Double-blind Comparison of Two Creams Containing Urea as the Active Ingredient, *Acta Derm Venereol* (Stockh.), Suppl. 177, 34–38, 1992.
14. Halkier-Sørensen L. and Thestrup-Pedersen K., The Efficacy of a Moisturizer (Locobase) Among Cleaners and Kitchen Assistants During Everyday Exposure to Water and Detergents, *Contact Dermatitis*, 29, 266–271, 1993.
15. Lane A. T. and Drost S. S., Effects of Repeated Application of Emollient Cream to Premature Neonates' Skin, *Pediatrics*, 92, 415–419, 1993.
16. Gabard B., Elsner P., and Treffel P., Barrier Function of the Skin in a Repetitive Irritation Model and Influence of 2 Different Treatments, *Skin Research and Technol*, 2, 78–82, 1996.
17. El Gammal C., Pagnoni A., Kligman A. M., and El Gammal S., A Model to Assess the Efficacy of Moisturizers — the Quantification of Soap-Induced Xerosis by Image Analysis of Adhesive-Coated Discs (D-Squames®), *Clin Exp Dermatol*, 21, 338–343, 1996.
18. Lodén M. and Andersson A. C., Effect of Topically Applied Lipids on Surfactant-Irritated Skin, *Br J Dermatol*, 134, 215–220, 1996.
19. Lodén M., Urea-containing Moisturizers Influence Barrier Properties of Normal Skin, *Arch Dermatol Res*, 288, 103–107, 1996.
20. Mao-Qiang M., Feingold K. R., Thornfeldt C. R., and Elias P. M., Optimization of Physiological Lipid Mixtures for Barrier Repair, *J. Invest Dermatol*, 106, 1096–1101, 1996.
21. Møss J., The Effect of 3 Moisturizers on Skin Surface Hydration, *Skin Res. Technol*, 2, 32–36, 1996.
22. Olivarius F. F., Hansen A. B., Karlsmark T., and Wulf H. C., Water Protective Effect of Barrier Creams and Moisturizing Creams: A New *In Vivo* Test Method, *Contact Dermatitis*, 35, 219–225, 1996.
23. Lodén M., Barrier Recovery and Influence of Irritant Stimuli in Skin Treated with a Moisturizing Cream, *Contact Dermatitis*, 36, 256–260, 1997.
24. Mortz C. G., Andersen K. E., and Halkier-Sørensen L., The Efficacy of Different Moisturizers on Barrier Recovery in Hairless Mice Evaluated by Non-Invasive Bioengineering Methods, *Contact Dermatitis*, 36, 297–301, 1997.
25. Ramsing D. W. and Agner T., Preventative and Therapeutic Effects of a Moisturizer, *Acta Derm Venereol* (Stockh.), 77, 335–337, 1997.
26. Bettinger J., Gloor M., Vollert A., Kleesz P., Fluhr J., and Gehring W., Comparison of Different Non-Invasive Test Methods with Respect to the Effect of Different Moisturizers on Skin, *Skin Res Technol*, 5, 21–27, 1999.

27. Michaels A.S., Chandrasekaran S. K., and Shaw J. E., Drug Permeation Through Human Skin: Theory and *In Vitro* Experimental Measuremnet, *AIChE J*, 21, 985–996, 1975.
28. Elias P. M., Brown B. E., et al., Localization and Composition of Lipids in Neonatal Mouse Stratum Granulosum and Stratum Corneum, *J Invest Dermatol*, 73**,** 339–348, 1979.
29. Elias P. M., Epidermal Lipids, Barrier Function, and Desquamation, *J Invest Dermatol*, 80, 44s-49s, 1983.
30. Williams M. I. and Elias P. M., The Extracullular Matrix of Stratum Corneum: Role of Lipids in Normal and Pathological Function, *CRC Crit Rev Therap Drug Carrier Systems*, 3, 95–122, 1987.
31. Friberg S. E. and Osborne D. W., Small Angle X-Ray Diffraction Patterns of Stratum Corneum and a Model Structure for Its Lipids, *J Dispersion Sci Technol*, 6, 485–495, 1985.
32. Forslind B., A Domain Mosaic Model of the Skin Barrier, *Acta Derm Venereol* (Stockh.), 74, 1–6, 1994.
33. Forslind B., Engström S., Engblom J., and Norlén L., A Novel Approach to the Understanding of Human Skin Barrier Function, *J Dermatol Sci*, 14,115–125, 1997.
34. Forslind B., Norlén L., and Engblom J., A Structural Model for the Human Skin Barrier, *Progr Colloid Polym Sci*, 108, 40–46, 1998.
35. Jackson E. M., Moisturizers: What's in Them? How Do They Work?, *Am J Contact Dermatitis*, 3, 162–168, 1992.
36. Wertz P. W. and Downing D. T., Metabolism of Topically Applied Fatty Acid Methyl Esters in BALB/C Mouse Epidermis, *J Dermatol Sci*, 1, 33–38, 1990.
37. Rhein L. D., Simion F. A., Froebe C., Mattai J., and Cagan R. H., Development of a Stratum Corneum Lipid Model to Study the Cutaneous Moisture Barrier Properties, *Colloid Surf*, 48, 1–11, 1990.

16 Emulsifiers

Patricia A. Aikens and Stig E. Friberg

CONTENTS

16.1 INTRODUCTION

Emulsifiers play several roles in skin care formulations. They modify the properties of the original formulations to ensure the stability of the original dispersion of different active components such as oil, fragrance, and preservatives; they make formulations esthetically attractive during application; and they serve an essential role to create optimal structures to facilitate the beneficial action of active components during the structural changes occurring after application.

Of these factors, the last one has received only scant attention. Because of the traditional opinion that the action on the skin is dominated by the chemical structure of the active substance, the remaining part of the formulation has been considered as a passive package, the function of which is limited to bringing the active substance to the skin surface.

This unfortunate perception has caused the attention to be centered on the original dispersion structures and attempts have been made to relate the action on the skin to the size and shape of the original dispersed particles. So a large part of the literature has become concerned with the beneficial action of vesicles or liposomes on the skin, because of an initial report that vesicles should penetrate the stratum corneum layer in intact form.[1] This notion is, to say the least, highly unlikely to be true. Aside from the fact that liposomes are of a size that makes the penetration in intact form physically virtually impossible, as has been well described "like forcing a basketball

0-8493-7520-7/00/$0.00+$.50

though a quarter inch mesh,"[2] it is obvious that the interaction between the amphiphiles in the vesicles and those in the stratum corneum would lead to structure changes.

Finally, and most importantly, a vesicular solution will inevitably change to a lamellar liquid crystal or an α-gel[3] within 15 minutes after application on the skin,[4] making the argument of size and structure a moot point.

In the same vein, microemulsion formulations have been met with hesitance, because a microemulsion is *a priori* a structure that will disorder a lamellar structure, such as that in the lipid part of the stratum corneum, into a more disordered liquid. This fact has caused concerns that such formulations should cause irritation.

Also in this case the perception per se is not based on facts. The microemulsion colloidal structure will disappear within the same time period as mentioned for vesicles, and the interaction with stratum corneum depends on the structures formed at low water concentrations. Those can only be known after information is obtained on the evaporation path through different phases. Obviously, if the microemulsion contains surface-active substances, which per se cause irritation, a problem should be anticipated, but microemulsion may be formulated from nonirritating substances.

The factors mentioned in this introduction reveal that emulsifiers play a more active role, not only in the formulation, but also in the function of skin care lotions as well as fragrances. They are, in fact, essential for their success and will be discussed more in detail in the following sections.

The complex function of emulsifiers can only be comprehended if the different surfactant association structures are known as well as their dependence of the total composition. With such knowledge available, the changes in structure during the evaporation of water and volatile organics may be estimated and the potential interaction with skin evaluated.

Realizing these relations, this chapter will give a brief review of emulsion stability and of surfactant amphiphilic structures and their appearance in different parts of a lotion system. This brief description will be followed by a simple evaluation of the conditions during evaporation. The final section gives a series of examples of surfactants for skin lotions.

16.2 STABILITY OF EMULSIONS

Stability of emulsions is an area where the literature is sometimes contradictory. The influence of added electrolytes on the stability may be mentioned as an illustrative example. The DLVO theory[5,6] states unequivocally, and in agreement with an overwhelming number of research results, that added electrolyte in excess of certain concentrations leads to cancellation of the electric double layer stabilization — the Schultze-Hardy rule. On the other hand, recent results by Cabane et al.[7] reveal that increased amounts of salt in excess of the Schultze-Hardy limit lead to enhanced stabilization.

The explanation of this and other "contradictions" is found in the facts that destabilization of an emulsion is a multistage process and that the stabilization mechanism is different for the consecutive processes. In short, the initial process is the flocculation (Figure 1A $\rightarrow$ B), in which the droplets aggregate. The stabilization is in the form of "long distance" repulsive forces and/or in the rheology of the continuous phase to retard the movement of droplets. For this step there is no doubt that addition of salt in excess of a certain level causes destabilization.

The second step in the total process is the coalescence (Figure 1B $\rightarrow$ C). The thin film between flocculated droplets bursts and a larger droplet is formed. In this step, the rheology of the medium has little importance; now the structure of the interfacial layers is paramount as illustrated by Cabane and co-workers'[7] results. Adding electrolyte reduces the repulsion between the surfactants in the interfacial layer. The packing is made more dense and stability is improved. This part of the destabilization process has been incompletely studied and Cabane and co-workers' contribution[7] is a valuable introduction to further studies.

In parallel with and following these two primary phenomena is the gravitational transport of droplets called sedimentation or creaming depending on the relative density of the dispersed and

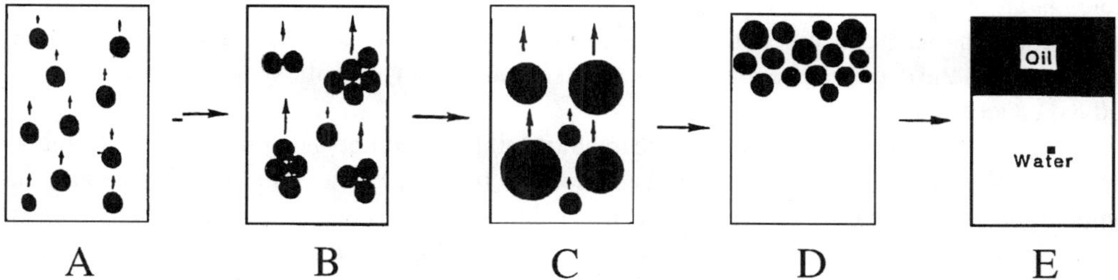

FIGURE 1 The destabilization of an emulsion includes several steps. Flocculation A → B, coalescence B → C, creaming (or sedimentation) B → D, C → D and phase separation D → E.

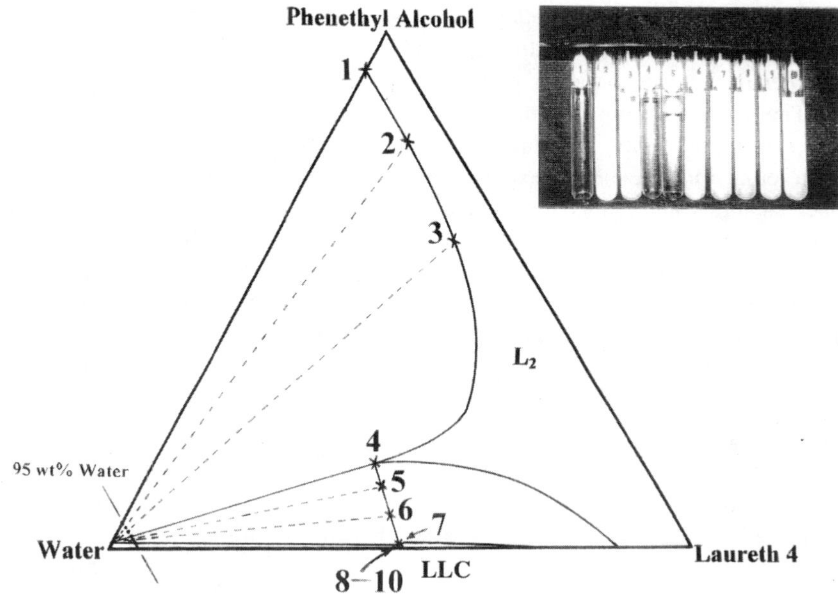

FIGURE 2 The stability of a phenethyl alcohol emulsion is influenced by several factors: (1) the relative density of the aqueous and oil phase giving maximum stability of emulsions 2 and 3 because the density ratio is close to 1.0; and (2) the presence of a lamellar liquid crystalline phase effective from emulsion 6 and on.

continuous phase (Figures 1B + 1C → 1D). It becomes important for macroemulsion droplets; for microemulsions, the Brownian movement is the dominant phenomenon and gravitational transport does not take place. For macroemulsions, the density difference is important, as demonstrated by fragrance emulsions. In a series with increased emulsifier content, a maximum of the stability was observed (Figure 2). The reason for this optimal ratio is that the phenethyl alcohol is more dense than water. The addition of a surfactant, Brij 30, gave reduced density, and the optimal stability was observed for equal values of density (emulsions 2 and 3 in Figure 2).

The creaming or sedimentation leads to a layer of more concentrated emulsion,[8] flocculated or not, with enhanced coalescence as a result. Finally, the coalescence becomes complete, and a phase separation takes place.

Because different applications require stabilization against different destabilization steps, the formulator must decide which step is essential in order to choose the optimal emulsifier. The choice is illustrated by two emulsions whose stabilization requires an entirely different approach. In the first case, a fluorocarbon-in-water emulsion for a blood substitute, the flocculation is the essential step to prevent aggregated droplets clogging the arteries and causing death. The second emulsion choice is an orange beverage, essentially a flavor emulsion in a suspension of orange pulp. Now the flocculation-coalescence is not a serious problem because the emulsion is very dilute. Instead, the creaming is the decisive phenomenon; a "crud" or an oily layer in the bottle neck will inevitably lead to reduced consumer acceptance.

The choice of emulsifier to obtain acceptable stability also depends on the type of emulsion. For the O/W emulsions the HLB value is a most useful concept, as long as it is realized that a combination of emulsifiers with an average HLB value in general gives improved stability compared to a single emulsifier. However, a combination also requires enhanced total emulsifier concentration.

The W/O emulsions are more difficult, and now polymeric emulsifiers are the preferred choice. The oil-soluble graft block co-polymers have become the stabilizer of choice. They are not only excellent stabilizers, but the degree of grafting may be utilized to monitor the type of emulsion, when salt content is also taken into consideration.[9]

Special kinds of emulsions are the double emulsions, the W/O/W type, which provide properties not found in simple systems.[10] Examples include formulations[11] with separated active ingredients, such as α-hydroxy acids in the inner droplets, and a fragrance in the oil phase with a polymeric rheology modifier in the outer aqueous phase, thus avoiding the interaction between the acid and the polymer. The separate compartments also allow a controlled release of water-soluble active components — an impossibility in a common O/W emulsion.

The double emulsions have been extensively investigated,[12] resulting in emulsifier selections giving enhanced stability and reduced leakage between the two aqueous phases. However, recently, a significant improvement has been achieved by the use of block co-polymer emulsifiers.[11] The key ingredient is a polyhydroxy stearic acid-polyethylene oxide-polyhydroxysteoric acid block co-polymer, which forms a lamellar liquid crystal in a hydrocarbon oil. This not only stabilizes the primary W/O emulsion, but actually reduces the interfacial tension to values close to zero, resulting in very small water droplets in the oil.

16.3 SURFACTANT ASSOCIATION STRUCTURES

The behavior of surfactants with water is related to the corresponding phenomenon, when water and an amphiphile in general are mixed. Two examples are useful to understand the phenomenon. Water and isopropanol are soluble in each other in all proportions, i.e., the entire phase diagram consists of one phase (Figure 3A), a liquid isopropanol-water solution. By replacing isopropanol with pentanol, one finds that the solubility of pentanol in water is limited to 2.6% by weight and, vice versa, the solubility of water in pentanol is limited to 8.0%. All formulations between these two values form an emulsion of the two mentioned compositions, which separates into two layers at standing (Figure 3B). In other words, these low molecular weight alcohols in combination with water form one simple solution within the solubility region and two simple solutions (aqueous and nonaqueous) once phase saturation occurs.

Sufacants such as octaethylene glycol dodecyl ether ($C_{12}E_8$) form simple aqueous solutions only at very low concentrations, < 0.1%. $C_{12}E_8$, however, can be solubilized in water to far greater amounts, up to approximately 30%. This high dissolution limit in water is due to the fact that contrary to pentanol the sufactant does not separate when its aqueous solution is saturated.

Instead, it forms an association structure, a micelle, and *this structure is soluble in water* (Figure 3C). With this in mind, the maximum solubility of the surfactant per se in water is called the critical micellization concentration (cmc). The micelles formed at concentrations in excess of this value are in most cases of spherical shape, but exceptionally the micelles may form long cylinders giving rise to viscoelastic solutions. The shape of the micelle has been related to the geometry of the surfactant by the Ninham-Israelachvili packing ratio:[13]

$$R = v_H/a_o\ell$$

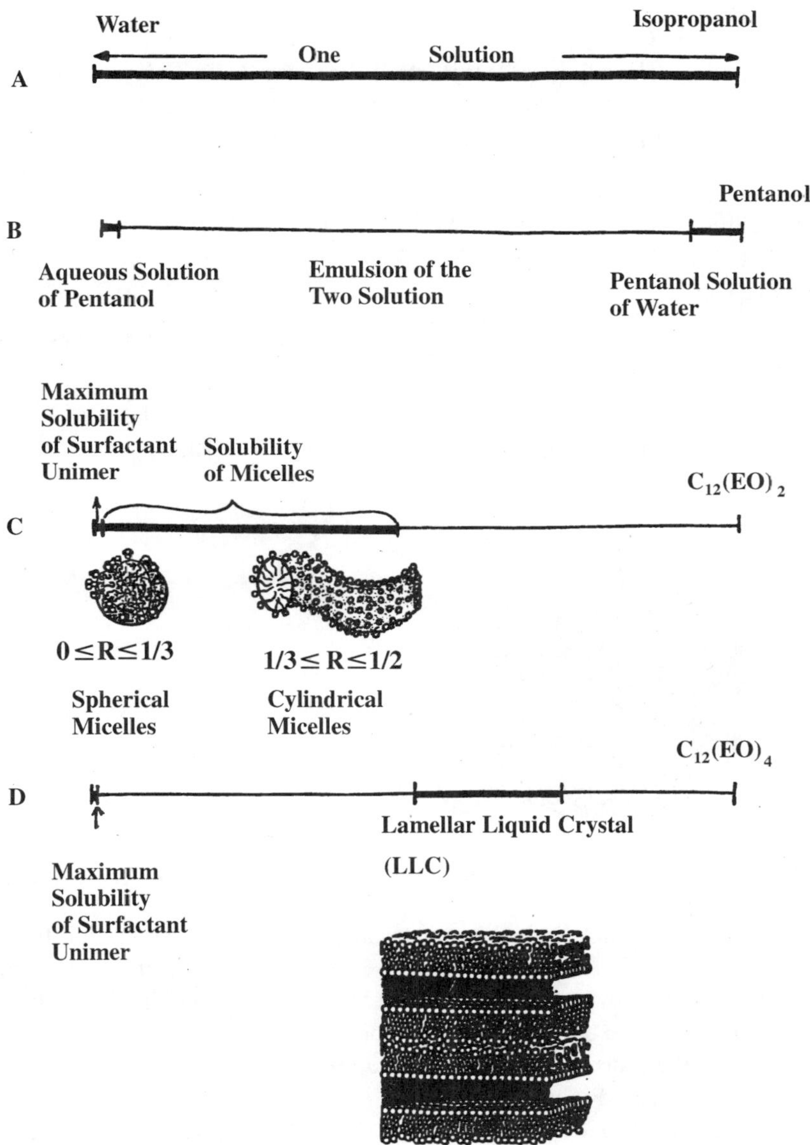

FIGURE 3 The structure of the amphiphilic decides its association structure with water (see text).

in which ν_H is the volume occupied by its hydrocarbon chain, a_o is the cross-sectional area occupied by the polar group in the association structure, and ℓ is approximately the length of the hydrocarbon chain.

In the simplest approximation, the shape of the association structure follows the limits in Table 1.

The most important consequence of this rule is that for R values <½ the "maximum" solubility of the surfactant will be in an isotropic liquid solution reaching several tens of percent.

For higher R values the surfactant becomes "insoluble" in water because additions of it to more than a few hundredths of a percent lead to a turbid liquid. Hence, one may feel that the behavior of that surfactant is fundamentally different from that of the micelle-forming ones.

It is not so; the principal behavior is identical. When exceeding its solubility limit, the surfactant molecule will form an association structure, as in micellization, but, contrary to that

TABLE 1
The Ninham-Israelachvili Packing Ratio Limits for Different Amphiphilic Association Structures (AAS)

R	O	⅓	½	1
AAS	Sphere	Cylinder	Lamella	Inverse

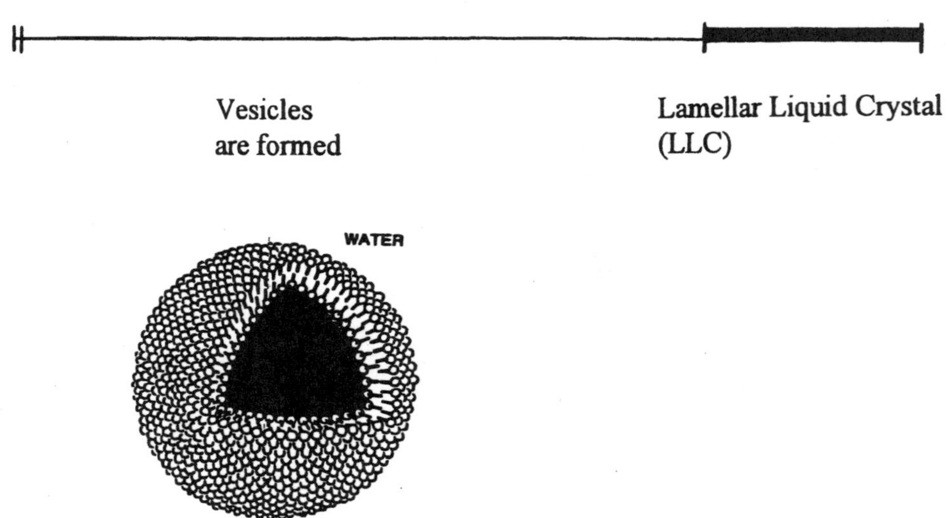

FIGURE 4 Vesicles are formed when a lamellar liquid crystal is dispersed in water.

structure, the association is not limited geometrically. In micellar association the geometry is naturally closed when a sphere is formed because the hydrocarbon chains are shielded from water by the polar groups. However, for the second kind of surfactant, the association takes place with the surfactants parallel to each other, the hydrocarbon chains are not shielded from exposure to water, and, hence, the association will continue "infinitely" and a lamellar liquid crystal is separated as a second phase (Figure 3D).

The two-phase range between the maximum solubility of unimers and the lamellar liquid crystal with maximum water content is an emulsion[14] and has semisolid lumps of the liquid crystal in water. However, with high water content under intensive dispersing action, the lamellar liquid crystal will form liposomes or vesicles (Figure 4). These structures are formed when the critical association concentration is exceeded and are developed only if there is no forced interaction between the colloidal structures.

Micellar, in the first case, and a lamellar liquid crystal, in the second case, are both formed because the molecular structure and the intermolecular interactions favor the respective packing and, hence, exist at low concentrations of the surfactant. However, when the amount of water becomes restricted at very high concentrations (>40%) of surfactant, the limited water volume leads to a crowding of colloidal structures. Now their increased mutual interaction causes a significant structure change or a phase separation. In the simplest case, that of a short chain ionic surfactant, sodium octanoate, the crowding in the micellar solution leads to a change from spherical micelles to cylindrical ones, a change that has been somewhat imprecisely termed a "second cmc." Further reduction in the water content leads to a phase separation at 46% surfactant of a liquid crystalline phase with a minimum surfactant content of 51% by weight. This liquid crystalline phase consists

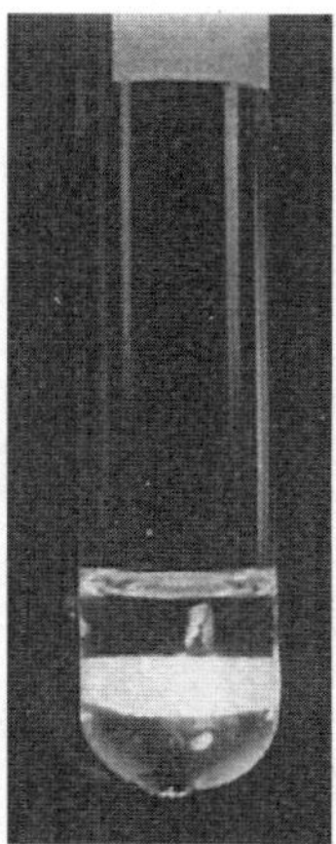

FIGURE 5 A liquid crystal (middle layer) is detected because it is birefringent, contrary to the two isotropic liquids (top and bottom layer).

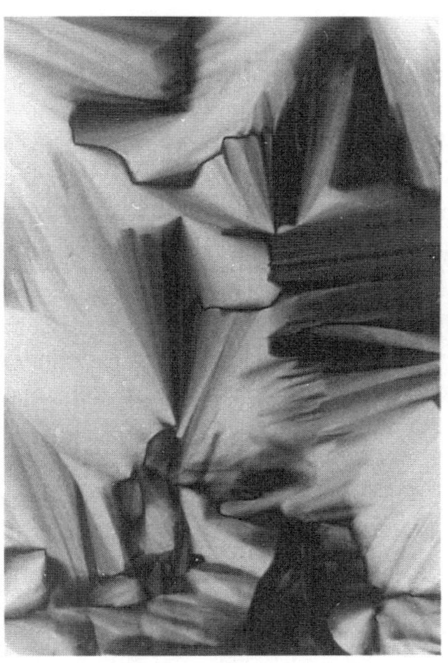

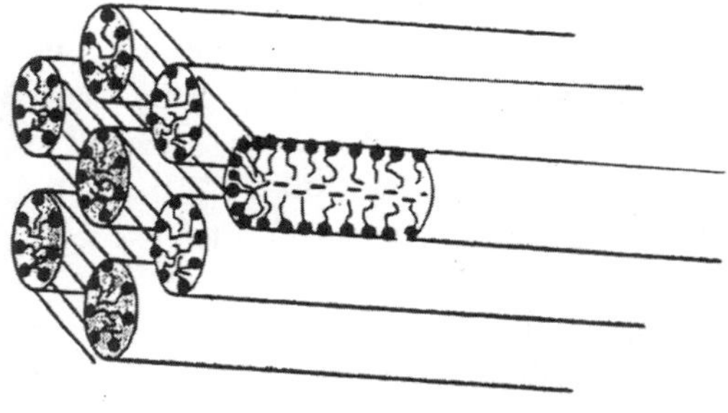

FIGURE 6 The hexagonal liquid crystal of hexagonally close-packed surfactant association cylinders is identified from its microscope pattern between crossed polarizers.

of close-packed cylinders of associated surfactants. It is easy to detect because of its birefringence (Figure 5) and also to identify from its optical microscopy pattern when viewed between crossed polarizers (Figure 6). Further reduction of water content leads, in this case, to a separation of a hydrated solid surfactant.

A surfactant with a longer chain such as an oleate also gives rise to these phases, but, in addition, when the water content is less than the limit for the stability of the liquid crystal of close-packed association cylinders, the hydrated solid surfactant is not separated. Instead, a lamellar liquid crystal is found (Figure 7). This phase is also birefringent like the hexagonal phase and is easily identified from its optical pattern when placed between crossed polarizers (Figure 7). The common non-ionic surfactants, the ethylene glycol adducts, show a similar behavior with sufficiently long polar chains.

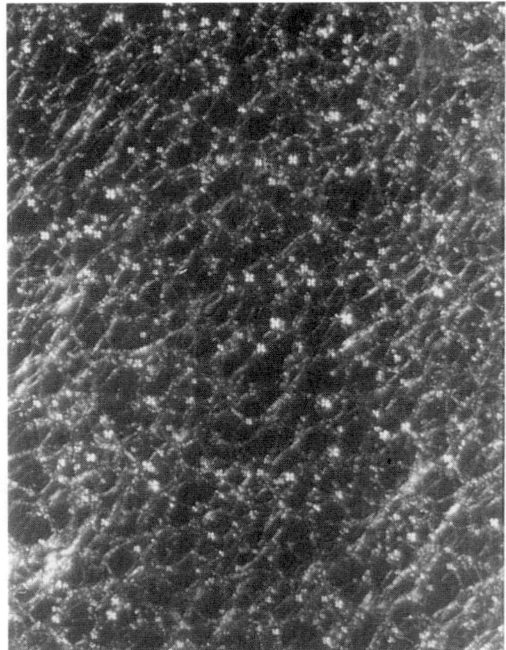
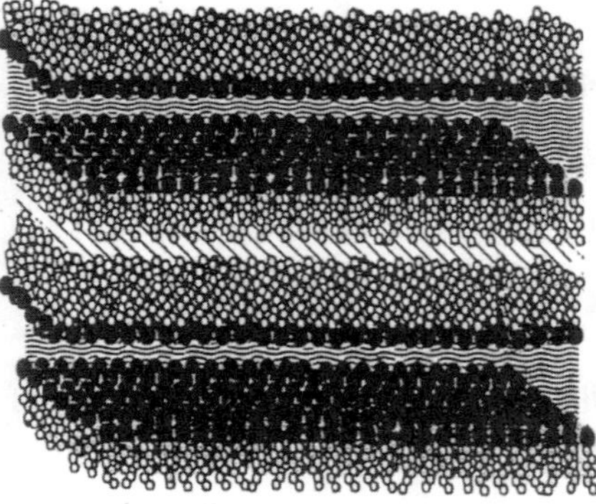

FIGURE 7 The lamellar liquid crystal is identified from its microscope pattern between crossed polarizers.

These structures are influenced by addition of a third substance,[15] with the same principles applying. In the simplest case, with water and a short chain ionic surfactant, one finds that addition of a hydrocarbon or a long chain ester has no structure-forming influence; the added substance is accepted into the water/surfactant association structures to the smallest extent the stability of the structure will allow. The location in the hydrocarbon part of the association structure does not change it, and after exceeding the solubility limit the added substance is separated in essentially pure form.

Addition of a long chain alcohol, on the other hand, leads to drastic changes. The polar group is small and the combination value of a_o in the Ninham-Israelivili packing ratio is strongly reduced; the R value is increased from less than ⅓ (spherical micelles) to the range ½ to 1 and a lamellar liquid crystal is formed at small additions of the alcohol. Greater additions lead to R values in excess of one, and inverse micelles are formed.

Both these structures are important. The inverse micellar liquid is the basis of W/O microemulsions, while the liquid crystal has a significant influence on the properties and action of cosmetic formulations. These phenomena are treated in a later section after a few words have been mentioned about the behavior of the polymeric surfactants the block co-polymers.

Their structures when combined with water are very similar to that of the common surfactants, e.g., the phase behavior depends on the relative length of the polar and nonpolar chains. An illustrative example is the series of block co-polymers of propylene oxide plus ethylene oxide.

The block co-polymer surfactants, because of the conformational freedom of their long chains, have the capacity to organize themselves into all possible patterns when combined with water and a hydrophobic short chain molecule. Figure 8 demonstrates all possible forms of association structures which have been found so far with these surfactants.

The variation of these structures with the water content have a decisive importance for the action of skin care formulations because they appear during evaporation of water and volatile organic substances. The following sections will exemplify this importance.

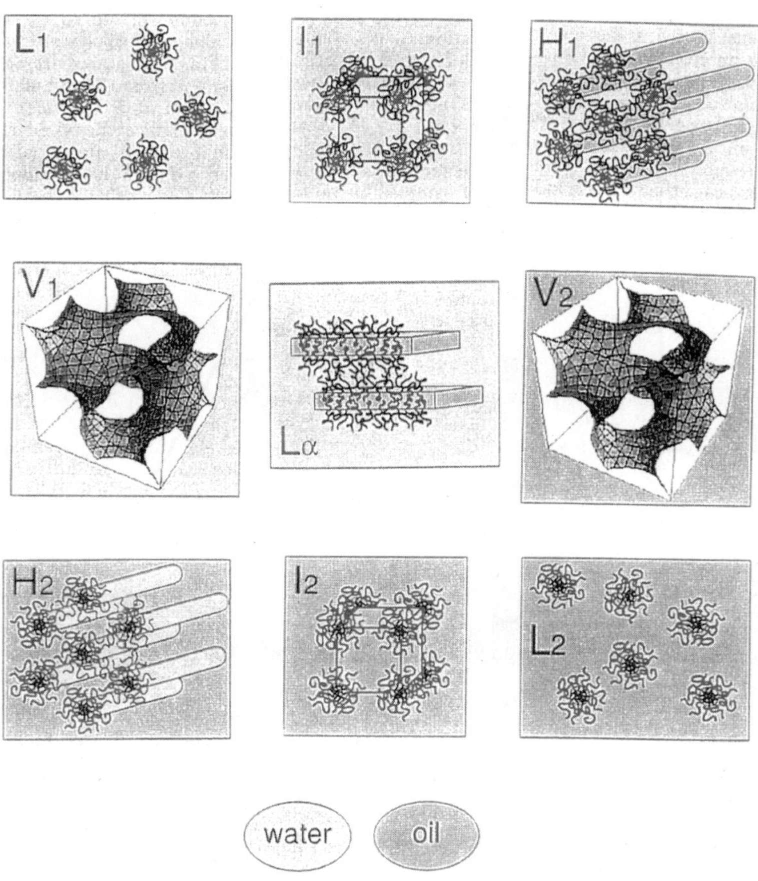

FIGURE 8 Micellar and lyotropic liquid crystalline structures.

16.4 STRUCTURE CHANGES AFTER APPLICATION OF SKIN CARE LOTIONS

The most important phenomenon after application of a skin care lotion is the fact that 90% of the water has evaporated within 20 minutes after application,[4] leading to pronounced structural changes. These are best illustrated from a phase diagram, such as that in Figure 9. In this example, the importance of relative oil and surfactant ratios is well illustrated for a system in which the oil combination has an insignificant vapor pressure in comparison with water. An example of an oil may be a paraffin oil-like hexadecane; its content in the vapor phase is approximately 0.2% by weight of the water content and hence without influence on the evaporation paths given in Figure 9.

The figure shows the compositions for emulsions with 5% of surfactant (dashed line) and the importance of the water-oil ratio for the final structure after evaporation. Emulsions with more than 5% oil will all finish as a homogenous W/O microemulsion, as demonstrated by the line marked as ____.____. Emulsions with oil content in the range of 0.6 to 5% end as a slurry of solid surfactant in the W/O microemulsion. The percentage of W/O microemulsion in this mixture is easily calculated as

$$p_{w/o} = 22.73p_o - 13,64$$

in which $p_{w/o}$ is percentage W/O microemulsion in the final slurry, and p_o is the percentage of oil in the original emulsion.

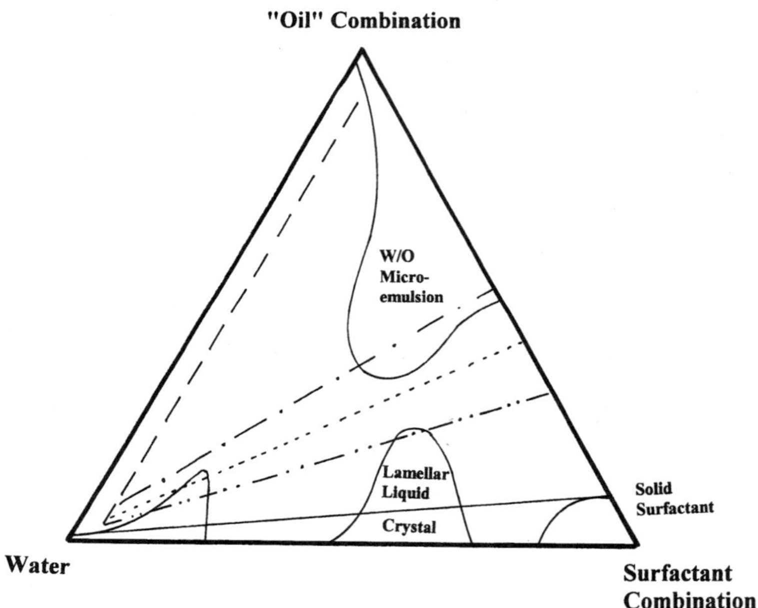

FIGURE 9 Evaporation paths from an emulsion with 5% emulsifier and varied amount of a non-evaporating oil (see text).

Intermediate emulsions show some peculiar behavior. An original emulsion with 3.6% oil is first transformed to an O/W microemulsion, e.g., it temporarily becomes transparent in the early stages of evaporation, but, at the end, after passing through a number of complex emulsions, finishes as a slurry of approximately 30% solid surfactant in a W/O microemulsion. An emulsion with 2.27% oil is also initially transformed to an O/W microemulsion, but during the continued evaporation passes through a lamellar liquid crystal, which is felt as a loose "gel." Its final composition is a very thick slurry of 60% solid surfactant and 40% of the W/O microemulsion.

This simplified approach to estimate the evaporation path is useful for the common skin care lotions because they usually do not contain volatile oils to a significant amount. For fragrances, on the other hand, a more exact treatment is needed, and the influence on the evaporation path by higher vapor pressure compounds will be discussed in a later section dealing with fragrance formulations.

For skin lotions, on the other hand, there are two essential points to be made. Both points are well illustrated by one system that reveals the rich variety of structural changes taking place during evaporation.[16] In the system of water — Laureth 4 (Brij 30)–glycolic acid–white oil (Figure 10) — a composition of 80% water, 8% glycolic acid, 8% Brij 30, and 4% white oil will pass through the following stages during evaporation. Initially, surfactant-water vesicles and oil droplets are found dispersed in an aqueous solution of glycolic acid. During the evaporation the vesicles and the droplets are dissolved into a one-phase isotropic liquid O/W microemulsion, which, in turn, is separated into a suspension of glycolic acid in an oil-surfactant solution (Figure 11).

The results illustrate the two essential aspects on the behavior and effect of skin lotions. At first they demonstrate that skin care formulations in general pass through a significant number of structural changes during evaporation. The entire picture is rather bewildering, and the practical relevance of studies such as these[16] may be questioned.

However, such a conclusion is not valid. For fragrances, on the other hand, a more exact treatment is needed, and the fact is that the value of results such as those of Reference 16 is not to evaluate the phase changes during the evaporation, although they may provide some pertinent information as to the esthetic qualities of the lotion and to one exceptional case in which the penetration of an active substance into the skin is drastically influenced by the shape of the phase areas.

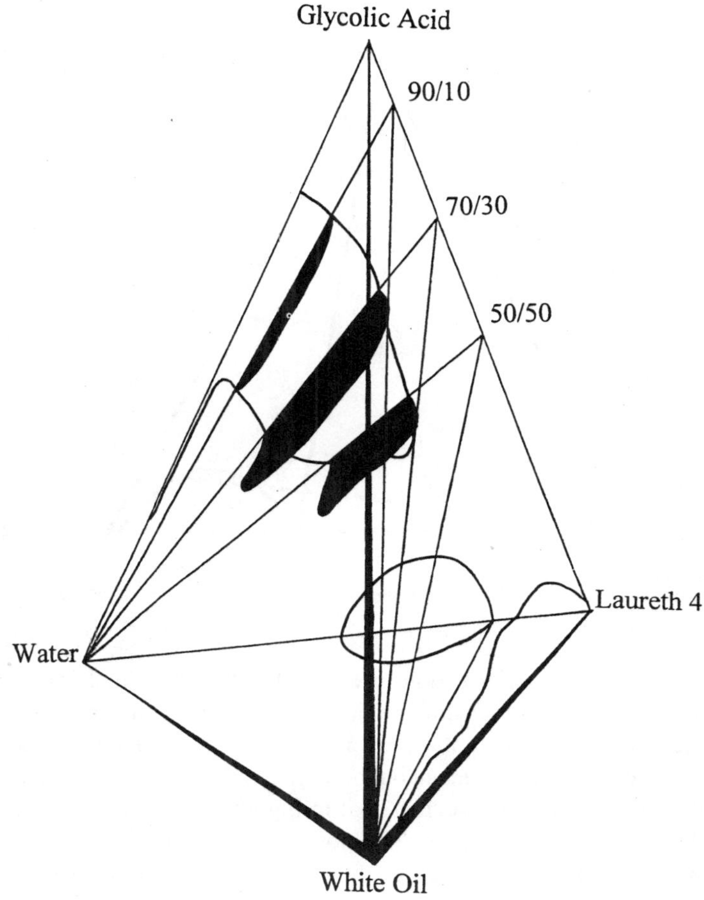

FIGURE 10 The phase areas in a typical skin lotion system.

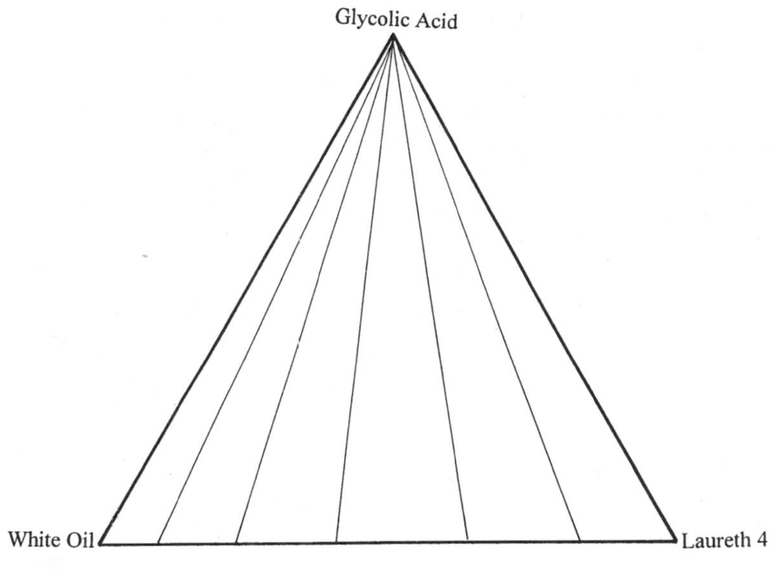

FIGURE 11 The phase diagram of three of the four components in Figure 10.

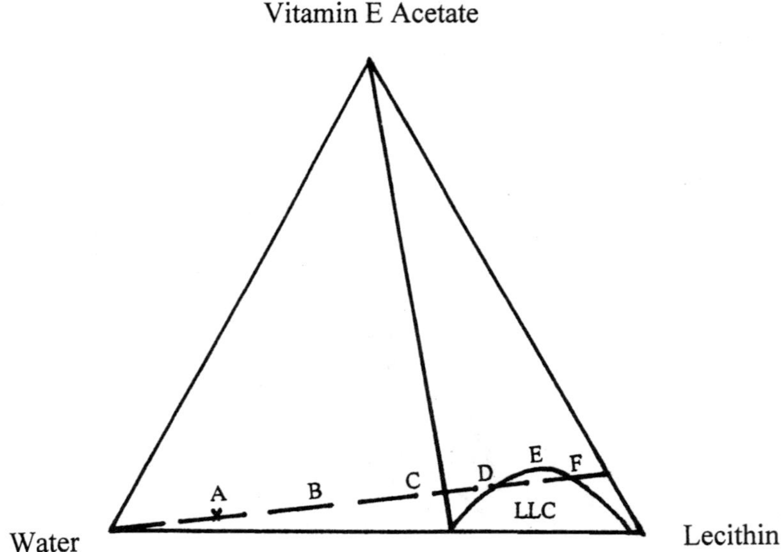

FIGURE 12 The phase diagram of the system water–lecithin–vitamin E acetate. The dashed line is an evaporation path.

The real relevance is in the information in Figure 10 about the final state after evaporation. Whatever stages the formulation passes through during the evaporation, the final state, as illustrated in Figure 11, is the agent that affects the properties of the skin. Hence, to obtain the relevant information on the influence of the surfactant on the action of the active substance, it is not necessary to determine the entire phase diagram such as that in Figure 10. A task of that kind is rather time consuming and the information obtained does not in general justify the effort. The essential information on the contribution by the emulsifier is instead gained by determining the phase conditions of the components minus the water and the volatile organics in Figure 11 — a laboratory effort of a few hours.

The structure changes *during* evaporation are extremely important in some cases, as illustrated by a simple model system (Figure 12). In this case, the consequences of evaporation of a dilute emulsion are drastic. They are, in short, a situation in which the tendency of an active substance to leave the formulation and, hence, to enter the skin is greater than that of the pure substance.*

The underlying phenomena are understood from the structures found during evaporation of an emulsion of water with dispersed vitamin E acetate (VEA) and surfactant in a ratio at the level of 1/18. An emulsion of this kind contains vitamin E acetate droplets as well as vesicles (VES) or particles of the lamellar liquid crystal (LLC) of the lecithin dispersed in water. Evaporation to point C in Figure 12 changes the emulsion from (VEA + VES)/W to VEA/LLC over a state (VEA+W)/LLC.[17] Evaporation of a few percent water from point C to point D causes the vitamin E acetate droplets to disperse into the lamellar liquid crystal, forming a molecular one-phase solution in it. The water evaporates from this phase, and when the composition reaches point F vitamin E acetate is no longer soluble and droplets of it should separate from the liquid crystal. However, no droplets are formed within hours[17] and, hence, further evaporation of water leads to a supersaturated solution of vitamin E acetate.

Hence, original emulsion of vitamin E acetate with a few percent of vitamin E acetate has reached a state in which the chemical potential (that is the tendency to leave the lotion to enter the skin) is now greater than that of the pure vitamin E acetate!

* At equilibrium such a state is impossible; thermodynamically, a pure substance has the highest possible chemical potential.

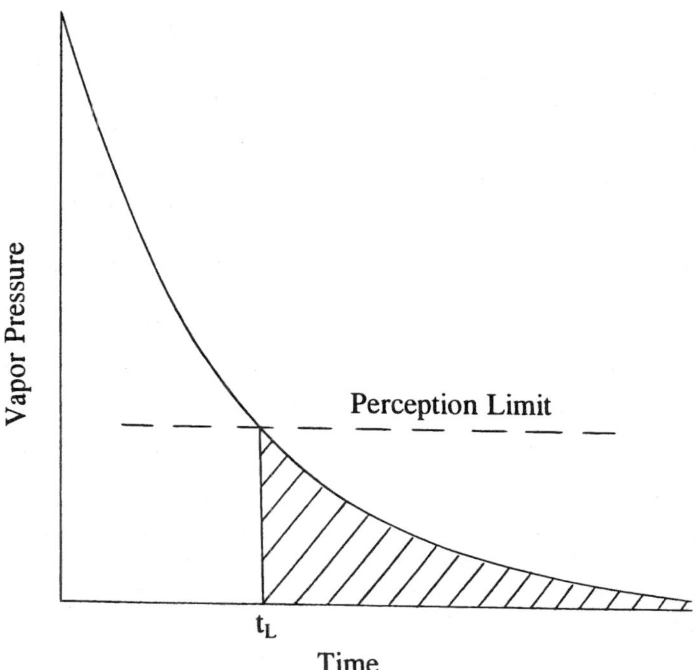

FIGURE 13 The fragrance vapor pressure from an alcohol-based formulation is reduced exponentially with time. The shaded area shows the amount of fragrance wasted because it cannot be perceived.

16.5 FRAGRANCE FORMULATIONS

Fragrances usually are not considered as skin care vehicles, but the recent ban on volatile organic compounds has forced formulators to consider amphiphilic solubilization, and a small but significant number of publications have described the phases formed by fragrance compounds when combined with surfactants and water.[18-28] This information is useful for the formulation of fragrances, but it does not provide knowledge about the most essential factor for the use of a fragrance: the variation with time of the vapor pressure of the fragrance compound after application.

This variation was well known for the traditional alcohol-based fragrances (Figure 13). The vapor pressure declined as an exponential function of time. The consequence is obvious:[29] all the fragrance evaporated after the limit of perception had been reached is wasted. This is a significant phenomenon because the cost of the fragrance is a large part of the total cost of a skin care formulation.

The formulations with surfactants will, as mentioned, give more[30] or less[31] complex phase behavior, but the vapor pressure variation with time is surprisingly constant.[32] Hence, it is possible to give a reasonably accurate estimate of the evaporation path in fragrance-water-surfactant systems with a simple iteration method.[33]

Such estimations show some unexpected features.[33] Among them is a most drastic relation between fragrance/surfactant weight ratio in an emulsion at constant surfactant concentrate and the relative vapor pressures of water and the fragrance compound. An example is useful to understand the phenomenon. The vapor pressure of benzaldehyde saturated with water is 0.7 mmHg at room temperature, while that of water is 19.8 mmHg. Hence, the vapor in equilibrium with an emulsion of the two will have a weight fraction of limonene 0.17 and water 0.83. The evaporation follows the equilibrium conditions[32] and, hence, one is able to indicate a likely evaporation path for an emulsion with 5% emulsifier with the following equation.

$$f_{BA} = \{f_w(f^o - 0.17) - (f^o_{BA} - 0.1615)\}/(0.12 - f^o_{BA}) \quad (1)$$

in which f° and f are initial and varying weight fractions, while subscripts W and BA denote water and benzaldyhyde.

The equation demonstrates the strong dependence of the final composition on the initial amount of benzaldehyde. With initial weight fraction of benzaldehyde equal to 0.17, its final weight fraction, when water is evaporated, is still 0.17. However, even a small reduction in the original weight fraction of benzaldehyde to 0.1615 leads to the benzaldehyde being completely depleted at the same time water is. A reduction of the initial weight fraction to 0.153 results in a complete depletion of the benzaldehyde, while water still remains at a weight fraction of 0.5. Values in excess of 0.17 do not lead to such pronounced results. The weight fraction of fragrance compounds goes toward 0.95 as a broken function

$$f^{\infty}_{BA} = (0.1615 - f^{o}_{BA})/(0.12 - f^{o}_{BA}) \quad (2)$$

16.6 INFLUENCE ON SKIN

The essential influence by the emulsifiers on the skin is found in the interaction with the stratum corneum lipids, whose lamellar structure is decisive per se for preventing excessive drying of the skin. For surfactants, which give rise to a final lamellar liquid crystal, the action on the skin should be beneficial, as pointed out by Junginger.[34] The interesting problem is, of course, what structures will be found if a lamellar structure such as that of the stratum corneum lipids encounters a liquid crystal of different structure.

One example gives some guidance. The emulsifier Tween 80 forms only one liquid crystal, a hexagonal array of cylinders, and the structural modifications, when this liquid crystal is mixed with a lamellar one, are of interest. The results[35] showed the lamellar structure to prevail. The bulky head group of Tween 80 was accommodated within the lamellar structure by an increased water layer thickness. It is obvious that the lamellar structure of stratum corneum is very resistant to changes.

This short review has thus far given a brief account of the fundamental phenomena of emulsifiers in skin formulations. The following sections will give examples of emulsifiers used and also some typical examples of formulations.

16.7 COMMONLY USED EMULSIFIERS FOR SKIN MOISTURIZING PREPARATIONS

16.7.1 Alkoxylated Fatty Alcohols

Fatty alcohols of longer chain lengths such as cetyl (C_{16}), cetosearyl ($C_{16,18}$), stearyl (C_{18}), isostearyl (branched C_{18}), and oleyl (C_{18} with double bond) treated with ethylene oxide to form ether ethoxylates are often used as emulsifiers in skin moisturizing products. Ceteareth-20 and oleth-10 are listed in the USP/National Formulary (NF, meaning they are used in pharmaceutical products). The length of the polyethylene oxide hydrophile can vary between 2 and 20 (or 21), and often the longer hydrophiles stabilize W/O emulsions, while the higher PEG derivatives (>10) are more water soluble and stabilize O/W emulsions. These non-ionic surfactants are rarely used alone; the best results with respect for emulsion stability are achieved when hydrophilic and hydrophobic surfactants are used in combination. The ratios of each depend on the oil used, known as the HLB system (Hydrophile Lipophile Balance). Ethoxylated surfactants become more hydrophobic as they are heated in water due to dehydration of the glycol ether characterizing the surfactant. In addition, fatty alcohols themselves are often used in combination with the ether ethoxylate surfactant to add structure to the emulsion. Compared to most anionic surfactants, they are nonirritating to the skin.

16.7.2 Alkoxylated Fatty Esters

A commonly used emulsifier for skin and pharmaceutical products is ethoxylated stearic or cetearic acid. The PEO-40, PEO-50, and PEO-100 stearates are listed in the NF. Like the alcohol ethoxylates, the ester ethoxylates are used in combinations of hydrophilic and lipophilic to best suit the oil phase.

16.7.3 Glycerol Fatty Esters

The glycerol ester of stearic acid, also USP and NF approved, is used as an emulsifier and thickening agent for moisturizing creams. Often this is supplied in combination with propylene glycol for a W/O emulsifier or in combination with PEG-100 stearate for O/W emulsifier (also called "self-emulsifying glycerol monostearate[11]). Mono- and diglycerides of fatty acids can be ethoxylated to make them more hydrophilic or converted to polyglycerol esters (up to four glycerol units).

16.7.4 Sorbitan Fatty Esters and Polysorbates

The hydrophilic portion of these surfactants are derived from sorbitol, a sugar product. Water is eliminated from sorbitol to form a cyclic structure called 1,4 sorbitan. The free hydroxyl groups form mono-, di-, and triesters when reacted with fatty acids. Cetearic, stearic, isostearic, and oleic acid, as well as beeswax and lanolin derivatives, are used for the hydrophobe. These sorbitan esters are fairly liphophilic with an HLB of around 5. The sorbitan esters can be ethoxylated, usually with either 4 or 20 mol of EO to form polysorbates which have higher HLBs between 10 and 15. Sorbitan esters and polysorbates are often used together as an emulsification system.

16.7.5 Glucosides and Sucrose Esters

Emulsifiers which are ethers or esters with polymeric sugar based hydrophile are good for skin care products because they are extremely mild. The headgroup contains many free hydroxyl groups which bind water, providing additional moisturization. Some sugar based surfactant systems such as sucrose cocoate in combination with sorbitan stearate form structured emulsions in water with or without oil.

16.7.6 Dimethicone Copolyols

The hydrophobic portion of these emulsifiers is a flexible siloxane polymer, and the hydrophilic portion is polyethlene oxide. They are most useful for providing emulsion stability to W/O emulsifiers for most oils including silicone.

16.7.7 Lecithin

Zwitterionic phospholipids from natural sources such as soybeans, as well as synthetically modified lecithins can emulsify many types of oils, especially vegetable oils, and are nonirritating to the skin due to their chemical similarity to skin lipids and ability to form lamellar phases. Lecithin is often advertised in the skin care market for its ability to form liposomes, however, it has been shown to be an excellent O/W emulsifier.

16.7.8 Polymeric Surfactants

Recently, polymeric surfactants of MW around 5,000 Da have been introduced to offer enhanced stability and low skin irritation potential to moisturizing lotions and creams. For W/O preparations, ethoxylated dipolyhydroxystearic acid is used for a wide variety of oils and is especially good for high internal phase systems and systems containing electrolytes. Acrylate polymers are used for O/W emulsions. They are not very surface active and help to stabilize the emulsion by increasing viscosity which slows down coalescence of the droplets. Block co-polymers (poloxymers) are also used in O/W emulsions.

16.7.9 Phosphate Esters

The cetyl and stearyl phosphate monoesters are anionic surfactants that are very good mild emulsifiers. The cationic counterion is either sodium, potassium, or triethanolamine. They are used in combination with low HLB emulsifiers or fatty alcohols to give structured W/O emulsions. Triethanolamine salts of oleth-3 or oleth-10 phosphate esters are also used as hydrophilic emulsifiers.

16.7.10 Carboxylate Salts (Soaps) and Carboxylic Acids

Carboxylic acid salts of aluminum, magnesium, sodium, potassium zinc, and triethanolamine are an older method of emulsification and are not used as commonly as many of the more mild anionic or nonionic surfactants. Carboxylic acids, particularly stearic and cetearic, are often used in combination with other emulsifiers to give body and structure to a skin care emulsion.

16.8 FORMULATIONS

Emollient oils typically used in skin moisturizing preparations are mineral oils, including petrolatum, triglyceride and ester vegetable oils, synthetic fatty esters, silicone polymers, and lanolin. In addition, other ingredients which might be included in a formulation to heal dry skin include α-hydroxy acids, lipids such as ceramides, natural moisturizing factors, and others. The emulsion may be W/O, O/W, or a W/O/W multiple emulsion.

Shown below are several formulations demonstrating the different types of formulations.[36,37]

I. DRY SKIN CARE LOTION
A formulation from Costec Inc. containing petrolatum and lanolin. This formulation was published in Reference 36, p. 103.

Phase	Ingredient	%
A	Deionized water	74.40
	Disodium EDTA	0.05
	Sorbitol (70% aq.)	3.00
	Triethanolamine	1.85
	Methylparaben	0.02
	Sodium chloride	0.02
B	Mineral oil	7.00
	Petrolatum	3.00
	Lanolin	3.00
	Lanolin alcohol	3.00
	Stearic acid, triple pressed	2.50
	Cetyl alcohol	1.75
	Propylparaben	0.10
C	Quaternium-15	0.20
D	Fragrance	qs

Procedure: Combine phase A with mixing and heat to 75°C in main vessel. In a separate vessel, combine phase B and heat with mixing to 75°C. Add phase B to A (both homogeneous and at 75°C) with strong mixing. Maintain at 70 to 75°C for 15 minutes and then start cooling with moderate agitation. At 40°C, add phase C and then D. Continue mixing and cooling until uniform and at 25°C.

II. HAND AND BODY CREAM
This formulation was provided by Penreco and published in Reference 37, p. 98.

Phase	Ingredient	%
A	Deionized water	70.60
	Carbomer	0.20
B	Prophylene glycol	7.00
	Methylparaben	0.20
	Panthenol	0.10
C	Mineral oil (and) hydrogenated butylene/ethylene/styrene co-polymer (and) hydrogenated ethylene/propylene/styrene co-polymer	7.00
	Propylene glycol dicaprylate/dicaprylate	5.00
	Isostearyl alcohol	2.00
	Proplyparaben	0.10
	Cetyl alcohol	2.00
	Glyceral stearate (and) PEG-100 stearate	2.50
	Potassium cetyl phosphate	1.75
	Tocopheryl acetate	0.10
D	Triethanolamine	0.15
E	Diazolidinyl urea	0.20
F	Soy lecithin	1.00
	Fragrance	0.10

Procedure: Disperse phase A. Add phase B. Heat to 75 to 80°C and mix until uniform and lump free. Combine C and heat to 80°C and mix until all the solids are dissolved. Add phase C to the A+B mixture. Mix for 30 minutes until good agitation. Add D. Mix until completely smooth and homogeneous. Cool to 50°C. Add E and cool to 40°C. Add F. Continue mixing and cooling to 30°C.

III. OIL-IN-WATER SILICONE OIL PROTECTIVE CREAM
This formula is from ICI Surfactants, Reference 36, p. 104.

Phase	Ingredient	%
A	Dmethicone (and) silicone oil, 350 cs	10.00
	Cetyl alcohol	4.00
	Isosorbide laurate	1.00
	Hybrid sunflower oil	1.00
	Lanolin	1.00
	Steareth-2	2.30
	Steareth-21	2.80
B	Deionized water	67.40
	Carbomer	0.20
	Sorbitol	5.00
	Glycerin	5.00
	10% aq. sodium hydroxide	0.20
	Quaternium-10	0.10

Procedure: Heat phase A to 70°C and phase B to 72°C. Add B to A and mix well. Add C at 50°C and stir. Add D at 35°C and stir until room temperature.

IV. SKIN THERAPY CREAM (F-668)

This is a substansive cream formulation containing the essential fatty acid γ-linolenic acid from Mona Industries, Reference 36, p. 101.

Phase	Ingredient	%
A	Borageamidopropyl phosphatdyl PG-dimonium chloride	1.50
	Stearamidopropyl PG-dimonium chloride phosphate (and) cetyl alcohol	2.20
	Cetyl phosphate	1.00
	Clycerin	2.00
	Titanium dioxide	0.50
	Proprylene glycol (and) diazolidinyl urea (and) methyl paraben (and) propyparaben	0.40
	Aminomethyl propanpl	0.40
	Deionized water	80.00
B	Cetyl alcohol	2.00
	Steareth-2	2.00
	Squalene	0.80
	Octyl stearate	4.00
	Isopropyl palmitate	2.40
	Dimethicone	0.80

Procedure: Heat phases A and B separately to 65°C. Slowly add B to A with homogenization and continue blending. Stir, cool to 40 to 45°C and add fragrance if needed.

V. MULTIPHASE EMULSION FROM ICI SURFACTANTS USING POLYMERIC SURFACTANTS[38]

Step 1: Primary Water-in-Oil Emulsion

Phase	Ingredient	%
A	Isohexadecane	15.00
	Caprylic/capric triglycerides	7.50
	PPG-15 stearyl ether	7.50
	Dipolyhydroxystearate	4.00
B	Water	65.60
	Sodium chloride	0.40
	Preservative	qs

Procedure: Heat phases A and B separately to 45°C. Add B to A with propeller stirring and homogenize thoroughly. Propeller stir for 30 minutes.

Step 2: Preparation of Multiple Emulsion

Phase	Ingredient	%
A	Primary emulsion from Step 1	70.0
B	Water	26.8
	Poloxymer 407	2.0
C	Carbomer	0.5
D	Sodium chloride	0.2
E	Preservative	qs
F	Triethanolamine	0.5

Procedure: Dissolve poloxymer in water at 20°C with stirring to form phase B. Sift C into B with fast stirring. Add D and E to (B+C) mixture with fast stirring. Slowly add A to this mixture followed by F with moderate stirring and continue stirring for 15 minutes.

REFERENCES

1. M.Mezei, L.Gulasekharem, *Life Sci.* 26, 1473 (1980).
2. K.Stanzl, *Novel Cosmetic Delivery Systems,* S.Magdassi and E.Touitou, eds., Marcel Dekker, New York, 1999, p.233.
3. K.Larsson, *Lipids-Molecular Organization, Physical Functions and Technical Applications,* The Oily Press, Dundee, Scotland, 1994.
4. T. Huang, Ph.D. thesis Microemulsions, Emulsions and Liquid Crystals — Implications in Cosmetics and Fragrances, Clarkson University, 1995.
5. B.Derjaguin, L.D.Landau, *Acta Physicochim. URSS,* 14, 633 (1941).
6. E.J.W.Verwey, J.T.G.Overbeek, *Theory of the Stability of Lyophobic Colloids,* Elsevier, Amsterdam, 1948.
7. O.Sonneville, B.Cabane, T.Gulik, *Proc. 2nd World Congress Emulsions.* 2, 3–7 (1998).
8. V.J.Purfield, E.Dickenson, M.J.W.Poney, *J. Colloid Interface Sci.* 166, 363 (1994).
9. P.Perrin, N.Monfreux, A.L.Dufour, F.Lafuma, *Colloid Polym. Sci.* 276, 945 (1998).
10. Th.F.Tadros, *Int. J. Cosmet. Sci.* 14, 93 (1992).
11. Th.F.Tadros, C.Dederen, M.C.Toelman, *Cosmetics & Toiletries.* 112, 75 (1997).
12. N.Garti, A.Aserin, *Adv. Colloid Interface Sci.* 65, 37 (1996).
13. D.J.Mitchell, B.W.Ninham, *J. Chem. Soc. Faraday Trans.* 2, 77, 601 (1981).
14. International Union of Pure and Applied Chemistry, *Manual on Colloid and Surface Science,* Butterworths, London, 1972.
15. P.Ekwall, *Advances in Liquid Crystals,* Vol. 1, G.H.Brown, ed., Academic Press, New York, 1975, p.1.
16. S.E.Friberg, A.Al-Bawab, J.L.Barber, P.A.Aikens, *J. Disp. Sci. Technol.* 19, 399 (1998).
17. S.E.Friberg, T.Moaddel, A.J.Brin, *J. Soc. Cosmet. Chem.* 46, 255 (1995).
18. R.Akahaski, S.Horike, S.Noda, *Nippon Kagaku Kaishi.* 1974 (1984).
19. R.Akahaski, S.Horike, S.Noda, *Nippon Kagaku Kaishi.* 943 (1985).
20. H.Uchiyama, S.D.Christian, J.F.Scamehorn, M.Abe, K.Ogino, *Langmuir.* 7, 95 (1991).
21. M.Abe, K.Mizuguchi, Y.Kondo, K.Ogino, H.Uchiyama, J.F.Scamehorn, E.E.Tucker, S.D.Christian, *J. Colloid Interface Sci.* 160, 16 (1993).
22. Y.Tokuoka, H.Uchiyama, M.Abe, S.D.Christian, *Langmuir.* 11, 725 (1995).
23. S.Horike, R.Akahoshi, *Nippon Kagaku Kaishi.* 12, 1033 (1996).
24. Y.Tokuoka, H.Uchiyama, M.Abe, *Nihan Yukagakaishi.* 45, 13 (1996).
25. J.Yang, G.Rong, S.E.Friberg, P.A.Aikens, *Int. J. Cosmet. Sci.* 18, 43 (1996).
26. S.E.Friberg, J.Yang, T.Huang, *Ind. Eng. Chem. Res.* 35, 2856 (1996).
27. S.E.Friberg, J.Yang, *Surfactants in Cosmetics,* Surfactant Series Vol. 68, M.M.Rieger and L.Rhein, eds., Marcel Dekker, New York, 1997, p.225.
28. S.E.Friberg, T.Huang, L.Fei, S.A.Vona, Jr., P.A.Aikens, *Prog. Colloid Lett.* 15, 1172 (1996).
29. S.E.Friberg, *Adv. Colloid Interface Sci.* 75, 181 (1998).
30. S.E.Friberg, T.Huang, L.Fei, S.A.Vona, Jr., P.A.Aikens, *Prog. Colloid Polym. Sci.* 101, 18 (1996).
31. S.E.Friberg, L.Fei, S.Campbell, H.Yang, Y.Lu, *Colloids Surf.* 127, 223 (1997).
32. S.E.Friberg, M.Szymula, L.Fei, J.Barber, A.Al-Bawab, P.A.Aikens, *Int. J. Cosmet. Sci.* 19, 259 (1997).
33. P.A.Aikens, Q.Yin, V.Marin, Z.Zhang, *J. Disp. Sci. Technol.* 20, 257 (1999).
34. H.E.Junginger, W.Hering, *Dtsch. Apoth. Ztg.* 130, 684 (1990).
35. G.Rong, H.Yang, S.E.Friberg, P.A.Aikens, J.Greenshields, *Langmuir.* 12, 4286 (1996).
36. *Cosmet. Toiletries* 112, 7/97 Skin-Care Formulary, 101–104.
37. *Cosmet. Toiletries* 112, 12/97 Creams and Lotions Formulary, 89–109.
38. ICI Americas Technical Bulletin 52-0034-520, 5/96 (ICI Americas, Wilmington, DE 19810 U.S.).

17 Hydrophilic Pastes

Bernard Gabard and Christian Surber

CONTENTS

17.1 INTRODUCTION

The majority of dermatological textbooks, even some newer ones, describe pastes as semisolid, stiff preparations containing a high proportion of finely powdered material, such as zinc oxide, titanium dioxide, starch, kaolin, and talc, incorporated at relatively high concentration in a suitable vehicle.* These vehicles are by the majority lipophilic or greasy, and the properties of the pastes are globally described as cooling, drying, exudate absorbing, and protecting.[1-7] In a recent publication, a critical review of the evidence available to assert these statements was conducted.[8] It was concluded that "serious doubts must arise from the available explanations and the various formulas of pastes and their absorptive features." Detailed investigations showed that first the powders themselves presented very different absorptive features, and further that two-phase, lipophilic pastes did not absorb moisture independently from the inner phase (powder). On the contrary, three-phase pastes consisting of an hydrophilic two-phase emulsion and a high concentration of powder (inner phase) showed considerable water uptake. It was concluded that not only the "active component(s)" of a paste, that means the powder itself or the mixture of several powders, but also the vehicle used to manufacture the paste is of major importance for the final effect on the skin. Based on these statements, a classification of the pastes was proposed[8] (Figure 1).

After a short reminder of the published results, we extend these *in vitro* experiments *in vivo,* and we investigate in a more detailed fashion the interaction of semisolid pastes with the skin. Emphasis was put on hydrophilic pastes, however, whenever necessary and for comparison purposes, results obtained with lipophilic pastes will be shown as well.

17.2 MATERIAL AND METHODS

17.2.1 TEST PRODUCTS

The test products are all commercially available and are shown in Table 1.

* Some textbooks (e.g., References 2 and 4) consider a concentration of at least 10% of solid material necessary for the product to be a paste. Others (References 3 and 7) require 20 to 50%.

0-8493-7520-7/00/$0.00+$.50

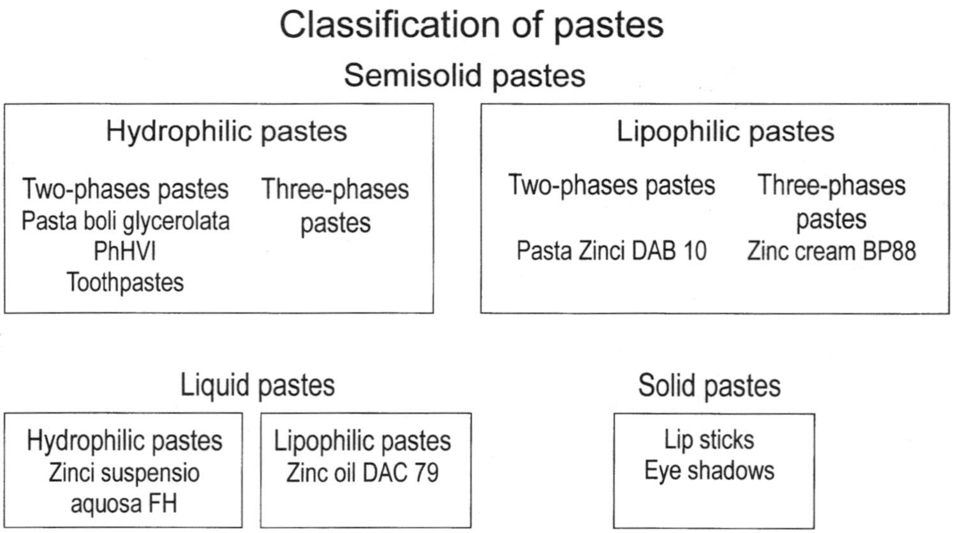

Classification of pastes

Semisolid pastes

Hydrophilic pastes

Two-phases pastes: Pasta boli glycerolata, PhHVI, Toothpastes

Three-phases pastes

Lipophilic pastes

Two-phases pastes: Pasta Zinci DAB 10

Three-phases pastes: Zinc cream BP88

Liquid pastes

Hydrophilic pastes: Zinci suspensio aquosa FH

Lipophilic pastes: Zinc oil DAC 79

Solid pastes

Lip sticks

Eye shadows

FIGURE 1 Classification of pastes. (Modified from Juch, R.D. et al., *Dermatology,* 189, 376, 1994. With permission.)

TABLE 1
Composition of the Test Products, as far as Known or Readable from the Packaging Declaration

	Tested Pastes and Their Main Components (%)							
	ZnO	**TiO_2**	**Talc**	**Kaolin**	**Starch**	**Water**	**Lipids**	**Glycerol**
Lipophilic								
LP1	46					(?)	(?)	
LP2	17				17	14	46	
Hydrophilic								
HP1	10	10	10	11		29	0	25
HP2	25		25			30 (?)	0	20
HP3		20				53	25	
HP4[x]		16				33	25	
HP5[xx]	25					25 (?)	(?)	25

Note: (?): Approximate or unknown; [x]: contains also 10% NMP; and [xx]: contains also 25% $CaCO_3$.

17.2.2 Methods

1. Evaluation of the absorptive features of different powders: these were quantified according to Enslin as previously described.[8,9] Briefly, a thermostated glass cylinder with a porous membrane on one end was filled with water and connected to a graduated capillary tube at the other end. The membrane was covered with the powder. Water absorption through the membrane was measured by the variation in the liquid level in the capillary tube.

2. Evaluation of water absorption properties of pastes *in vitro*: this experiment was conducted as described in Reference 8. Briefly, 10 g of each paste were uniformly distributed on the bottom of a Petri dish, thereby ensuring that the surface of the paste was absolutely plain and unruffled. The preparation was covered with 20 ml of distilled water and left for 30 min at 20°C. The water was removed, and the surface of the product was dried with a soft tissue. The absorptive feature of the paste preparation was calculated from the weight difference before and after incubation. In a second step, considering that some pastes may be dry after being on the skin for a while, the absorptive features of the same test products were measured in a similar way after pre-drying the preparations at 50°C to weight constancy.
3. Evaluation of the occlusive properties of different pastes *in vitro*: 2 g of test product were carefully spread over the surface of agar-filled Petri dishes. The dishes were weighed and kept at room temperature in a box covered by a protecting cloth (start values). Further weighings were taken at days 1, 2, and 5 thereafter. For control purposes, white petrolatum and a plate without any test product were included in the test. Each experiment was conducted in triplicate.
4. Evaluation of the occlusive properties of different pastes *in vivo*: these were evaluated *in vivo* on tape-stripped skin exactly as described in Reference 10. Briefly, the stratum corneum of the forearm of healthy volunteers was tape stripped until the transepidermal water loss (TEWL) attained values between 40 and 50 g/m^2/h. After a rest period of 1 h, 2.5 mg/cm^2 of the test products were carefully applied on the stripped sites using a gloved finger, and the TEWL was measured at different times until 120 min after application. Percent changes relative to a nontreated control site were calculated over time. Positive control was white petrolatum.
5. Interactions of the pastes with the skin *in vivo*: all *in vivo* measurements were conducted in a climatized room under standardized temperature and humidity conditions (22°C, 45 ± 5% rh). Six healthy volunteers participated in the study. In the first part, after measurement of skin hydration with the NOVA DPM 9003,[11] the pastes were randomly applied at a rate of 10 mg/cm^2 on different areas (2 × 2 cm; including one untreated control area) of the ventral forearms for 5, 30, and 120 min. Thereafter, the pastes were removed with a soft paper tissue and skin hydration was measured at 1, 2, 3, 4, 5, and 15 min. The second part of this study was conducted on the same volunteers following exactly the same procedures, but the skin was preliminary hydrated by an occlusive application of a moisturizer (an O/W lotion containing 5% urea and 10% glycerol) for 1 h. This was intended to mimic a clinical situation where the pastes are applied on wet skin states with the explicit goal of drying the skin.

17.3 RESULTS AND DISCUSSION

The absorptive properties of commonly used powders such as titanium dioxide (TiO_2), zinc oxide (ZnO), kaolin, cornstarch, and methylcellulose were shown to differ considerably when evaluated under standardized conditions (Figure 2). The highest water absorption was shown with ZnO and kaolin, followed by cornstarch and TiO_2. Methylcellulose formed a gel with water that prevented the entire soaking of the powder, and thus water absorption remained low.

The paramount role of the vehicle in modulating the absorptive properties of a paste is shown by the results on water absorption *in vitro* (Figure 3). First, lipophilic pastes did not absorb water significantly even after previous drying to constant weight. This confirms our former results.[8] Second, hydrophilic pastes absorbed water in significant amounts. Most of them absorbed more water after than before drying to weight constancy. Based on these results, one may distinguish the following categories:

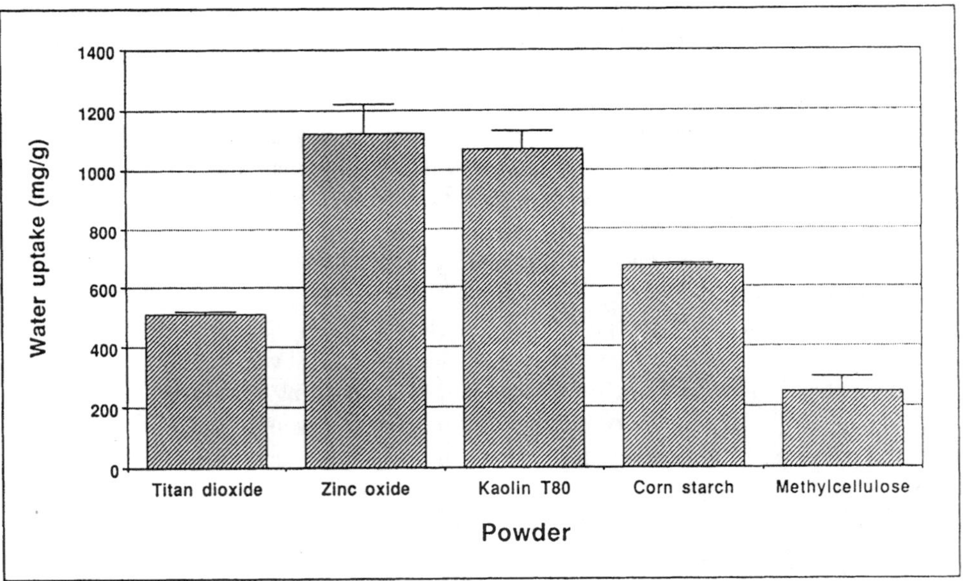

FIGURE 2 Absorptive features of commonly used powders determined by the method of Enslin[8]; n = 3, means ± SD. (From Juch, R.D., et al., *Dermatology,* 189, 375, 1994. With permission.)

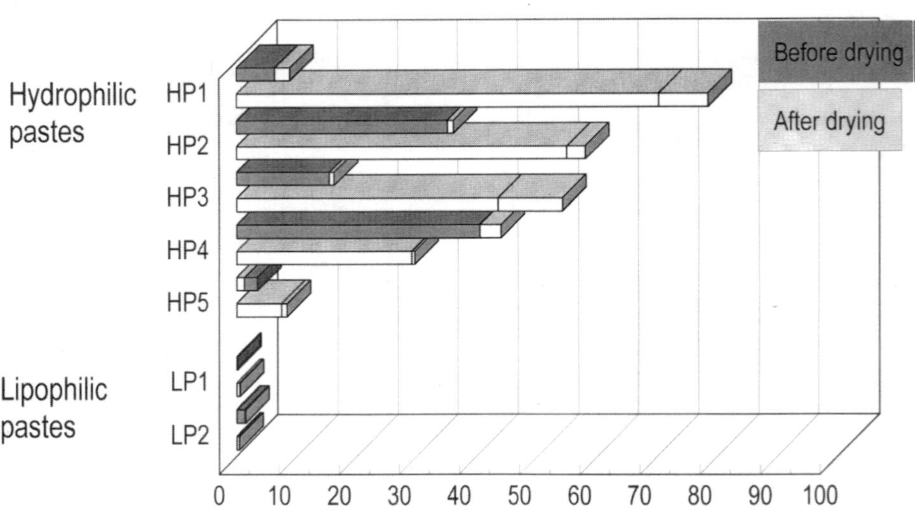

FIGURE 3 Water absorption properties of five hydrophilic (HP1 to HP5) and two lipophilic (LP1, LP2) pastes *in vitro* before and after drying to weight constancy; n = 3, means + ½SD.

- Pastes showing poor absorptive features in wet state, but strongly absorbing in the dry state (HP1, HP3 to a lesser extent)
- Pastes showing relatively good absorptive features in wet and dry states (HP2)
- Pastes showing poor absorptive features (HP5)
- Pastes showing better water absorption in the wet state than in the dry state (HP4)

TABLE 2
Occlusion *In Vitro*: Water Loss at Day 5 (g; Means ± SD)

	Water Loss (g)	% from Untreated Control
Controls		
Untreated	12.2 ± 1.1	100.0
White petrolatum	1.6 ± 1.2	13.1
Lipophilic pastes		
LP1	0.05 ± 0.01	0
LP2	0.22 ± 0.02	1.3
Hydrophilic pastes		
HP1	11.6 ± 0.5	95.2
HP2	10.7 ± 0.8	87.8
HP3	9.1 ± 0.4	74.5
HP4	8.8 ± 0.1	72.7
HP5	11.4 ± 0.5	93.8

Note: Means ± SD (n = 3) of water loss at day 5.

From this, it is obvious that it is not possible to use any hydrophilic paste in any given dermatologic situation. Apart from water (exudate) absorption, which may be a significant (and/or desirable) component of a paste's action on the skin, occlusion is another factor of importance in situations where skin protection is required.

The results of the *in vitro* occlusion tests are given in Table 2. They are, at a first glance, in accordance with what would be expected from the composition of the pastes. The hydrophilic pastes were not or only slightly occlusive; on the contrary, the lipophilic pastes show strong occlusive properties. A closer look reveals that differences were measured among the hydrophilic pastes, at least concerning their capacity to interfere with water loss from the agar plate. The pastes formulated with a small percentage of lipids in the vehicle (HP3, HP4; see Table 1) showed a slight occlusive effect. This was confirmed *in vivo* (Figure 4). However, compared to the occlusive effect of the lipophilic pastes, the diminution of TEWL seen after application of a hydrophilic paste such as HP3 is of questionable physiological significance. As expected, in both *in vitro* and *in vivo* models, a strong occlusion was seen after application of white petrolatum. This strong occlusive effect as observed with the lipophilic pastes led to a diminution of the TEWL because of the concomitant increase in the barrier function of the stratum corneum and despite an accumulation of moisture in the horny layer. This justifies the use of such pastes for skin protection, but not for drying the skin.

Summarizing, the results mean that besides using powder with strong absorptive features such as ZnO or, on a second line, TiO_2, pastes purposed to dry the skin should be of the hydrophilic type. Not only were these shown to significantly absorb water *in vitro*, but they lack a significant occlusive effect which is detrimental in a situation where water evaporation should not be impaired.

The *in vivo* investigations were conducted with three representative hydrophilic pastes: HP1 (poor absorption in the wet state, strong in the dry), HP2 (good absorption in both states), and HP3 (the only paste without addition of a humectant or any other substance; see Table 1). The results are shown in Figure 5. After a 5-min application of the pastes on normal skin, hydration was significantly higher than in control skin. However, as soon as 2 min after removal of the products, two groups were characterized, enclosing test products not statistically different from each other: HP2/HP1 on one side and HP3/control on the other. The same situation was encountered after application of the pastes during 30 min; after 120 min application time, HP2 hydration values were still high and significantly

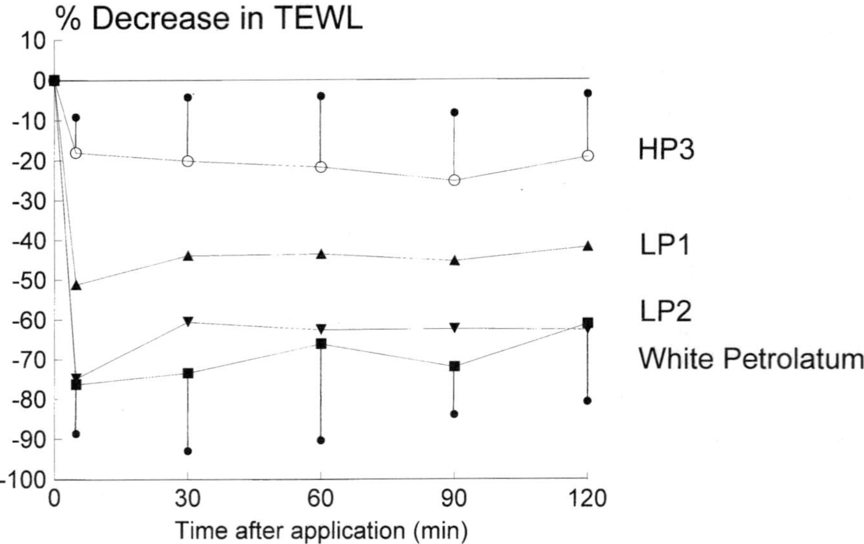

FIGURE 4 Occlusive properties of different pastes on stripped skin *in vivo* (percent decrease in transepidermal water loss) of n = 6 healthy volunteers. HP3: hydrophilic paste; LP1 and LP2: lipophilic pastes. For the sake of clarity, means are shown + ½SD (HP3) or –½SD (white petrolatum) only.

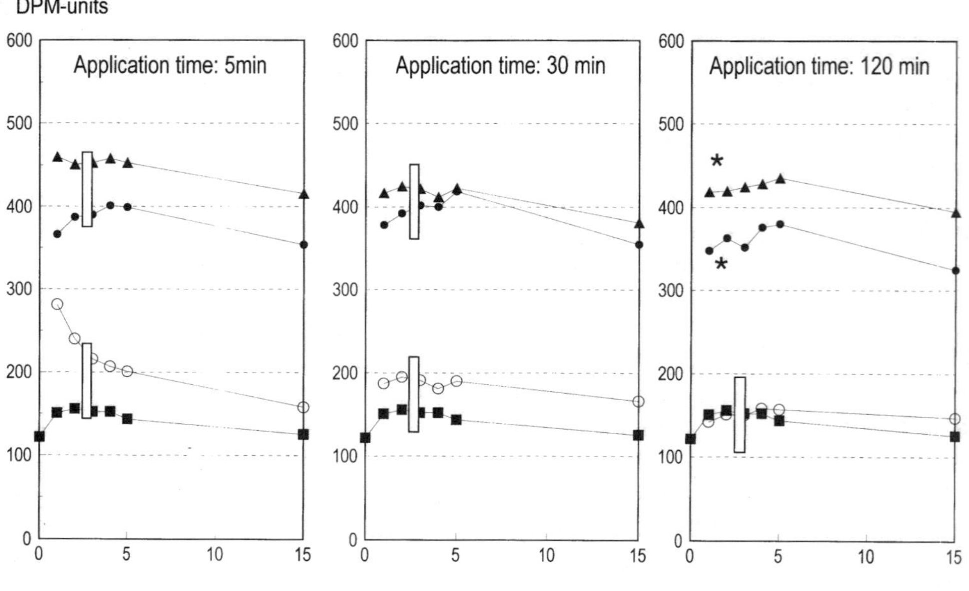

FIGURE 5 DPM measurements of skin hydration after application of pastes (10 mg/cm²) during 5 (left), 30 (middle), or 120 min (right) on normal skin of n = 6 healthy volunteers. The measurements were done 1, 2, 3, 4, 5, and 15 min after removal of the pastes. For the sake of clarity, only means are indicated. Squares: control, normal skin; closed circles: HP1; triangles: HP2; open circles: HP3; *: statistically significant differences with the control group and beween each other group. □ indicates homogenous subsets.

higher compared to HP1. HP3 and control values were no different than before. Thus, after application on normal skin, some pastes significantly and durably enhanced skin moisturization.

As seen in Figure 6, application of a moisturizer containing humectants such as urea and glycerol for 1 h under occlusion significantly increased the measured values. There was a gradual decrease in this exaggerated hydration over time, but even after 120 min normal control skin values were not totally recovered. After applying the pastes on this hydrated skin for 5 min, measured values remained high in all groups. However, as soon as 2 min after removing the paste, HP3 values were significantly lower than the other ones and also lower than control values. If the pastes remained on the skin for 30 min, a significant drying effect was measured for HP3 only. For both other pastes, hydration values remained higher than the control ones. After application for 120 min, the situation was even more obvious: HP1 and HP2 did not change the hydration values of the skin, whereas HP3 and control values showed no significant differences. Thus, we were not able to show any drying of the skin surface with hydrophilic pastes containing humectants, even if the skin was preliminary hydrated by occlusive application of a moisturizer. On the other hand, a more simple hydrophilic paste was indeed able to induce a faster dehydration after treatment than measured on a nontreated control zone left open. It is not possible to clearly prove that these results are due to the presence of humectants in the pastes. We consider it likely and see the measured values as the results of a competition between water absorption (which indeed was measured *in vitro*, see Figure 3) and water binding in the stratum corneum by the humectants. On the other hand, these differences could also have been due to a different water evaporation from the skin surface. Therefore, we measured the skin surface water loss with an evaporimeter after application of HP2 and HP3 on hydrated skin for 30 min, following the guidelines of the European Society of Contact Dermatitis.[12] The results (Figure 7) show that the water loss after HP3 was always higher than after HP2. However, this effect remained for short duration. Therefore, it is likely that the differences in water content of the vehicles themselves might have been at the origin of the differences in water evaporation.

17.4 CONCLUSION

In conclusion, after investigating *in vitro* the water absorption capacities of the main "active" component(s) of pastes, the powder(s), we showed that hydrophilic, but not lipophilic, pastes absorb water to a significant degree. This pointed out a paramount role for the vehicle incorporating the powder. Different categories were noticed, particularly when considering the absorptive capacities after predrying of the pastes. Drying is a phenomenon occurring on the skin possibly after a certain time that thus may contribute to drastic changes of the water-absorbing properties of a paste. Further, hydrophilic pastes showed no or only a slight occlusion, whereas highly occlusive properties were confirmed *in vitro* and *in vivo* for lipophilic pastes.

In vivo, hydrophilic pastes showed different interactions with the skin. Some pastes clearly hydrated the skin, others could indeed remove water from a preliminary hydrated horny layer. Elements contributing to these properties may be the presence of humectants such as glycerol, contributing to a long-lasting presence of water on the skin in the first case, or the acceleration of skin surface water loss, contributing to an accelerated removal of water from a hydrated horny layer in the second case. However, this represents, in our opinion, at most one of the elements contributing to the measured events and may simply be due to a different water content of the pastes.

We conclude that pastes cannot be pooled in a single group and be generally characterized as "drying" and "exudate binding." Lipophilic pastes did not bind any water at all and were highly occlusive. Thus, they are likely to hydrate the skin through an impairment of the transepidermal water loss. They should be preferably used for skin protection. Hydrophilic pastes, on the other hand, hydrated the skin or maintained an elevated hydration state if they contained humectants. Only an hydrophilic paste without any additional component was able to reduce a hydrated state and led to measurably decreased skin hydration values.

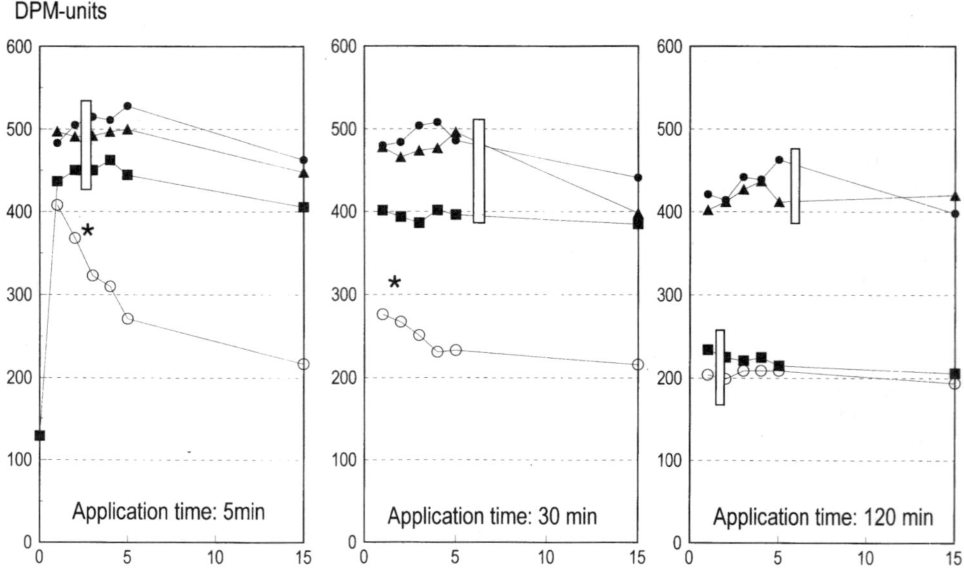

FIGURE 6 DPM measurements of skin hydration after application of pastes (10 mg/cm^2) during 5 (left), 30 (middle), or 120 min (right) on previously hydrated skin of n = 6 healthy volunteers. The measurements were done 1, 2, 3, 4, 5, and 15 min after removal of the pastes. For the sake of clarity, only means are indicated. Squares: control, hydrated skin; closed circles: HP1; triangles: HP2; open circles: HP3; *: statistically significant differences with the control group. □ indicates homogenous subsets.

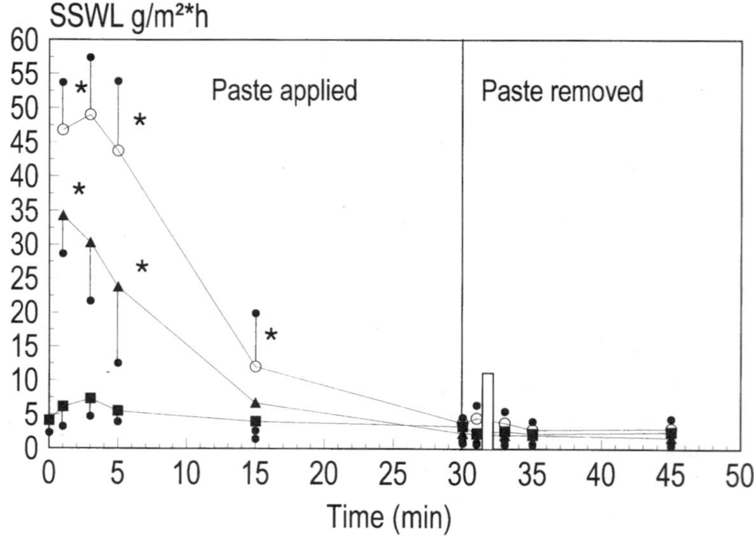

FIGURE 7 Measurement of skin surface water loss (Evaporimeter EP-1, Servomed, Stockholm) during application and after removal of two hydrophilic pastes for 30 min on previously hydrated skin of n = 6 healthy volunteers. Means ± ½SD for the sake of clarity. Closed squares: control, hydrated skin; triangles: HP2; open circles: HP3; *: statistically significant differences with the control group. □ indicates homogenous subsets.

REFERENCES

1. Thoma, K., *Dermatika*, Werbe- und Vertriebsgesellschaft Deutscher Apotheker, München, 1983.
2. Hornstein, O. P. and Nürnberg, E., *Externe Therapie von Hautkrankheiten*, Georg Thieme Verlag, Stuttgart, 1985.
3. Arndt, K. A., *Manual of Dermatologic Therapeutics*, 4th ed., Little, Brown & Co., Boston, 1989.
4. Braun-Falco, O., Plewig, G., and Wolff, H. H., *Dermatologie und Venerologie*, 4th ed., Springer-Verlag, Berlin, 1995.
5. Jung, E. G., *Dermatologie*, 3rd ed., Hippokrates Verlag, Stuttgart, 1995.
6. Korting, H. C., *Dermatotherapie*, Springer-Verlag, Berlin, 1995.
7. Altmeyer, P., *Therapielexikon Dermatologie und Allergologie*, Springer-Verlag, Berlin, 1997.
8. Juch, R. D., Rufli, Th., and Surber, C., Pastes: What do they contain? How do they work?, *Dermatology*, 189, 373, 1994.
9. Nürnberg, E. and Surmann, P., *Hagers Handbuch der Pharmazeutischen Praxis*, Vol. 2, Springer-Verlag, Berlin, 1991, 60.
10. Gabard, B., Testing the efficacy of moisturisers, in *Bioengineering of the Skin: Water and the Stratum Corneum*, Elsner, P., Berardesca, E., and Maibach, H. I., Eds., CRC Press, Boca Raton, FL, 1994, chap. 13.
11. Gabard, B. and Treffel, P., Hardware and measuring principles: the NOVA DPM 9003, in *Bioengineering of the Skin: Water and the Stratum Corneum*, Elsner, P., Berardesca, E., and Maibach, H. I., Eds., CRC Press, Boca Raton, FL, 1994, chap. 15.
12. Pinnagoda, J., Tuoker, R. A., Agner, T., and Serup, J., Guidelines for transepidermal water loss measurement: a report from the standardization group of the European Society of Contact Dermatitis, *Contact Dermatitis*, 22, 164, 1990.

18 Glycerine: A Natural Ingredient for Moisturizing Skin

Donald S. Orth and Yohini Appa

CONTENTS

18.1 INTRODUCTION

Glycerine is one of the best natural moisturizers in living systems and has been used in skin care products for preventing and treating skin dryness because it moisturizes/plasticizes the stratum corneum (SC). Until recently, the moisturizing benefits were attributed to its humectant action; however, it is now known that the skin care benefits of glycerine include attraction of moisture, osmoregulation of the intracellular milieu, maintenance of liquid crystallinity/fluidity of cell membranes and intercellular lipids (ICLs), and normalization of desquamation by hydrating enzymes involved with desmosome digestion.[1-5] The goals of this chapter are to discuss the need for moisturizing skin, to review the use of glycerine in skin care formulations, and to describe methods for evaluating skin moisturization.

0-8493-7520-7/00/$0.00+$.50

18.2 THE ROLE OF GLYCERINE AS A HUMECTANT FOR COSMETIC PRODUCTS

18.2.1 Moisturizers in Cosmetic Products

The commonly used skin moisturizers are oil-in-water (o/w) emulsions such as creams and lotions and water-in-oil (w/o) emulsions such as hand creams. Waxes, pastes, salves, and ungents are used infrequently because they lack "cosmetic elegance." One problem with emulsion formulations is that they tend to dry out over time, which results in the formation of a crust on the surface of products in jars or plugging of pump dispensers. Cosmetic formulators have used 1 to 3% humectants (glycerine, sorbitol, propylene glycol, etc.) to retain moisture and prevent these products from drying up and plugging pumps. Many early formulations used humectants primarily for maintaining product integrity, with little thought about skin moisturizing benefits.

18.3 THE ROLE OF GLYCERINE IN MOISTURIZING SKIN AND MAINTAINING MEMBRANE FLUIDITY

18.3.1 The Need for Skin Moisturization

The SC provides a barrier to the evaporation of water from the viable epidermis. Many factors work to compromise this barrier and increase the rate of water loss from the skin. Exposure to harsh environmental conditions including cold, dry winter weather; frequent washing with soap and hot water; exposure to surfactants (i.e., dishwashing liquid or laundry detergents); or irritating chemicals/solvents may cause skin dryness. Solvent extraction of the skin removes lipids and has been shown to cause severe barrier damage.[6] Feingold[7] reviewed the biochemical basis and regulation of permeability barrier function. He indicated that repair of barrier function involves secretion of preformed lamellar bodies; increased epidermal cholesterol, fatty acid, and sphingolipid synthesis; formation and secretion of new lamellar bodies; return of lipid to the SC; and extracellular processing of secreted lipid.

It is believed that dry skin is a subtle disorder which affects desquamation.[8] The SC continually sheds clusters of corneocytes (squames) from the surface of the skin while continually replenishing them from underlying layers. Normally, the clusters are very small and the process is imperceptible; however, in dry skin, the larger aggregates of squames are shed as flakes or scales. Dry skin is characterized by a rough, dry feel and "flaky" appearance due to uplifted corneocytes. Dry skin may itch and become red and irritated, and persons suffering from very dry skin (xerosis) may scratch affected areas repeatedly. If left untreated, severely dry skin may crack and bleed. Skin dryness may be graded using a 5-point scale with descriptions for dryness, roughness, redness, itching, cracking, softness, and tightness, as follows:

Skin Dryness Grading Scale

0 = Smooth, no evidence of dryness
1 = Slightly dry skin; occasional scale, not necessarily uniformly distributed
2 = Moderately dry skin; fairly uniformly distributed scale, but no widespread uplifting flaking
3 = Severely dry skin; pronounced scaling visible with the naked eye, definite uplifting of edges or scale sections — skin surface may have a whitish appearance
4 = Extremely dry skin; more scale and pronounced separation of scale edges, some evidence of cracking (for hands, the skin looks abraded)

Use of a grading scale such as this is of value in assessing dry skin on the initial visit of a patient to the dermatologist's office or in selecting panelists to participate in skin moisturization studies. Effective moisturizers decrease the dryness grade. Expert grader evaluation during the course of treatment enables the dermatologist to evaluate a patient's progress in a semiquantitative manner, to compare the performance of different products in treating dry skin, and to measure healing of skin dryness during the course of treatment with topical moisturizing products.

18.3.2 Skin Moisturization

Glycerine is used in a diverse range of living organisms to maintain the correct osmotic pressure within living cells. Many genera of microorganisms including bacteria and yeasts accumulate neutral amino acids (proline, glycine) and polyols (glycerine, trehalose, etc.) in response to osmotic stress. Glycerine is known to cross all biological membranes by passive diffusion, and it has been reported to have both active and facilitated transport systems in yeast.[9,10]

Mast[11] reviewed the use of glycerine in cosmetic products, noting that it was compatible with human skin and that it was an ideal compliment to water in cosmetic practice because it is completely water miscible and has some oil/water compatibility.

The SC serves as the primary barrier against excess water loss from the body. Osmoregulation in humans involves accumulation of *protective solutes* such as glycerine, which is supplied via glycolysis (dephosphorylation and enzymatic oxidation of glyceraldehyde-3-phosphate), or the action of lipases that hydrolyze fats. Osmoregulation is essential for maintenance of the hydration of enzymes critical for maintenance of normal cellular functions. Rawlings et al.[5] reported that one of the primary effects of applying glycerine to dry skin is the hydration of proteolytic enzymes required for desmosome degradation. Impairment of enzyme action due to lack of sufficient available water results in decreased enzyme action and sloughing of visible "clumps" of corneocytes (squames). These squames cause the skin to appear rough and dry due to visible, whitish "flakes." Normalization of desquamation due to hydration of proteolytic enzymes results in normal, imperceptible exfoliation of corneocytes.

Elias and Menon[12] and Downing[13] suggested that the cutaneous barrier to water loss was attributable to the SC lipids. Imokawa et al.[14] reported that ICLs, especially ceramide, play a critical role in water-holding properties of the SC. Several workers have reported that mixtures of ceramides with cholesterol, cholesteryl sulfate, and fatty acids are important components in protecting and/or restoring damaged skin barrier function.[15-18]

Skin moisturizers are used to help prevent skin from becoming dry and to return dry skin to its normal condition. Rieger[19] observed that the benefits of moisturizing dry skin are evident to everyone — the use of moisturizers or emollients is the remedy for dry skin. Until the 1980s, cosmetic products intended to moisturize dry skin contained humectants (i.e., glycerine, propylene glycol, or sorbitol) or occlusive moisturizers (i.e., petrolatum, mineral oil, lanolin, dimethicone, etc.) to maintain the hydration state of the SC. Many earlier workers thought that humectants merely attracted moisture to the surface of the skin and that occlusive moisturizers merely "trapped" moisture by forming an anhydrous film that prevented water from evaporating from the skin. We have learned a great deal since these early concepts were stated.

Mixtures of glycerine in water such as "glycerine and rosewater" contained rose-scented water and glycerine. Originally, these systems contained equal parts of glycerine and rose water, but later were diluted to about 20 to 25% glycerine. Simple glycerine and rose water products are not popular today because of their stickiness and inability to heal dry skin compared to therapeutic glycerine-containing moisturizers. The lack of cosmetic elegance has prevented many manufacturers from developing formulas that contain more than the customary 3 to 10% glycerine; however, exceptional "high glycerine" formulations with up to 40% glycerine are available today (see Section 18.4).

Besides maintaining proper osmotic pressure across cell membranes, the protective solutes maintain the normal liquid crystallinity (i.e., "fluidity") of cell membranes and ICLs. Liquid crystallinity of cell membranes is necessary for lateral phase separation and translocation of molecules within and through cell membranes (i.e., membrane transport). Froebe et al.[2] reported that addition of glycerine to a mixture of SC lipids (i.e., artificial sebum) *in vitro* inhibited the lipid

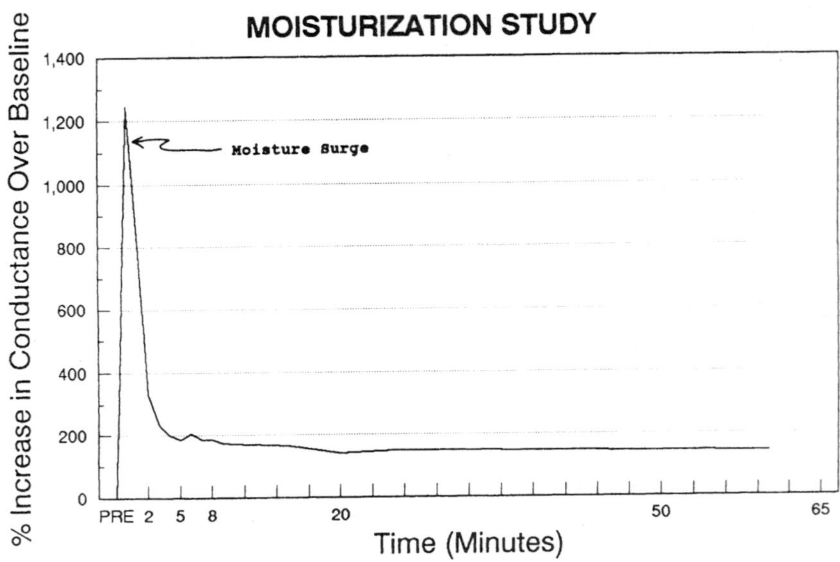

FIGURE 1 Time course of moisturization study showing moisture surge.

phase transition from liquid to solid crystals when water evaporated at low (6%) relative humidity. These workers concluded that glycerol maintains the liquid crystalline state and prevents crystal formation in dry ambient conditions. This demonstrates that glycerine helps maintain membrane fluidity and, as such, is very important for use in treating dry skin.

The addition of 1 to 10% glycerine to model ICLs markedly decreased the energy (heat flow) required for melting and heat of crystallization.[4,20] These workers observed sharp melting curves when 10% of a high glycerine product was blended with the model ICLs and broader melting curves when low glycerine products were blended with the model ICLs. These differential scanning calorimetry data suggested that high glycerine products maintain cohesiveness and liquid crystallinity of the ICLs better than the low glycerine products.

Elias et al.[16] proposed that the ICLs form multiple layers alternating with water to form a lamellar liquid crystalline arrangement. This multilayer structure of the ICLs is supported by the work of Friberg and Osborne,[21] who used X-ray crystallography to demonstrate that lipid bilayers were formed by free fatty acids when they were adjusted to the pH of the skin (pH 4.5 to 6). The fatty acids are partially converted to the corresponding soaps in this pH range, and this acid/soap combination forms a lamellar liquid crystal with water.[2] The balance between the liquid crystalline and the solid crystal phases is established by the type and composition of lipids, including the degree of fatty acid unsaturation, the amount of water, and other factors.[1]

Friberg et al.[22] studied a model lipid system *in vitro* and proposed that the physical state of the lipids is important in maintaining proper skin hydration and that a mixture of both solid and liquid crystalline states produces the optimal barrier to water loss. More recent reports indicate that specific ratios of ceramides, cholesterol, cholesteryl sulfate, and fatty acids provided optimal barrier repair, as determined by decrease in trans epidermal water loss (TEWL) in animal models.[12]

Moisturization studies revealed a "moisture surge" immediately after applying an emulsion to dry skin, followed by a decrease to a fairly constant level after 10 to 20 min. The time course of skin moisturization was determined by taking conductance measurements every 5 min after application (Figure 1). After this moisture surge, skin treated with products that contain more hygroscopic moisturizers (such as glycerine) return to a new, higher level of moisturization than skin treated with lower levels of glycerine.

18.4 HIGH GLYCERINE THERAPEUTIC MOISTURIZERS

High glycerine (>25%) therapeutic moisturizers have been reported to heal dry skin faster and give significantly better relief of dryness than low glycerine (<10%) moisturizers.[3-5]

18.4.1 Healing of Dry Skin During Winter Clinicals

Appa et al.[23] summarized findings from clinical studies that were conducted from 1991 to 1996 to compare 2 high glycerine therapeutic moisturizers with 16 other therapeutic moisturizers. Test products were selected because they were recommended by dermatologists, popular with consumers, and/or examination of the ingredient statements revealed that they contained materials believed to be most effective in moisturizers (e.g., petrolatum, ICLs, silicone, AHAs, urea, and glycerine).

18.4.1.1 Test Products

All products tested were commercially available dry skin treatments except for one prototype formula. Besides water, oils (other than mineral oil), and emollient esters typically contained in these products, the primary moisturizing ingredients included the following.

Product		Moisturizing Ingredients
A	40%	Glycerine
B	25%	Glycerine, dimethicone, and petrolatum
C	3%	Glycerine, 12% ammonium lactate, mineral oil, and propylene glycol (Rx product)
D	2%	Glycerine, Aloe vera gel, mineral oil, and dimethicone
E	6%	Glycerine, potassium lactate, lactic acid, urea, amino acids, and sodium PCA
F	5%	Glycerine, dimethicone, petrolatum, potassium lactate, and urea
G	3%	Glycerine, mineral oil, sodium lactate, urea, and panthenol
H	0%	Glycerine, sodium lactate, lactic acid, and mineral oil
I	9.5%	Glycerine, silicones, dipropylene glycol, ICL analogs, lactic acid, and lactate salts
J	7.6%	Glycerine, petrolatum, mineral oil, ICL analogs, and silicones
K	4%	Glycerine, ICLs, and dimethicone
L	5%	Glycerine, silicones, petrolatum, and EFA
M	6%	Glycerine, dimethicone, and petrolatum
N	5%	Glycerine, mineral oil, and dimethicone
O	0%	Glycerine, mineral oil, glyceryl lanolate, sorbitol, and propylene glycol
P	0%	Glycerine, petrolatum, lanolin, sorbitol, and lanolin alcohol
Q	5.6%	Glycerine, dimethicone, and petrolatum
R	5%	Glycerine, mineral oil, petrolatum, cholesteryl esters, and dimethicone

18.4.1.2 Study Design

Each annual study was a controlled, double-blind clinical trial designed to compare the efficacy of test samples on severe winter dry skin under supervised normal use conditions. Tests were done in Winnipeg, Canada, or in Colorado during January or February.

Treatment conditions (test products and an untreated control) were randomly assigned to test subjects so that the entire outer aspect of each lower leg was treated with a single product in the Winnipeg studies and the backs of both hands were treated with a single product in the Colorado studies.

The 1991 study involved a 1-week washout period and a 3-week treatment phase. The 1993/1996 studies involved a 1-week washout period, a 1-week treatment phase, and a 1-week regression phase during which product applications were discontinued. The 1993 study treated hands; the other studies treated the outer aspect of the lower legs. During the washout period, the subjects abstained from moisturizer use on the treatment sites and used Ivory soap in place of their usual cleansing products.

18.4.1.3 Test Subjects

The 394 panelists who completed the testing in the five clinicals were between 25 and 55 years of age. Subjects selected had severely dry skin (dryness grade 3 or 4) at the test sites at baseline (day 0).

18.4.1.4 Test Protocol

Each subject was shown the correct application technique, which involved application of ~1 g of test material to the assigned test site (to one leg or to both hands) twice a day, at least 8 h apart during the application phase. One application was done under supervision of the clinical center each day. Subjects were also instructed not to wet the test sites for at least 4 h prior to evaluations. On evaluation days, test materials were applied following the evaluation.

18.4.1.5 Evaluations

Expert: All visual/tactile evaluations were performed by the same trained grader in each study, with the aid of a 3-diopter illuminating magnifying lens. Visual evaluations were conducted in a blinded manner, such that the evaluator was unaware of the test sample distribution. Evaluations included dryness, roughness, erythema, and microfissures.

18.4.1.6 Self Evaluations

Subjects in the leg studies assessed their skin condition at 10 to 17 h after the initial application and on days 7 and 14. They used a 5-point scale with descriptions similar to the expert grader scale for dryness, roughness, redness, itching, cracking, softness, and tightness. Subjects in the hand studies examined their hands for these attributes at 2 and 8 h after the initial application and on days 1, 7, and 14. Grading of skin dryness used the 5-point scale (discussed earlier).

18.4.1.7 Instrumental Measurements

Skin moisture levels were measured with a Skicon Meter (IBS, Japan). The means of three readings for each leg were used in the calculations. Skin barrier competency was evaluated by TEWL measurements at baseline, 12 h, and on days 7 and 14 with an Evaporimeter (Servomed, Sweden).

18.4.1.8 Statistical Analysis

The differences from baseline were used for statistical analysis with $p \leq 0.05$. A binomial analysis was employed to evaluate within treatment dryness, erythema and roughness scores, and the instrumental ratings. For comparison of samples, an analysis of variance (ANOVA) with repeated measures was used to test the effect of sample and subject. The samples were also compared at each evaluation day whenever significant interaction of sample and day was detected. The ANOVA was used to compare the magnitude of self-assessed attributes on days 0, 7, and 14.

18.4.1.9 Discussion of Clinical Data

This 5-year retrospective analysis was done to summarize findings that were obtained during controlled, double-blind winter clinicals conducted from 1991 to 1996 to evaluate the benefits of high glycerine therapeutic moisturizers. A total of 394 panelists with severely dry skin (grade 3 or 4) participated in the studies.

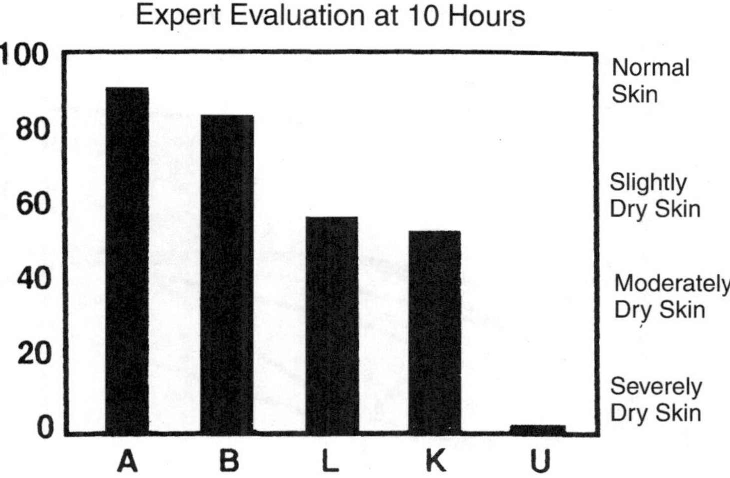

FIGURE 2 Healing skin dryness (percent healing).

The most significant finding was that the high glycerine products were superior to all other products tested in all five clinicals for rapidly restoring skin dry skin to a maintenance of normal hydration during treatment, and for helping prevent the return to dryness following termination of treatment in the four studies in which there was a regression phase. This level of sustained improvement was not observed with the low glycerine formulations with or without petrolatum, AHAs, ICLs, silicones, or the 12% AHA prescription product. After 1 week of treatment, TEWL measurements demonstrated that the skin barrier continued to improve for at least 1 week after use of the high glycerine products was discontinued (regression phase). Furthermore, the test subjects' assessments of their skin dryness were in excellent agreement with expert grader evaluations.

Skin treated with the two high glycerine moisturizers showed a rapid improvement in dryness and was transformed from severely dry, flaking, peeling skin (grade 3) to essentially normal skin, as determined by expert grader evaluation and skin moisture levels. The rapid healing of dryness observed in all studies is illustrated in comparisons of products A and B with products K and L in the 1994 clinical (Figure 2).

The findings of the 1996 study (products A/O and U = untreated control) are representative and illustrate how the high glycerine moisturizers were significantly better than low glycerine moisturizers for rapid healing of dryness and roughness 12 h after the first application, for maintenance of healing during the treatment phase, and for continued healing that was demonstrated by only slight increases in dryness during the regression phase (Figure 3). These studies establish the high glycerine therapeutic moisturizers as new benchmarks for the treatment of xerosis.

The prescription AHA product (C) did not improve skin dryness below a grade of 1 during the entire study. Although product O provided relief of the signs and symptoms of xerosis during the treatment phase, the apparent benefits (masking of dryness) decreased rapidly during the regression phase. In contrast, the healing benefits of the two high glycerine products continued for the duration of the regression phase because skin dryness scores remained in the 1 to 2 range (slightly to moderately dry).

There was an excellent agreement between panelists' self-assessment of skin dryness and expert grader scores for all studies, as illustrated in the 1992 study using products A, B, O, P, Q, and R (Figure 4).

The remarkable visual improvement 10 to 12 h after the first application was corroborated by conductance measurements, which showed very high levels of skin moisture produced by use of the two high glycerine products. The 1992 study data in Figure 5 show the dramatic increase in skin moisturization index (increase in conductance/baseline conductance × 100%) 17 h after initial

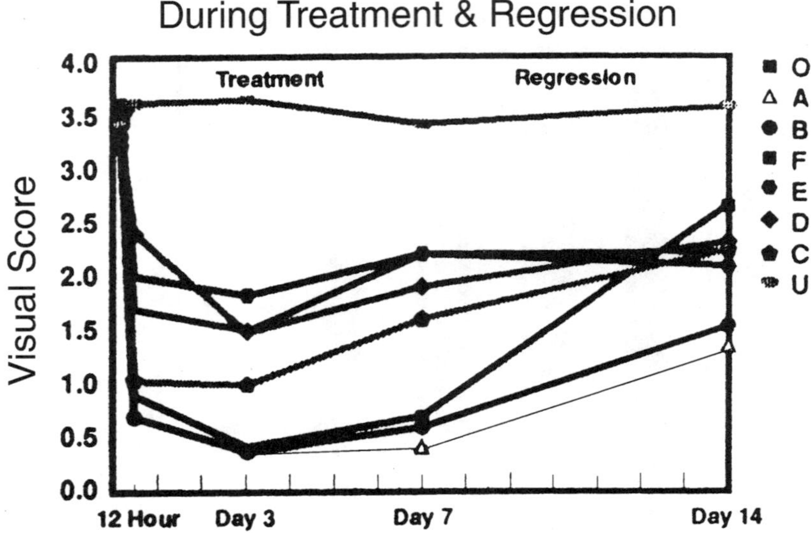

FIGURE 3 Expert evaluation of skin dryness during treatment and regression.

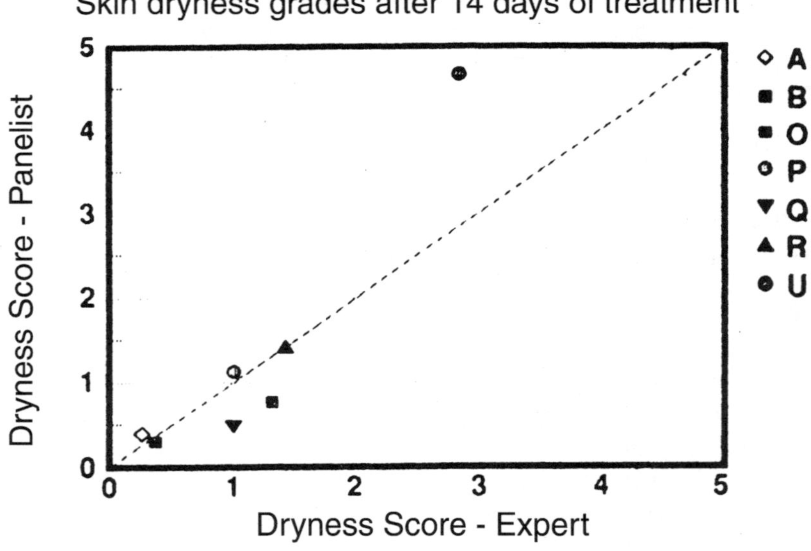

FIGURE 4 Panelist and expert evaluation of skin dryness.

application of products A and B. These products rapidly hydrated dry skin and maintained a high level of skin hydration throughout the treatment phase of all studies.

Signs of xerosis include tightness, erythema, itching, cracking, and soreness. Ratings of each of these attributes for the panelists was summed and normalized (relative to the untreated control site) to arrive at a quantitative measure of skin comfort for each product. Mean values for skin comfort for products A, B, H, I, and J obtained in the 1995 study are presented in Figure 6. It is evident that the high glycerine products gave much more relative skin comfort than the low glycerine products in the leg studies. This corroborated data from the 1993 study on hands in which subjective self-assessment showed that many dry skin attributes improved at least one unit with a single application of products A and B; whereas, panelists treated with products M and N did not obtain

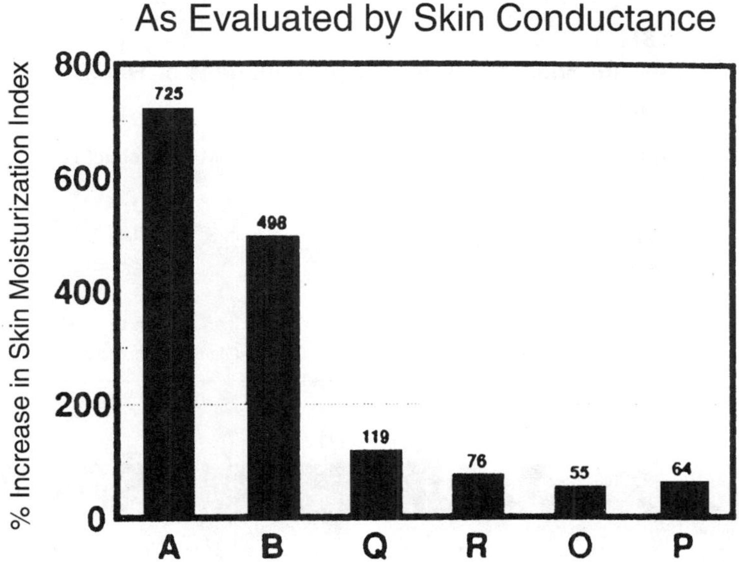

FIGURE 5 A 17-h moisturizer efficacy study.

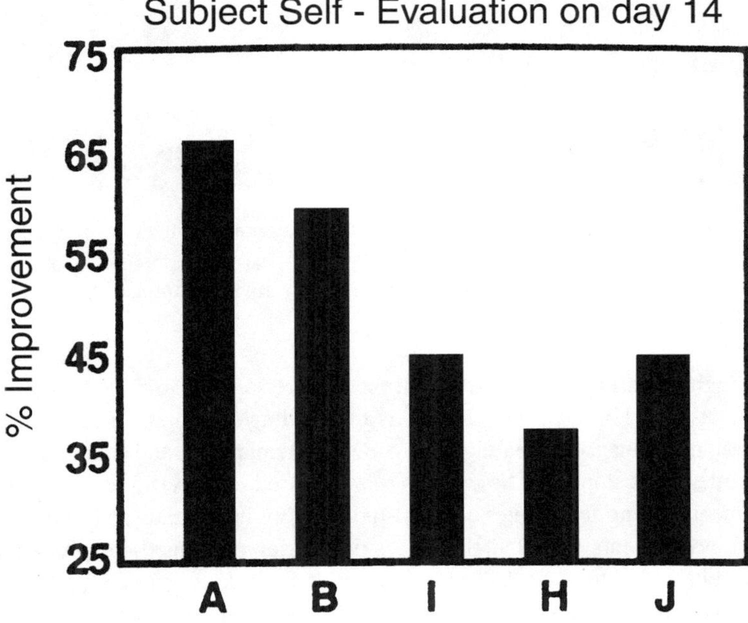

FIGURE 6 Relative skin comfort.

relief for 7 days (or not at all) during the treatment phase (Table 1). The visual improvement in hands treated with product A is shown in Figures 7a and 7b.

Persistent dry skin is associated with impaired skin barrier function. Effective products should do more than retain moisture — they should correct/normalize impaired barrier function as a primary mechanism of action to help control moisture loss. TEWL measurements at baseline, day 7, and day 14, demonstrated that the high glycerine products improve skin barrier. A remarkable finding revealed by the 1994/1996 studies was that improvement in barrier function, as determined by >35% decrease in TEWL, continued for up to one week after product use was discontinued.

TABLE 1
Time for Subject Self-Assessed Evaluations of Hands to Improve One Unit or More

Attribute	Product A	Product B	Product M	Product N
Dryness	2 Hours	2 Hours	Not reached	7 Days
Roughness	2 Hours	2 Hours	Not reached	7 Days
Redness	2 Days	8 Hours	7 Days	Not reached
Cracking	2 Days	2 Hours	7 Days	7 Days
Tightness	1 Day	2 Hours	7 Days	Not reached
Softness	2 Hours	7 Days	Not reached	Not reached

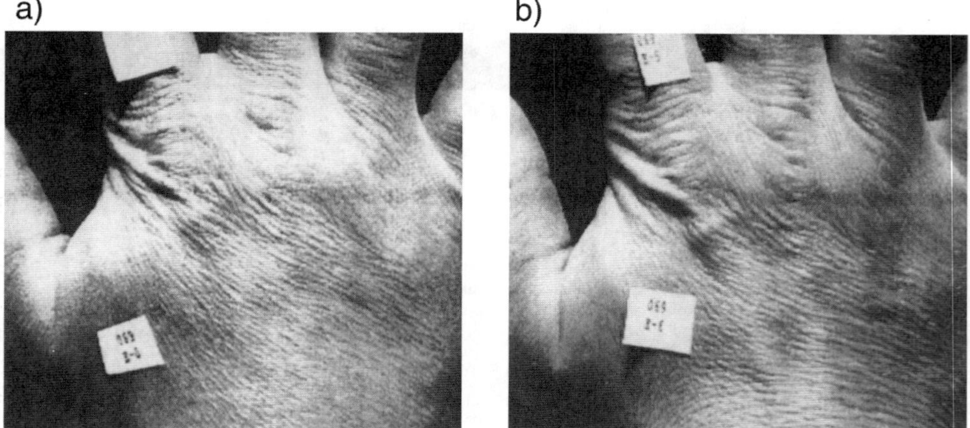

FIGURE 7 (a) Baseline (day 0) and (b) after 7 days of treatment with product A.

The retrospective analysis of the treatment of dry skin during winter clinicals by Appa and co-workers[23] revealed the following:

- The two high glycerine therapeutic moisturizers were superior to all low glycerine competitive products tested because they provided rapid healing of dryness in 10 to 17 h after initial application, maintenance of healing during the treatment phase, and continued improvement after treatment was stopped. These findings were based on expert grading and conductance measurements during five winter clinical studies using both hands or legs for test sites.
- TEWL measurements revealed that the skin barrier continued to improve during the treatment phase (up to 3 weeks) and for at least 1 week after use of the high glycerine products was discontinued (regression phase). This was corroborated by expert grader evaluation and panelists' self-assessment. Continued improvement in barrier function was not observed during the regression phase with the low glycerine formulations or the 12% AHA prescription product.
- Subjects applying the high glycerine products were able to see/feel improvement in many dry skin attributes in 2 h; whereas, subjects receiving some low glycerine products did not obtain relief during the treatment phase.
- It is believed that the superior clinical performance of the high glycerine formulations is due to their ability to deliver glycerine to the skin and create a glycerine reservoir throughout the SC. This provides an additional barrier and moisture-retaining properties while encouraging natural restoration of xerotic skin.

18.5 EFFECT OF HIGH GLYCERINE THERAPEUTIC MOISTURIZERS ON ULTRASTRUCTURE OF THE STRATUM CORNEUM

Orth et al.[24] reported the effects of high glycerine products on the ultrastructure of the SC *in vivo* in human skin. Clinical studies involved three Caucasian female panelists, 25 to 45 years old, with normal skin. Test materials included glycerine, 99.7% white petrolatum, USP, hand and body lotion with 25% glycerine, and hand cream with 40% glycerine. Volar forearms of subjects were treated twice daily with 2 to 3 μl/cm² with two test materials for 5 days. Two-millimeter-diameter punch biopsies of each test site and the untreated control site on the volar forearm were taken at least 4 h after the morning application on the last day of product use. The biopsies were immediately placed in Karnovsky's fixative and processed for electron microscopy. This included postfixation osmium tetroxide, staining *en block* with phosphotungstic acid and 2% uranyl acetate, dehydration in graded ethanols, and embedding in Spurr's resin in flat embedding molds. Semithin and ultrathin sections were cut using a Sorval MT-2b Ultramicrotome, and the sections were examined using a Phillips EM 300 electron microscope. Photos of representative fields of each treatment were prepared.

Figure 8 shows the appearance of the SC and suprabasal layers of human skin treated with 99.7% glycerine for 5 days. The layers of the SC appeared to be closely packed and were not visibly different form the untreated control. No alterations were evident in the suprabasal layers. Figure 9 shows the appearance of the SC and suprabasal layers of skin treated with petrolatum for 5 days. Some separation of the upper layers is evident, but no expansion of the SC is evident. Figure 10 shows the appearance of the SC and suprabasal layers of skin treated with the 25% glycerine lotion. The entire SC had an expended appearance, which is due to both increased thickness of corneocytes as well as increased spaces between successive layers of corneocytes. No identifiable alterations were noted in the suprabasal layers. Similar changes were observed in punch biopsies of skin treated with the 40% glycerine cream. These findings were corroborated with *in vitro* data obtained by treating a fully differentiated SC surface fo Skin ZK1300 skin model (Advanced Tissue Sciences, La Jolla, CA) twice a day for 5 days, followed by processing and electron microscopy studies.

The ultrastructural studies of Orth and co-workers show that application of two high glycerine therapeutic moisturizers produced significant expansion throughout the entire thickness of the SC of human skin *in vivo* and in an *in vitro* skin model. Application of pure glycerine or petrolatum

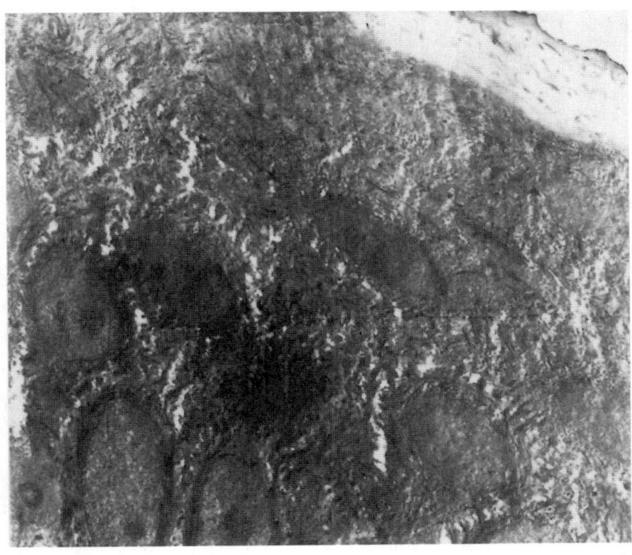

FIGURE 8 Human skin treated *in vivo* with glycerine for 5 days, (10,500 × magnification at original size).

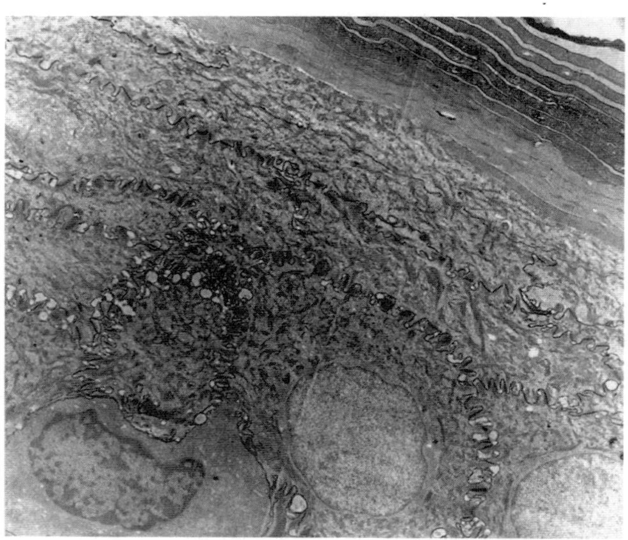

FIGURE 9 Human skin treated *in vivo* with petrolatum for 5 days (12,250 × magnification at original size).

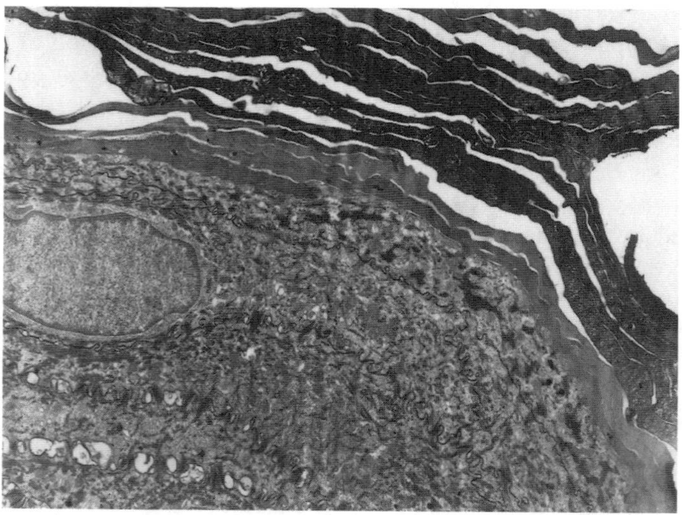

FIGURE 10 Human skin treated *in vivo* with test lotion C for 5 days (12,000 × magnification at original size).

in a similar manner produced only minimal or superficial changes in the appearance of the SC. The expansion of corneocytes and the intracellular spaces between corneocytes is believed to be due to the glycerine delivered into the SC by the high glycerine products. Enhancement of the SC barrier and the moisture-retaining properties as a result of the accumulation of glycerine throughout the SC — without disruption of the liquid crystalline/lamellar structure — is believed to encourage natural repair of xerotic skin and provide the basis for the superior clinical performance of these high glycerine products.

Wintertime clinical studies conducted during the past several years demonstrated that high glycerine (25 and 40%) therapeutic moisturizers healed clinically dry skin faster and better than low glycerine products that contained <6% glycerine.[20,23,24] Furthermore, the panelists' skin did not revert back to baseline for more than 1 week after product use was discontinued. These findings suggested that use of the high glycerine products caused some change in the skin that enabled it to better withstand the cold, dry weather conditions than untreated skin.

Electron microscopic examination of the SC following use of high glycerine moisturizers revealed that the high glycerine therapeutic moisturizers affected the full thickness of the SC, as evidenced by the expanded appearance of corneocytes and ICLs.[24] It is believed that the superior clinical performance of the high glycerine formulations observed in double-blind winter clinicals over several years is due to their ability to create a glycerine reservoir throughout the SC which provides moisturization and enhanced barrier properties.[25]

18.6 METHODS FOR EVALUATING MOISTURIZATION OF COSMETICS

The SC functions to provide a barrier to the evaporation of water from the viable epidermis. Normal SC contains 10 to 30% water, and the water content is regulated by the barrier properties and water-holding capacity of the SC. The basic tenet is that dry skin results from low water content. The prevalence of dry skin in exposed body sites and not in protected areas supports this belief.[8] However, equating moisturization with skin hydration alone is inadequate, and in some instances erroneous. In practical terms, a moisturizer will maintain or restore the flexibility and suppleness of the SC, while decreasing surface roughness and scaliness. Assessments of moisturization must include clinical (visual and palpable improvements) and sensory (subject self-assessements and/or trained practitioners') evaluations correlated with instrumental readings. Several noninvasive measurement techniques are available for measuring changes in skin hydration, moisture loss, moisture-holding capacity, desquamation, and mechancial properties.[26–28] Here we will touch on two basic techniques, with the caveat that relying only on a single technique could lead to false conclusions.

18.6.1 Transepidermal water loss (TEWL)

TEWL may be defined as insensible water loss through the skin. It is not the same thing as active perspiration. TEWL measurements determine the water flux through the SC, thereby providing a measure of the barrier integrity and an indirect assessment of water holding capacity. TEWL measurements are made with an evaporimeter and are used widely to determine changes in the hydration state of the skin and to monitor the effects of topically applied moisturizers. As noted by Appa, measurements must be done in controlled environmental conditions which include restricting air currents about the skin surface being measured.[8]

The interpretation of TEWL results must be done with caution. It is apparent that application of an occlusive material to the skin surface will, at least in part, physically block the surface and lower the TEWL. However, occlusive moisturizers actually may cause the TEWL to rise above baseline values after several hours because of the increased diffusion of water through the skin that results from hydration. Thus, there are opposing mechanisms at work, and some occlusive materials may actually increase TEWL, depending on the time measurements made after application of the test materials. Therefore, while TEWL measurements are widely accepted for determining barrier competency at the time of measurement, it is not good clinical or laboratory practice to use only TEWL measurements to assess skin moisturization.

18.6.2 Electrical Measurement of Skin Moisturization

The skin exhibits complex electrical properties which may be related to its physical and chemical state. Leveque et al.[26] reported that skin conductance is inversely related to the degree of typical winter xerosis of the face. Many moisturizing claims have been made by relating measured values of skin conductance (or impedance) to skin permeability increase induced by hydration following application of topical moisturizers. Measurements made with conductance meters such as the Skicon 200 (IBS Labs) or capacitance devices such as the Corneometer (Courage & Khazaka) are highly sensitive, easy to perform, and noninvasive.[29] The interpretation of conductance readings requires knowledge of the type of products applied to skin. For example, glycerine placticizes the skin and affects skin conductance independently of the water content. However, increases in skin conductance following application of topical products containing glycerine accomplish the intended objective — to moisturize skin. Appa[8] pointed out that the observed changes in conductance following topical application of a product containing glycerine are not due entirely to changes in water content. This is true of other plasticizers including salts, urea, and proteins which can alter the ratio between water molecules tightly bound and "free" without changing the water content of the SC. Inflammation of the skin may be accompanied by an increase in conductivity. Also, barrier function of skin damaged by repeated soap washing can increase both TEWL and conductance values. This highlights the need to use more than one method (i.e., TEWL, conductance, or elasticity measurements) to assess skin moisturization.

Aesthetic evaluation of skin moisturization is useful for determining clinical efficacy of moisturizing products. Grading skin dryness by trained graders using a scale provides confirmatory semiquantitative data that may corroborate the quantitative measurements obtained using instrumental techniques. Also subjective (consumer) evaluation of panelists is valuable to determine how the product has performed when used. Although each instrument generally measures a single physical/chemical property, human perception is the result of multiple sensory inputs. Thus, a much better understanding of the skin's response to topical application of products may be gained using a battery of tests rather than relying on any one technique.[8]

18.7 SUMMARY

Glycerine has been used as a cosmetic ingredient for more than 50 years. Glycerine is natural, so it is consumer acceptable for the newly emerging class of "natural" products. It has a long history of use and is safe at the concentrations used. It is a cost-effective moisturizer that has numerous beneficial effects when applied to the skin via topical products. High glycerine products are able to heal skin dryness. They moisturize (hydrate) the full thickness of the SC without causing apparent changes in the suprabasal layers. The high glycerine therapeutic moisturizers appear to create a "reservoir" of moisture-holding ability in the skin which makes the skin more resistant to drying conditions than untreated skin. Glycerine functions to stabilize/fluidize cell membranes and ICLs and normalize sloughing of corneocytes by hydrating enzymes needed for desmosome degradation. Although glycerine is an "old" ingredient, research has revealed multiple mechanisms of action, and it appears that it will have a bright new future in skin care products.

REFERENCES

1. Klingman, A.M., Lavker, R.M., Grove, G.L., and Stoudemayer. Some aspects of dry skin and its treatment. In: A.M. Kligman and J.J. Leyden (Eds.). *Safety and Efficacy of Topical Drugs and Cosmetics*. Grune and Stratton, New York, pp. 221–238 (1982).
2. Froebe, C.L. et al. Prevention of stratum corneum lipid phase transitions *in vivo* by glycerol — an alternate mechanism for skin moisturization. *J. Soc. Cosmet. Chem.* 41:41–65 (1990).
3. Appa, Y., D.S. Orth and L. Lewis. Clinical evaluation of hand and body moisturizers that heal skin dryness. Poster presentation at the 51st Annual Meeting of the American Academy of Dermatology, December 1992.
4. Appa, Y., D.S. Orth, J. Widjaja and A. Asuncion. Effect of glycerin on energy requirements and liquid crystallinity of model intercellular lipids. *J. Invest. Dermatol.* 100:587 (1993).
5. Rawlings, A. et al. The biological effects of glycerol. *J. Invest. Dermatol.* 100:526 (1993).
6. Imokawa, G. and M. Hattori. A possible function of structural lipids in the water-holding properties of the stratum corneum. *J. Invest. Dermatol.* 84:282–284 (1985).

7. Feingold, K.R. Biochemical basis and regulation of permeability barrier homeostasis. Oral presentation at the Advanced Technology Conference held in Miami, FL. *Advanced Technology Conference Proceedings*, Allured Publishing, Carol Stream, IL, pp. 7–12 (1998).
8. Appa (Appapillai), Y. Methods for evaluating the efficacy of cosmetics containing glycerine. In: E. Jungermann and N.O.V. Sonntag (Eds.). *Glycerine. A Key Cosmetic Ingredient.* Marcel Dekker, Inc., New York, pp. 277–309 (1991).
9. Sutherland, F.C.W., F. Lages, C. Lucas, K. Luyten, J.H. Albertyn, S. Hohmann, B.A. Prior and S.G. Kilian. Characteristics of Fps1-dependent and -independent glycerol transport in Saccharomyces cerevisiae. *J. Bacteriol.* 179:7790–7795 (1997).
10. Reizer, J., A. Reizer and M.H. Saier. The MIP-family of integral membrane channel proteins: sequence comparisons, evolutionary relationships, reconstructed pathway of evolution, and proposed functional differentiation of the two repeated halves of the proteins. *Crit. Rev. Biochem. Mol. Biol.* 28:235–257 (1993).
11. Mast, R. Functions of glycerine in cosmetics. In: E. Jungermann and N.O.V. Sonntag (Eds.). *Glycerine. A Key Cosmetic Ingredient.* Marcel Dekker, Inc., New York, pp. 223–275 (1991).
12. Elias, P.M. and G.K. Menon. Structural and lipid biochemical correlates of the epidermal permeability barrier. *Adv. Lipid Res.* 24:1–26 (1991).
13. Downing, D.T. Lipid and protein structures in the permeability barrier of mammalian epidermis. *J. Lipid Res.* 33:301–313 (1992).
14. Imokawa, G., S. Akasaki, A. Kawamata, S. Yano and N. Takaishi. Water-retaining function in the stratum corneum and its recovery properties by synthetic pseudoceramides. *J. Soc. Cosmet. Chem.* 40:273–285 (1989).
15. Man, M., K.R. Feingold and P.M. Elias. Exogenous lipids influence permeability barrier recovery in acetone-treated murine skin. *Arch. Dermatol.* 129:728–738 (1993).
16. Elias, P.M., B.E. Brown, P. Fritsch, J. Goerke, G.M. Gray and R.J. White. Localization and composition of lipids in the neonatal mouse stratum granulosum and stratum corneum. *J. Invest. Dermatol.* 73:339–347 (1979).
17. Conti, A., J. Rogers, P. Verdejo, C.R. Harding and A.V. Rawlings. Seasonal influences on stratum corneum ceramide 1 fatty acids and the influence of topical essential fatty acids. *Int. J. Cosmet. Sci.* 18:1–12 (1996).
18. Downing, D.T., M.E. Stewart, P.W. Wertz, S.W. Colton, VI, W. Abraham and J.S. Strauss. Skin lipids: a review. *J. Invest. Dermatol.* 88:2s–6s (1987).
19. Rieger, M. Water, water, everywhere. Some thoughts on skin moisturization. *Cosmet. Toiletries* 113(9):75, 76, 78, 80–87 (1998).
20. Shapiro, W.B., D.S. Orth, Y. Appa, P.C. Contard and L.A. Rheins. Glycerin moisturizers. *Cosmet. Dermatol.* 9(11):26s–30s (1996).
21. Friberg, S.E. and D.W. Osborne. Small angle X-ray diffraction patterns of stratum corneum and a model structure its lipids. *J. Disp. Sci. Technol.* 6:485–495 (1985).
22. Friberg, S.E., I. Kayali and L.D. Rhein. Direct role of linoleic acid in barrier function: effect of linoleic acid on the crystalline structure of oleic acid/oleate model stratum corneum lipid. *J. Disp. Sci. Technol.* 11(1):31–47 (1990).
23. Appa, Y., R. Thomas and D.S. Orth. High glycerine therapeutic moisturizers — a retrospective analysis of treating dry skin during winter clinicals: 1991–1996. Poster presentation at the 55th Annual Meeting of the American Academy of Dermatology in San Francisco, CA, March 21–26, 1997.
24. Orth, D.S., Y. Appa, P. Contard, E. Siegel, T.A. Donnelly and L.A. Rheins. Effect of high glycerin therapeutic moisturizers on the ultrastructure of the stratum corneum. Poster presentation at the 53rd Annual Meeting of the American Academy of Dermatology, February 1995.
25. Appa, Y., L. Hemingway, D.S. Orth, W. Lazer and L. Lockhart. Healing of dry skin with high glycerine therapeutic moisturizers. Poster presentation at the 53rd Annual Meeting of the American Academy of Dermatology, February 1995.
26. Leveque, J.L., G. Grove, J. de Rigal, P. Corcuff, A.M. Kligman and D. Saint Leger. Biophysical characterization of dry facial skin. *J. Soc. Cosmet. Chem.* 82:161–166 (1987).
27. Serup, J. and G. Jemec (Eds.). *Handbook of Noninvasive Methods and the Skin*, CRC Press, Boca Raton, FL, pp. 1–702 (1995).

28. Elsner, P., E. Berardesca and H.I. Maibach. *Bioengineering of the Skin: Water and Stratum Corneum.* CRC Press, Boca Raton, FL, pp. 1–296 (1994).
29. Fluhr, J.W., M. Gloor, S. Lazzerini, P. Kleesz, R. Grieshaber and E. Berardesca. Comparative study of five instruments measuring stratum corneum hydration (corneo-) meter CM 820 and CM 825, Skicon 200, Nova DPM 9003, DermaLab). II. In vivo. *Skin Res. Technol.* 5:171–178 (1999).

19 Effects of Natural Moisturizing Factor and Lactic Acid Isomers on Skin Function

Clive R. Harding, John Bartolone, and Anthony V. Rawlings

CONTENTS

19.1 INTRODUCTION

Dry, flaky skin remains one of the most common and vexing of human disorders. Although there is no unambiguous definition of this dermatosis, it is characterized by a rough, scaly, and flaky skin surface that often becomes fissured, particularly during the winter months of the year. However, research by Irwin Blank in the 1950s[1] demonstrated that the low moisture content of the skin is a prime factor causing this condition, and in many respects these pioneering studies heralded the dawn of moisturization research. During the past 40 years many scientists have investigated the complex process of stratum corneum (SC) maturation in both normal and dry skin and have begun to unravel the biological and physical implications of SC moisturization.

In order to maintain water within the skin the epidermis undergoes a process of maturation or terminal differentiation to produce a thin, inert, water-retaining barrier, the SC. This heterogeneous structure has been likened to a brick wall in which the anucleated nonviable cells, termed corneocytes (bricks), are embedded in a continuous matrix of specialized intercellular lipids (mortar).[2] Each individual corneocyte can be viewed simplistically as a highly insoluble protein complex, consisting primarily of a keratin macrofibrillar matrix, stabilized through inter- and intrakeratin chain disulfide bonds, and encapsulated within a protein shell called the cornified cell envelope. This latter structure is composed of a number of specialized proteins[3] which are extensively cross-linked through the action of at least two members of the transglutaminase family.[4] Given that elements of the internal keratin matrix are also linked to the interior aspect of the cornified envelope

0-8493-7520-7/00/$0.00+$.50

(through both disulfide linkages and the action of transglutaminase[5]), each corneocyte can be likened to a single, intricately cross-linked "macro-protein." This extensive protein interaction imparts great strength to the corneocyte. The overall integrity of the SC itself is achieved primarily through specialized intercellular protein structures called corneodesmosomes,[6,7] which effectively rivet the corneocytes together, but which ultimately must be degraded to facilitate desquamation.

In order to maintain its flexibility and integrity the SC must remain hydrated, and in healthy skin the tissue contains greater than 10% water.[1,8] In the absence of water the SC is an intrinsically fragile structure which readily becomes cracked, brittle, and rigid. The maintenance of water balance in the SC is therefore vital to this tissue and is preserved through two major biophysical mechanisms. The first of these is the intercellular lamellar lipids which provide a very effective barrier to the passage of water through the tissue.[9,10] The second mechanism is provided by the natural moisturizing factor (NMF), a complex mixture of low molecular weight, water-soluble compounds which is present within the corneocytes.[11] Collectively, the NMF components have the ability to bind water against the desiccating action of the environment and thereby maintain tissue hydration. The highly structured intercellular lipid lamellae fulfill a further function in that, as well as restricting water movement through the SC, they also effectively prevent the highly water-soluble NMF from leaching out of the surface layers of the skin.

Usually these two biophysical mechanisms interact precisely to provide a highly efficient barrier against water loss and retain water within the tissue to maintain flexibility. Nevertheless, this barrier is continually prone to damage by external forces, and with its failure increased loss of water from the tissue ultimately leads to the formation of dry skin. The dry appearance of skin is now generally accepted to be the consequence of the scattering and reflection of light off the rough skin surface resulting from abnormal desquamation. This perturbation to the ultimate step of terminal differentiation emphasizes a critical and often overlooked role of water in the SC, namely, its importance for the activity of a variety of hydrolytic enzymes involved in various aspects of SC maturation and desquamation.[12-14] When the tissue is desiccated a loss of hydrolytic enzyme activity leads to ineffective corneodesmosomal degradation and consequently skin scaling.

For a proper appreciation of the underlying biochemistry of dry skin we should consider this condition as a dysfunction of one or more of the vital processes that generate and protect the water-holding capacity of the SC. With this concept in mind, in this chapter we will first describe the generation and critical importance of the NMF to SC function and then consider the effects of topically applied NMF components, particularly the effects of lactic acid and its isomers, on the alleviation of dry skin symptoms.

19.2 NATURAL MOISTURIZING FACTOR (NMF)

19.2.1 The Role of the NMF in the Stratum Corneum

The NMF consists primarily of amino acids or their derivatives such as pyrrolidone carboxylic acid (PCA) and urocanic acid (UCA) together with lactic acid, urea, citrate, and sugars[15] (Table 1). These compounds are collectively present at high concentrations within the cell and may represent 20 to 30% of the dry weight of the SC.[16] The importance of the NMF lies in the fact that its constituent chemicals, particularly its PCA and lactic acid salts, are intensely hygroscopic. These salts absorb atmospheric water and dissolve in their own water of hydration, thereby acting as very efficient humectants. In essence the amount of NMF in the SC determines how much water it can hold for any given relative humidity. In the absence of NMF the SC can only absorb significant amounts of water at 100% humidity, a situation which seldom occurs.

The properties of the individual components of the NMF have been studied extensively. Fox et al.,[17] investigating the humectancy capabilities of sodium lactate, demonstrated a 60% increase in water content at 60% relative humidity (RH), whereas, in contrast under the same conditions, glycerol only provided a 38% increase. Laden and Spitzer,[18] after studying the composition of

TABLE 1
The Chemical Composition of NMF

	%
Free amino acids	40.0
Pyrrolidone carboxylic acid	12.0
Lactate	12.0
Sugars, organic acids, peptides, unidentified materials	8.5
Urea	7.0
Chloride	6.0
Sodium	5.0
Potassium	4.0
Ammonia, uric acid, glucosamine creatine	1.5
Calcium	1.5
Magnesium	1.5
Phosphate	0.5
Citrate, formate	0.5

NMF, concluded that since amino acids are relatively nonhygroscopic at skin pH, PCA itself must also contribute significantly to the SC water binding capacity. Although it has been demonstrated that sodium lactate is slightly more hygroscopic than sodium PCA at 50% RH,[19,20] both of these salts contribute significantly to the hygroscopicity of the SC. Biologically, this property allows the outermost layers of the SC to maintain liquid water against the desiccating action of the environment.

Traditionally, it was felt that this liquid water plasticized the SC, keeping it resilient by preventing cracking and flaking which might occur due to mechanical stresses. However, under conditions of reduced RH, when water can only provide a transient effect, topically applied lactic acid achieves a long-term plasticization of the SC. Similarly, while developing a skin cream designed to reduce dry and flaky skin, Middleton measured changes in SC extensibility and water-holding capacity and showed that at 81% RH sodium lactate and sodium PCA were as effective as other moisturizing agents. Although their benefits were essentially lost on rinsing the SC with water,[21] lactic acid-treated skin retained some residual plasticization benefit.

Urea, another principle component of the NMF, has also been demonstrated to have similar effects,[22] although no direct comparison with either PCA or lactic acid has been reported.

The precise mechanisms by which these NMF components influence SC functionality have been studied extensively. From a physical chemistry perspective the specific ionic interaction between keratin and NMF, accompanied by a decreased mobility of water, leads to a reduction of intermolecular forces between the keratin fibers and increased elastic behavior. Recent studies have emphasized that it is the neutral and basic free amino acids[23] in particular which are important for helping keratin acquire and maintain its elastic properties.

However, as our understanding of the terminal differentiation and SC maturation process has increased, it has become clear that by maintaining free water in the SC, the NMF also facilitates critical biochemical events. The coordinated activity of specific proteases is essential for optimum SC function, and these hydrolytic processes can only function in the presence of water which is effectively maintained by the water-retaining capacity of the NMF. Perhaps the most striking example of this is the regulation of a number of proteases within the corneocyte which, as we discuss in the next section, are ultimately responsible for the very generation of the NMF itself.

19.2.2 The Origin of the Skin's NMF

The precise origin of the lactic acid and urea components of the NMF remain ill defined. In contrast, the source of the amino acids and their derivatives within the SC, which together represent over

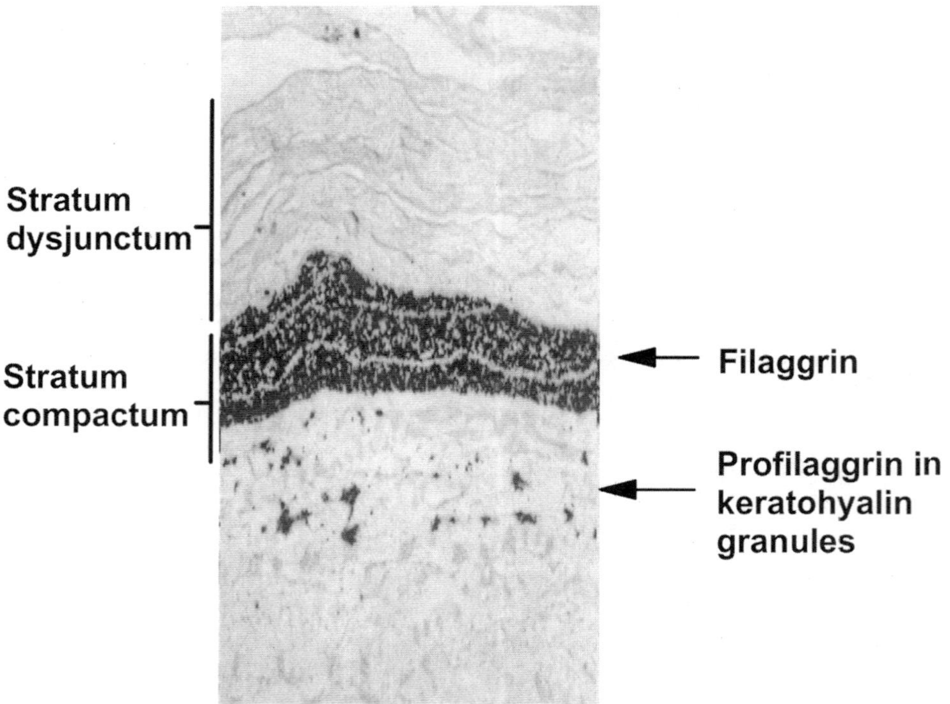

FIGURE 1 Distribution of filaggrin in human stratum corneum. Immunoelectron micrograph of human facial skin (9-year-old male). Ultrathin sections were incubated with rabbit-antihuman filaggrin followed by incubation with goat-antirabbit/colloidal gold (5 nm diameter).

50% of the NMF, was elucidated through studies conducted by Scott and co-workers during the early 1980s.[24-26] These investigations lead to the conclusion that all of the amino acid components of the NMF were derived specifically from a single, high molecular weight, histidine-rich protein, which represented the major component of the F-type keratohyalin granules.[27] Studies indicated that this protein was rapidly dephosphorylated during the transition of the mature granular cell into the corneocyte and then underwent selective proteolytic processing to form lower molecular weight basic species within the SC.[28] Based upon their ability to aggregate keratin fibers *in vitro* into macro-structures reminiscent of the keratin pattern seen in the SC *in vivo*, Dale and co-workers named this class of basic proteins filaggrins,[29] and the phosphorylated precursor protein subsequently became known as profilaggrin.

However, regardless of the putative structural function proposed for this family of proteins within the SC, it soon became clear that this was, at best, a transient role. Radiolabel pulse chase,[26] immunohistochemical,[30] and biochemical studies[28] confirmed that filaggrin, with the exception of a minor incorporation into the cornified cell envelope,[4,31] did not persist beyond the deepest two or three layers of the SC (Figure 1). First, it became extensively deiminated through the activity of the enzyme peptidyl deiminase, which served to reduce the affinity of the filaggrin/keratin complex. Second, it was rapidly and completely degraded through small peptides to free amino acids. Finally, specific constituent amino acids were catabolized further to form specialized components of the NMF.

Foremost among these catabolites is PCA itself (derived primarily by the nonenzymatic cyclization of glutamine[24]), and UCA, a natural UV absorber[32] formed by the action of the enzyme histidase on histidine[33] (filaggrin catabolism summarized in Figure 2).

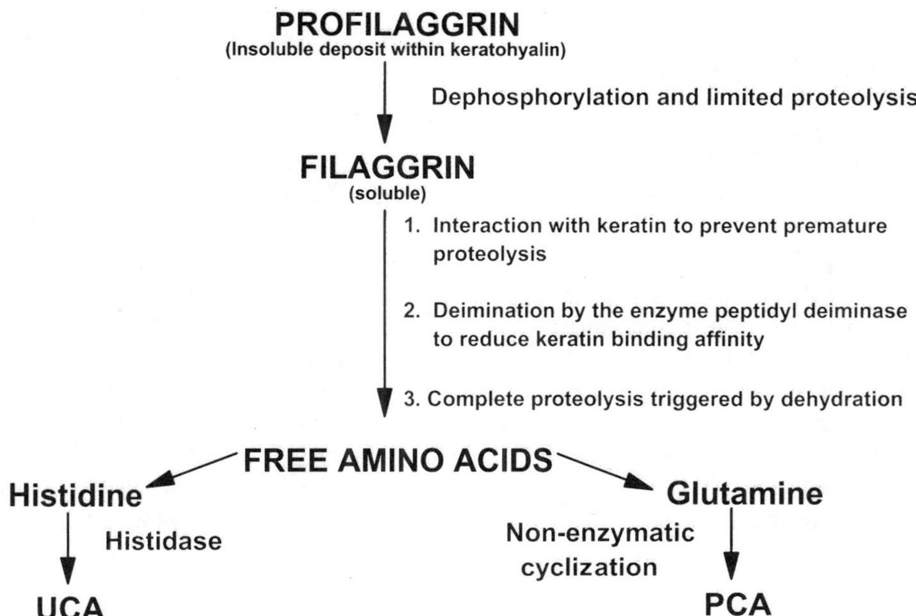

FIGURE 2 Schematic representation of profilaggrin catabolism during terminal differentiation.

19.2.3 Control of Filaggrin Hydrolysis

Although the precise nature of the protease systems catalyzing filaggrin breakdown remains to be identified, the "trigger" which initializes the proteolysis at a defined stage of SC maturation was elucidated following careful observation of changes in filaggrin distribution during SC maturation of fetal and newborn rat skin.[34] In normal adult skin filaggrin is only detected in the innermost layers of the SC (as in Figure 1), whereas in newborn and fetal tissue there is no indication of any proteolytic breakdown of filaggrin in the outer regions. However, within a few hours of birth, the breakdown of filaggrin is initiated in these regions. This triggering could be prevented in a very humid environment, which indicates the possibility that water content of the SC is a critical factor. Subsequent studies on filaggrin breakdown in isolated SC revealed that hydrolysis only occurred if the SC was maintained within a certain RH range (70 to 95%). Similarly, if the skin was occluded for a long period[35] filaggrin hydrolysis was blocked, the corneocytes remained filled with the protein, and the NMF level of the SC fell close to zero. These observations suggest strongly that filaggrin hydrolysis is initiated by changes in water activity within the SC itself.

It is now appreciated that the water activity within the SC and the water flux through this tissue are intimately involved in several aspects of tissue homeostasis, notably in relation to water barrier repair.[36] However, the observations on the control of filaggrin catabolism, originally made over a decade ago, represent some of the earliest studies to indicate and emphasize the dynamic nature of SC maturation.

At first sight the process by which the skin generates the NMF within the SC seems an absurdly complex one. However, the rationale of nature's complexity becomes apparent once it is appreciated that the epidermis cannot afford to generate NMF, either within the viable layers or within the newly formed immature corneocyte itself, due to the risk of osmotic damage. It is imperative that the activation of the filaggrin protease systems is delayed until the corneocyte has flattened and strengthened and moved far enough out into the dryer areas of the SC to be able to withstand the osmotic effects of the concentrated NMF pool. The epidermis circumvents the potentially harmful effects of osmotic pressure resulting from the inappropriate hydrolysis of filaggrin through two strategies. First, profilaggrin, once synthesized, is precipitated within the keratohyalin granule where it acts as an insoluble and, most importantly, an osmotically inactive repository of the NMF. Second, the interaction between keratin and filaggrin forms a proteolytically resistant complex which prevents premature proteolysis of the filaggrin (an intrinsically labile protein containing some 10 to 15 mol% arginine residues[26]) during the intensely hydrolytic processes which accompany SC formation.

In summary, these mechanisms are part of a subtle process which ensures that it is only as filaggrin containing corneocytes migrate upward from the deepest layers and begin to dry out (and the water activity within the cell decreases) that the proteases, by a poorly understood mechanism, are activated and the NMF is produced. The point at which this hydrolysis is initiated is independent of the age of the corneocyte[30] and is dictated ultimately by the environmental humidity. When the weather is humid the proteolysis occurs almost at the outer surface. In conditions of extreme low humidity the proteolysis is initiated deep within the tissue so that all but the deepest layers contain the NMF required to prevent desiccation. Thus, SC has developed an elegant self-adjusting moisturization mechanism to respond to the different climatic conditions it is exposed to.

19.2.4 NMF Levels and Dry Skin Conditions

The failure to either make or process (pro)filaggrin is a major problem for the skin and is associated with various dermatological disorders. The symptoms of ichthyosis vulgaris[37] are closely associated with an inability or failure to make profilaggrin. The absence of keratohyalin granules histologically has been known for many years, and the NMF content of corneum in ichthyotic vulgaris patients is close to zero. Likewise, in psoriatics there is again a paucity of keratohyalin granules and the associated SC is essentially NMF deficient.[38] Subjects with atopic dermatitis also have decreased levels of NMF.[39]

Although it is clear that in all these disorders several aspects of keratinization are impaired, the inability to produce or retain NMF within the SC appears to be a significant factor contributing to the overall manifestation of the skin problem.

Reduced NMF levels are also implicated in the more common dry skin conditions. Free amino acid levels have been reported to decrease significantly in dry, scaly skin induced experimentally by repetitive tape stripping.[40] Additionally, a significant correlation exists between the hydration state of the SC and its amino acid content in elderly individuals with skin xerosis.[41] Indeed, the subtleties of the NMF generating mechanism outlined earlier in this chapter offer an explanation for the transient reduced water-holding capacity of the SC of newborn infants.[42]

In this laboratory we have studied some of the factors influencing SC NMF levels using PCA as a marker of NMF levels. Typical SC depths vs. NMF concentration profiles obtained by sequential tape stripping of young and old individuals are shown in Figure 3. These profiles indicate that the levels of NMF decline markedly toward the surface of the skin. This is typical of normal skin exposed to routine soap washing where much of the readily soluble NMF is washed out from the superficial SC.[43]

The data also illustrate that there is a significant age-related decline in the level of NMF. Taken together with electron microscopy studies which report decreased numbers of keratohyalin granules in senile xerosis,[44] these results suggest that the intrinsically lower NMF levels present in aged skin, compared with young skin, reflects a general reduced synthesis of profilaggrin. In addition, it is likely that in aged skin the loss of NMF becomes more pronounced as elderly individuals also show an age-related decline in water barrier repair.[45] The decline in NMF production probably reflects the cumulative effects of actinic damage as it was observed in SC recovered from the back of the hand (photodamaged), but not from the inner aspect of the biceps (photoprotected).

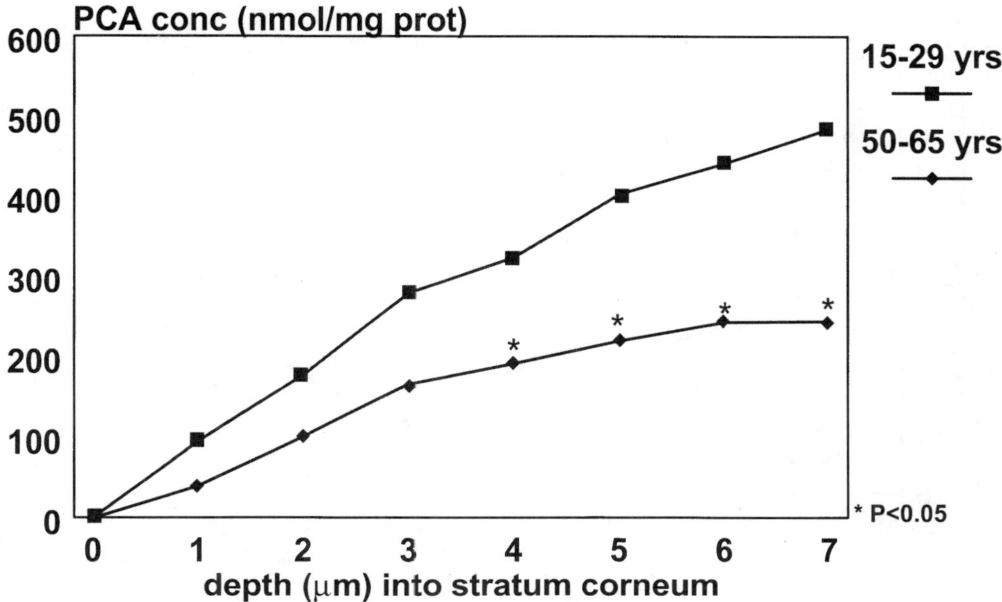

FIGURE 3 Profile of mean PCA concentration distribution vs. SC depth in hand skin of young and old individuals.

In summary, the various processes leading from profilaggrin synthesis to conversion to filaggrin and then to NMF are under tight control. However, these controls are perturbed in different ways by a range of factors including UV light,[30] exposure to surfactants, and, of course, rapid changes in environmental humidity. These very different causes can all lead to reduced NMF and contribute to the complex phenomenon known as dry skin.

19.3 THE EFFECT OF TOPICALLY APPLIED NMF

Moisturizing ingredients have been used widely in skin care products for the treatment of dry skin for many years. In fact the use of oils for smoothing skin is reported as early as 2300 B.C., although it was not until the work of Blank in the 1950s[1] that research focused on water-imbibing substances to retain moisture in the SC. This section will discuss briefly the effects of PCA, urea, and lactic acid on human SC function *in vivo*.

19.3.1 Pyrrolidone Carboxylic Acid

A considerable amount of work has been performed evaluating the effects of PCA and its salts *in vitro*. However, surprisingly only a limited amount of work has been reported on the influence of PCA topically applied on human skin. In one such study Middleton and Roberts[46] demonstrated that lotions containing PCA were more effective at treating dry skin compared to a placebo lotion.

19.3.2 Urea

Urea is a major component of the NMF, and it has been used in hand creams since the 1940s. This unique physiological substance has proven to be a potent skin humidifier and descaling agent[47] and in high concentrations it has been shown to be an effective treatment for dry skin, being more efficacious than salicylic acid and petroleum jelly.[48] Urea containing moisturizers are also reported

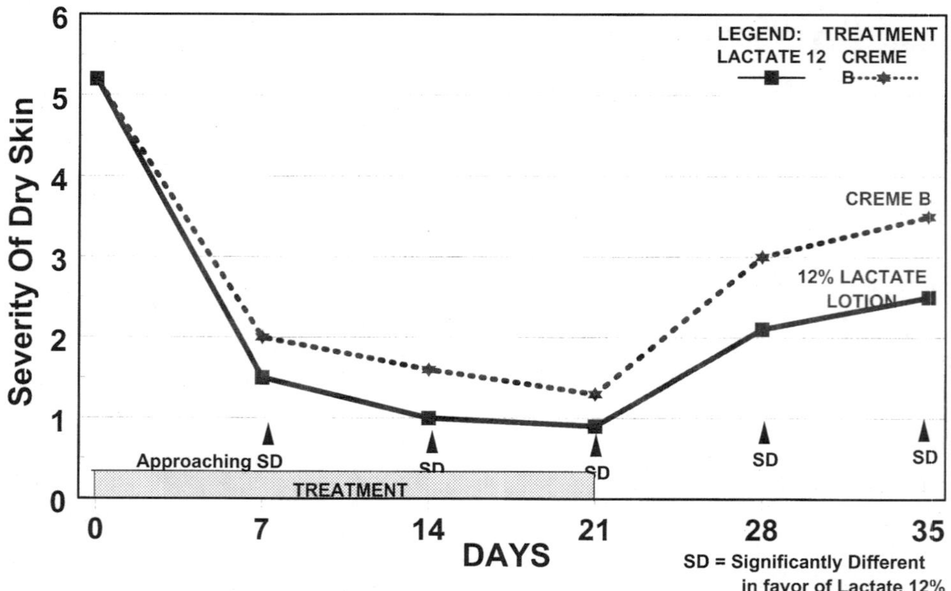

FIGURE 4 Improvement in dry skin condition following twice daily applications of a 12% lactic acid formulation. (Reprinted by permission of publisher from Wehr, R., Krochmal, L., Bagatell, F. and Ragsdale, W. A. Controlled 2 center study of lactate 12% lotion and a petrolatum based cream in patients with xerosis, *Cutis*, 23, 205, 1986. Copyright 1999 by Quadrant Healthcom Inc.)

to influence barrier properties of the skin, reducing TEWL,[49-52] increasing skin capacitance, and reducing irritant reactions Corresponding lotions containing glycerol as the humectant had no comparable effect on reducing TEWL. Although the precise mode of action of urea is unknown, the improved barrier function may be related to increased corneocyte size resulting from reduced keratinocyte proliferation. High concentrations of urea have also been reported recently to enhance lipid biosynthesis.[53] Finally, in combination with lactic acid, urea has also been shown to be an effective treatment of ichthyosis[54] and in combination with polidocanol urea is reported to improve juvenile atopic dermatitis.[55]

19.3.3 Lactic Acid

Lactic acid, as well as being a component of the NMF, is also a member of the class of molecules called alpha hydroxy acids (AHAs) which exert specific and unique benefits on skin structure and function. Although originally described for the treatment of dry skin-related disorders, their pleiotropic properties include influencing skin cell renewal and other anti-ageing benefits which have become the focus of considerable interest in recent years (see later).

The first recorded use of lactic acid was in 1943 by Stern who used it for the treatment of ichthyosis,[56] and in the early 1970s and 1980s Middleton[57] and Van Scott and Yu[58,59] demonstrated the efficacy of these short chain AHAs in ameliorating dry skin in moisturization efficacy studies.

Other researchers[60-62] have also shown that racemic mixtures of lactic acid ameliorate the common problem of winter xerosis. Typical effects of lactic acid in moisturization efficacy studies are shown in Figure 4.[62] Recently, Berardesca et al. have also reported the ability of a number of AHAs to improve SC barrier and prevent skin irritation.[63]

However, as is the case with other humectants, application of lactic acid alone fails to ameliorate the symptoms of dry skin, and co-formulation with occlusive agents is required to help retain the humectant bound water within the surface layers of the SC. Typically, we have found that lotions containing barrier lipids (ceramides) and lactic acid provide synergistic relief of dry skin.[64] These

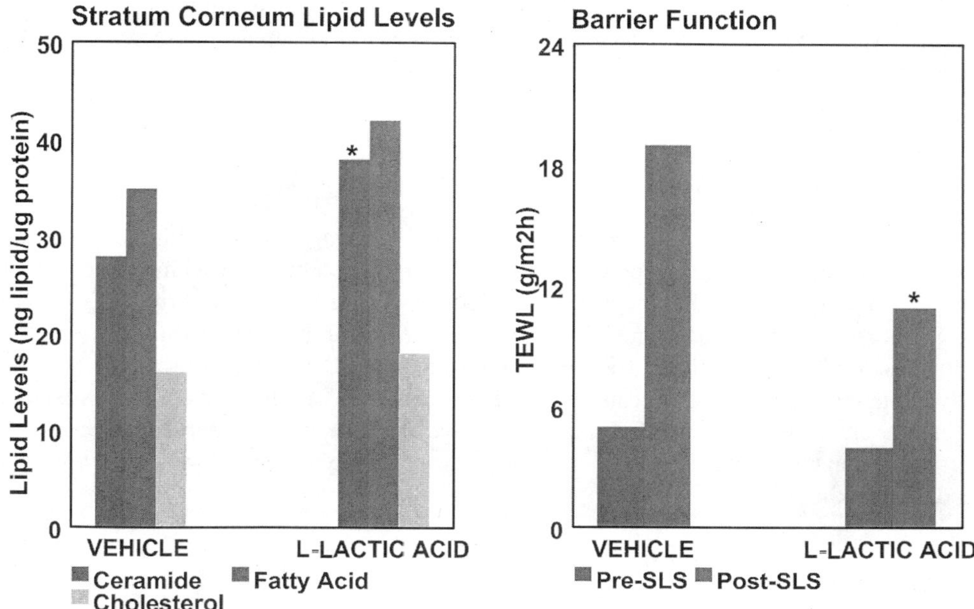

FIGURE 5 Effect of lactic acid on SC lipid levels and barrier function following a 1-month topical application of 4% lactic acid in an aqueous vehicle. TEWL evaluated before application of SLS patch and 24 h after removal (*p <0.05). (Reprinted with permission by publisher from Rawlings, A. V., Davies, A., Carlomusto, M., Pillai, S., Zhang, K., Kosturko, R., Verdejo, P., Feinberg, C., Nguyen, L. and Chandar, P. Keratinocyte ceramide synthesis, effect of lactic acid isomers on stratum corneum lipid levels and stratum corneum barrier function, *Arch. Dermatol. Res.*, 288, 383, 1996. Copyright 1999 by Springer-Verlag, New York.)

results are similar to those found with lotions containing barrier lipids and glycerol[65] and we believe that these lotions then act by increasing enzymatic activity within the SC leading to corneodesmolysis.

More recently, the relative efficacy of the different isomers of lactic acid have been studied to help decipher its mode of action in improving SC resilience. *In vitro* lactic acid increased the production of ceramides by keratinocytes, and the L-isomer was found to be more effective than the D-isomer.[66] Similar effects were observed *in vivo* where in a 4-week study topically applied lactic acid increased SC ceramide levels and L-lactic acid was seen to be the most active isomer. These changes were associated with improvements in SC barrier performance measured by changes in TEWL following a challenge to skin with sodium lauryl sulfate (Figure 5) and by a decrease in the expression of dry skin in the regression phase of a moisturization efficacy study. Significant improvements in these parameters were observed following application of lotions containing L-lactic acid and D,L-lactic acid but not D-lactic acid. In the studies outlined previously a significant increase in the ratio of ceramide 1 linoleate to ceramide 1 oleate may also have contributed to the improvements in SC performance. Ceramide 1 linoleate is of critical importance to the SC, where it functions as an important modulator of lipid phase behavior.[67]

In a pivotal clinical study evaluating the effects of lactic acid on photodamaged skin,[68] an 8% L-lactic acid formula was found to be statistically significantly superior to the vehicle cream in reducing the overall severity of photodamage, mottled hyperpigmentation, sallowness, and skin roughness. Furthermore, the benefit of lactic acid on skin roughness was confirmed instrumentally following laser profilometry of silicone replicas taken from the cheek area. The results indicated that the L-lactic acid formula substantially reduced the roughness of the skin compared to the vehicle cream regardless of the roughness parameter calculated. Generally, the improvement in skin roughness was of the order of 25 and 10% compared to baseline values for the lactic and vehicle creams, respectively. Although the exact mechanisms which explain these observations are not known, we have shown that lactic acid imparts changes to SC lipids and increases epidermal turnover rates which should reveal smaller corneocytes. Further studies are in progress to understand more clearly the mode of action of lactic acid in the effective treatment of photodamaged skin.

19.4 FINAL COMMENTS

The NMF is essential for normal functioning of the SC. Working together with the SC lipids this pool of low molecular weight compounds assists in the retention of water within the corneocytes, a capacity which is vital for the integrity of this barrier, and its mechanical properties. Hydration of the SC is also essential for normal functioning of enzymatic processes which are pivotal, not only for desquamation, but also for the generation of the NMF itself. Perturbations to either of these two biophysical mechanisms can lead to xerotic problems. Applications of lotions containing a variety of the constitutive NMF components have been shown to improve SC extensibility properties, desquamation performance, and water barrier quality and to alleviate the symptoms of dry and aging skin.

REFERENCES

1. Blank, I. H. Factors which influence the water content of the stratum corneum, *J. Invest. Dermatol.*, 18, 483, 1952.
2. Elias, P. M. Epidermal lipids, barrier function and desquamation, *J. Invest. Dermatol.*, 80 (Supp 1), 44, 1983.
3. Steinert, P. M. and Marekov, L. N. The proteins elafin, filaggrin, keratin intermediate filaments, loricrin, and small proline-rich proteins are isodipeptide cross-linked components of the human cornified cell-envelope, *J. Biol. Chem.*, 270, 17702, 1995.
4. Reichert, U., Michel, S. and Scmidt, R. The cornified envelope: a key structure of terminally differentiating keratinocytes, in *Molecular Biology of the Skin: The Keratinocyte,* Darmon, M. and Blumberg, M. Eds., Academic Press, New York, 1994, chap 2.
5. Candi, E., Tarcsa, E., Digiovanna, J. J., Compton, J. G., Elias, P. M., Marekov, L. N. and Steinert, P. M. A highly conserved lysine residue on the head domain of type II keratins is essential for the attachment of keratin intermediate filaments to the cornified cell envelope through isodipeptide crosslinking by transglutaminase, *Proc. Natl. Acad. Sci. U.S.A.*, 95, 2067, 1998.
6. Skerrow, C. J., Clelland, D. G. and Skerrow, D. Changes to desmosomal antigens and lectin-binding sires during differentiation in normal epidermis: A quantitative ultrastructural study, *J. Cell Sci.*, 92, 667, 1989.
7. Chapman, S. and Walsh, A. Desmosomes, corneosomes and desquamation. An ultrastructural study of adult pig epidermis, *Arch. Dermatol. Res.*, 282, 304, 1990.
8. Blank, I. H. Further observations on factors which influence the water content of the stratum corneum, *J. Invest. Dermatol.*, 21, 259, 1953.
9. Elias, P. M. and Menon, G. K. Structural and lipid biochemical correlates of the epidermal permeability barrier, *Adv. Lipid Res.*, 24, 1–26, 1991.
10. Wertz, P. W., Miethke, M. C., Long S. A. et al. Composition of ceramides from human stratum corneum and comedones, *J. Invest. Dermatol.*, 84, 410, 1985.
11. Tabachnick, J. and Labadie, J. H. Studies on the biochemistry of epidermis. IV. The free amino acids, ammonia, urea and pyrrolidone carboxylic acid content of conventional and germ free albino guinea pig epidermis, *J. Invest. Dermatol.*, 54, 24, 1970.
12. Egelrud, T. Purification and preliminary characterization of stratum corneum chymotryptic enzyme-A proteinase that may be involved in desquamation, *J. Invest. Dermatol.*, 101, 200, 1993.
13. Suzuki, Y., Nonura, J., Hori, J., Koyama, J., Takahashi, M. and Horii, I. Detection and characterization of endogenous proteases associated with desquamation of stratum corneum, *Arch. Dermatol. Res.*, 285, 327, 1993.

14. Rogers, J. S., Watkinson, A. and Harding, C. R. Characterization of the effects of protease inhibitors and lipids on human stratum corneum chymotrytic-like enzyme supports a role in desquamation, *J. Invest. Dermatol.,* 110, 672, 1998.
15. Cler, E. J. and Fourtanier, A. L'acide pyrrolidone carboxylique (PCA) et la peau, *Int. J. Cosmet. Sci.,* 3., 101, 1981.
16. Trianse, S. J. The search for the ideal moisturizer, *Cosmet. Perfum.,* 89, 57, 1974.
17. Fox, C., Tassoft, I., Rieger, M. M. and Deem, D. F. Modifications of the water holding capacity of callus by pre-treating with additives, *J. Soc. Cosmet. Chem.,* 13, 263, 1962.
18. Laden, K. and Spitzer, R. Identification of a natural moisturising agent in skin, *J. Soc. Cosmet. Chem.,* 18, 351, 1967.
19. Jacobi, O. K. Humectants vs. moisturizers, *Am. Cosmet. Perfum.,* 87, 35, 1972.
20. Takahashi, M., Yamada, M. and Machida, Y. A new method to evaluate the softening effect of cosmetic ingredients on the skin, *J. Soc. Cosmet. Chem.,* 35, 171, 1984.
21. Middleton, J. D. Development of a skin cream designed to reduce dry and flaky skin, *J. Soc. Cosmet. Chem.,* 25, 519, 1974.
22. Takahashi, M., Kawasaki, K., Tanaka, M., Ohra, S. and Tsuda, Y. The mechanism of stratum corneum plasticisation with water, in *Bioengineering and the Skin*, Marks, R. and Pine, P. A. Eds., MTP Press, Lancaster, England, 1981, 67.
23. Jokura, Y., Ishikawa, S., Tokuda, H. and Imokawa, G. Molecular analysis of elastic properties of the stratum corneum by solid-state C-13-nuclear magnetic resonance spectroscopy, *J. Invest. Dermatol.,* 104, 806, 1995.
24. Barrett, J. G. and Scott, I. R. Pyrrolidone carboxylic acid synthesis in guinea pig epidermis, *J. Invest. Dermatol.,* 81, 122, 1983.
25. Scott, I. R. and Harding, C. R. Studies on the synthesis and degradation of a histidine rich phosphoprotein from mammalian epidermis, *Biochim. Biophys. Acta*, 669, 65, 1981.
26. Scott, I. R., Harding, C. R. and Barrett, J. G. Histidine rich proteins of the keratohyalin granules: source of the free amino acids, urocanic acid and pyrrolidone carboxylic acid in the stratum corneum, *Biochim. Biophys. Acta*, 719, 110, 1982.
27. Steven, A. C., Bisher, M. E., Roop, D. R. and Steinert, P. M. Biosynthetic pathways of filaggrin and loricrin — two major proteins expressed in terminally differentiated epidermal keratinocytes, *J. Struct. Biol.,* 104, 150, 1990.
28. Harding, C. R. and Scott, I. R. Histidine-rich proteins (filaggrins). Structural and functional heterogeneity during epidermal differentiation, *J. Mol. Biol.*, 170, 651, 1983.
29. Steinert, P. M., Cantieri, J. S., Teller, J. D., Lonsdale-Eccles, J. D. and Dale, B. A. Characterisation of a class of cationic proteins that specifically interact with intermediate filaments, *Proc. Natl. Acad. Sci. U.S.A.,* 78, 4097, 1981.
30. Scott, I. R. Alterations in the metabolism of filaggrin in the skin after chemical and ultraviolet induced erythema, *J. Invest. Dermatol.,* 87, 460, 1986.
31. Richards, S., Scott, I. R., Harding, C. R., Liddell, E. and Curtis, G. C. Evidence for filaggrin as a component of the cell envelope of the newborn rat, *Biochem. J.,* 253, 153, 1988.
32. Angelin, J. H. Urocanic acid a natural sunscreen, *Cosmet. Toiletries,* 91, 47, 1976.
33. Scott, I. R. Factors controlling the expressed activity of histidine ammonia lyase in the epidermis and the resulting accumulation of urocanic acid, *Biochem. J.,* 194, 829, 1981.
34. Scott, I. R. and Harding, C. R. Filaggrin breakdown to water binding components during development of the rat stratum corneum is controlled by the water activity of the environment, *Dev. Biol.,* 115, 84, 1986.
35. Harding, C. R., Ellis, K. and Scott, I. R. Alterations in the processing of human filaggrin following skin occlusion *in vitro* and *in vivo*, *J. Invest. Dermatol.,* 100, 579, 1993.
36. Hanley, K., Jiang, Y., Elias, P. M., Feingold, K. R. and Williams, M. L. Acceleration of barrier ontogenesis *in vitro* through air exposure, *Pediatr. Res.,* 41, 293, 1997.
37. Sybert, V. P., Dale, B. A. and Holbrook, K. A. Ichthyosis vulgaris: identification of a defect in filaggrin synthesis correlated with a an absence of keratohyalin granules, *J. Invest. Dermatol.,* 84, 191, 1985.
38. Marstein, S., Jellum, E. and Eldjarn, L. The concentration of pyroglutamic acid (2- pyrrolidone-5-carboxylic acid) in normal and psoriatic epidermis determined on a microgram scale by gas chromatography, *Clin. Chim. Acta,* 49, 389, 1973.

39. Seguchi,T., Chang, Y. C., Kusuda, S., Takahashi, M., Aisuy, K. and Tezuka, T. Decreased expression of filaggrin in atopic skin, *Arch. Dermatol. Res.,* 288, 442, 1996.
40. Denda, M., Hori, J., Koyama, J., Yoshida, S., Nanba, R., Takahashi, M., Horii, I. and Yamamoto, A. Stratum corneum sphingolipids and free amino acids in experimentally-induced scaly skin, *Arch. Dermatol. Res.,* 284, 363, 1992.
41. Horii, I., Nakayama, Y., Obata, M. and Tagami, H. Stratum corneum hydration and amino acid content in xerotic skin, *Br. J. Dermatol.*, 121, 587, 1989.
42. Senji, S. and Tagami, H. Dry skin of newborn infants: functional analysis of the stratum corneum, *Pediatr. Dermatol.,* 8, 155, 1991.
43. Scott, I. R. and Harding, C. R. A filaggrin analogue to increase natural moisturising factor synthesis in skin, *Dermatology 2000,* p. 773, 1993.
44. Tezuka, T. Electron microscopal changes in xerotic senilis epidermis. Its abnormal membrane coating granule formation, *Dermatologica,* 166, 57, 1983.
45. Ghadially, R., Brown, B. E., Sequeiramartin, S. M., Feingold, K. R. and Elias, P. M. The aged epidermal permeability barrier-structural, functional, and lipid biochemical abnormalities in humans and a senescent murine model, *J. Clin. Invest.,* 95, 2281, 1995.
46. Middleton, J. D. and Roberts, M. E. Effect of a skin cream containing the sodium salt of pyrrollidone carboxylic acid on dry and flaky skin, *J. Soc. Cosmet. Chem.*, 29, 201, 1978.
47. Rattner H. Use of urea in hand cream, *Arch. Dermatol. Siph.,* 48, 47, 1943.
48. Fredrikkson, T. and Gip, L. Urea creams in the treatment of dry skin and hand dermatitis, *Int. J. Dermatol.*, 14, 442, 1975.
49. Serup, J. A. 3 hr test for rapid comparison of effects of moisturisers and active constituents (urea), *Arch. Derm. Venereal.* (*Stockholm*), Suppl. 1, 177, 29–33, 1997.
50. Serup, J. A. double blind comparison of 2 creams containing urea as the active ingredient, *Acta Derm. Venereol.* (*Stockholm*), Suppl. 77, 34, 1992.
51. Loden, M. Urea containing moisturisers influence barrier properties of normal skin, *Arch. Dermatol. Res.,* 288, 103, 1996,
52. Loden, M., Biophysical methods of providing objective documentation of the effects of moisturising creams, *Skin Res. Technol.*, 1, 101, 1995.
53. Pigatto, P. D., Bigardi, A. S., Cannistraci, C. and Picardo, M. 10% Urea cream (Laceran) for atopic dermatitis: a clinical and laboratory evaluation, *J. Dermatol. Treat.*, 7, 171, 1996.
54. Swanbeck, G. Treatment of dry hyperkeratotic, itchy skin with urea containing preparations, *Dermatol. Dig.* 11, 39, 1972.
55. Hauss, H., Proppe, A. and Matthies, C. A formulation for the treatment of dry, itching skin in comparison-results from therapeutic use, *Dermatosen Beruf Umwelt.*, 41, 184, 1993.
56. Stern, E. C. Topical application of lactic acid in the treatment and prevention of certain disorders of the skin, *Urol. Cutaneous Rev.,* 50, 106, 1943.
57. Middleton, J. D. Sodium lactate as a moisturiser, *Cosmet. Toiletries*, 93, 85, 1978.
58. Van Scott, E. and Yu, R. Hyperkeratinisation, corneocyte cohesion, and alpha hydroxy acids, *J. Am. Acad. Dermatol.*, 11, 867, 1984.
59. Van Scott, E. and Yu, R. J. Control of keratinisation with a-hydroxy acids and related compounds, *Arch. Dermatol.,* 110, 586, 1974.
60. Bagatell, F. K. and Smoot, W. Observations on a lactate containing emollient cream, *Cutis,* 18, 591, 1976.
61. Dahl, M. V. and Dahl, A. C. 12% Lactate lotion for the treatment of xerosis, *Arch. Dermatol.,* 119, 27, 1983.
62. Wehr, R., Krochmal, L., Bagatell, F. and Ragsdale, W. A controlled 2 center study of lactate 12% lotion and a petrolatum based cream in patients with xerosis, *Cutis*, 23, 205, 1986.
63. Berardesca, E., Distante, F., Vignoli, G., Oresajo, C. and Green, B. Alpha hydroxy acids modulate stratum corneum barrier function, *Br. J. Dermatol.,* 137, 934, 1997.
64. Bowser, P., Evenson, A. and Rawlings, A. V. 1997. Cosmetic Composition Containing a Lipid and a Hydroxyacid, European Patent Appl. EP058788B1.
65. Summers, R. S., Summers, B., Chander, P., Feinberg, C., Gursky R. and Rawlings, A.V. The effect of lipids with and without humectant on skin xerosis, *J. Cosmet. Chem.,* 47, 27, 1998.

66. Rawlings, A. V., Davies, A., Carlomusto, M., Pillai, S., Zhang, K., Kosturko, R., Verdejo, P., Feinberg, C., Nguyen, L. and Chandar, P. Keratinocyte ceramide synthesis, effect of lactic acid isomers on stratum corneum lipid levels and stratum corneum barrier function, *Arch. Dermatol. Res.,* 288, 383, 1996.
67. Critchley, P., Tiddy, G. and Rawlings A. V. Specialized role for ceramide one in the stratum corneum water barrier, *J. Invest. Dermatol.,* 102, 525, 1994.
68. Stiller, M. J., Bartolone, J., Stern, R., Smith, S., Kollias, N., Gillies, R. and Drake, L. A. Topical 8% glycolic acid and 8% lactic acid creams for the treatment of photodamaged skin — a double-blind vehicle controlled clinical study, *Arch. Dermatol.,* 132, 631, 1996.

20 Urea

Marie Lodén

CONTENTS

20.1 INTRODUCTION

Urea is a physiological substance occurring in human tissues, blood, and urine. The amount in urine is of the order of 2%. The extraction of pure urea from urine was first accomplished by Proust in 1821, and it was first synthesized by Wöhler in 1828.[1] Urea is also a major constituent of the water-soluble fraction of the stratum corneum, as a component of the natural moisturizing factor (NMF).[2] The level of urea in the stratum corenum is significantly reduced in patients with atopic dermatitis.[3]

Folklore is rich in references to the healing properties of urea. The Babylonians of about 800 B.C. are known to have used it.[4] In the beginning of this century, urea was employed in the treatment of infections, particularly infected wounds and ulcers, infection of the ears, infected tooth sockets, and infected malignant growths, and of burns.[4-6] Solutions containing 20% urea have been proposed to reduce experimentally induced itching,[7] but the effect appears too weak to justify the use of more dilute preparations as antipruritics on their own.[4-8]

The most well-known dermatologic effects from urea appear to stem from its generally accepted property of unfolding proteins, thus solubilizing them and/or denaturing them.[6,9,10] Pieces of upper epidermis kept in saturated urea solutions change mechanically and lose their original quaternary structure.[9] Urea can also be used for avulsing dystrophic nails, and a preparation with 40% urea has been shown to be slightly more effective in removing the nail than a formulation with 22%, but it was also more irritating.[11] Urea is also used as a keratoplastic agent (at 40%) to increase the bioavailability of the drug in the treatment of onychomycosis.[12] Concern has been expressed about the use of urea in moisturizers, with reference to the risk of reducing the chemical barrier function of the skin to toxic substances.[9]

0-8493-7520-7/00/$0.00+$.50

Urea has also been used for treatment of a variety of dermatoses. For example, 10% urea in a nongreasy base showed good results in an open study on patients with ichthyosis and other hyperkeratotic conditions; only fair results in atopic dermatitis, disseminated neurodermatitis, hand dermatitis, and seborrheic dermatitis; and no improvement in psoriasis, pustular psoriasis, solar keratosis, and perioral dermatitis.[1] Another trial could not demonstrate any difference in the therapeutic effect between a urea cream (10%) and an aqueous cream when cracked chapped hands (18 patients), atopic eczema (18 patients), hyperkeratosis of the feet (8 patients), ichthyosis (7 patients), and psoriasis (4 patients) were treated for 3 weeks in a double-blind manner.[13]

However, several other clinical studies have shown urea-containing moisturizers to be useful in the treatment of dry and hyperkeratotic skin. In this chapter these studies will be reviewed along with data on the influence of urea on the barrier function of the skin.

20.2 CHEMISTRY AND *IN VITRO* BEHAVIOR

Urea (carbamide, carbonyl diamide, CAS no 57-13-6, molecular weight 60.08) is a white, crystalline, and quite inexpensive powder. The substance is hygroscopic, freely soluble in water, slightly soluble in alcohol, and practically insoluble in ether.[14] Urea in solution hydrolyzes slowly to ammonia and carbon dioxide.[14]

Urea is readily incorporated in topical formulations by virtue of its solubility. However, preparations may need to be stored in a refrigerator because of decomposition of urea. In one patent it is claimed that lactic acid retards the decomposition of urea.[15] Immersion of psoriatic and ichthyotic scales in 5 *M* urea show that they will absorb 38% of water at 85% relative humidity.[16] Addition of equal concentration of sodium chloride claims to give a synergistic effect in regard to the water-retaining property of human skin than for any of the compounds alone at a comparable concentration.[17]

20.3 EFFECTS OF UREA ON THE SKIN BARRIER FUNCTION

20.3.1 Normal Skin

Urea is easily absorbed into the skin[18-20] and has been proposed to influence epidermal proliferation in healthy human skin and in guinea pig ear.[20,21] Incorporation of ^{3}H-thymidine in DNA was reduced and a thinning of epidermis was found after short-term contact with a saturated urea solution. After long-term exposure to urea, lasting more than 2 to 6 weeks, no further thinning occurred, and there was no tendency for atrophy during this period.[20,21] No changes in the binding forces within stratum corneum have been found after 6 h occlusive exposure of normal skin to 10%.[18]

Several studies have shown that urea is an efficient accelerant for the penetration of different substances.[22-27] Increased levels of hydrocortisone, triamcinolone acetonide,[23] dithranol,[24] and retinoic acid[22] were found in various layers of isolated human skin after 1000 min of exposure time to creams containing 10 to 12% urea. The penetration of ketoprofen through isolated rat skin was also enhanced by the addition of urea.[27] Furthermore, it has been shown that the time of onset of erythema, induced by hexyl nicotinate, is significantly reduced by the addition of urea to an oily cream.[25] However, not all studies support the belief that urea is an effective penetration promoter.[28-32] For instance, the latency time to induce erythema by another nicotinate was not changed by pretreatment of forearm skin with an aqueous solution of 10% urea.[30] Moreover, urea (10%) had a minimal effect on the penetration of hydrocortisone through excised human and guinea pig skin.[28] Hydrocortisone acetate was even retarded through hairless mouse skin with increasing concentrations of urea (up to 12%).[31] This could be due to an increased binding capacity within the stratum corneum, which is due to an alteration of the surface structure of keratin.[29] Urea does not seem to influence the lipid matrix of the skin, since the transition temperatures of mouse skin lipids were not significantly changed by exposure to 12% urea.[31]

Measurement of transepidermal water loss (TEWL) is another way to study the skin barrier function. *In vitro* measurements on piglet stratum corneum suggest that urea markedly decreases TEWL.[32] *In vivo* TEWL measurements have also been combined with challenge of the skin with an irritant (sodium lauryl sulfate, SLS) to elucidate possible changes in susceptibility to irritation.[33,34] Results indicate that treatment for a limited number of days (1 to 2 days) with 5 to 10% urea appears to increase TEWL, whereas longer treatment times (10 to 20 days) decrease TEWL.[33,35] Furthermore, the irritant reactions after exposure to SLS were significantly lower after treatment for 20 days than in the untreated skin.[33,34] A decreased susceptibility to SLS was noticed also after three applications of both 5 and 10% urea moisturizers, although this decrease in susceptibility was not preceded by a reduction in TEWL.[33] The improvement in skin barrier function due to the inclusion of urea in the formulation has recently been confirmed in a placebo-controlled study.[36] A significantly lower TEWL and subsequently lower skin susceptibility to SLS were found in the urea-treated skin compared to the placebo-treated skin.[36]

20.3.2 Diseased Skin

Topical treatment of psoriasis by 10% urea cream has been found to reduce epidermal DNA synthesis and induce epidermal proliferation, without influencing TEWL.[37] The number of stratum corneum cell layers was reduced in 6 of 11 patients with ichthyosis after treatment with 10% urea (Calmuril®, Pharmacia & Upjohn, Sweden).[38] TEWL in ichthyotic skin was slightly reduced by the application of 10% urea for 3 weeks.[39] After 2 days of treatment of atopic patients with 10% urea cream (Laceran, Beiersdorf), TEWL tended to increase, but after 7 days of treatment a significant decrease was noted in the atopic patients.[35] Furthermore, the urea treatment increased the level of certain extractable lipids from the skin, which was suggested to be due to enhanced skin lipid synthesis, but might also have been derived from applied cream lipids.

In patients with atopic dermatitis, a 5% urea cream (Canoderm®, ACO Hud AB, Sweden) has been found to reduce TEWL on the back of the hands,[40] whereas the other test cream (4% urea combined with sodium chloride as actives; Fenuril®, Pharmacia & Upjohn AB, Sweden) did not change TEWL.[40] Moreover, the 5% urea cream reduced TEWL on the volar aspect of the forearm in atopics and made the skin less susceptible to the surfactant SLS.[41] The irritant reaction was measured using a laser Doppler flowmeter and an Evaporimeter.

In dry skin, no influence on TEWL was noted after treatment with a 3% urea cream, whereas TEWL decreased in skin treated with 10% urea cream.[42] In surfactant-damaged skin a 5% urea cream has been shown to promote barrier recovery.[34,36] The acceleration in barrier recovery was mainly observed as a decrease in TEWL. Furthermore, a recent placebo-controlled study proved that urea was responsible for the accelerated barrier recovery and that the improved barrier function appeared to be of clinical relevance, since the susceptibility to SLS also was decreased.[36] Twice daily exposure to 15% SLS (except weekends) and the 5% cream for 15 days induced a slight but significant barrier damage, measured as TEWL, but urea-treated sites appeared less damaged than the vehicle treated.

20.4 CLINICAL STUDIES ON UREA-CONTAINING MOISTURIZERS (TABLE 1)

20.4.1 Psoriasis

Urea treatment has been found to reduce epidermal DNA synthesis and induce epidermal differentiation.[35] Five psoriatic patients with chronic therapy-resistant lesions obtained soft and pliable skin after treatment with 10% urea, but no effect on erythema was observed.[16] Psoriatic lesions on the extremities (at least 5 cm in diameter in size) showed clinical improvement after 2 weeks of treatment with an ointment containing 10% urea (Basodexan® S ointment) in a placebo-controlled study on 10 patients.[37] Higher values of skin capacitance (suggested to reflect skin hydration) were noted on urea-treated areas.

TABLE 1
Summary of Clinical Data on the Treatment of Diseased Skin with Urea Preparations

Diagnosis	No. of Patients	Concentration (%)	Design	Results	Ref.
Psoriasis	5	10	Open	Softening effects	16
	10	10	Double-blind, placebo controlled	Better than placebo	37
Ichthyosis	7	10	Open	Improvement	16
	84	10	Double-blind	Better than placebo	44
	14	10	Double-blind, placebo controlled	Better than placebo	39
	60	10	Double-blind, placebo controlled, bilateral	Better than placebo	45
Ichthyosis associated with atopic dermatitis	30	10	Double-blind, bilateral, reference cream	Urea cream pH 6 better than urea cream pH 3	43
Atopic dermatitis	12	1	Open	Improvement, burning sensation in one patient	16
	40	10	Single-blind, "placebo" controlled	Clinical improvement, decreased TEWL	35
	50	4, 5	Double-blind, 4% to 5%	Clinical improvements, no difference between products	40
	1905	10	Open, uncontrolled	?	46
Atopic skin	15	5	Blind evaluation, untreated control	Reduced susceptibilility to SLS induced irritation	41
Dry skin, hands	250	3	Bilateral placebo	Urea cream better	5
Hand eczema	30	10	Double-blind, bilateral, reference cream with 10% urea	Both creams effective, the one with pH 6 preferred to the one with pH 3	43
Asteatosis	26	4 Urea + 4 sodium chloride	Double-blind, placebo controlled	Clinical improvement, urea cream better than placebo	17
Dry skin	47	3, 10	Blind evaluation, untreated control	Less scaling, improved hydration	42
Various dermatoses	58	10	Open	Ichthyosis — improvement, atopic dermatitis, hand dermatitis — fair	1
Hyperkeratosis (e.g., chapped hands, atopic eczema)	55	?	Double-blind, bilateral	No difference in effect compared with aqueous cream BP; 3 patients (5%) reported stinging	13
Dry senescent skin	60	10	Double-blind, bilateral, placebo controlled	Differences in skin capacitance, not clinically	8
Surfactant damaged skin	13	5	Blind evaluation, untreated control	Accelerated barrier recovery	34

20.4.2 Ichthyosis

The use of high concentrations (about 10%) of urea in creams has been suggested for the therapy of ichthyosis and other hyperkeratotic conditions.[16] The water-holding capacity of the scales is increased by 100%, from 9 to 18% by the treatment with an urea cream (10%).[39] In seven patients with severe ichthyosis a pronounced keratolytic effect was noticed and the skin became soft and pliable.[16]

A 10% urea cream (Calmuril) was statistically significantly better in controlling the clinical signs of ichthyosis than three other preparations (salicylic acid ointment, an oily cream, and E45 cream, Boots) in a double-blind trial on 84 outpatients with ichthyosis vulgaris or X-linked ichthyosis.[44] The patient's assessment did not reveal any statistically significant difference between the groups.

Significant clinical improvement was also noted in 14 patients with ichthyosis after treatment for 3 weeks with 10% urea compared with treatment with the base. None of the patients complained of irritation.[39] Also in 60 children with ichthyosis the improvement was stronger in the extremity treated with a 10% urea lotion than in corresponding placebo-treated extremity.[45]

When comparing two preparations containing 10% urea on 30 patients with ichthyosis associated with atopic dermatitis, both investigators and patients preferred a cream containing multisterols, phospholipids, and fatty diols (pH about 6) to the other cream (Calmuril) containing betaine and lactic acid (pH about 3).[43]

20.4.3 Atopic Dermatitis

Treatment with 10% urea cream containing hydrocortisone has been shown to be clinically better than treatment with other hydrocortisone preparations in a single-blind and bilateral study on 12 patients with atopic eczema.[16] All patients became more soft and smooth in the skin. One patient reported a burning sensation after application of the urea cream to freshly excoriated lesions, but no other side effects were noted.[16] A combination of 10% urea moisturizer (Basodexan) and one 1% hydrocortisone preparation with 10% urea was evaluated in an open, uncontrolled, multicenter study on 1905 patients with atopic dermatitis.[46] Over the 12-month observational period, a total of 84% of the patients were exclusively treated with the two trial preparations and only 16% required additional treatment with other corticosteroids. Some patients experienced smarting sensations and itching, but the underlying skin disease may well have accounted for some of these problems.

A 10% urea cream (Laceran, Beiersdorf, Germany) produced improvement of the xerosis and the pruritus, but somewhat less of the erythema compared to those of a base cream (Essex base cream, Schering-Plough).[35] No results from treatment of the cream base were reported. Two patients felt irritation during treatment with the urea cream and therefore dropped out of the study.

A 5% urea cream (Canoderm) showed similar efficacy as a 4% urea cream also containing 4% sodium chloride as active ingredient (Fenuril) in a double-blind, randomized, and parallel study on 50 atopic patients.[40] The assessment showed improvements in both groups during the treatment period.[40]

20.4.4 Hand Dermatitis

One of the first clinical studies on urea in a cream was published 1943.[5] Two hundered and twenty-five hospital personnel were given two jars of cream, one with 3% urea and one without urea, and were requested to use one on each hand. Both the investigators and the patients experienced better results with the urea cream, in that the skin seemed softer, smoother, and even whiter.[5] Patches of slight dermatitis were reported to improve by the application of urea cream.[5]

Two preparations containing 10% urea were found to be helpful therapeutic agents in a double-blind, bilateral study.[43] Both investigators and patients expressed preference for the cream containing multisterols, phospholipids, and fatty diols (pH of about 6) to the other cream (Calmuril) containing betaine and lactic acid (pH about 3). Some patients noted burning sensations after treatment with the latter cream (Calmuril).

20.4.5 Dry Skin

A cream containing 4% urea (Fenuril, also containing sodium chloride as active humectant) was significantly better than corresponding placebo in reducing dryness and scaling on 26 patients with asteatosis.[17] The effect of active treatment was excellent on dryness and scaling, as judged by the doctor as well as by the patients. The urea concentration did not seem to be high enough to exert a keratolytic effect.

A 10% urea lotion proved to be more effective than its vehicle in another placebo-controlled bilateral study on 60 elderly volunteers, as evaluated by capacitance measurements.[8] No difference between the treatments was noted by the patients, although both lotions reduced skin dryness and itching. Six patients reported erythema from treatment of the urea-containing lotion and two of these also experienced erythema from the vehicle. Two patients reported pruritus from the urea lotion and one from the vehicle. One patient also reported skin exfoliation.

Creams containing 3% urea (n = 23) or 10% urea (n = 24) were applied to one of the volar forearms on individuals with some evidence of dry skin for 3 weeks.[42] Both creams improved the skin with respect to dryness characteristics, as evaluated by a dermatologist, measurements of electrical capacitance and conductance, and tape assessments of scaling. Both creams were considered equally effective, but the 3% urea cream turned the skin color golden.

20.5 SIDE EFFECTS

Urea is a normal physiological metabolite and is generally regarded as nontoxic. No report on sensitization has been found, despite its wide use in dermatological preparations. In 1943, Rattner patch tested 500 hospital patients, 66 of whom had skin disease, with a 3% urea cream and found no adverse reaction.[5] Clinical and patient assessments of the use of creams with 10% area or lower give no evidence of skin irritation with inflammation and barrier damage,[42] although occlusive exposure to 20% urea in petrolatum for 24 h causes significant inflammation (i.e., increase in blood flow and skin thickness) and also increases TEWL.[47]

However, some patients report disagreeable skin sensations from urea treatments, like redness, stinging, and smarting sensations.[1,16,17,35,41-43,46] Application of urea to freshly excoriated areas and to lesioned skin can give burning sensations.[48] This is not irritation in the ordinary sense and usually does not cause clinically noticeable damages to the skin, but the disagreeable sensations will hamper compliance, especially in children.[1] Furthermore, it may be difficult to treat sensitive body areas, for example, the face, since stinging and other side effects from topical treatment are mainly perceived in the face.[49,50]

20.6 CONCLUSION

Data from the literature shows that urea increases the water-binding properties of scales from ichthyotic and psoriatic patients and that high concentrations of urea have keratolytic properties. However, the keratolytic effects are dose-dependent, and it seems that in hyperkeratotic skin a decrease in the number of cell layers can be expected after treatment with 5 to 10%, whereas in normal skin levels exceeding 10 to 20% are needed to obtain keratolysis.

Several studies demonstrate beneficial effects of urea-containing moisturizers in the treatment of different dry skin conditions such as ichthyosis, psoriasis, asteatosis, atopic dermatitis, and chapped hands. In some studies the treatment effects could be attributed to urea. A 5% urea cream has also been found to promote late barrier recovery in experimentally induced irritation. Furthermore, in diseased as well as in normal skin a lowering of TEWL has been found after treatment for some days with urea formulations (5 to 10%). In normal skin this has been linked to a decreased skin susceptibility to surfactant-induced irritation. A possible explanation for the observed lowering of TEWL might be an increased size of the corneocytes, since larger corneocytes will decrease skin permeability.[51]

REFERENCES

1. Rosten, M., The treatment of ichthyosis and hyperkeratotic conditions with urea. *Aust. J. Dermatol.,* 11, 142–144, 1971.
2. Jacobi, O. K., Moisture regulation in the skin. *Drug Cosmet. Ind.,* 84, 732–812, 1959.
3. Wellner, K., Wohlrab, W., Quantitative evaluation of urea in stratum corneum of human skin. *Arch. Dermatol. Res.,* 285, 239–240, 1993.
4. *Drugs Ther. Bull.,* 9, 29–30, 1971.
5. Rattner, H., Use of urea in hand creams. *Arch. Dermatol. Syph.,* 48, 47–49, 1943.
6. Ashton, H., Frenk, E., Stevenson, C. J., Therapeutics. XIII. Urea as a topical agent. *Br. J. Dermatol.,* 84, 194–196, 1971.
7. Swanbeck, G., Rajka, G., Antipruritic effect of urea solutions. *Acta Derm. Venereol. (Stockholm),* 50, 225–227, 1970.
8. Schölermann, A., Banké-Bochita, J., Bohnsack, K., Rippke, F., Herrmann, W. M., Efficacy and safety of Eucerin 10% urea lotion in the treatment of symptoms of aged skin. *J. Dermatol. Treatm.,* 9, 175–179, 1998.
9. Hellgren, L., Larsson, K., On the effect of urea on human epidermis. *Dermatologica,* 149, 289–293, 1974.
10. Kuntz, D., Brassfield, T. S., Hydration of macromolecules. II. Effects of urea on protein hydration. *Arch Biochem. Biophys.,* 142, 660–664, 1971.
11. Farber, E. M., South, D. A., Urea ointment in the nonsurgical avulsion of nail drystrophies. *Cutis,* 22, 689–692, 1978.
12. Fritsch, H., Stettendorf, S., Hegemann, L., Ultrastructural changes in onchomycosis during the treatment with bifonazole/urea ointment. *Dermatology,* 185, 32–36, 1992.
13. General practitioner research group, Carbamide in Hyperkeratosis. Report No. 179, 294–296, 1973.
14. Reynolds, J. E. F., *Martindale, The extra pharmacopoeia.* London: The Pharmaceutical Press, 1993.
15. Swanbeck, G. P. E., Skin-Treating Composition and Vehicle for Skin-Treating Agents, U.S. Patent 3,666,863, May 30, 1972.
16. Swanbeck, G., A new treatment of ichthyosis and other hyperkeratotic conditions. *Acta Derm. Venereol. (Stockh),* 48, 123–127, 1968.
17. Frithz, A., Investigation of cortesal, a hydrocortisone cream and its water-retaining cream base in the treatment of xerotic skin and dry eczema. *Curr. Ther. Res.,* 33, 930–935, 1983.
18. Lodén, M., Boström, P., Kneczke, M., Distribution and keratolytic effect of salicylic acid and urea in human skin. *Skin Pharmacol.,* 8, 173–178, 1995.
19. Wellner, K., Wohlrab, W., Quantitative evaluation of urea in stratum corneum of human skin. *Arch. Dermatol. Res.,* 285, 239–240, 1993.
20. Wohlrab, W., Schiemann, S., Untersuchungen zum Mechanismus der Harnstoffwirkung auf die Haut. *Arch. Dermatol. Res.* 255, 23–30, 1976.
21. Wohlrab, W., Böhm, W., Epidermisreaktion nach Langzeiteinwirkung von Harnstoff. *Dermatologica,* 151, 149–157, 1975.
22. Wohlrab, W., The influence of urea on the penetration kinetics of vitamin-A-acid into human skin. *Z. Hautkr.,* 65, 803–805, 1990.
23. Wohlrab, W., The influence of urea on the penetration kinetics of topically applied corticosteroids. *Acta Derm. Venereol. (Stockh),* 64, 233–238, 1984.
24. Wohlrab, W., Bedeutung von Harnstoff in der externen Therapie. *Hautarzt* 40, Suppl. 9, 35–41, 1989.
25. Beastall, J., Guy, R. H., Hadgraft, J., Wilding, I., The influence of urea on percutaneous absorption. *Pharm. Res.,* 3, 294–297, 1986
26. Allenby, A. C., Creasey, N. H., Edginton, J. A. G., Fletcher, J. A., Chock, C., Mechanism of action of accelerants on skin penetration. *Br. J. Dermatol.,* 81, Suppl. 4, 47–55, 1969.

27. Kim, C. K., Kim, J.-J., Chi, S.-C., Shim, C.-K., Effect of fatty acids and urea on the penetration of ketoprofen through rat skin. *Int. J. Pharm.,* 99, 109–118, 1993.
28. Wahlberg, J. E., Swanbeck, G., The effect of urea and lactic acid on the percutaneous absorption of hydrocortisone. *Acta Derm. Venereol. (Stockh),* 53, 207–210, 1973.
29. Stüttgen, G., Penetrationsförderung lokal applizierter Wirkstoffe durch Harnstoff. *Hautarzt,* 40, Suppl. 9, 27–31, 1989
30. Lippold, B. C., Hackemüller, D., The influence of skin moisturizer on drug penetration *in vivo*. *Int. J. Pharm.,* 61, 205–211, 1990.
31. Bentley, M. V. L. B., Kedor, E. R. M., Vianna, R. F., Collett, J. H., The influence of lecithin and urea on the *in vitro* permeation of hydrocortisone acetate through skin from hairless mouse. *Int. J. Pharm.,* 146, 255–262, 1997.
32. McCallion, R., Po, A. L. W., Modelling transepidermal water loss under steady-state and non-steady-state relative humidities. *Int. J. Pharm.* 105, 103–112, 1994.
33. Lodén, M., Urea-containing moisturizers influence barrier properties of normal skin. *Arch. Dermatol. Res.,* 288, 103–107, 1996.
34. Lodén, M., Barrier recovery and influence of irritant stimuli in skin treated with a moisturizing cream. *Contact Dermatitis,* 36, 256–260, 1997.
35. Pigatto, P. D., Bigardi, A. S., Cannistraci, C., Picardo, M., 10% urea cream (Laceran) for atopic dermatitis: a clinical and laboratory evaluation. *J. Dermatol. Treatm.,* 7, 171–175, 1996.
36. Lodén, M., Bárány, E., Mandahl, P., Wessman, C., Differences between a urea-containing emulsion and its placebo in affecting skin susceptibility to surfactant-induced irritation. Submitted.
37. Hagemann, I., Proksch, E., Topical treatment by urea reduces epidermal hyperproliferation and induces differentiation in psoriasis. *Acta Derm. Venereol. (Stockh),* 76, 353–356, 1996.
38. Blair, C., The action of urea-lactic acid ointment in ichthyosis. *Br. J. Dermatol.,* 94, 145–155, 1976.
39. Grice, K., Sattar, H., Baker, H., Urea and retinoic acid in ichthyosis and their effect on transepidermal water loss and water holding capacity of stratum corneum. *Acta Derm. Venereol. (Stockh),* 53, 114–118, 1973.
40. Andersson, A. C., Lindberg, M., Lodén, M., The effect of two urea-containing creams on dry, eczematous skin in atopic patients. I. Expert, patient and instrumental evaluation. *Dermatol. Treatm.,* 10, 165–169, 1999.
41. Lodén, M., Andersson, A.-C., Lindberg, M., Improvement in skin barrier function in patients with atopic dermatitis after treatment with a moisturising cream (Canoderm®). *Br. J. Dermatol.,* 140, 264–267, 1999.
42. Serup, J., A double-blind comparison of two creams containing urea as the active ingredient. Assessment of efficacy and side-effects by non-invasive techniques and a clinical scoring scheme. *Acta Derm. Venereol. (Stockh),* Suppl. 177, 34–38, 1992.
43. Fredriksson, T., Gip, L., Urea creams in the treatment of dry skin and hand dermatitis. *Int. J. Dermatol.,* 14, 442–443, 1975.
44. Pope, F. M., Rees, J. K., Wells, R. S., Lewis, K. G. S., Out-patient treatment of ichthyosis: a double-blind trial of ointments. *Br. J. Dermatol.,* 86, 291–296, 1972.
45. Kuster, W., Bohnsack, K., Rippke, F., Upmeyer, H. J., Groll, S., Traupe, H., Efficacy of urea therapy in children with ichthyosis. A multicenter randomized, placebo-controlled, double-blind, semilateral study. *Dermatology,* 196, 217–222, 1998.
46. Burkard, G., Schmitt, S., Langzeitstudie Neurodermitis-Therapie mit harnstoffhaltigen externa. *Hautarzt,* 43, 13–17, 1992.
47. Agner, T., An experimental study of irritant effects of urea in different vehicles. *Acta Derm. Venereol. (Stockh),* Suppl. 177, 44–46, 1992.
48. Gabard, B., Nook, T., Muller, K. H., Tolerance of the lesioned skin to dermatological formulations. *J. Appl. Cosmetol.,* 9, 25–30, 1991.
49. Frosch, P. J., Kligman, A. M., A method for appraising the stinging capacity of topically applied substances. *J. Soc. Cosmet. Chem.,* 28, 197–209, 1977.
50. DeGroot, A. C., Nater, J. P., Lende, R., Rijcken, B., Adverse effects of cosmetics and toiletries: a retrospective study in the general population. *Int. J. Dermatol. Sci.,* 9, 255–259, 1988.
51. Potts, R. O., Francoeur, M. L., The influence of stratum corneum morphology on water permeability. *J. Invest. Dermatol.,* 96, 495–499, 1991.

21 Petrolatum

David S. Morrison

CONTENTS

21.1 INTRODUCTION

"The secret to younger-looking skin!" "The best moisturizer there is!" These statements are often heard when consumers talk about various cosmetic products, but it is surprising that this high praise also refers to the very common and not-so-elegant material known as petroleum jelly, or petrolatum. So, what exactly is this decades-old ingredient which elicits such comments from people?

Petrolatum is a purified material consisting of a complex combination of hydrocarbons with an ointment-like consistency and is derived from petroleum (crude oil). Based on its origin, it would seem that the properties of petrolatum would vary dramatically depending on the type of crude oil used. However, since different types of crude oils have widely differing properties (depending on the source of the oil), only certain waxy crudes are suitable for the manufacture of petrolatum.

Petrolatum has been used as a skin care product since its discovery by Robert A. Chesebrough in 1872.[1] In his patent, Chesebrough stated that this material is useful as a chapped hand treatment. At that time, one of the main benefits of petrolatum was that it did not become rancid (oxidize) as did the commonly used fats of that day. While the refining (and thus purity) of petrolatum has been improved over time, its form remains essentially unchanged from the original. Not long after Chesebrough's discovery, the moisturizing benefits of petrolatum were more widely recognized, primarily in terms of its medical applications.[2]

These days, the many benefits of petrolatum (petroleum jelly) are still being touted in the media around the globe, mainly for the treatment of dry, chapped skin.[3-6] In addition, petrolatum has been cited as useful for adding shine to the lips,[3] cheeks,[3] and eyelids;[7] moisturizing the feet;[8] conditioning eyelashes;[9] stopping cuts from bleeding;[4] as a makeup remover;[4] and as a facial moisturizer.[10] Presumably because of petrolatum's newly recognized properties as a skin treatment product, it was included in the 1880 edition of the *U.S. Pharmacopoeia*[2] and is still listed today. In the modern-day Pharmacopoeia, there are actually two listings for this material, "Petrolatum" and "White Petrolatum," with the differences being the colors and ignition residues of the two products.

0-8493-7520-7/00/$0.00+$.50

21.2 SKIN MOISTURIZATION BY PETROLATUM ALONE

Petrolatum's skin moisturization properties are clearly due to its occlusivity.[11] The petrolatum blocks the evaporation of water from the skin (transepidermal water loss, TEWL), thus keeping the stratum corneum well hydrated.[12] It should be noted that the term "moisturization" is commonly used to describe the action of occlusive agents on skin, even though water is not actually added to the skin.

The lack of oxidation of petrolatum is due to the nature of the hydrocarbon molecules which are present in this substance. During the oil refining process, the hydrocarbon material is hydrogenated (saturated) to create oxidation-resistant molecules throughout, from the liquid oil to the solid waxes. This property enables pure petroleum jelly to be marketed with the benefit of a long shelf life. The lack of rancidity also gave early cosmetic formulators a new ingredient which could be processed with little regard to possible degradation.

As technology progressed over the years, scientific techniques were developed to quantify the ability of various ingredients to "moisturize" the skin. Cutaneous impedance is one method which has been used to determine how well certain products moisturize the skin, with a decrease in impedance typically indicating an increase in skin hydration. Interestingly, measurements made after application of petrolatum show an initial *increase* in impedance, due to the resistance of petrolatum, and thus its occlusivity, rather than being due to dehydration of the skin.[13] Results from a later study by Lodén and Lindberg[14] revealed the drawbacks associated with electrical skin measurements. It was noted that this method should not be solely relied upon to determine skin moisture content; thus, other methods also should be used to verify (and possibly support) the findings of skin moisturization studies. Recently, skin capacitance values have been compared with skin hydration as determined by ultrasonography (echographic image analysis).[15]

The moisturizing ability of petrolatum also has been determined with a spectroscopic technique for evaluating skin hydration, opto-thermal transient radiometry (OTTER).[16] These authors reported that the hydration level of *in vivo* skin increased from 45% (initially) to approximately 80% at 2 h after application of petroleum jelly.

One of the most popular and commonly used methods for determining the effectiveness of skin moisturizers is by grading the xerosis on the lower legs of panelists with both visual and tactile assessments.[17,18] Using this method, Kligman determined that petrolatum was an extremely effective moisturizer.[18]

Another very practical and useful method for evaluating skin moisturizers is by the direct measurement of TEWL on human skin.[19] Not surprisingly, several studies which incorporate this test method have proven that petrolatum is an excellent moisturizer.[20-22] It should be noted that in many studies on TEWL, petrolatum is used as a positive standard when evaluating other cosmetic emollients, since petrolatum is nearly always the most occlusive TEWL barrier material tested. It is often the standard by which other ingredients and formulations are judged.

In a recent study on gelled mineral oils by our laboratory, petrolatum was evaluated in a clinical TEWL study and compared to light mineral oil and a gelled light mineral oil.[23] The study panel consisted of 15 subjects who had extremely dry skin (baseline TEWL > 7.0 $g/m^2/h$). Application of the test materials occurred three times (at 1-h intervals) to the volar surface of the subjects' forearms, with TEWL measurements taken 1 h after each application. The results (Figure 1) clearly indicate that the improvement in TEWL by petrolatum is superior to that of both the light mineral oil and the gelled light mineral oil, with petrolatum reducing TEWL by an average of 33% over 3 h.

Similar studies of moisture transport across a barrier also have been done using *in vitro* methods, which determine the movement of water vapor across a film which has been coated with a measured amount of the material to be tested. These are rapid methods for rough determinations of occlusivity and work very well for screening several ingredients at a reasonable cost. Once again, petrolatum's occlusivity has been shown in tests of this nature.[24,25]

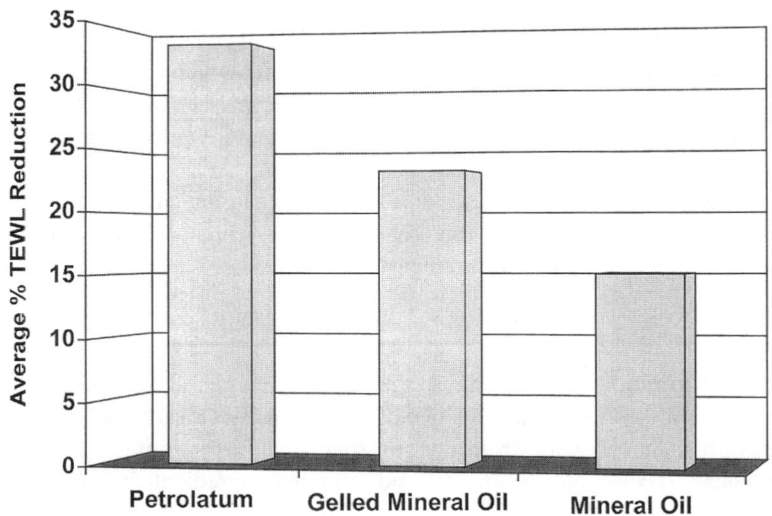

FIGURE 1 The average percent reduction in TEWL compared to untreated skin (over 3 h) for some hydrocarbon ingredients.[23]

21.3 SKIN MOISTURIZATION — PETROLATUM IN COSMETIC COMPOSITIONS

The use of petrolatum in cosmetic compositions is evident simply by looking at the ingredient listings on commercially available skin creams and lotions. While new ingredients which are beneficial to skin are always being discovered and incorporated into skin care products, petrolatum seems to be a material which never falls out of favor.

Most investigations on skin moisturization evaluate petrolatum alone. The moisturizing efficacy of a petrolatum-containing cream was reported by Prall and co-workers in one study and compared to two other creams, one containing urea and one containing alpha-hydroxy acids.[26] In both cases, the petrolatum-containing product was found to be comparable to the other formulations as judged by skin dryness.

Numerous patents have been issued over the years for topical cosmetic products which contain petrolatum. Of course, the owners of a patent wish to protect as many ingredients in a formulation as possible, and when hydrocarbons are suitable ingredients, petrolatum is invariably one of the ingredients covered by the patent. In no way does this diminish the importance of petrolatum as an ingredient (whether it is a preferred ingredient or not); rather, it supports the frequent use of petrolatum as a skin care ingredient for cosmetic formulations and recognizes its application in many different types of cosmetic compositions. Examples of recent patents include a diaper rash treatment for patients of all ages which can incorporate petrolatum as the composition's base,[27] an improved ointment base which utilizes a high molecular weight petrolatum fraction for skin moisturization and other applications,[28] and a moisturizing bar soap with petrolatum as a key ingredient.[29] Petrolatum also has been claimed in skin care products designed to reduce wrinkles,[30,31] in products for moisturization and skin conditioning,[32-36] and as a base for dispersing other skin care ingredients.[37,38]

21.4 SKIN MOISTURIZATION — PETROLATUM IN DERMATOLOGICAL APPLICATIONS

Despite the effectiveness of petrolatum at moisturizing dry skin, some critics would charge that petrolatum should not be used on skin and certainly not recommended by medical doctors for their patients. It is purported that petrolatum is comedogenic ("clogs the pores"), as evidenced by its greasy, ointment-like consistency. However, petrolatum actually is noncomedogenic,[39-41] which is unrelated to its physical properties.[42] In fact, some ingredients which are drier feeling on the skin and less greasy than petrolatum are actually highly comedogenic when tested neat.[39,40] Nevertheless, these products are likely used as ingredients (at low concentrations) in various formulations which are then determined to be noncomedogenic.

Petrolatum continues to be used quite extensively in dermatological applications, primarily for three purposes: (1) as an inert patch testing base, (2) as a vehicle in the dermal application of pharmaceuticals, and (3) as a treatment product itself.

21.4.1 Patch Testing

Petrolatum's lack of irritation[43] explains its frequent use as a suitable vehicle for patch testing of contact allergens[44,45] and irritants. Since this material is unreactive, various substances can be tested with no concern about interference from the substrate. It is a traditional patch testing base for anhydrous materials, especially for fragrances and fragrance ingredients.[46] Advantages include the uniform suspension of powders in petrolatum, the holding of test material in place very well, the lack of evaporation, and good solubility properties. Tests for photoallergy, phototoxicity, irritation, allergic reaction (repeat insult patch test), and diagnostic testing for allergic contact dermatitis are some of the types of studies which frequently use petrolatum as the test vehicle. Petrolatum also has been compared with an aqueous system when evaluating a water-soluble allergen.[47]

21.4.2 Drug Delivery

Petrolatum can be used in the delivery of pharmaceuticals to the skin. While petrolatum itself does not penetrate below the stratum corneum, its ability to solubilize lipophilic materials and suspend hydrophilic solids has made it a commonly used transdermal drug delivery vehicle. Liposomal formulations incorporating petrolatum also have been studied as part of topical drug delivery systems.[48]

21.4.3 Treatment Products

Probably the most widely reported information concerning petrolatum's effect on damaged skin was a 1992 article by Ghadially and co-workers.[49] Newspapers across the U.S. reported the results of this study which showed that, when applied to skin which had been damaged by acetone, petrolatum accelerated the recovery of the skin's normal barrier properties. It was noted that this is in contrast to materials which are highly impermeable to water vapor (such as polyethylene films) which hinder barrier repair. However, another publication has indicated that the repair of the permeability barrier in human skin is *not* delayed by occlusion.[50]

Although the permeability barrier can be repaired to a presumably greater extent using a complete mixture of physiologic lipids, petrolatum, which remains restricted to the stratum corneum, provides a more rapid barrier repair. This delay in barrier repair when using the physiologic lipids has been attributed to the time necessary for lipid uptake and processing by the skin.[51] Recently, a petrolatum-based cream gave positive results when used for the treatment of hand dermatitis.[52]

In addition to the repair of the epidermal barrier, petrolatum has been used in other types of dermatological treatments. It has been reported that a petrolatum-based ointment provides favorable treatment for premature infants: bacterial colonization of the treated skin was decreased, and the frequency of dermatitis was reduced.[53] In another article, petrolatum was shown to inhibit tumorigenesis in skin irradiated with UVB light, and petroleum jelly even reduced tumor yield when applied after irradiation.[54] Other uses include postlaser skin resurfacing treatment;[55] application to burns, cuts, and abrasions;[56] and use as a wound care ointment.[57,58] In one study, the use of white petrolatum in postsurgery wound care showed an infection rate similar to patients who used bacitracin ointment, thus prompting the authors to refer to petrolatum as "an effective, safe wound care ointment."[58] These authors also estimated the dramatic cost savings which would be realized by switching from antibacterial ointments to white petrolatum. Finally, petrolatum has been cited as major ingredients in patents which describe products for topical skin treatment.[59,60]

21.5 SKIN MOISTURIZATION — PETROLATUM IN PAPER PRODUCTS

During the past several years, the market has seen "new and improved" facial tissue products which are softer than the standard facial tissue or which contain lotion to "soothe sore noses" and the surrounding skin. Constant wiping with a facial tissue can irritate the skin, so a product containing emollients is likely to reduce irritation. Petrolatum may be used as an inexpensive, yet effective emollient in tissue products of these types.

Diapers are another type of paper product which benefits from the addition of emollients such as petrolatum. Not only can petrolatum reduce the adherence of bodily waste to the skin, it also provides emolliency.[61]

21.6 CONCLUSION

It is clear that petrolatum is widely used as a classic skin moisturizer.[62] Its uses range from cosmetic skin care products to dermatological treatments to patch test substrates to tissue paper emollients. As long as people require soft, supple, moisturized skin, petrolatum will be a key ingredient in meeting that requirement.

REFERENCES

1. Chesebrough, R. A., Improvement in Products from Petroleum, U.S. Patent 127,568, June 4, 1872.
2. Schindler, H., Petrolatum for drugs and cosmetics, *Drug Cosmet. Ind.*, 89, 36, 1961.
3. Cohen, J., *Telegraph Magazine*, September 19, 1998, p. 120.
4. Nelson, J., *Washington Post Magazine*, January 11, 1987, p. w27.
5. Petroleum Jelly Still a Trusty Moisturizer, *Daily News of Los Angeles*, January 23, 1989, p. L10.
6. Skin-Care Secret: Petroleum Jelly, *Chicago Tribune*, January 9, 1991, Style Section, p. 4.
7. Rourke, M., *Los Angeles Times*, May 21, 1993, View Section, p. 1.
8. Fox, M., *New Woman*, May 1995, p. 112.
9. PR Newswire, August 27, 1985 (*Harper's Bazaar*).
10. Shannon, S., *Woman's Day*, July 18, 1989, p. 42.
11. Lazar, A. P., Lazar, P., Dry skin, water, and lubrication, *Dermatol. Clin.*, 9, 45, 1991.
12. Rieger, M., Skin care: new concepts vs. established practices, *Cosmet. Toiletries*, 106, 55, 1991.
13. Wepierre, J., Study of the hydrating effect of cosmetic preparations by measuring cutaneous impedance in the hairless rat, *Soap Perfum. Cosmet.*, 50, 506, 1977.
14. Lodén, M., Lindberg, M., The influence of a single application of different moisturizers on the skin capacitance, *Acta Derm. Venereol. (Stockh.)*, 71, 79, 1991.
15. Pellacani, G., Belletti, B., Seidenari, S., Evaluation of the short-term effects of skin care products: a comparison between capacitance values and echographic parameters of epidermal hydration, in *Skin Bioengineering Techniques and Applications in Dermatology and Cosmetology*, 26, Elsner, P., Barel, A. O., Berardesca, E., Gabard, B., Serup, J., Eds., Karger, Basel, 1998, 177.
16. Bindra, R. M. S., Imhof, R. E., Andrew, J. J., Cummins, P. G., Eccleston, G. M., Opto-thermal measurements for the non-invasive, non-occlusive monitoring of *in vivo* skin condition, *Int. J. Cosmet. Sci.*, 17, 105, 1995.
17. Grove, G. L., Noninvasive methods for assessing moisturizers, in *Clinical Safety and Efficacy Testing of Cosmetics*, Waggoner, W. C., Ed., Marcel Dekker, New York, 1990, chap. 7.

18. Kligman, A. M., Regression method for assessing the efficacy of moisturizers, *Cosmet. Toiletries*, 93, 27, 1978.
19. Morrison, Jr., B. M., ServoMed evaporimeter: precautions when evaluating the effect of skin care products on barrier function, *J. Soc. Cosmet. Chem.*, 43, 161, 1992. (The frequently used ServoMed EP1 evaporimeter also has its drawbacks when used to measure TEWL.)
20. Tsutsumi, H., Utsugi, T., Hayashi, S., Study on the occlusivity of oil films, *J. Soc. Cosmet. Chem.*, 30, 345, 1979.
21. Lodén, M., The increase in skin hydration after application of emollients with different amounts of lipids, *Acta Derm. Venereol. (Stockh.)*, 72, 327, 1992.
22. Frömder, A., Lippold, B. C., Water vapour transmission and occlusivity *in vivo* of lipophilic excipients used in ointments, *Int. J. Cosmet. Sci.*, 15, 113, 1993.
23. Morrison, D. S., The effects of petrolatum, mineral oil and other hydrocarbons on the stratum corneum, *Cosmet. Dermatol., Suppl.*, p. 26, November 1997.
24. Tranner, F., Berube, G., Mineral oil and petrolatum: reliable moisturizers, *Cosmet. Toiletries*, 93, 81, 1978.
25. Obata, M., Tagami, H., A rapid *in vitro* test to assess skin moisturizers, *J. Soc. Cosmet. Chem.*, 41, 235, 1990.
26. Prall, J. K., Theiler, R. F., Bowser, P. A., Walsh, M., The effectiveness of cosmetic products in alleviating a range of skin dryness conditions as determined by clinical and instrumental techniques, *Int. J. Cosmet. Sci.*, 8, 159, 1986.
27. Pichierri, V., Diaper Rash Treatment, U.S. Patent 5,194,261, March 16, 1993.
28. Gans, E. H., Süess, H. R., Ointment Base and Method of Use, U.S. Patent 5,336,692, August 9, 1994.
29. Schuler, W. H., Moisturizing Soap Bar, U.S. Patent 5,547,602, August 20, 1996.
30. Barker, D. E., Human Skin Cleansing and Wrinkle-Reducing Cream, U.S. Patent 5,360,824, November 1, 1994.
31. Blank, R. L., Use of Salicylic Acid for Regulating Skin Wrinkles and/or Skin Atrophy, U.S. Patent 5,780,456, July 14, 1998.
32. Rentsch, S. F., Non-Greasy Petrolatum Emulsion, U.S. Patent 5,387,417, February 7, 1995.
33. Znaiden, A. P., Rose, W., Cheney, M. C., Petroleum Butter, U.S. Patent 5,595,745, January 21, 1997.
34. Fishman, Y., Skin Lotion Composition and Softgel Filled Therewith and Methods for Making and Using Same, U.S. Patent 5,824,323, October 20, 1998.
35. Scott, I. R., Cosmetic Composition, European Patent 0 342 056 B1, August 17, 1994.
36. Geria, N. M., Skin Moisturizing Composition and Method of Preparing Same, European Patent 0 336 899 B1, March 30, 1994.
37. Znaiden, A. P., Cheney, M. C., Rose, W., Petroleum Jelly with Alpha Hydroxy Carboxylic Acids, U.S. Patent 5,552,147, September 3, 1996.
38. Znaiden, A. P., Crotty, B., Johnson, A., Petroleum Jelly with Inositol Phosphates, U.S. Patent 5,552,148, September 3, 1996.
39. Lanzet, M., Comedogenic effects of cosmetic raw materials, *Cosmet. Toiletries*, 101, 63, 1986.
40. Fulton, Jr., J. E., Pay, S. R., Fulton, III, J. E., Comedogenicity of current therapeutic products, cosmetics, and ingredients in the rabbit ear, *J. Am. Acad. Dermatol.*, 10, 96, 1984.
41. Kligman, A. M., Petrolatum is not comedogenic in rabbits or humans: a critical reappraisal of the rabbit ear assay and the concept of "acne cosmetica," *J. Soc. Cosmet. Chem.*, 47, 41, 1996.
42. American Academy of Dermatology Invitational Symposium on Comedogenicity, *J. Am. Acad. Dermatol.*, 20, 272, 1989.
43. Motoyoshi, K., Toyoshima, Y., Sata, M., Yoshimura, M., Comparative studies on the irritancy of oils and synthetic perfumes to the skin of rabbit, guinea pig, rat, miniature swine and man, *Cosmet. Toiletries*, 94, 41, 1979.
44. Heikkilä, H., Stubb, S., Reitamo, S., A study of 72 patients with contact allergy to tioconazole, *Br. J. Dermatol.*, 134, 678, 1996.
45. Johansen, J. D., Andersen, K. E., Rastogi, S. C., Menné, T., Threshold responses in cinnamic-aldehyde-sensitive subjects: results and methodological aspects, *Contact Dermatitis*, 34, 165, 1996.
46. Stephens, T. J., Personal communication, 1999.
47. Gammelgaard, B., Fullerton, A., Avnstorp, C., Menné, T., *In vitro* evaluation of water and petrolatum as vehicles in chromate patch testing, *Contact Dermatitis*, 27, 317, 1992.

48. Foldvari, M., Effect of vehicle on topical liposomal drug delivery: petrolatum bases, *J. Microencapsulation*, 13, 589, 1996.
49. Ghadially, R., Halkier-Sorensen, L., Elias, P. M., Effects of petrolatum on stratum corneum structure and function, *J. Am. Acad. Dermatol.*, 26, 387, 1992.
50. Welzel, J., Wilhelm, K. P., Wolff, H. H., Skin permeability barrier and occlusion: no delay of repair in irritated human skin, *Contact Dermatitis*, 35, 163, 1996.
51. Mao-Qiang, M., Brown, B. E., Wu-Pong, S., Feingold, K. R., Elias, P. M., Exogenous nonphysiologic vs. physiologic lipids, *Arch. Dermatol.*, 131, 809, 1995.
52. Schleicher, S. M., Milstein, H. J., Ilowite, R., Meyer, P., Response of hand dermatitis to a new skin barrier-protectant cream, *Cutis*, 61, 233, 1998.
53. Nopper, A. J., Horii, K. A., Sookdeo-Drost, S., Wang, T. H., Mancini, A. J., Lane, A. T., Topical ointment therapy benefits premature infants, *J. Pediatr.*, 128, 660, 1996.
54. Kligman, L. H., Kligman, A. M., Petrolatum and other hydrophobic emollients reduce UVB-induced damage, *J. Dermatol. Treatment*, 3, 3, 1992.
55. McDaniel, D. H., Ash, K., Lord, J., Newman, J., Zukowski, M., Accelerated laser resurfacing wound healing using a triad of topical antioxidants, *Dermatol. Surg.*, 24, 661, 1998.
56. Kligman, A. M., Why cosmeceuticals?, *Cosmet. Toiletries*, 108, 37, 1993.
57. Phan, M., Van der Auwera, P., Andry, G., Aoun, M., Chantrain, G., Deraemaecker, R., Dor, P., Daneau, D., Ewalenko, P., Meunier, F., Wound dressing in major head and neck cancer surgery: a prospective randomized study of gauze dressing vs. sterile vaseline ointment, *Eur. J. Surg. Oncol.*, 19, 10, 1993.
58. Smack, D. P., Harrington, A. C., Dunn, C., Howard, R. S., Szkutnik, A. J., Krivda, S. J., Caldwell, J. B., James, W. D., Infection and allergy incidence in ambulatory surgery patients using white petrolatum vs. bacitracin ointment, *J. Am. Med. Assoc.*, 276, 972, 1996.
59. Flender, G., Topical Ointment, U.S. Patent 5,179,086, January 12, 1993.
60. Shin, J. S., Medicament for the Topical Treatment of Skin, U.S. Patent 5,330,980, July 19, 1994.
61. Roe, D. C., Bakes, F. H., Warner A. V., Diaper Having a Lotioned Topsheet, U.S. Patent 5,643,588, July 1, 1997.
62. Morrison, D. S., Petrolatum: a useful classic, *Cosmet. Toiletries*, 111, 59, 1996.

22 Lanolins

Ian Harris and Udo Hoppe

CONTENTS

22.1 INTRODUCTION

Lanolin has been used by man as a skin emollient for thousands of years.[1] Lanolin (from the Latin *lana* for wool and *oleum* for oil) is another name for wool wax, which is secreted by the sebaceous glands of the sheep (*ovis aries*) to soften the fleece and protect it against the elements. Lanolin was used by the ancient Greeks (*circa* 700 B.C.), and a method of recovering lanolin from wool washings was described by the Greek physician Dioscorides (60 A.D.) in his *De materia medica*.[2]

Lanolin and its numerous derivatives have been widely used in the pharmaceutical and cosmetic industries for many years as vehicles for active ingredients and for their beneficial effects on skin function.[3] Although purified lanolin is used without incident by millions of people, confusion still exists concerning the possible allergenic potential of lanolin. The extremely low incidence of sensitization of healthy individuals to purified lanolin used in the cosmetic and pharmaceutical industries has been comprehensively reviewed.[4-6]

22.2 PURIFICATION OF LANOLIN (WOOL WAX)

Lanolin is a very complex mixture of esters, diesters, and hydroxy esters of high molecular weight lanolin alcohols and lanolin acids. Being a complex natural product, the method of refinement for lanolin is very important, as this determines the composition, properties, and quality of the purified lanolin.[1,7,8] It is necessary, therefore, to bear in mind that not all refined lanolins are the same. The incredibly complex composition of lanolin also means that it cannot be synthesized.[1]

Wool wax, unlike human sebum, contains no triglycerides and is chemically a wax rather than a fat.[8,9] The wool wax of newborn lambs is thought to consist almost entirely of esters which are very pale in color. These esters are hydrolyzed in the alkaline secretions by bacteria and the environment. The products can undergo further oxidation and degradation. The yield and composition of the secreted wool wax depend on physiological and environmental factors, such as the age of the sheep, the time of year, the use of pesticides, and the presence of airborne pollutants.[1,7] Therefore, some producers of lanolin use raw material from countries such as New Zealand, which have strict laws on the use of pesticides and which are relatively free from industrial pollution. The crude lanolin is also blended to overcome the problem of variability.

0-8493-7520-7/00/$0.00+$.50

The ancient Greeks (*circa* 700 B.C.) extracted lanolin by boiling the fleece in water. Methods of recovering and refining have been improved to remove dirt, detergents, and other unwanted contaminants.[10] The degradation products of wool wax esters such as oxidized material are undesirable and are the source of color and free acidity. The oxidized material is more polar and more readily emulsifies in the wool washings. As a result the degradation products remain in the aqueous phase and can be removed by centrifuging.[11,12] This process is relatively inefficient, with yields of less than 50%. However, the quality is superior to the older method of acid cracking. The resultant product is refined, and the remaining water and associated detergents are removed to produce anhydrous lanolin.[1]

22.3 COMPOSITION OF LANOLIN

The purity of lanolin and standard tests have been described in the *European Pharmacopoeia* (EP), in *The United States Pharmacopoeia* (USP), and according to other national standards.[13,14] Lanolin is a semisolid with a melting point of approximately 40 ± 6°C and has a molecular weight in the range of 790 to 880 Da. Lanolin is a complex and variable mixture of mainly esters diesters, hydroxy esters (87.0 to 93.5%, w/w),[7,8,15] lanolin alcohols (6.0 to 12.5%, w/w), lanolin acids (< 0.5%, w/w), and lanolin hydrocarbons (<1.0%, w/w). The latter are also called "paraffins" and "petrolatum" by the EP and USP, respectively.[13,14,16-18] Approximately 40% of the esters are α-hydroxy esters. Due to the extremely complex nature of lanolin, the true number of different esters present is unknown. Barnett calculated the theoretical number of monoester combinations from random combinations of 69 aliphatic lanolin alcohols, 6 sterols, and 138 saturated lanolin acids to total 10,350.[8] This is most probably an underestimate of the total number of esters, as dibasic acids and dihydric alcohols also occur naturally in lanolin.[19] Further combinations of cyclic mono- and diesters may be formed by dehydration and from inter- and intra-esterification due to heating during the manufacturing process.[7,8]

The analysis of lanolin has concentrated on the lanolin alcohols (the unsaponifiable fraction of lanolin) and lanolin acids produced by hydrolysis rather than the esters in lanolin itself.[20] Lanolin alcohols belong to three major groups: (1) 69 aliphatic alcohols from C_{12} to C_{36}, (2) sterols (cholesterol and dihydrocholesterol), and (3) trimethyl sterols (lanesterol, dihydrolanesterol, agnosterol, and dihydroagenosterol).[21] The latter have been incorrectly termed triterpenoids. The relative proportion of each group is 22% (w/w) aliphatic alcohols, 35% (w/w) sterols, and 38% (w/w) trimethyl sterols.[8]

The nature of the substance that is responsible for sensitization to lanolin is not clear, but it has a high affinity for the natural free alcohols.[1] Clark has proposed that the incidence of adverse reactions can be virtually eliminated by reducing the level of lanolin alcohols to no more than 3% (w/w).[1] Alternatively, the lanolin alcohols can be intensively purified to eliminate traces of the compounds which may cause sensitization.[22]

The reported number of lanolin acids (C_7 to C_{41}) varies dramatically from 32 to 138.[17,18,21,23-26] The possible explanation for this discrepancy is that different methods were used to produce the alcohols.[8] The lanolin acids comprise four major classes: normal, iso (ω-1-methyl substituted), anteiso (ω-2-methyl substituted), and α- and ω-hydroxy acids. The relative proportions are 12.1% normal acids, 22.1% iso acids, 26.3% anteiso, 27.1% α-hydroxy acids, and 5.1% ω-hydroxy acids.[27,28] Minor constituents include polyhydroxy acids (4.7%) and unsaturated acids (2.1%).[23-25]

22.4 COMPARISON OF LANOLIN TO SEBUM AND STRATUM CORNEUM LIPIDS

Although lanolin and human sebum are both products of sebaceous glands, their compositions are very different.[9] Lanolin contains sterol esters, unlike human sebum, which contains mainly triglycerides, and squalene, which is a precursor of cholesterol.

Cholesterol is a major component of the alcoholic fraction of lanolin.[15] It is also an essential constituent of the lipids of the stratum corneum which form the epidermal permeability barrier.[29,30] However, the other stratum corneum lipids (ceramides and fatty acids) are different from those of lanolin. Clark and Steel have suggested that the α-, β-, and ω-hydroxy lanolin acids are esterified with diols to form diesters with two long acyl chains which are similar to those found in ceramides.[16,31,32]

Stratum corneum lipids and lanolin share an important physical characteristic in that they can coexist as solids and liquids at physiological temperatures.[33] A differential scanning calorimetry thermogram of lanolin is similar to that of stratum corneum lipids, showing two broad (heterogenous) phase transitions with midpoint melting temperatures at 21.9 and 38.3°C.[16] The lower temperature peak may represent the transition from a liquid crystal to a gel phase, which has also been described for lanolin alcohols.[34]

22.5 LANOLIN AS A MOISTURIZER

Apart from being a lubricant which reduces friction and roughness, lanolin is an effective moisturizer. That is, when lanolin is applied to dry or inflexible stratum corneum it becomes hydrated and more supple, overcoming the signs and symptoms of dry skin.[35]

Kligman demonstrated that hydrous lanolin, like petrolatum, was able to improve mild to moderate winter xerosis in ten white, young-adult females using a visual scoring system in a double-blind study.[35] A twice daily application to the lower leg produced a successive improvement in the xerosis over a 21-d period. Application of lanolin four times daily was also demonstrated to be superior to twice daily applications. The water in the hydrous lanolin is unlikely to be responsible for the moisturizing as repeated immersion of dry legs in water for 5 minutes, 6 times a day, for 2 weeks had no effect in relieving xerosis.[35] The beneficial effects of lanolin and petrolatum are not due to the greasy nature of the substances as neither mineral oil, olive oil, nor goose grease had significant moisturizing effects.[35]

Powers and Fox demonstrated that lanolin is semi-occlusive and can reduce TEWL.[36] The application of lanolin and lanolin oil (5.0 to 6.25 mg/cm^2, equivalent to a film thickness of 54 to 68 μm) to the inner surface of the forearm reduced the TEWL by 32 and 22%, respectively.[36] This is in comparison with petrolatum which reduced the TEWL by 48%. Spruits reported a 20 to 30% reduction in TEWL using a 50-μm lanolin film.[37] The clinical improvement in xerotic skin is not simply due to a transient reduction in TEWL, because a completely impermeable plastic film applied twice a day had no beneficial effects.

Lanolin appears to penetrate into the stratum corneum, but remains in the more superficial layers.[38,39] Using the tape stripping technique, Clark demonstrated the penetration of anhydrous lanolin (2 mg/cm^2) applied to the flexor aspect of the inner forearm.[40] Almost all of the applied lanolin was recovered and most was removed in the first 15 strippings. Although the bulk of lanolin may remain in the superficial layers, electron-dense lead linoleate and lead oleate topically applied in lanolin were observed by transmission electron microscopy to be localized in intracellular spaces as far down as the stratum granulosum.[40]

Anhydrous lanolin appears to trap some of the water which is moving through the stratum corneum and spontaneously forms emulsions when placed on the skin for only 5 min.[16,31] Cryo-SEM of skin samples following application of lanolin shows vesicles ranging from 0.5 to 300 nm in diameter, which are presumably water droplets that have passed through the skin, subsequently forming a water-in-oil emulsion.[16,31,32]

Many moisturizers can provide instant relief from xerosis, although the effects are short lived.[35] Lanolin and petrolatum can be distinguished from other moisturizers in that their effects are long lived. After application of lanolin or petrolatum for 21 d, the time taken to regress from the improved state back to the original state was 14 and 21 d, respectively.[35] The time taken for lanolin and petrolatum to improve xerotic skin and then, when application is stopped, to regress is approximately equivalent to the turnover time of the stratum corneum. This implies that lanolin and petrolatum

TABLE 1
Effect of Topically Applied Substances on Barrier Recovery

Treatment	n	TEWL (%) 45 min	TEWL (%) 4 h
Vehicle	10	106.9 ± 5.2	69.6 ± 5.5
Stratum corneum lipids (optimal molar ratio)	10	81.7 ± 5.4[a]	44.5 ± 5.3[a]
3% Lanolin	20	81.3 ± 4.1[a]	45.4 ± 3.1[a]
15% Lanolin	10	—	21.7 ± 1.7[a]
2% Petrolatum	10	—	51.7 ± 3.6[a]
10% Petrolatum	9	58.2 ± 10.5[a]	—

Note: TEWL measurements were taken following acetone perturbation of the stratum corneum of hairless mice and following application of substances in a propylene glycol-ethanol vehicle. The initial transepidermal water loss is 100%.

[a] Statistically significant relative to vehicle (p <0.001).

Source: Adapted from Elias, P. et al., The epidermal permeability barrier: effects of physiologic and non-physiological lipids, in *The Lanolin Book,* Beiersdorf AG, Hamburg, 1999. With permission.

may affect not only the anucleated horny layer, but may also change the physiology of the nucleated layers of the epidermis.[35]

In addition to restoring the clinical appearance of xerotic skin, lanolin can also accelerate the restoration of normal barrier function to normal skin that has been acutely perturbed. Elias and colleagues have demonstrated that lanolin accelerated epidermal barrier recovery following perturbation with acetone.[41] Three percent lanolin not only significantly (p <0.001) decreased the TEWL at 45 min, but also after 4 h compared to vehicle-treated sites (Table 1). However, the rate of barrier recovery of lanolin-treated sites between 45 min and 4 h was not significantly different compared to vehicle treatment. This indicates that lanolin has an immediate effect on restoring a permeability barrier and does not interfere with the process of lamellar body extrusion and lipid synthesis, which are required for continued recovery. The effect of 3% lanolin on barrier recovery was very similar to that of the optimized ratio of stratum corneum lipids (ceramides, cholesterol, and fatty acids).[42,43]

Other physical methods of assessment of the stratum corneum, such as corneometry and microprofilametry, demonstrate a statistically significant effect of lanolin.[16] The parameters of skin roughness, Rz and Ra, determined by microprofilametry, can be reduced by 2 mg/cm^2 lanolin alcohol or lanolin for at least 8 h after application. [16]

Lanolin and lanolin alcohols are more commonly used in a more complex formulation which provides a cream or lotion of a more acceptable consistency. Figure 1 shows that increasing levels of lanolin alcohol in a water-in-oil cream progressively decreased the roughness of xerotic skin in 24 elderly volunteers over a 14-d period, in a dose-dependent manner.[44] Lanolin alcohols also reduced the TEWL of the same volunteers over a 28-d period (Figure 2).[44] Petersen demonstrated that the hydration of stratum corneum was higher after application of a cream containing lanolin (oil-in-water formulation) than after application of petrolatum, using optothermal infrared spectrometry.[45] By measuring electrical conductance, Moss demonstrated that preparations containing lanolin increased the surface hydration.[46] Lanolin can also act as a barrier to the entry of virus particles and irritants into the skin.[44,47]

Lanolin does not have a detrimental effect on epidermal homeostasis of clinically normal skin or healing of wounds. In contrast to oils, such as olive oil and mineral oil, lanolin does not have adverse effects on the homeostasis of normal epidermis.[48] Butcher found that repeated application

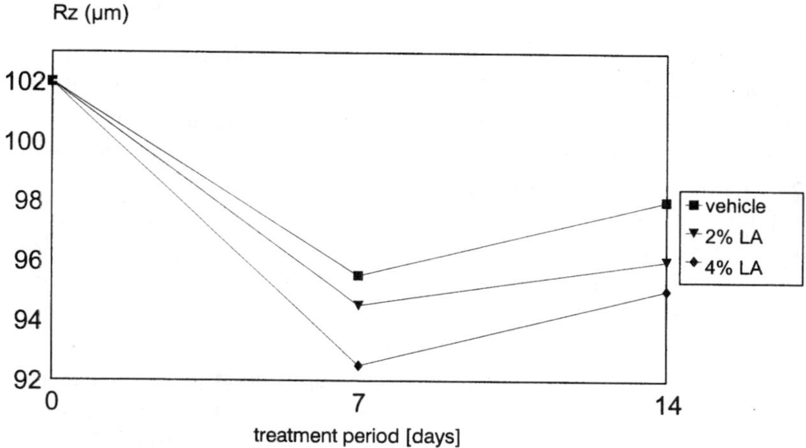

FIGURE 1 Lanolin alcohol (Eucerit®, Beiersdorf AG, Hamburg, Germany) reduces skin roughness, as measured by microprofilometry. Lanolin alcohol (2 and 4%, w/w; LA) in a water-in-oil cream containing petrolatum was applied twice daily to the volar aspect of the arm. (Adapted from Sauermann, G., Schreiner, V., The skin caring effects of topical products containing lanolin alcohols, *The Lanolin Book,* Beiersdorf AG, Hamburg, 1999. With permission.)

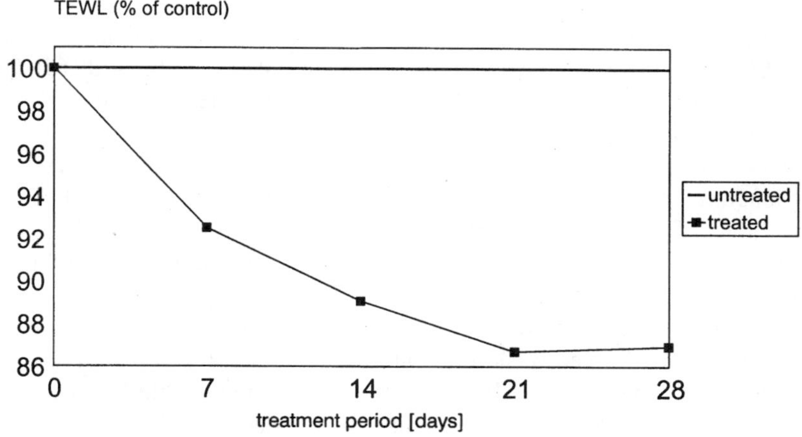

FIGURE 2 Lanolin alcohol (Eucerit) reduces TEWL over time. Lanolin alcohol in a water-in-oil cream containing petrolatum (Nivea®, Beiersdorf, AG, Hamburg, Germany) was applied twice daily to dry skin of the lower leg of 24 elderly volunteers relative to the untreated control site. TEWL was measured under controlled conditions 14 h after application of the cream using an evaporimeter. (Adapted from, Sauermann, G., Schreiner, V., The skin caring effects of topical products containing lanolin alcohols, *The Lanolin Book,* Beiersdorf AG, Hamburg, 1999. With permission.)

of olive oil and mineral oil resulted in acanthosis and parakeratosis, which is abnormal proliferation and differentiation.[48]

Chvapil et al. investigated the effects of epidermal growth factor (EGF) in a lanolin vehicle on partial thickness wounds.[49] A beneficial effect of lanolin vehicle was observed with little additional benefit from EGF. Lanolin statistically increased the rate of reepithelialization, the thickness of the dermis, and the number of cells in the dermis. Lanolin is likely to promote wound healing by maintaining a moist environment.[50,51]

22.6 LANOLIN AS AN EMULSIFIER AND A VEHICLE FOR DRUG DELIVERY

Lanolin and lanolin alcohols are excellent emulsifiers, giving oil-in-water emulsions, and can be combined with additional emulsifiers such as cetearyl alcohol to improve stability.[8] The ability of anhydrous lanolin and especially lanolin alcohols to form stable emulsions with up to 300% (w/w) of water distinguishes lanolin from petrolatum in its physical properties.[1] The chemical compositions of lanolin and petrolatum are also very different, as petrolatum is composed completely of hydrocarbons.[16] Lanolin alcohols and petrolatum can be combined to form cholesterized petrolatum, which also has the capacity to form emulsions. For example, a mixture of 65% (w/w) lanolin, 20% (w/w) water, and 15% (w/w) petrolatum can incorporate an equivalent weight of water without changing its consistency.[15,52]

The ability of lanolin alcohols to deliver active substances to the skin is partly due to their surface activity.[15] Lanolin alcohols, which contain a high proportion of cholesterol, have a high surface activity and are able to reduce the interfacial tension of a mineral oil-water system from 52.5 to 5.0 dyn/cm.[8,53] Even at low levels, cholesterol can reduce the interfacial tension of emulsions and dispersed systems.[8,54]

Lanolin has been used for many years as a vehicle for pharmacologically active substances in ophthalmic ointments and topical formulations.[55-60] In addition to being a vehicle for penicillin and other antimicrobial substances, lanolin contains lipids such as 10-methyldodecanoic acid and 12-methyltridecanoic acid which have antimicrobial activity.[61,62]

22.7 LANOLIN DERIVATIVES

The highly complex nature of lanolin makes it a rich source for fractionation and producing derivatives.[8,16] Lanolin, a semisolid of liquid and solid wax esters, can be further fractionated into lanolin oil and lanolin wax.[63,64] The solid esters of lanolin can be removed using low temperature fractional solvent crystallization. The liquid esters contain a higher concentration of lower molecular weight, branched-chain, hydroxy compounds. Lanolin oil is reported to possess the emollient properties of lanolin with the benefits of being fluid at room temperature and the ability to be spread to form thinner films.[65] It can be solubilized in clear detergent systems to give conditioning properties.[8] The hard lanolin wax esters are used to improve the consistency and to add stability to lip glosses and lipsticks.[8]

The extremely large number of lanolin derivatives has been reviewed by Barnett[8] and Steel.[16] Lanolin derivatives can be formed by acetylation, ethoxylation, propoxylation, alkoxylation, and isobutylation of hydroxy groups, as well as hydroxylation of the double bond in the sterol ester component. Hydrolysis of lanolin can also produce lanolin alcohols and lanolin acids, which like lanolin can be ethoxylated, acetylated, and hydoxylated.

Although cholesterol is essentially insoluble in water, a soluble cholesterol derivative can be formed by reacting it with high levels of ethylene oxide.[66,67] This ethoxylated product has balanced hydrophobic and hydrophilic properties. The increased hydrophilicity makes it useful as an oil-in-water emulsifier or as a stabilizer. Ethoxylated lanolin is used for viscosity regulation, pigment dispersion, and as a solubilizer. Less than 1% ethoxylated cholesterol is effective at reducing the viscosity of anionic lotions to make them easier to pour. Non-ionic systems require more ethoxylated cholesterol for this purpose.[68]

Lanolin has stood the test of time as an emulsifier and skin emollient. Its complex nature has been a rich resource of derivatives formed from fractionation and chemical reactions. Although the composition of lanolin is different from the lipids found on the surface of human skin, lanolin has been demonstrated to be equivalent in its ability to restore barrier function. In addition to the beneficial effects attributable to its physical properties, lanolin may also have a pharmacological effect on the epidermis.

REFERENCES

1. Clark, E. W., The history and evolution of lanolin, in *The Lanolin Book,* Beiersdorf AG, Hamburg, 1999, 15.
2. Dioscorides, *De materia medica*, Frellonii, Lyons, 1543.
3. *CTFA Cosmetic Ingredient Dictionary, 2nd ed.*, The Cosmetic, Toiletry and Fragrance association Inc., Washington, D.C., 1976.
4. Kligman, A. M., Lanolin allergy: crisis or comedy?, *Contact Dermatitis*, 9, 99, 1983.
5. Clark, E. W., Estimation of the general incidence of specific lanolin allergy, *J. Soc Cosmet. Chem.*, 26, 323, 1975.
6. Kligman, A. M., The myth of lanolin allergy, in *The Lanolin Book*, Beiersdorf AG, Hamburg, 1999, 161; also *Contact Dermatitis,* 39, 103, 1998.
7. Truter, E. V., *Wool Wax Chemistry and Technology*, Cleaver-Hume Press Ltd., London, 1956.
8. Barnett, G., Lanolin and derivatives, *Cosmet. Toiletries*, 101, 21, 1986.
9. Proserpio, G., Lanolides: Emollients or moisturizers?, *Cosmet. Toiletries*, 93, 45, 1978.
10. Clark, E. W., A brief history of lanolin, *Pharm. Hist.*, 10, 5, 1980.
11. Anderson, C. A., Wood, G. F., Fractionation of wool wax in the centrifugal recovery process, *Nature,* 193, 742, 1962.
12. Clark, E. W., Kitchen, G. F., Centrifugal fractionation of wool wax, *Nature*, 194, 572, 1962.
13. *European Pharmacopeia, 3rd ed.*, Council of Europe, Strasboug, France, 1997, 1726.
14. *The National Formulary, 6th ed., The United States Pharmacopeia,* United States Pharmacopeial Convention, Inc., Rockville, MD, 1985, 583.
15. Jacob, J., The chemical composition of wool wax, in *The Lanolin Book*, Beiersdorf AG, Hamburg, 1999, 53.
16. Steel, I., Lanolin and derivatives, in *The Lanolin Book*, Beiersdorf AG, Hamburg, 1999, 85.
17. Fawaz, F., Chaigneau, M., Giry, L., Pusieux, F., *CR Acad. Sci. Paris,* 270-C, 1577, 1970.
18. Fawaz, F., Choix, M., Miet, C., Pusieux, F., Analysis of ointments, oils and waxes. IX. Application of molecular sieves to the analysis of hydrocarbons, *Ann. Pharm. Francaises,* 29, 179, 1971.
19. Bertram, S. H., The constitution of wool waxes, *Am. Perfum.*, 55, 115, 1950; also in *J. Am. Oil Chem. Soc.*, 26, 454, 1949.
20. Motiuk, K., Wool wax alcohols: A review, *J. Am. Oil Chem. Soc.*, 56, 651, 1979.
21. Fawaz, F., Chaigneau, M., Pusieux, F., XV. Composition chimiques de la lanoline total et de ses différentes fractions, *Ann. Pharm. Francaises*, 32, 215, 1974.
22. Clark, E. W., Cronin, E., Wilkinson, D. S., Lanolin with reduced sensitising potential: A preliminary report, *Contact Dermatitis*, 3, 69, 1977.
23. Motiuk, K., Wool wax acids: a review, *J. Am. Oil Chem. Soc.*, 56, 91, 1979.
24. Fawaz, F., Chaigneau, M., Pusieux, F., XIII. Composition de la lanoline. 2. Ètude des acides non hydroxylés de la lanoline total et des ses différentes fractions, *Ann. Pharm. Francaise,* 31, 217, 1973.
25. Fawaz, F., Miet, D., Pusieux, F., XIV. Composition de la lanoline. 3. Ètude des acides hydroxylés de la lanoline total et de ses différentes fractions, *Ann. Pharm. Francaises,* 32, 59, 1974.
26. Fawaz, F., Chaigneau, M., Pusieux, F., XVI. Composition chimiques de la lanoline. 5. Ètude des sterols et des alcools triterpéniques de la lanoline total et de ses différentes fractions, *Ann. Pharm. Francaises*, 32, 301, 1974.
27. Downing, D. T., Kranz, Z. H., Murray, K. E., Studies in waxes. XIV. An investigation of the aliphatic constituents of hydrolyzed wool wax by gas chromatography, *Aust. J. Chem.*, 13, 80, 1960.
28. Downing, D. T., Solvent fractionation of wool wax acids, *Aust. J. Appl. Sci.*, 14, 50, 1963.
29. Harris, I. R., Cholesterol and the skin, in *The Lanolin Book*, Beiersdorf AG, Hamburg, 1999, 135.
30. Schurer, Y., Elias, P. M., The biochemistry and function of stratum corneum lipids, *Adv. Lipid Res.*, 24, 27, 1991.
31. Clark, E. W., Steel, I., Investigations into biomechanisms of the moisturising function of lanolin, *J. Soc. Cosmet. Chem.*, 44, 181, 1993.
32. Clark, E. W., Steel, I., Microstructure of Human Stratum Corneum Treated with Lanolin, Poster #2, American Academy of Dermatology, Washington, D. C., 1993.
33. White, S. H., Mirejovsky, D., King, G. I., Structure of lamellar domains and corneocyte envelopes of murine stratum corneum: An X-ray diffraction study, *Biochemistry*, 27, 3725, 1988.

34. Hoppe, U., Larsson, K., Water-in-oil emulsions — a study of wool-wax alcohols systems, *J. Despersion Sci. Technol.*, 2, 433, 1981.
35. Kligman, A., Regression method for assessing the efficacy of moisturizers, *Cosmet. Toiletries*, 93, 27, 1978.
36. Powers, D. H., Fox, C., A study of the effect of cosmetic ingredients, creams and lotions on the rate of moisture loss from the skin, *Proc. Sci. Sect. Toilet Goods Assoc.*, 28, 21, 1957.
37. Spruits, D., Interference of some substances with water vapour loss from human skin, *Am. Perfum. Cosmet.*, 86, 27, 1971.
38. Harry, R. G., Skin penetration, *Br. J. Dermatol. Syph.*, 53, 65, 1941.
39. MacKee, G. M., Sulzberger M. B., et al., Histologic studies on percutaneous penetration with special reference to the effect of vehicles, *J. Invest. Dermatol.*, 6, 43, 1945.
40. Clark, E. W., Short term penetration of lanolin into human stratum corneum, *J. Soc. Cosmet. Chem.*, 43, 219, 1992.
41. Elias, P., Man, M.-Q., Thornfeldt, C. R., Feingold, K. R., The epidermal permeability barrier: effects of physiologic and non-physiological lipids, in *The Lanolin Book*, Beiersdorf AG, Hamburg, 1999, 253.
42. Man, M.-Q., Feingold, K. R., Elias, P. M., Exogenous lipids influence permeability barrier recovery in acetone-treated murine skin, *Arch. Dermatol.*, 129, 728, 1993.
43. Mao-Qiang, M., Feingold, K. R., Thornfeldt, C. R., Elias, P. M., Optimization of physiological lipid mixtures for barrier repair, *J. Invest. Dermatol.*, 106, 1096, 1996.
44. Sauermann, G., Schreiner, V., The skin caring effects of topical products containing lanolin alcohols, in *The Lanolin Book*, Beiersdorf AG, Hamburg, 1999, 217.
45. Peterson, E. N., The hydrating effect of a cream and white petrolatum measured by optothermal infrared spectrometry *in vivo*, *Acta Derm. Venereol.*, 71, 373, 1991.
46. Moss, J., The effect of three moisturisers on skin surface hydration, *Skin Res. Technol.*, 2, 32, 1996.
47. Oz, M. C., Newbold, J.E., Lemole, G. M., Prevention of radioactive indicator and viral particle transmission with an ointment barrier, *Infect. Control Hosp. Epidemiol.*, 12, 93, 1991.
48. Butcher, E. O., The penetration of fat and fatty acid into the skin of the rat, *J. Invest. Dermatol.*, 21, 43, 1953.
49. Chvapil, M., Gaines, J. A., Gilman, T., Lanolin and epidermal growth factor in healing of partial pig wounds, *J. Burn Care Rehabil.*, 9, 279, 1988.
50. Hinman, C. D., Maibach, H. L., Effects of air exposure and occlusion on experimental skin wounds, *Nature*, 200, 377, 1963.
51. Steel, I., Marks, R., The Effect of Lanolin on Wound Healing in Normal Human Volunteer Subjects, Poster #342, American Academy of Dermatology, Washington, D.C., 1996.
52. Falbe, J., Regitz, M., *Römpp Chemie Lexikon*, 9. Aufl., G. Thieme Verlag, Stuttgart, New York, 1995, 2445.
53. Lower, E. S., Wool wax alcohols in cosmetics, *Am. Perfum.*, 49, 659, 1947.
54. Truter, E. V., The activities of some water-in-oil emulsifying agents, *J. Soc. Cosmet. Chem.*, 13, 173, 1962.
55. von Sallmann, L., Grosso, A., Marsh, M. G., Ophthalmic penicillin ointments, *Ophthalmology*, 36, 284, 1946.
56. Sitruk-Ware, R., Trans-dermal application of steroid hormones for contraception, *J. Steroid Biochem. Mol. Biol.*, 53, 247, 1995.
57. Prout, W. A., Strickland, M. A., A comparison of the antiseptic properties of certain ointments employing various bases, *J. Am. Pharm. Assoc.*, 26, 730, 1937.
58. Iyer, B. V., Vasavada, R. C., Evaluation of lanolin alcohol films and kinetics of release of triamcinolone acetonide release, *J. Pharm. Sci.*, 68, 782, 1979.
59. Bottari, F., di Colo, G., Nannipieri, E., Saettone, M. F., Serafini, M. F., Influence of drug concentration on *in vitro* release of salicylic acid from ointment bases, *J. Pharm. Sci.*, 63, 1779, 1974.
60. Khan, A. R., Iyer, B. V., Cirelli, R. A., Vasavada, R. C., *In vitro* release of salicylic acid from lanolin alcohols-ethylcellulose films, *J. Pharm. Sci.*, 73, 302, 1984.
61. Wolf, F., Antimicriobial properties of wool wax acids, in *The Lanolin Book*, Beiersdorf AG, Hamburg, 1999, 237.
62. Goodrich, B. S., Roberts, D. S., Antimicrobial factors in wool wax, *Aust. J. Chem.*, 24, 153, 1971.

63. Clark, E. W., Liquid lanolin — development, production, properties and uses, *Am. Perfum.*, 77, 89, 1962.
64. Clark, E. W., Liquid derivatives of lanolin, *Soap Perfem. Cosmet.*, 36, 981, 1963.
65. Russell, K. L, Hoch, S. G., Clear detergent solutions containing lanolin oil, *Drug Cosmet. Ind.*, 90, 294, 1962.
66. Saad, H. Y., Higuchi, W. I., Water solubility of cholesterol, *J. Pharm. Sci.*, 54, 1205, 1965.
67. Petit, A., The chemistry and cosmetological uses of cholesterol, *Perfum. Essent. Oil Rec.*, 47, 102, 1956.
68. Conrad, L. I., Maso, H. F., Functional properties of lanolin derivatives in formulations, *Am. Perfum.*, 77, 97, 1962.

23 Skin Moisturizers: Development and Clinical Use of Ceramides

Genji Imokawa

CONTENTS

23.1 INTRODUCTION

The flexibility of the stratum corneum (SC) plays an important role in keeping the skin supple and giving it a radiant appearance. Water is essential for flexibility of the SC, and its amount is primarily associated with the water-holding function within the SC. Evidence has suggested that water-soluble materials such as free amino acid, organic acid, urea, and inorganic ions are primarily responsible for the water-holding properties of the SC and these materials have been termed the natural moisturizing factor.[1] Based upon this mosturizing theory, many moisturizers have been designed

0-8493-7520-7/00/$0.00+$.50

and developed in the cosmetic fields. Since, despite their poor ability to remove water-soluble materials, well-known removers of lipids, such as organic solvents, induce dry skin which is characterized specifically by reduced water-holding function of the SC, we hypothesized that the structural lipids play a considerable role in the water-holding potential of the SC. In this chapter, we introduce clarification of new mechanisms underlying the water-holding properties of the SC and present a brief review for development of new moisturizers and their clinical use.

23.2 MOISTURIZING MECHANISMS IN THE STRATUM CORNEUM

23.2.1 Role of the Stratum Corneum Lipids in the Water-Holding Properties

23.2.1.1 Effects of Removal of Lipids by Solvent

In order to clarify roles of lipids in holding water in the SC, we have tried to remove lipids specifically from the SC and to assess their effects on the water-holding properties.[2-5] Application of acetone/ether (1:1) to human forearm skin for periods of 5 to 20 min induces an enduring (more than 4 days), chapped, and scaly appearance of the SC with no inflammatory reaction, as compared to the usual procedure for the extraction of skin surface lipids. Under these conditions, a significant decrease in the water content within the treated areas is observed, as evidenced by the conductance value (Figure 1). The decreasing conductance barely returns to the normal level until more than 4 days after treatment, with the exception of the 5-min treatment in which the previous normal level of conductance value was almost attained by 4 days with disappearance of scaly skin. In contrast, such a persistent scaly skin, accompanied by a significant decrease in the conductance value, was not induced after the 1-min treatment. Of considerable interest is the fact that acetone/ether treatment could not induce a substantial release from the SC of any hygroscopic materials such as free amino acids or lactic acid,[3] suggesting a deep involvement of structural lipids in induced deficiency of water content. In order to clarify the mechanisms involved in the decrease of the conductance value, we compared the composition of extracted lipids after the solvent treatment for varying periods.[2-5] The one-dimensional thin-layer chromatography (TLC) analysis (Figure 2) shows that even after 1 min of treatment the amounts of sebaceous gland lipids such as squalene, triglycerides, and wax

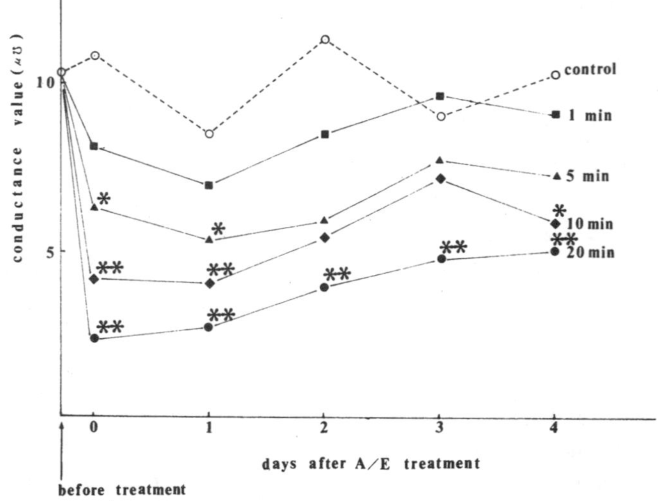

FIGURE 1 A 4-day marked decrease in water content measured by Impedance meter after different times of treatment of human forearm skin with acetone/ether (1:1) (*: $p < 0.05$; **: $p < 0.01$).

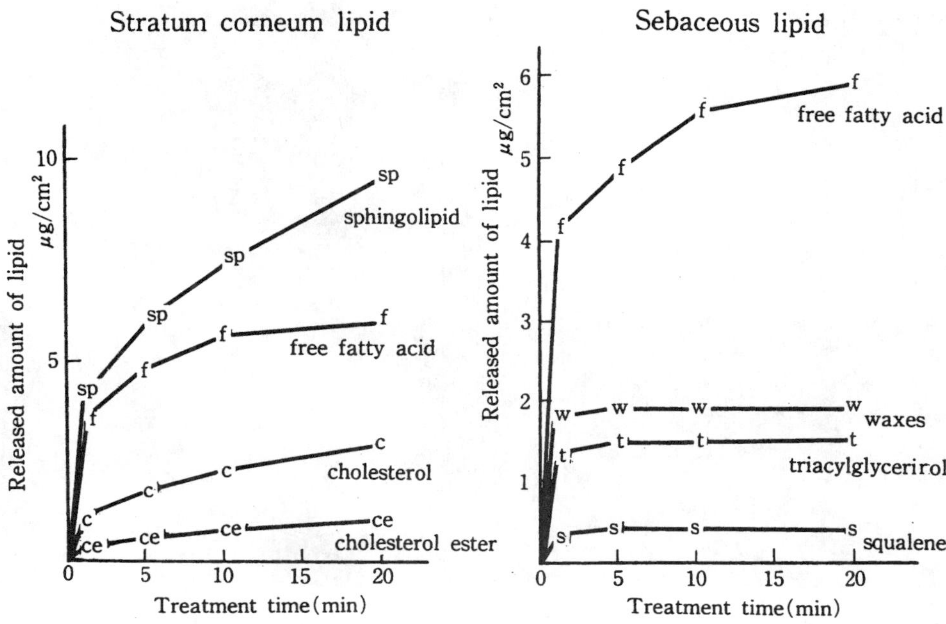

FIGURE 2 Analysis by TLC of lipids released after different times of treatment of human forearm skin with acetone/ether (1:1).

esters almost reach a plateau. Additional or prolonged treatments induce no substantial release of these lipids. On the other hand, SC lipids such as cholesterol, cholesterol esters, and sphingolipids are successively solubilized from the SC by the solvent treatment in a time-dependent manner. These findings reveal that the defect in water-holding properties in acetone/ether-induced dry skin is directly involved in the depletion of intercellular lipids, especially sphingolipids which comprise more than 50% of intercellular lipids.

23.2.1.2 Ultrastructural Changes in the Lipid Conformation

Electron microscopic observations from GTA-ruthenium tetroxide fixation of intact SC (Figure 3) demonstrates that there is preservation of intercellular spaces, which means there is the presence of multiple lamellae consisting of alternating electron-dense and electron-lucent bands filling intercellular spaces.[4-7] In contrast, electron microscopic observation from acrolein vapor fixation of the aceton/ether-treated SC (Figure 4) reveals that the intact intercellular lamellae are absent in many intercellular spaces.[2] These intercellular impairments continue even up to day 4 post-treatment, having not yet been filled by lamella-constructing lipids. Similarly, in GTA-ruthenium tetroxide fixation from SDS-treated SC,[6,7] there are areas that appear to be vacant space and amorphous electron-dense materials adhering to the partially remaining dense and lucent bands, representing some removal or impariment of major segments of the intercelluar lamelae by surfactant treatments.

23.2.1.3 Changes in the Amounts of Bound Water

In order to examine changes in the amounts of bound water in the SC which is responsible for the water-holding properties, an SC sheet was taken from the human forearm skin using a surgical knife, with the help of a tweezer, and subjected to differential scanning calorimetry

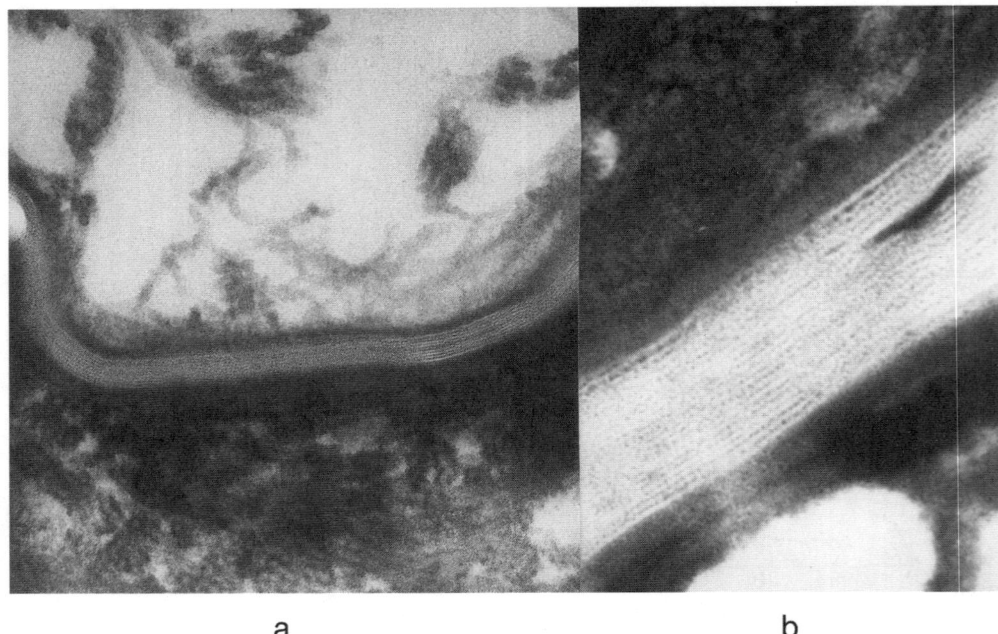

FIGURE 3 Observation of stratum corneum lipids (SCL) by electron microscopy after ruthenium tetroxide fixation in human forearm skin. Magnification (a) ×7000, (b) ×50,000.

(DSC) by which the amounts of the unfreezable water are calculated based on the melting behavior of the water in the SC. The DSC curve of the intact SC sheet shows one endothermic peak at –17 to –6°C, with a much lower melting temperature of ice than 0°C (freezing-point depression behavior) (Figure 5).[8-9] Treatment of the SC sheet with acetone/ether can selectively deplete SCLs and demonstrate a marked difference in DSC thermograms where an endothermic peak appears even at 30% of water content, indicating a decrease in the bound-water content (Figure 6). However, the melting temperature around which the endothermic peak is observed does not change even after acetone/ether treatment, which suggests that acetone/ether treatment releases no water-soluble materials like amino acids. The plot of calculated transition enthalpy against the total water content in the SC sheet demonstrates that the intact SC sheet possesses approximately 33.3% bound water that never freezes, even below –40°C (Figure 7). The depletion of stratum correum lipids by acetone/ether treatment causes the SC bound-water content to decrease from 33.3 to 19.7%.

23.2.1.4 Effects of Lipid Replenishment

23.2.1.4.1 Dryness and Water-Holding Properties

It is well known that the intercellular lipids comprise several components such as cholesterol, sphingolipids, and fatty acids, which by themselves possess no substantial capacity for holding water in extracted *in vitro* situations.[4] Therefore, it seems reasonable to assume that these lipids are sepcifically compartmentalized into the intercellular spaces to exert their water-holding properties. This led us to discover which lipid components are primarily responsible for their water-holding properties. Hence, we tried to measure the recovery potential of an extracted lipid for the water-holding properties after topical application on the lipid-depleted SC in which a marked decrease in the water-holding properties is found. Two daily topical applications of 10% stratum corneum lipid (SCL) fraction in alkyl glycery ether (GE)/squalane base on the

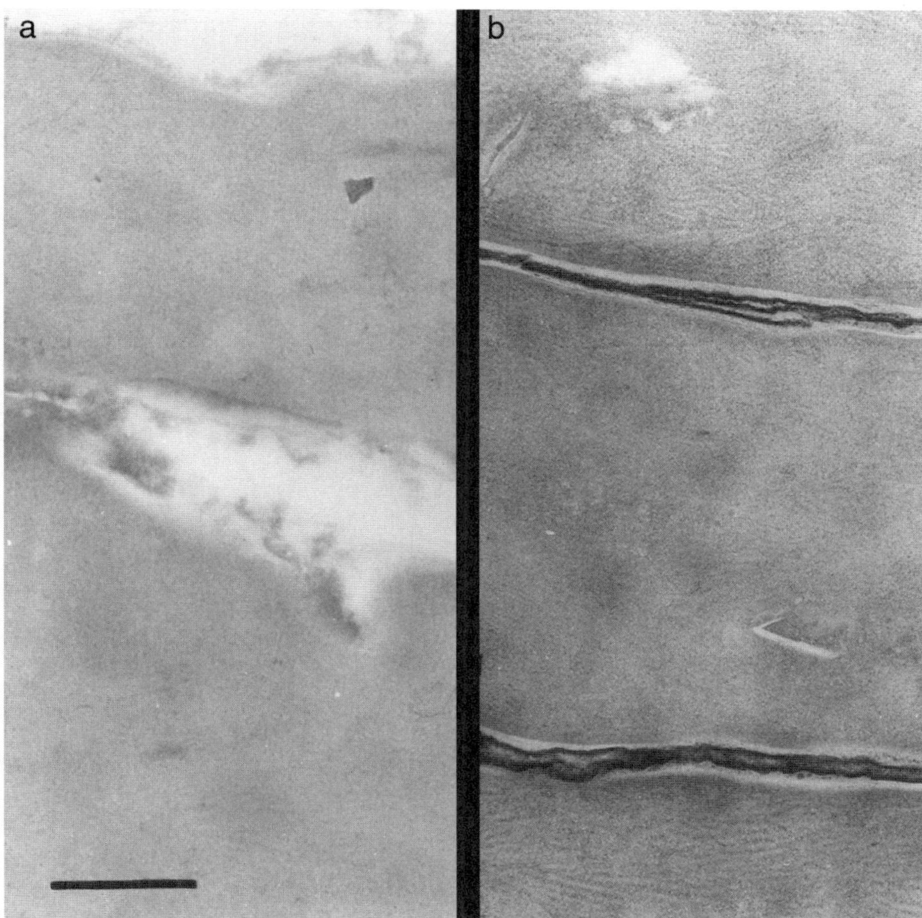

FIGURE 4 Ultrastructure of the SC of acetone/ether (20 min) (a) untreated and (b) treated areas of human forearm skin. Biopsy specimens taken 24 h after treatment were fixed with acrolein vapor/osmic acid and embedded in Spurr's resin.

acetone/ether-treated sebaceous lipid (SC) induce a significant recovery of the decreased conductance value as compared with nontreatment or GE/squalane base only, whereas the SL does not show any significant recovery even when compared to GE/squalane (Figure 8).[9-11] The recovery level by the SCL is significantly higher in comparison with 10% glycerin in the same GE/squalane system. Nevertheless, when GE is not added to this system, there is no significant recovery detectable with any of the lipid fractions. The observed recovery is specific for a combination with GE among the several surfactants employed. This is based on the fact that GE has potential as a penetration enhancer. Consistent with changes in the conductance value, the scaling that occurs after acetone/ether treatment significantly decreases after the two daily applications with SCL as compared with no application, while SL and glycerin do not show any recovery in the same system.

23.2.1.4.2 Ultrastructural Changes

In the lipid-depleted SC sheet followed by the application of isolated SCLs, intercellular lamellae reappear (Figure 9).[8,9] These seem to consist of alternating electron-dense and electron-lucent bands filling the intercellular space, although the detailed lamellar structure is not identical to that of intact lamellae.

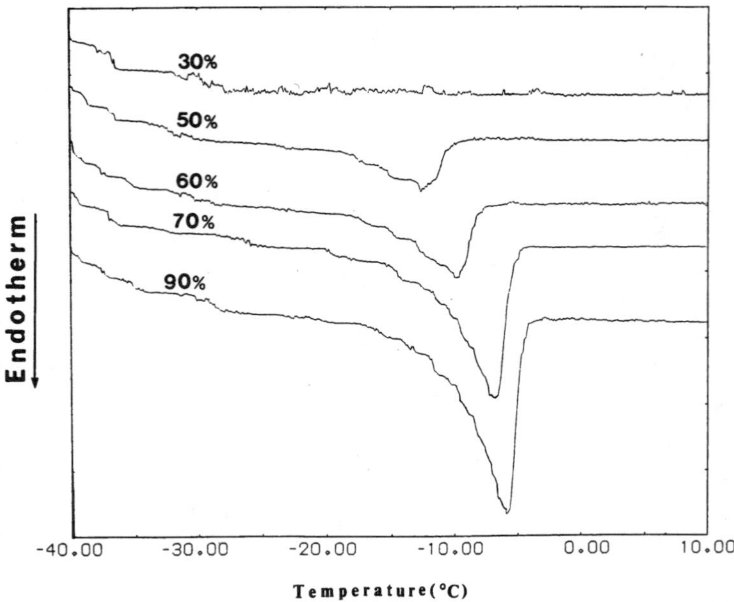

FIGURE 5 DSC thermal profiles obtained for intact human SC sheet with various levels of water contents.

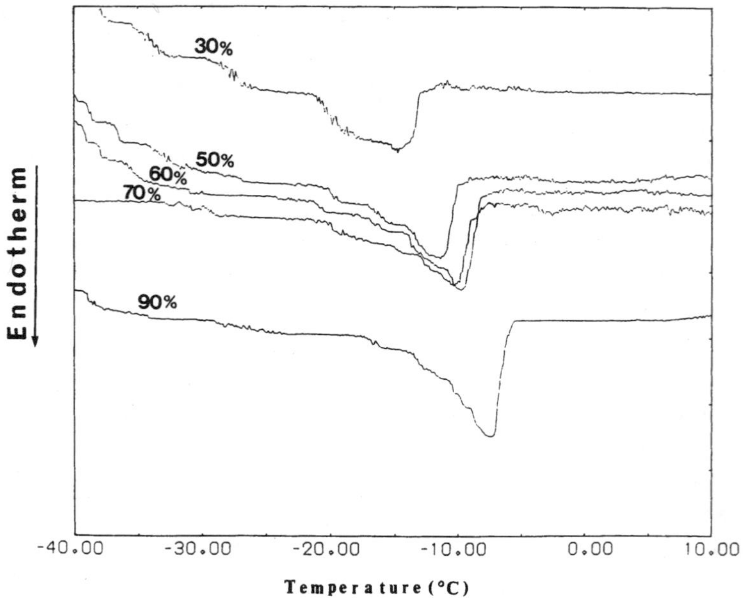

FIGURE 6 DSC thermal profiles obtained for aetone/ether-treated (20 min) human SC sheet with various levels of water contents.

23.2.1.4.3 Amounts of Bound Water

The application of isolated SCLs to the lipid-depleted SC sheet restores the DSC thermograms almost to the levels of those of the intact SC sheet (Figure 10).[8,9] The plot of calculated transition enthalpy against the total water content in the lipid-treated SC sheet demonstrates a marked increase in the bound-water content, from 19.7 to 26.8%, whereas the control solution composed of squalane

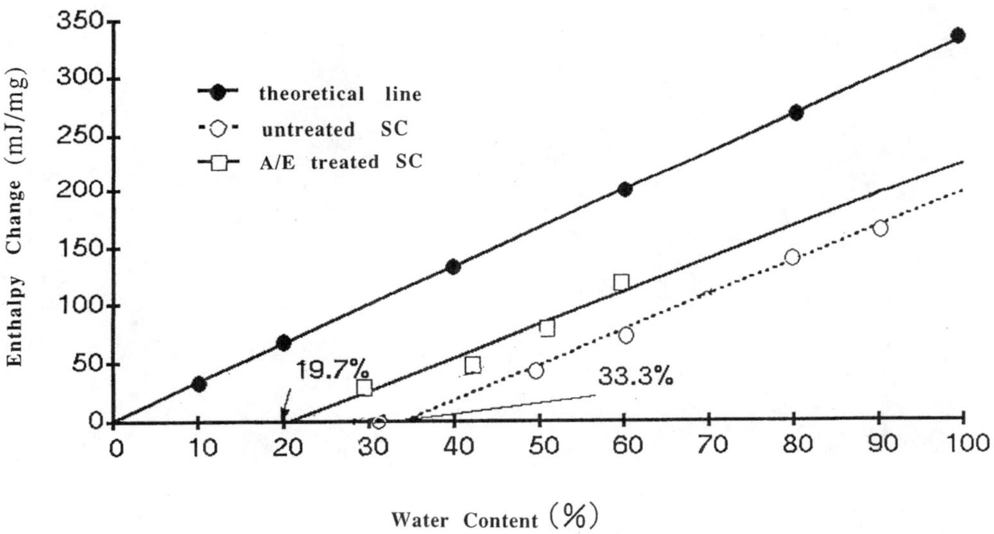

FIGURE 7 Calculation of bound water by plotting the melting enthalpy of ice against the total water content in intact and acetone/ether-treated human SC sheets. SC: stratum corneum sheet.

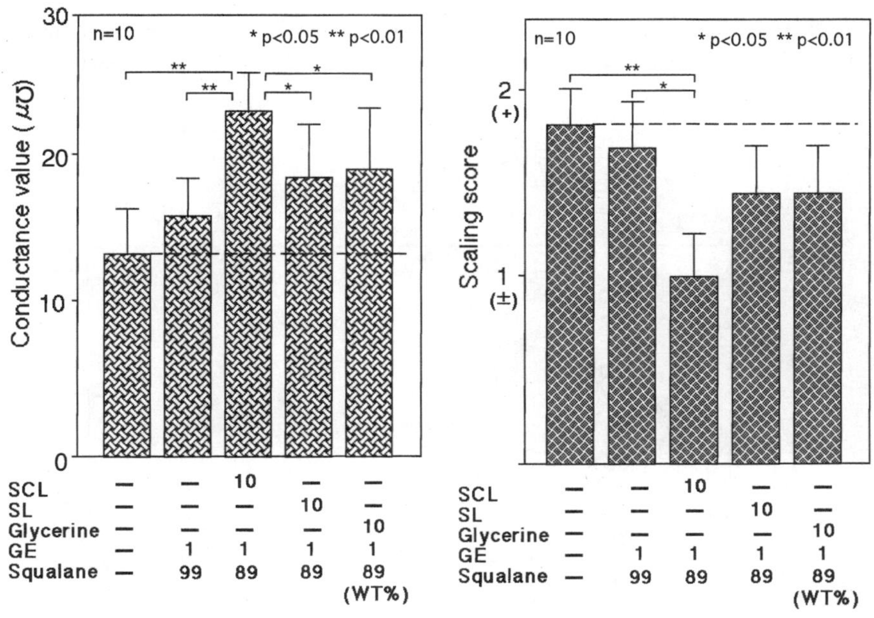

FIGURE 8 The recovery effect of isolated SC lipids on the forearm skin roughened by 30 min of treatment with acetone/ether (1/1) as assessed by water content and scaly score on day 4 following daily treatment for 3 days. (a) Water content measured by impedance meter, and (b) the intensity of scaly appearance. SCL: stratum corneum lipid; SL: sebaceous lipid; GE: glyceryl ether; *: $p < 0.05$; **: $p < 0.01$.

and 1% GE exhibits no influence on the bound-water content of the SC sheet (Figure 11). Taken together, all the previous evidence suggests that intercellular lipids in the SC serve as a bound-water modulator, providing it with radiancy.

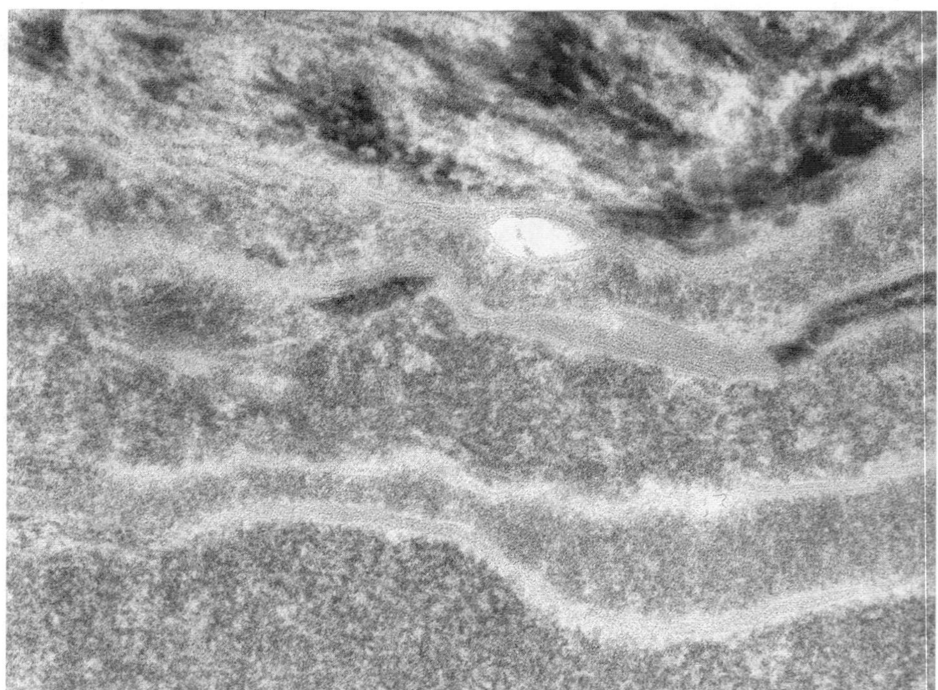

FIGURE 9 Reappearance of lamella structure between intercellular spaces in acetone/ether-treated SC sheet after treatment with SCLs as observed by electron microscopy after ruthenium tetroxide fixation. Magnification ×100,000.

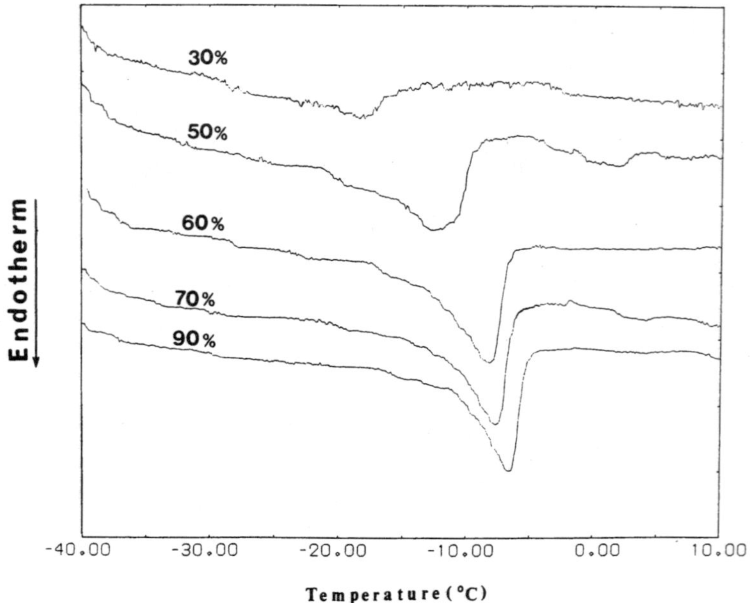

FIGURE 10 DSC thermal profiles obtained for SCL-treated human SC sheet after acetone/ether treatment.

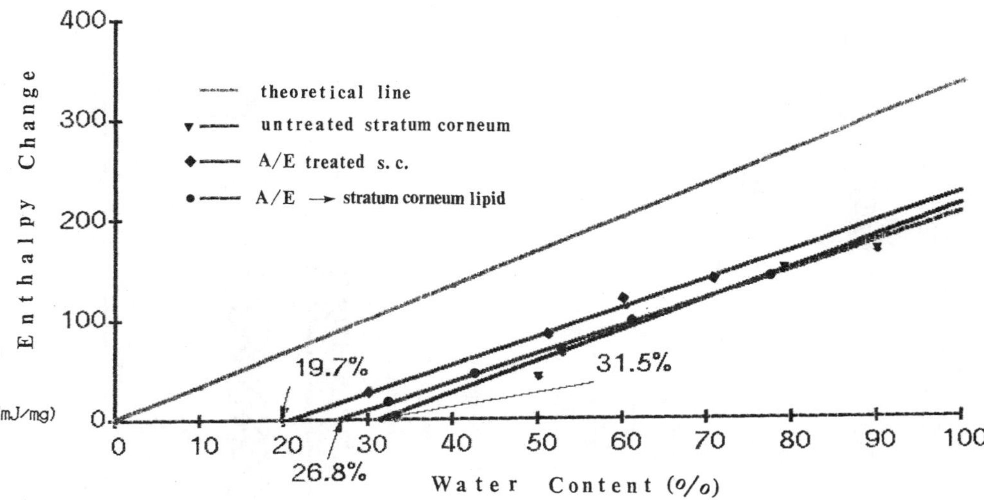

FIGURE 11 Calculation of bound water by plotting the melting enthalpy of ice against the total water content in SCL-treated human SC sheet after acetone/ether treatment. A/E: acetone/ether; SC: stratum corneum.

23.2.1.5 Identification of Lipids Essential for the Water-Holding Function

In order to determine which components are crucial for the water-holding function of intercellular lipids, the *in vivo* potential of each lipid component to repair dry skin induced by acetone/ether treatment was examined.[9-11] Two daily topical applications of five chromatographic separated lipid fractions (cholesterol ester, free fatty acid, cholesterol, ceramide, glycolipid) from the SCL at 10% concentration are carried out in the same system after a 30-min treatment of acetone/ether. Of five lipid fractions, the ceramide fraction induces a significant increase in the conductance value as compared with the GE/squalane base (Figure 12). Furthermore, the glycolipid and cholesterol fractions also exhibit a significant recovery when compared with no application. In contrast, the free fatty acid and cholesterol ester do not show any significant increase in their conductance value. The marked recovery effect of ceramide fraction on the water-holding function and scaly dry skin is also demonstrated by applying W/O emulsion containing ceramide fraction to lipid-depleted forearm skin (Figure 13).[14] Thus, ceramides play a central role in serving as water modulator in the SC because of their predominant abundancy and relatively high capacity of holding water.

23.2.2 Role of Water-Soluble Materials in the Water-Holding Properties

Treatment of the lipid-depleted SC sheet with water releases amino acid amounting to 0.13 mg/mg SC. In accordance with the release of amino acids, water treatment causes DSC thermograms to delete the freezing-point depression behavior (Figure 14).[8,9] Even under this condition, there is no substantial change in the degree of endothermic peak with various water content, suggesting no involvement of water-soluble materials such as amino acids in the capacity of the SC to hold water. Furthermore, our ^{13}C-NMR study demonstrated that the depletion of water-extractable materials from the SC caused marked increases in molecular interaction between 10-nm filaments of keratin fibers.[12] This induced increase of molecular interaction was reversed by the application of water-extractable materials such as amino acids. Based on these facts, it is conceivable that water-extractable materials play an important role in curtailing the intermolecular force between nonhelical regions of 10-nm filaments through interaction with water molecules, probably providing keratin fiber assembly with a high molecular mobility rather than retaining water molecules.

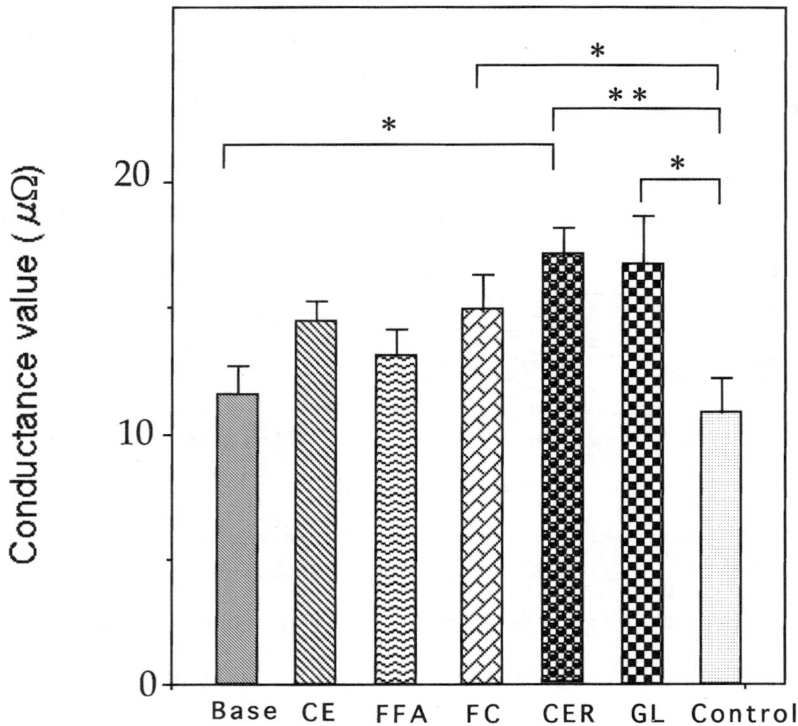

FIGURE 12 The recovery effect of isolated SCL components on the forearm skin roughened by 30 min of treatment with acetone/ether (1:1) as assessed by water content on day 4 following daily treatment for 3 days. Base: squalane (containing 1% glyceryl ether [GE]); CE: cholesterol fraction; FFA: free fatty acid fraction; CER: ceramide fraction; GL: glycolipid fraction; control: nontreatment; *: $p < 0.05$; **: $p < 0.01$.

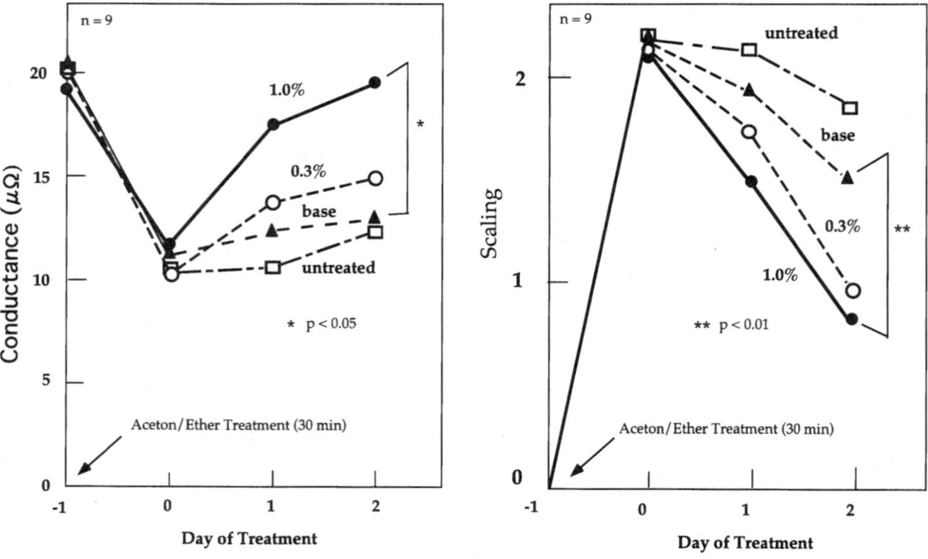

FIGURE 13 The recovery effect of isolated ceramide fraction on the forearm skin roughened by 30 min of treatment with acetone/ether (1:1) as assessed by water content and scaling during the course of daily treatment for 3 days. Base: O/W cream containing 1% GE; *: $p < 0.05$; **: $p < 0.01$.

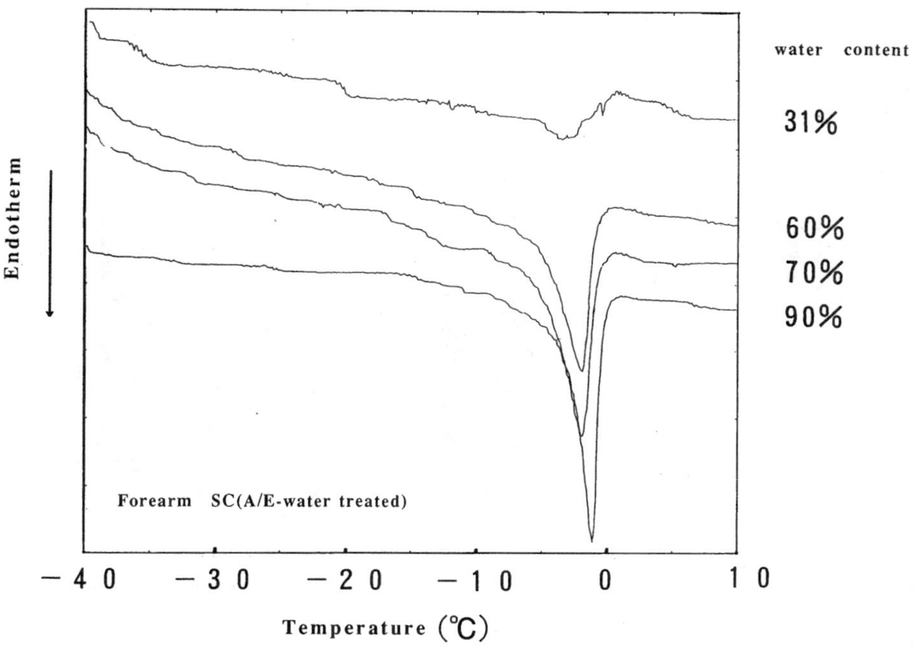

FIGURE 14 DSC thermal profiles obtained for water-treated human SC sheet after acetone/ether treatment. SC: stratum corneum sheet; AE: acetone/ether.

23.2.3 Dry Skin Mechanism in Xerosis and Atopic Dry Skin

23.2.3.1 Xerosis

Asteatotic eczema and its prototype, xerosis, have been thought to be associated with deficient skin surface lipids, which are mainly supplied by sebaceous glands. This hypothesis is based on the fact that sebum-derived lipids play an important role in preventing the skin from water loss by forming lipid films on the surface. In contrast, the previous evidence has demonstrated that SCLs produced by keratinocytes through the keratinization process serve as water modulators, trapping pertinent moisture as bound water to the SC, as well as acting as permeability barriers by forming a multilamellar structure between the SC cells. Of these lipids, ceramides comprise major constituents of the stratum corneum lipids performing both functions. Thus, quantitative analysis of ceramides in the SC provides useful information about etiological involvement of sphingolipids in such dry skin disorders. Ceramides were quantified by TLC after n-hexan/ethanol extraction of resin-stripped SC and evaluated as micrograms per multigram of SC.[13] In healthy leg skin (n = 49), there was age-related decline in the total ceramide, while xerosis (n = 25) suffering significantly reduced water-holding properties, exhibited still decreased level of ceramides as compared to healthy young control, but no definite decrease as compared to healthy age-matched control (Figure 15). These data indicate that the seemingly slight increase in ceramide is an artificial effect due to inflammatory processes or scratching which results from susceptibility to dryness or itchiness. It is very likely that the observed decrease in the SCLs explains the high incidence of winter dry skin in older people. The progression toward severe xerosis and asteatotic eczema can be ascribed to inflammation due to scratching or environmental stimuli which are triggered by dry, itchy skin resulting from ceramide deficiency.

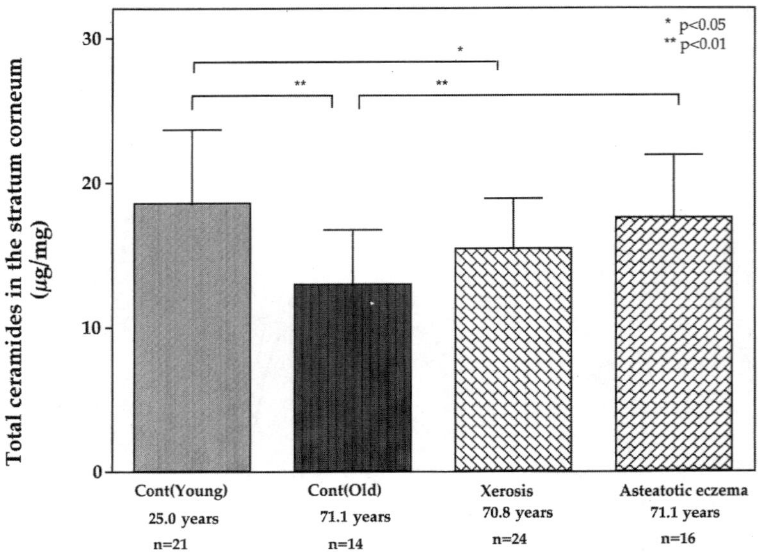

FIGURE 15 Quantitation of ceramide in the SC of patients with xerosis. Cont: healthy control.

23.2.3.2 Atopic Dry Skin

Atopic dry skin is characterized by the diminished water permeability barrier and deficient water-holding properties, as revealed by an evaporimeter for transepidermal water loss and by a capacitance conductance meter for skin surface water content, respectively (Figure 16).[5,14,15] Based upon the established relationship between ceramides and water-holding properties in the SC, we have tried removing SC layers to assess the quantity of ceramides per unit mass of the SC. In atopic dermatitis (n = 32 to 35), there was a marked reduction in the amount of ceramides in the lesional forearm skin compared with those of healthy individuals of the same age (Figure 17).[16] Interestingly, the nonlesional skin also exhibited a similar and significant decrease of ceramides. Among six ceramide fractions, ceramide 1 was most significantly reduced in both lesional and nonlesional skin. These findings suggest that an insufficiency of ceramides in the SC is an etiologic factor in atopic dry skin.

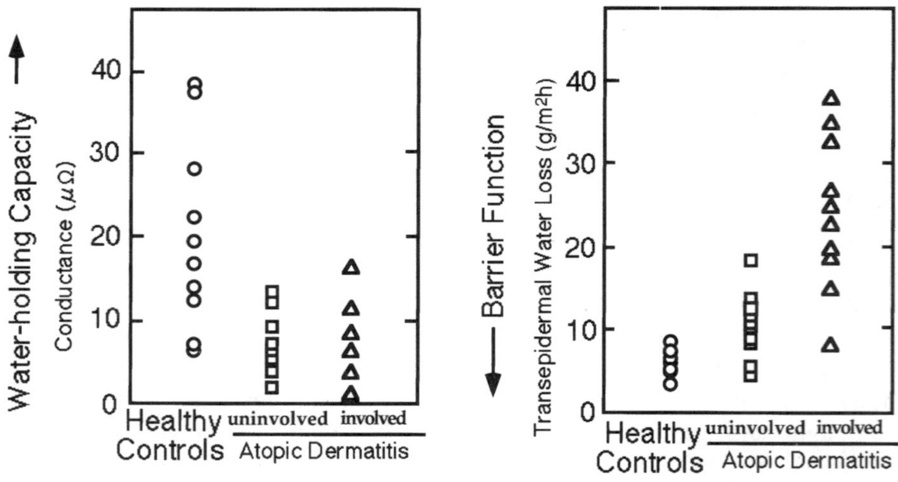

FIGURE 16 Characteristics of the skin with atopic dermatitis as demonstrated by decreased water-holding capacity and barrier function.

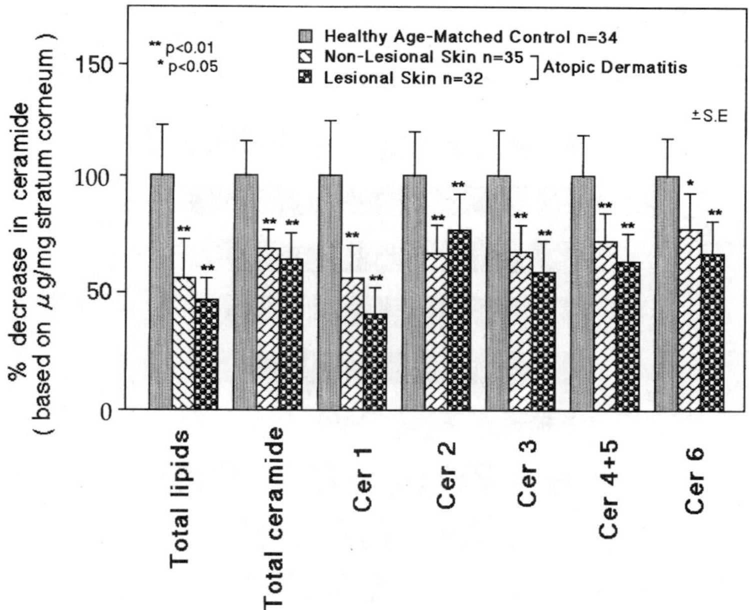

FIGURE 17 Quantitation of ceramides in the SC of patients with atopic dermatitis. Cer: ceramide.

23.3 DESIGN OF PSEUDO-CERAMIDE AS A MOISTURIZER

23.3.1 Structural Analysis of Water-Holding Function through *in vivo* Application of Synthetic Pseudo-Ceramides to Experimentally Induced Dry Skin

Since ceramides are found to be essential in providing the SC with water by forming a lipid multilayer, it is ideal to use ceramides as a new moisturizer. However, natural ceramides themselves or their synthesis are too expensive to make them commercially available. With reference to the chemical structures of natural ceramides (Figure 18), we have tried to synthesize

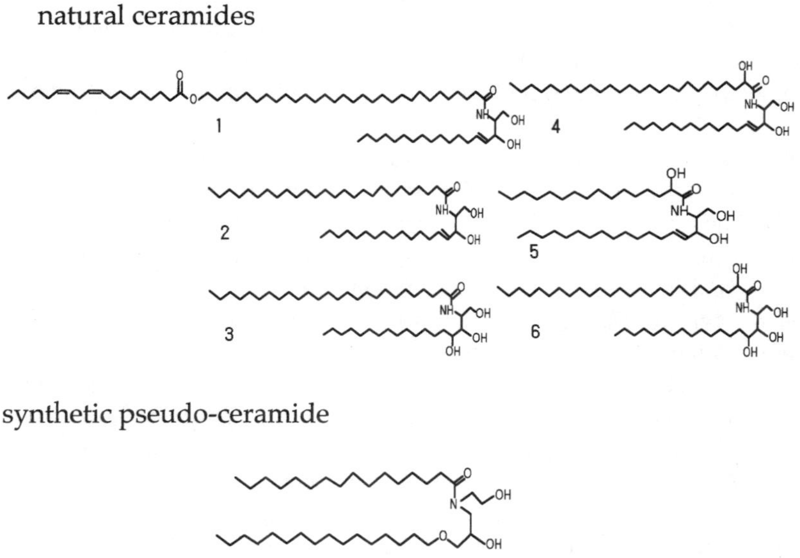

natural ceramides

1 2 3 4 5 6

synthetic pseudo-ceramide

FIGURE 18 Species and structures of ceramide and synthetic pseudo-ceramide.

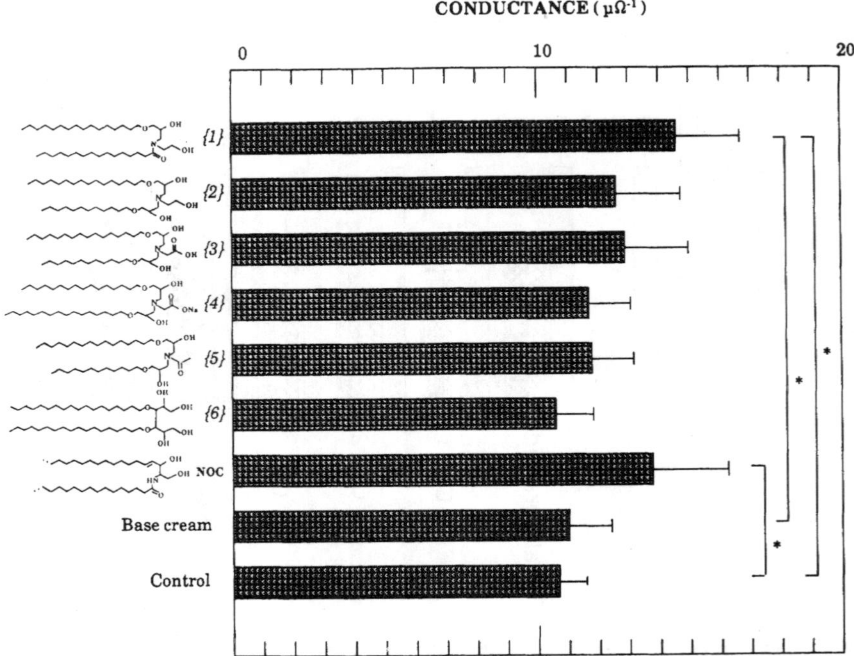

FIGURE 19 The recovery effect of various synthetic amide or amine derivatives on acetone/ether (1:1)-treated human forearm skin as measured by conductance value after 2 days of treatment. Synthetic compounds were emulsified at 1% in W/O cream for their usage. NOC: naturally occurring ceramide; *: $p < 0.05$.

various pseudo-ceramides with a simple process and low cost to develop a new moisturizer.[17,18] Following trials of synthesis, their efficacy was assessed using experimentally induced dry skin. Two daily applications of the synthetic pseudo-ceramides having different polar groups with the same alkyl chain length, emulsified at 1% in W/O cream to acetone/ether-induced dry skin, show a significant recovery of the decreased conductance value as compared with nontreated control or base cream when the polar group has an amide bond (Figure 19).[19,20] However, the single application of base cream or glycerin causes no significant recovery. The application of naturally occurring ceramide from calf brain (NOC) also shows a significant recovery as compared with nontreated control. Among three different structures with an amide bond in the main linkage, a structure with two hydroxyl groups is found to exhibit the highest potential for improving water-holding properties (Figure 20). This result is accompanied by a significant improvement of scaling induced by actone/ether treatment. Comparing compound {9} with compound {1} in Figure 21, it is clear that the substitution of a carbon–carbon bond for the ether bond found near the polar end of alkyl chain provides a less efficient recovery effect. This suggests that the ether bond in this pseudo-ceramide structure is similar to a double bond in natural ceramide and helps to promote water-retaining capacity. With respect to the properties of attached hydroxyl groups, a structure with hydroxyethyl group at the amide residue {1} is found to be most suitable for acquiring the water-retaining properties in comparison to structures with hydroxypropyl {10}, hydroxyhexyl {11}, hydroxyethoxy ethyl {12}, and dihydroxy propyl {13} groups (Figure 21). Since a structure consisting of a polar amide bond and hydroxyethyl groups in a structure like {2} is found to have potential for repairing the water-retaining function and is apparently a good substituent for naturally occurring ceramides, this basic pseudo-ceramide frame in the polar tail allows for the subsequent quantitation of the influence by alkyl chain properties that are basically linked to the water-holding function of the SC. The alkyl chain properties as seen in double-bonded or methy-branched lipids provide marked influences

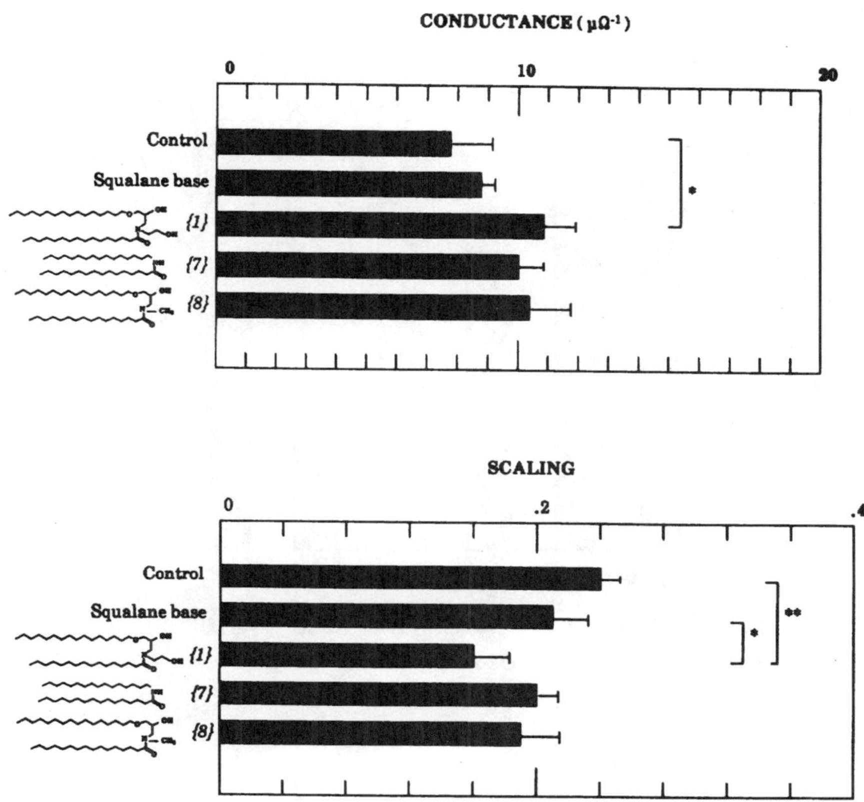

FIGURE 20 The recovery effect of various synthetic pseudoceramides with different polar groups on acetone/ether (1:1)-treated human forearm skin as measured by conductance value after 2 days of treatment. Synthetic compounds were emulsified at 1% in W/O cream for their usage. (*: $p < 0.05$; **: $p < 0.01$.)

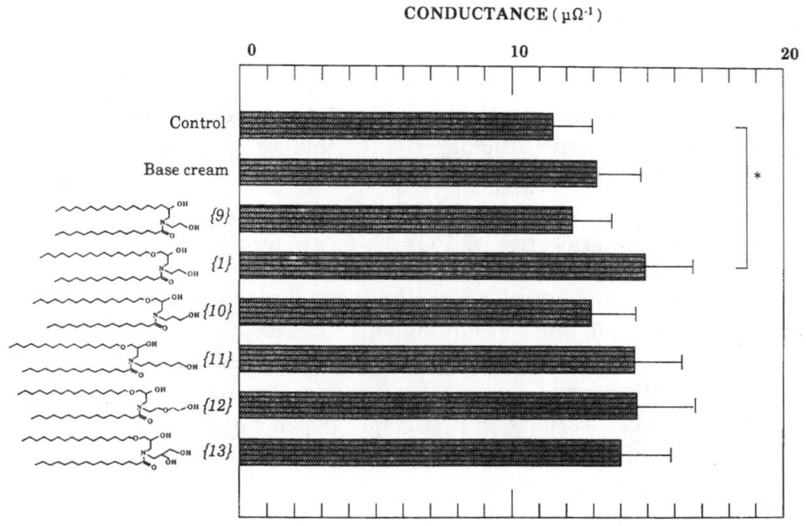

FIGURE 21 The recovery effect of various synthetic pseudo-ceramides with different hydroxyl groups on acetone/ether (1:1)-treated human forearm skin as measured by conductance value after a 2 days of treatment. Synthetic compounds were emulsified at 1% in W/O cream for their usage. (*: $p < 0.05$.)

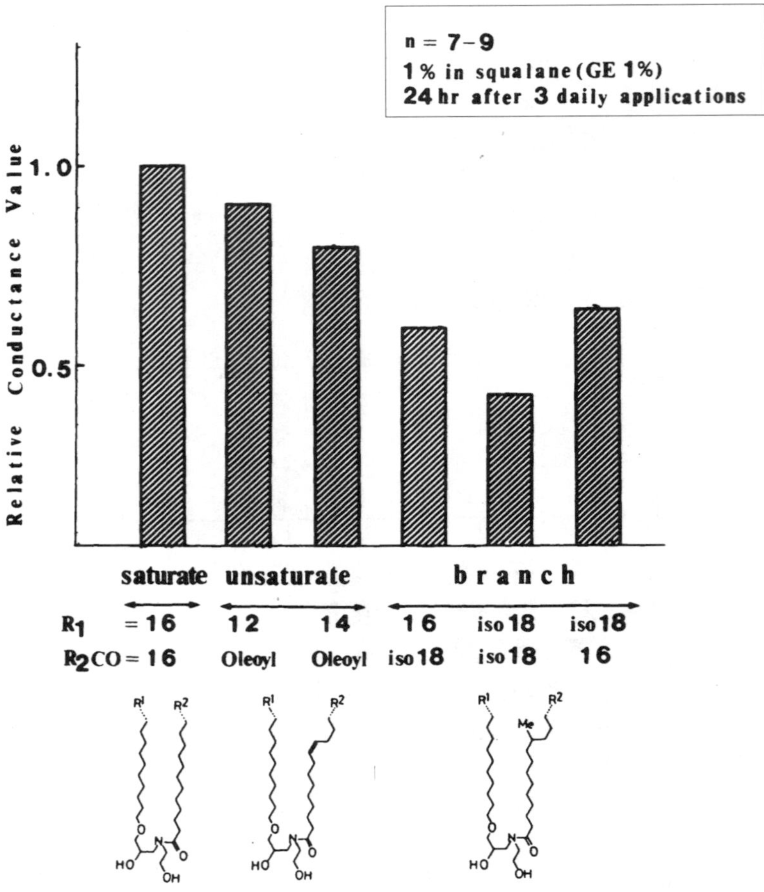

FIGURE 22 The recovery effect of various synthetic pseudo-ceramides with different alkyl properties on acetone/ether (1:1)-treated human forearm skin as measured by conductance value after 2 days of treatment. Synthetic compounds were emulsified at 1% in W/O cream for their usage.

on the recovery potential (Figure 22).[19,20] This indicates that one of the structural requirements for the water-holding function may be the presence of two saturated alkyl chains. Analysis of the alkyl chain length shows that the structure having a total of 31 carbons is the best requirement for water-holding properties (Figure 23).[7,18]

23.3.2 Physicochemical Properties of Pseudo-Ceramides

When mixed with a certain amount of water, the intercellular lipids isolated from human SC exhibited the capacity for formation of multilamellar vesicles as revealed by the appearance of optical texture under cross-polarized light (Figure 24).[7] In analogy to the phenomena of SC intercellular lipids, synthetic pseudo-ceramides in combination with other neutral lipids revealed the potential of multilamellae vesicles in a structure-dependent manner (Figure 25). It is well known that the formation of mutilamella vesicles is accompanied by the incorporation of water into the lamellae as bound water which serves as a water-holding property of the SC. In an attempt to clarify the water-holding mechanims, we measured the DSC thermograms of the SCL containing different amounts of water.[19,20] When the water content exceeded 15%, a small endothermic peak appeared around –5°C (Figure 26). Both the size of the endothermic peak and the peak temperature increased with increasing water content. DSC was also applied to mixtures of pseudo-ceramide and other neutral lipids involving stearic acid, cholesterol, and stearyl

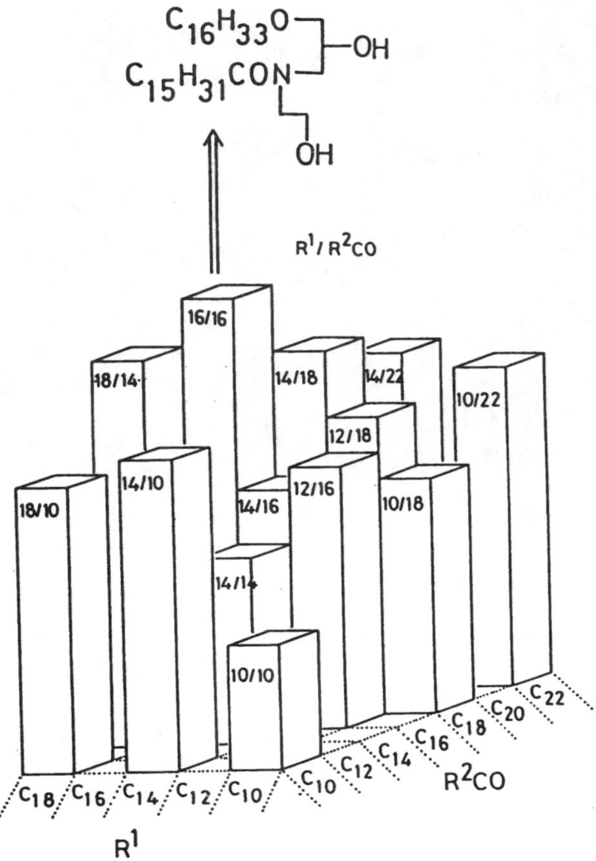

FIGURE 23 The recovery effect of various synthetic pseudo-ceramides with different alkyl chain lengths on acetone/ether (1:1)-treated human forearm skin as measured by conductance value after 2 days treatment. Vertical axis represents conductance values measured after 2 days of treatment. Synthetic compounds were emulsified at 1% in W/O cream for their usage.

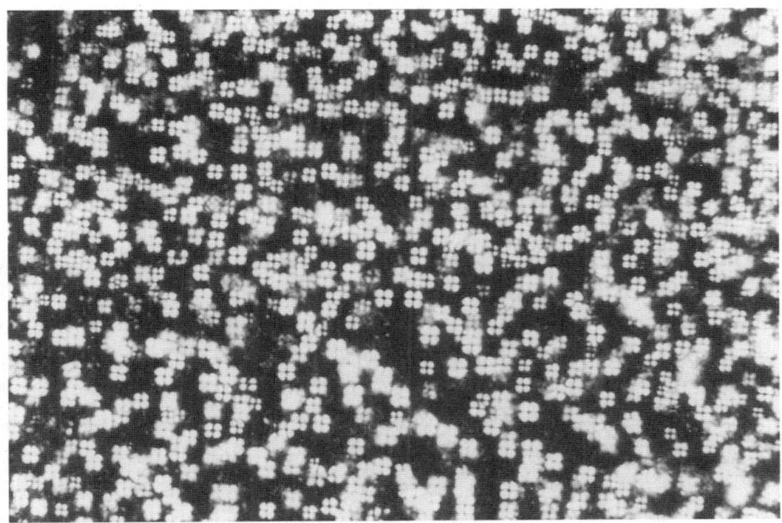

FIGURE 24 Observation of human SCLs dispersed in water under a cross-polarized light microscopy.

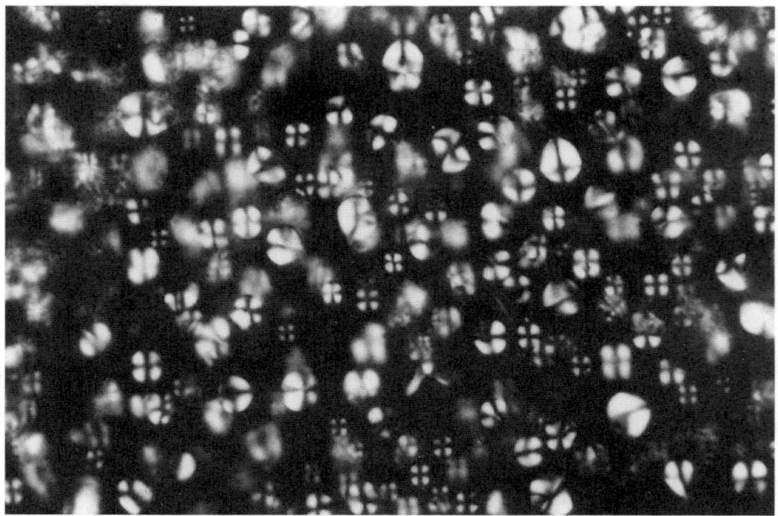

FIGURE 25 Observation of synthetic pseudo-ceramide dispersed in water in combination with other lipids under a cross-polarized light microscopy.

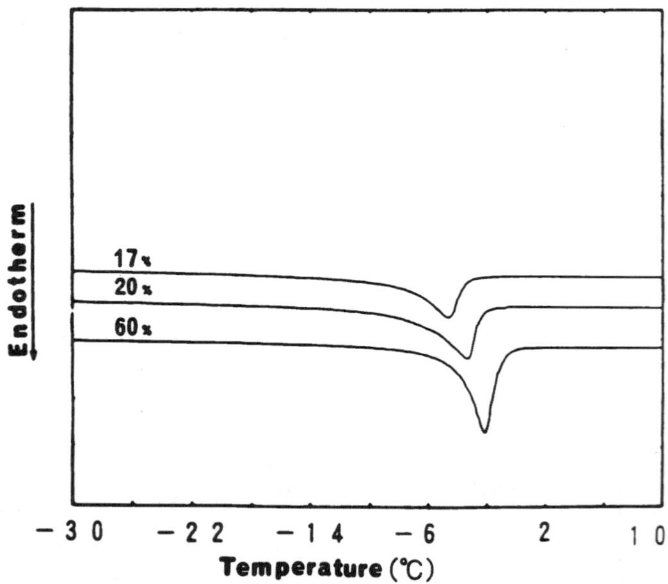

FIGURE 26 DSC of human SCLs dispersed in water at different total water contents.

cholesterol containing different amouts of water. Similar to extracted SCLs, a small endothermic peak appeared at about –2°C when the water content exceeded 10% (Figure 27). The peak size and peak temperature also increased with increasing water content. Next, the transition enthalpy was calculated from the peak area of each thermogram. Figures 28 and 29 show the values of transition enthalpy of the lipid mixture samples of different water content. The experimental data are compared to a theoretical curve which assumes that all the water present in the sample is unbound water. The transition enthalpy was detectable at the water contents of 4.34 and 3.68% for the SCLs and pseudo-ceramide-containing lipid, respectively, and increased linearly parallel to the theoretical lines. Values of the water content, 4.34 and 3.68%, represent the maximum quantity of bound water that may strongly interact with the lipid molecules. The formation of

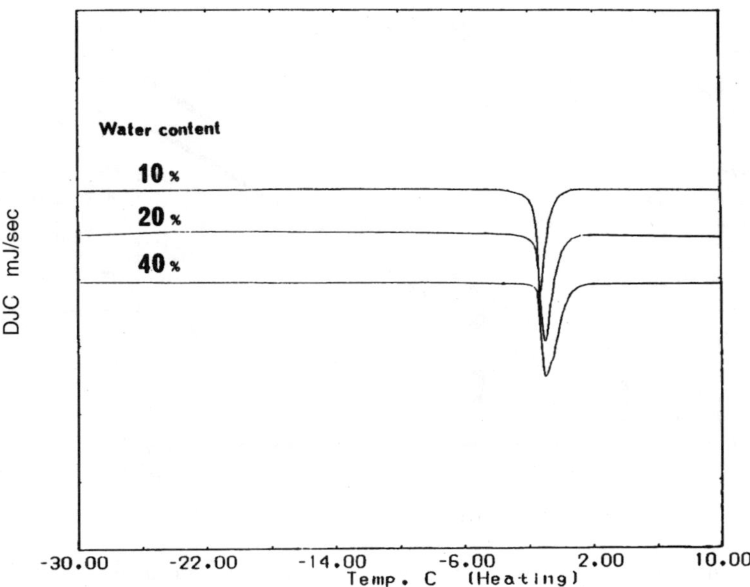

FIGURE 27 DSC of synthetic pseudo-ceramide dispersed in water in combination with other lipids at different total water contents.

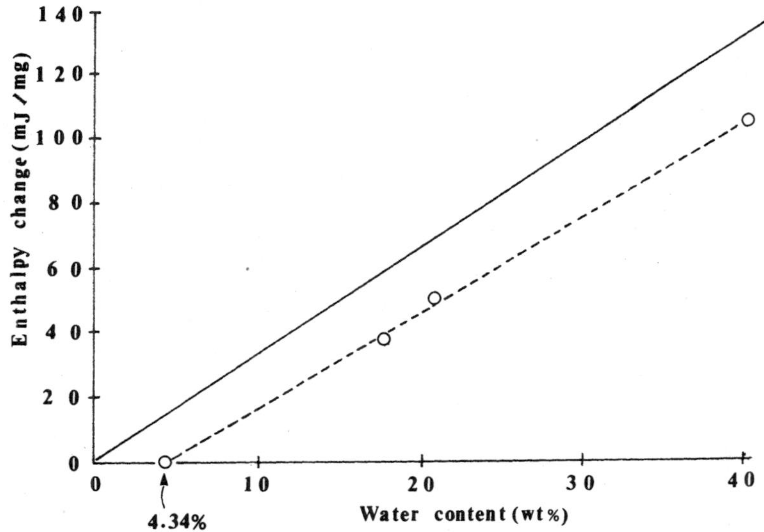

FIGURE 28 The melting enthalpy of ice plotted against the total water content in the SCLs after DSC analysis.

multilamella vesicles is associated with the ability to form the bound water which reflects the *in vivo* water-holding potential of the SC. Accordingly, the capacity to form multiconcentric lamella vesicles requires the water-holding function of the intercellular lipids. Therefore, we measured the recovery potential for the water-holding properties of several synthetic pseudo-ceramides. Figure 30 shows that there is a close relationship between the ability of forming the multiconcentric lamella and the recovery potential of water-holding properties which were obtained *in vivo* using acetone/ether-treated skin.

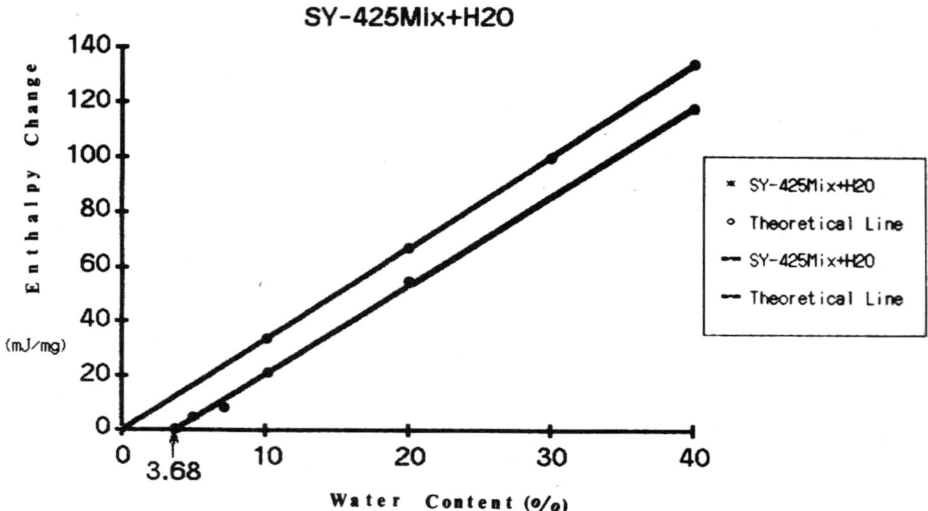

FIGURE 29 The melting enthalpy of ice plotted against the total water content in synthetic pseudo-ceramide in combination with other lipids after DSC analysis.

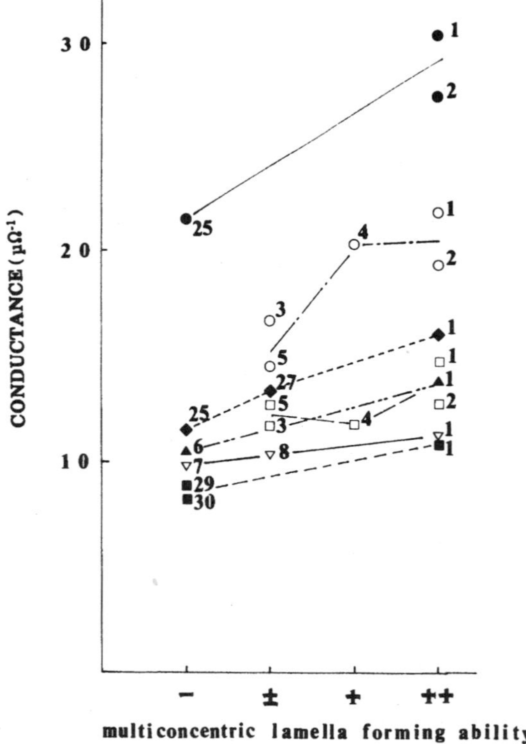

FIGURE 30 The relationship between water-holding potential and multilamellae vesicle-forming ability of pseudo-ceramides. Synthetic pseudo-ceramides/cholesterol/cholesterol stearate/stearic acid were mixed in a weight ratio of 50:15:5:30 on a cover glass and, after an addition of distilled water, heated and cooling process was repeated several times and the sample was applied under a cross-polarized microscope to evaluate the potential of the formation of multilamellae vesicles. The degree of the potential was evaluated according to the following criteria on the basis of the observed optical texture: –, no formation; ±, slight formation; +, moderate formation; ++, marked formation.

23.3.3 Bound Water-Holding Capacity of Pseudo-Ceramides in the Stratum Corneum Sheet

The application of synthetic pseudo-ceramides in combination with other intercellular lipids to the lipid-depleted SC sheet restored the DSC thermograms almost to the levels of those of the intact SC sheet (Figure 31).[20] The plot of calculated transition enthalpy against the total water content in the SC sheet demonstrates that application of the synthetic pseudo-ceramide in combination with other intercellular lipids induces a marked increase in the bound-water content from 19.7 to 26.8%, whereas the control solution composed of squalane and 1% GE exhibits no influence on the bound-water content of the SC sheet (Figure 32).[20] Tables 1 and 2 show the amounts of bound water of different pseudo-ceramides which were calculated by DSC analysis,[20] indicating that a best-suited pseudo-ceramide has the highest water-holding capacity when applied to the SC sheet.

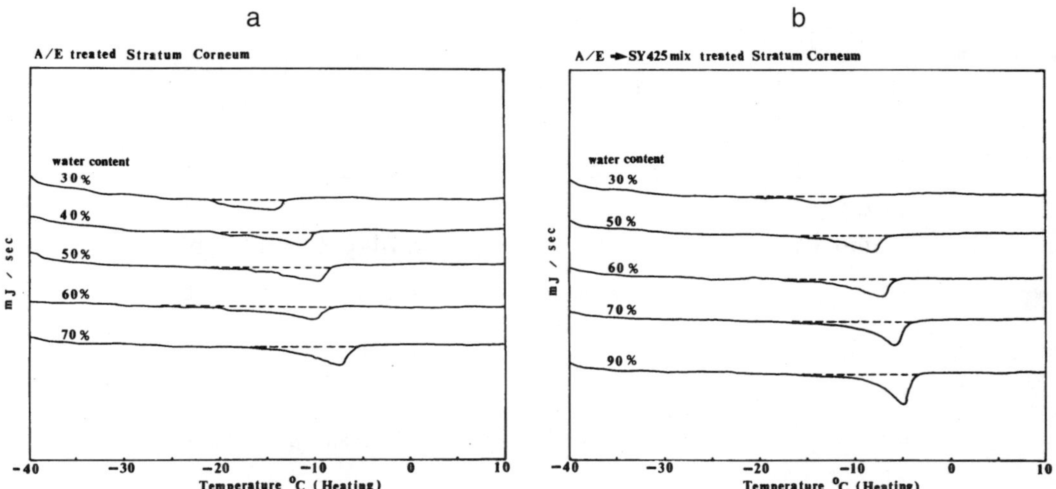

FIGURE 31 DSC thermal profiles obtained for synthetic pseudo-ceramide-treated human SC sheet after acetone/ether treatment. (a) Acetone/ether-treated SC sheet; (b) pseudo-ceramide-treated SC sheet after acetone/ether treatment.

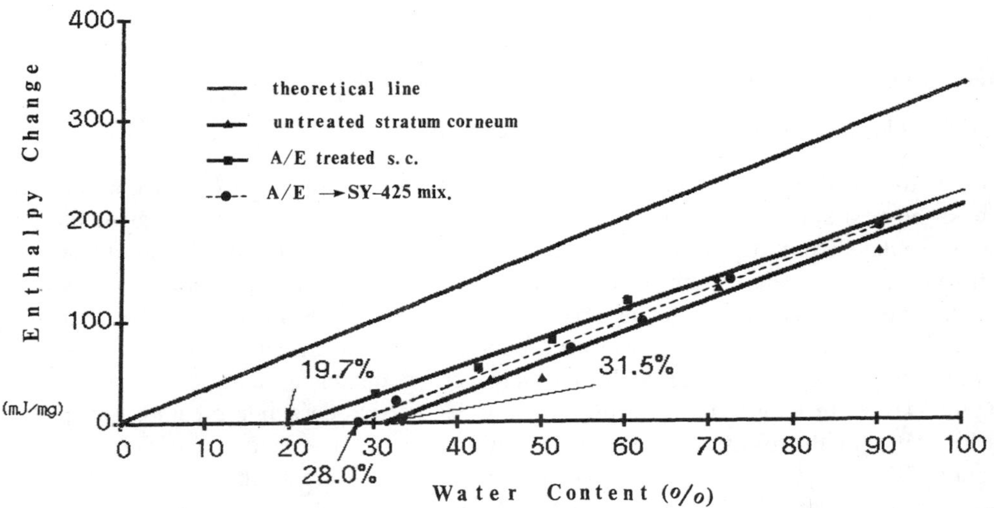

FIGURE 32 The melting enthalpy of ice plotted against the total water content in the SC sheet treated with lipid mixture including synthetic pseudo-ceramide based upon DSC analysis.

TABLE 1
Bound Water Content in SC Sheet and Pseudo-Ceramide Structure

Structure	Bound Water (%)	Recovered Bound Water (%)
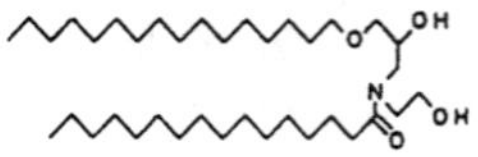	28.0	8.3
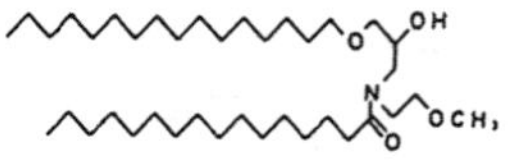	22.5	2.8
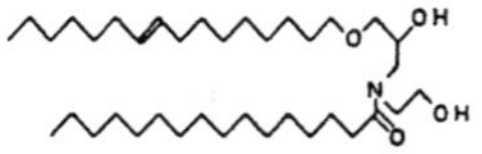	25.2	5.5

Note: Bound water % in acetone/ether-treated SC sheet: 19.7%.

TABLE 2
Bound Water Content in the SC Sheet and Alkyl Chain Length

The structure of pseudo-ceramides

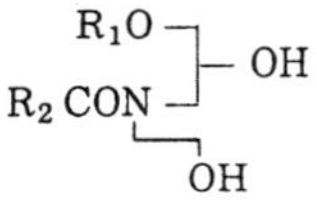

R_1O – OH
R_2 CON
OH

R_1/R_2	Bound Water (%)	Recovered Bound Water (%)
C_{10}/C_9 CO	26.5	6.8
C_{16}/C_{15}CO	28.0	8.3
C_{16}/C_{29}CO	17.0	—
C_{32}/C_{15}CO	19.9	—

Note: Bound water % in acetone-ether-treated SC sheet: 19.7%.

23.4 CLINICAL USE

23.4.1 Use in Experimentally Induced Dry Skin

In order to clarify the time course and dose dependency of the recovery in the conductance values, the best-suited pseudo-ceramide at 3 and 5% concentrations was applied daily for 3 successive days (from day 0 to day 2) and its effect was evaluated daily. A significant increase relative to the base cream (control) was observed with 3 and 5% pseudo-ceramide within 2 days after the first application, with the 5% application showing a higher recovery than the 3% (Figure 33).[18] The best compound was also found to exhibit a similar significant recovery effect on SDS-induced skin, as revealed by an increased conductance value and improved scaling (Figure 34).[18,19] In long-term experiments using 8% pseudo-ceramide cream on soap-induced dry forearm skin, the results of the visual evaluations (Figure 35A) and the instrumental readings (Figure 35B) indicate that both samples (8% pseudo-ceramide cream and commercially available anti-aging cream in U.S.) showed significant improvement from baseline. In addition, 8% pseudo-ceramide-containing sample is a significantly better moisturizer for dry skin than commercially available moisturizer cream.

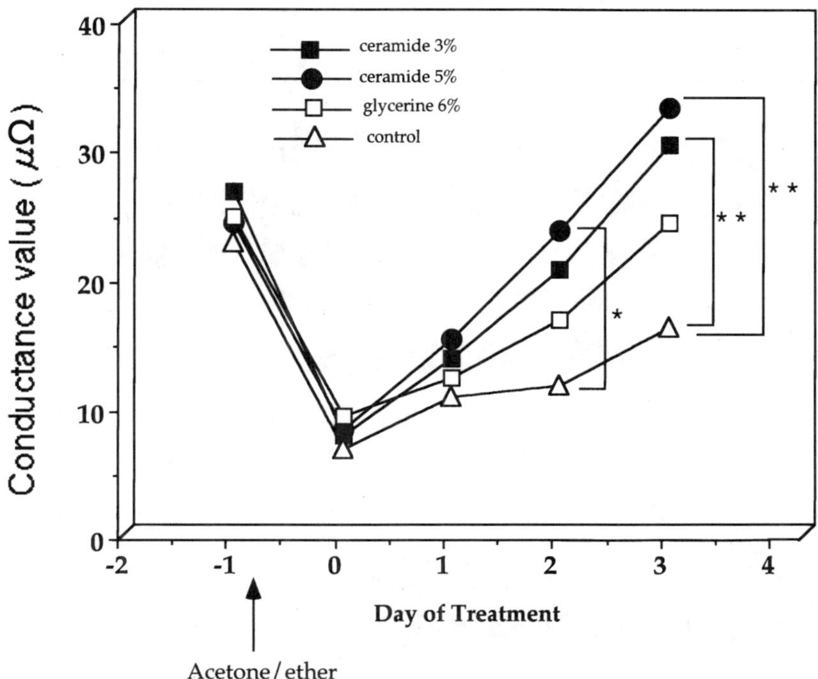

FIGURE 33 The time course and dose dependency of the recovery effect by the best-suited ceramide {1}. The forearm skin of healthy male volunteers was treated with acetone/ether for 30 min (day –1). The sample emulsified in W/O base cream at the indicated concentrations was applied daily from day 0 to day 2. Conductance value was measured daily in comparison with base only. (*: $p < 0.05$; **: $p < 0.01$.)

The within-treatment binomial analysis of the dryness scores indicated that both samples showed significant improvement from baseline throughout the entire study, including the regression phase. The within-treatment binomial analysis of the dry scores showed both samples to be significantly better than baseline on day 21 and 28. The between-treatment binomial analysis of the dryness scores indicated that pseudo-ceramide-containing cream was assigned the lower score significantly more often than control cream on days 2, 7, 19, 21, 26, and 28. The analysis of variance on the dryness scores indicated a significant difference between the two samples. The overall sample mean for pseudo-ceramide-containing cream was significantly lower, that is, less dryer, than for the control cream. The impedance readings reflect the skin's water content; therefore, the higher the value obtained, the moister the skin. Pseudo-ceramide-containing cream impedance readings near the elbow were significantly higher on study days 2 through 23 than those values for the control cream. Similarly, pseudo-ceramide-containing cream impedance readings taken near the wrist were significantly higher than for control cream on study days 2 through 26.

23.4.2 Clinical Use in Xerosis

Five percent pseudo-ceramide-containing cream was applied twice daily for 3 weeks to aged face skin (n = 35, female) which exhibits xerosis in comparison with typical American commercial available anti-aging cream G (Figure 36).[19,20] The within-treatment binomial analysis of the dryness scores indicated that both samples showed significant improvement from baseline throughout the entire study. The between-treatment binomial analysis of the dryness scores indicated that pseudo-ceramide-containing cream was assigned the lower score significantly more often than control cream on weeks 1, 2, and 3. The analysis of variance on the dryness

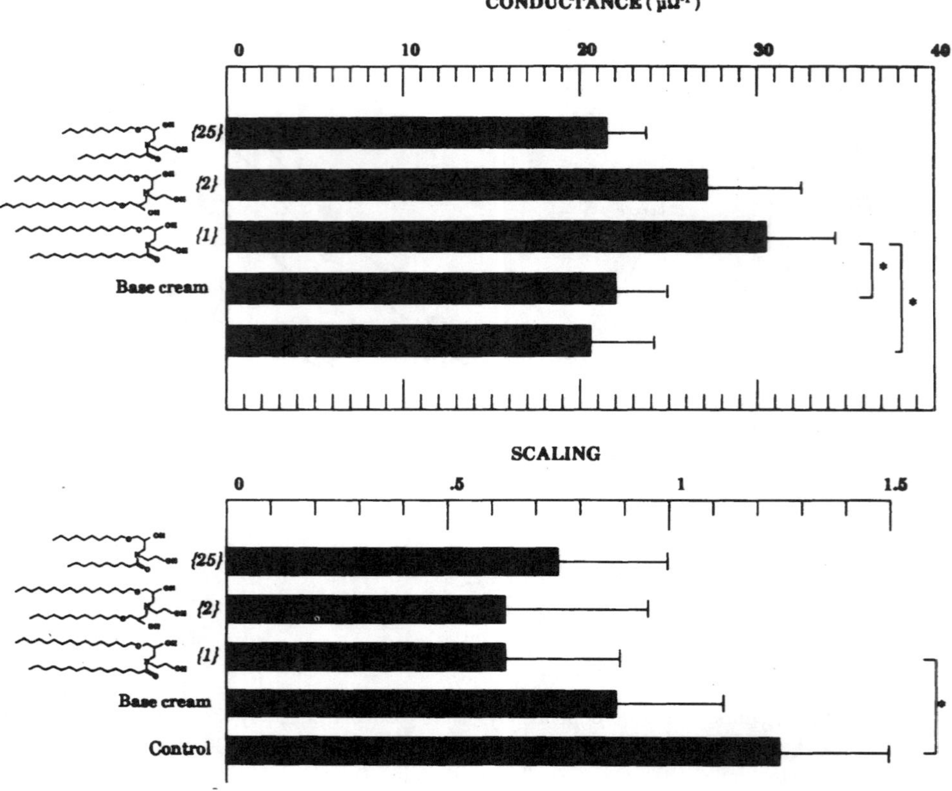

FIGURE 34 The recovery effect of synthetic pseudo-ceramides on SDS-induced dry skin. One day (day 0) following 5% SDS treatment (day –1), each pseudo-ceramide emulsified in W/O cream at 3% concentration was applied daily for 2 days. Bar represents standard error. *: $p < 0.05$ between samples and base cream or nontreated control. n = 7. (A) Evaluation by conductance measurement. Conductance was measured 24 h (day 3) after the last application of samples (day 2). (B) Evaluation by skin reaction. Scaling was evaluated 24 h (day 3) after the last application of samples (day 2).

socres indicated significant difference between the two samples. The overall sample mean for pseudo-ceramide-containing cream was significantly lower, that is, less dryer, than for the control cream. The impedance readings in another xerotic skin study using American anti-aging cream E as a control indicated that pseudo-ceramide-containing cream impedance readings on the cheek were significantly higher on study weeks 1 through 3 than those values for the control cream (Figure 37).[21]

23.4.3 Clinical Use in Atopic Dry Skin

When 8% pseudo-ceramide-containing cream was applied for 6 weeks to dry skin of forearm of atopic dermatitis patients (n = 18) in comparison with control cream excluding pseudo-ceramide which was applied to forearm skin of another arm, clinical appearances including dryness, scaling, and itching were improved, with the ceramide cream being significantly more effective than the control cream (Figure 38A).[21]

Comparison of clinical improvement between ceramide and control cream (Figure 38B) reveals that treatment with ceramide cream provides a better clinical improvement than that with control. Figure 39 shows different clinical studies applying 5% pseudo-ceramide-containing cream on the dry skin (cheek) of atopic dermatitis patients (n = 20) in Germany.[21] The treatment for 3 weeks

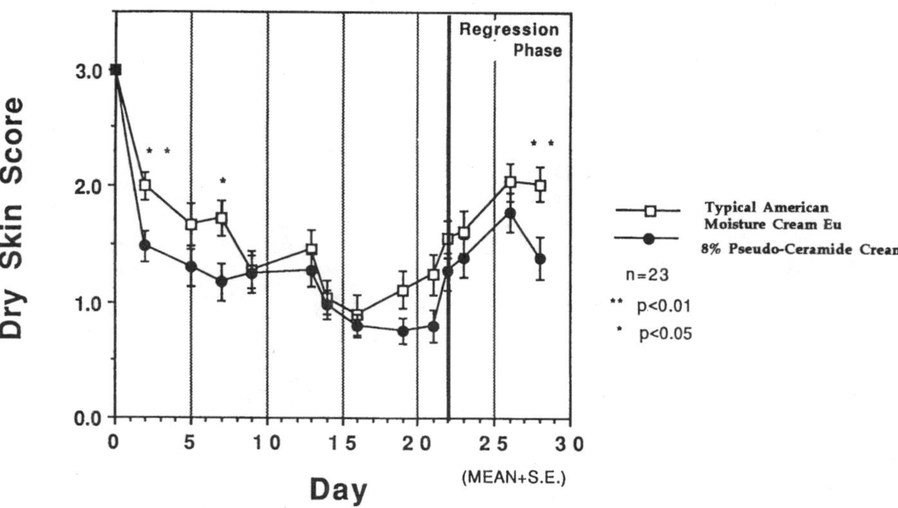

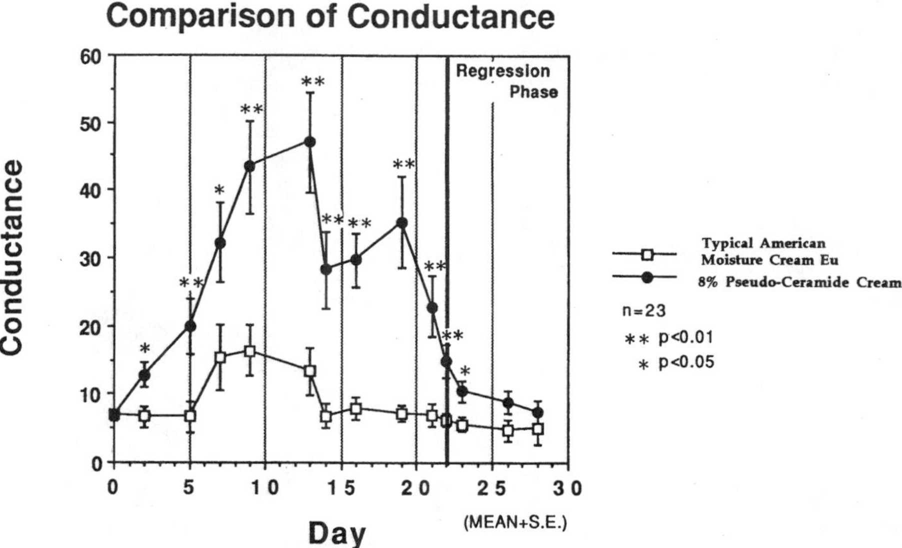

FIGURE 35 The application of 8% pseudo-ceramides cream to soap washing-induced dry skin for 28 days. Candidates with dry skin on the forearms were selected from volunteers who had undergone a 1-week conditioning period using Ivory soap exclusively on the test areas. Test materials were assigned to the right and left arms according to a predetermined randomization. Test materials were applied twice daily for 21 consecutive days. A regression period of 1 week without moisturizer use followed. On days 0, 2, 5, 7, 9, 13, 14, 16, 19, 21, 22, 23, 26, and 28 (A) visual evaluations were conducted by the same evaluator with the aid of a 7 diopter illuminated magnifying lense and (B) instrumental evaluations were done with a Skicon 200 impedence meter.

with the ceramide cream caused a marked declination in scaling with efficacy similar to 8.6% urea ointment, but urea treatment elicited some sensation side effects such as biting, burning, and redness. Consistent with clinical improvements, treatment with the ceramide cream increased water content in the skin surface to a greater extent than urea treatment. Figure 40 shows clinical data when

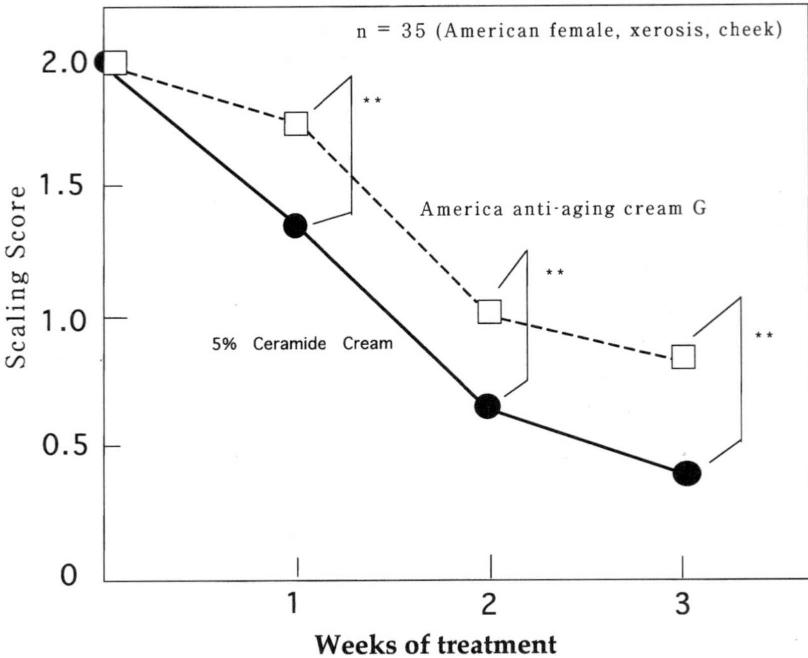

FIGURE 36 Clinical effects of 5% pseudo-ceramide cream on xerosis (cheek) in comparison with American anti-aging cream G during 3 weeks of treatment as demonstrated by scaling score. n = 35; **: $p < 0.01$.

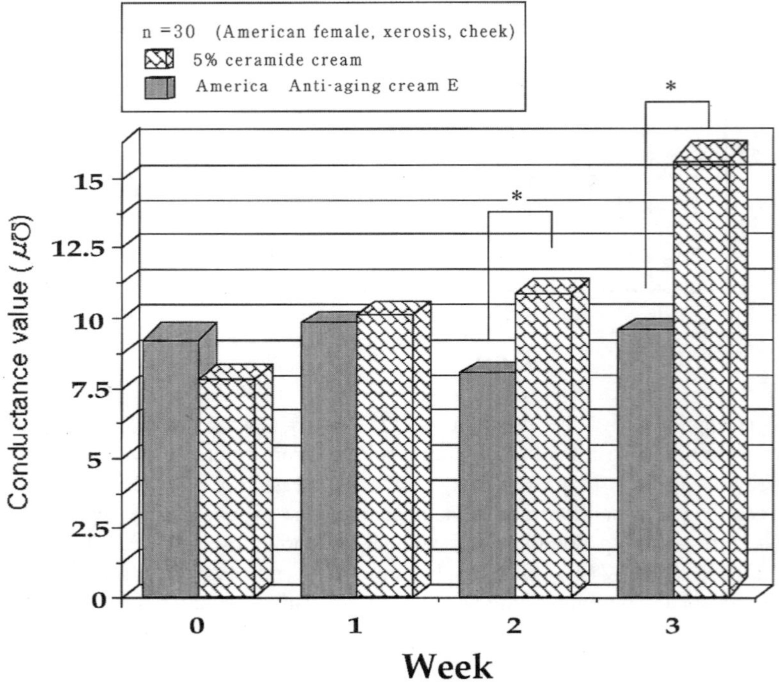

FIGURE 37 Clinical effects of 5% pseudo-ceramide cream on xerosis (cheek) in comparison with American anti-aging cream E during 3 weeks of treatment as demonstrated by conductance value. n = 30; *: $p < 0.05$.

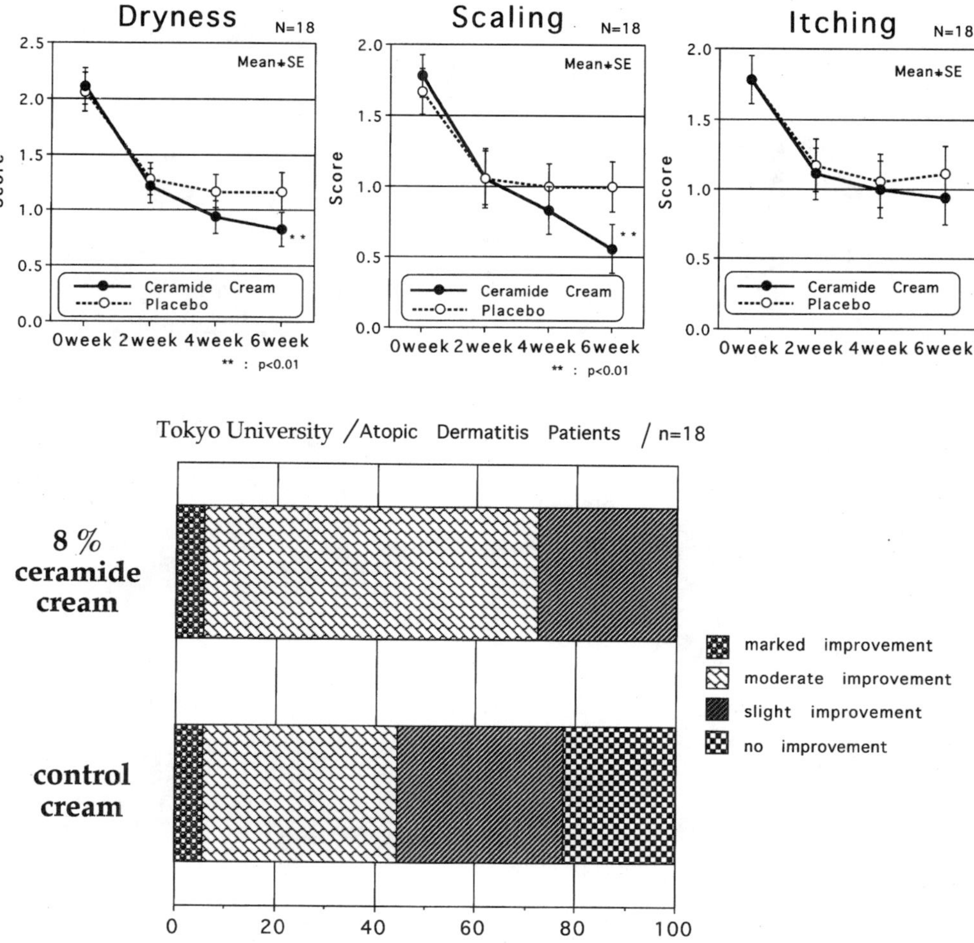

FIGURE 38 Clinical effects of 8% pseudo-ceramide cream on dry forearm skin of atopic dermatitis patients in comparison with control cream only excluding pseudoceramide as demonstrated (A) by clinical scores and (B) by comparison of clinical improvement between 8% pseudo-ceramide and control creams.

applying 8% pesudo-ceramide-containing cream for 4 weeks on dry skin of atopic dermatitis patients from different dermatological facilities in Japan.[21] Many clinical appearances were improved to the healthy control levels following 4 weeks of treatment with 8% pseudo-ceramide.

23.5 SUMMARY

After several efforts to clarify a new mechanism involved in holding water within the SC, we reached a distinct principle by which the SC acquires the capacity of retaining moisture. This is due to the intercelluar lipids comprising multilamellae which are located between the SC cells. Thus, water molecules are incorporated into the multilamella structure as a bound form which plays an essential role in retaining moisture in the SC. Ceramide is a major component of the intercellular lipids and plays a main role in generating multilamella architecture. With an idea that ceramides are an ideal moisturizer if available, we have made a great effort to synthesize various pseudo-ceramides which exhibit water-holding properties to an extent similar to natural ceramides. Since in several dry skin symptoms there is ceramide deficiency in the SC and it plays an essential role in eliciting dry skin, it is concievable that the application of pseudo-ceramides to dry skin is an

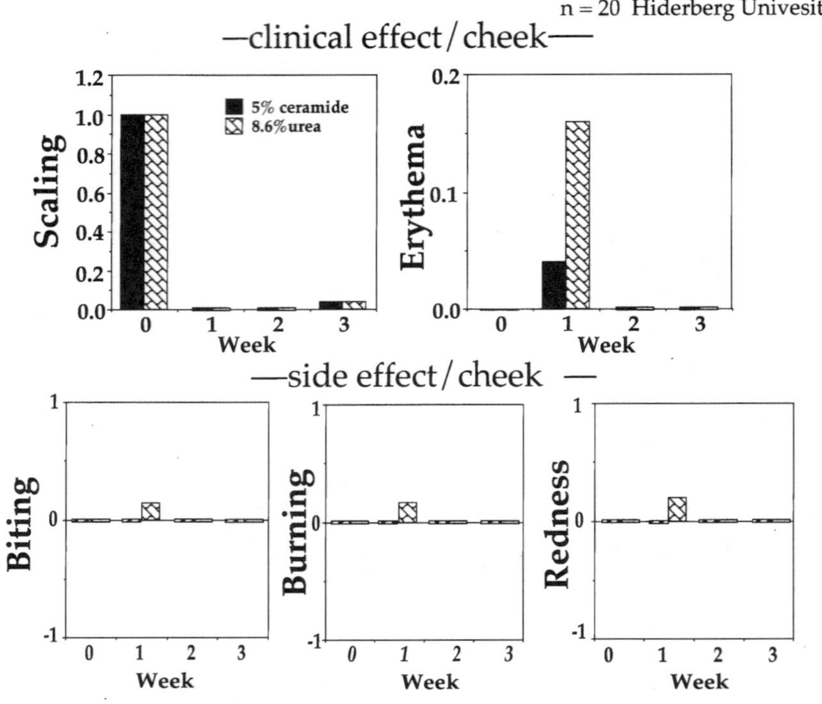

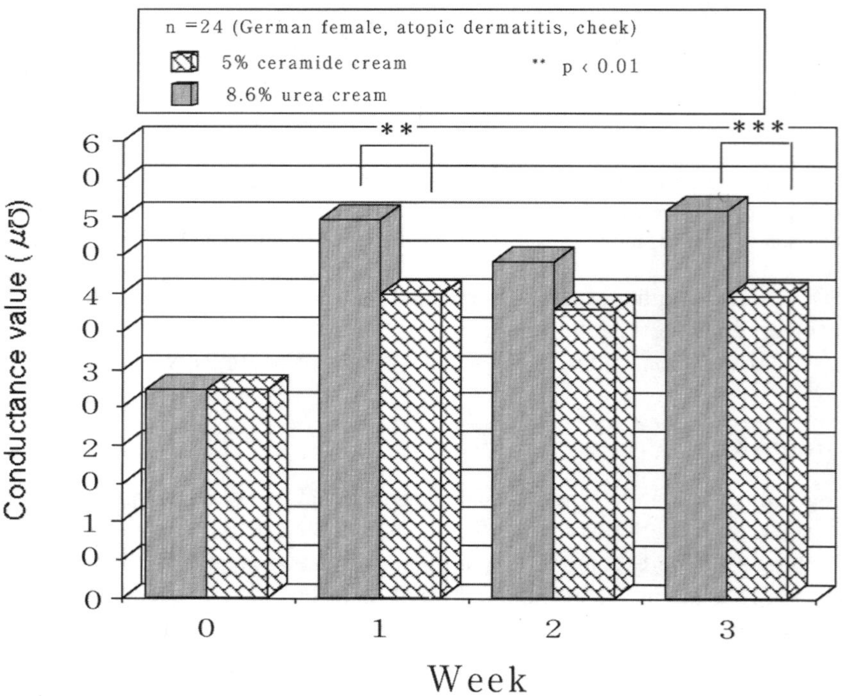

FIGURE 39 Clinical effects of 5% pseudo-ceramide cream on dry cheek skin of atopic dermatitis patients in Hiderberg University in comparison with 8.6% urea cream as demonstrated (A) by clinical scores and (B) by conductance values.

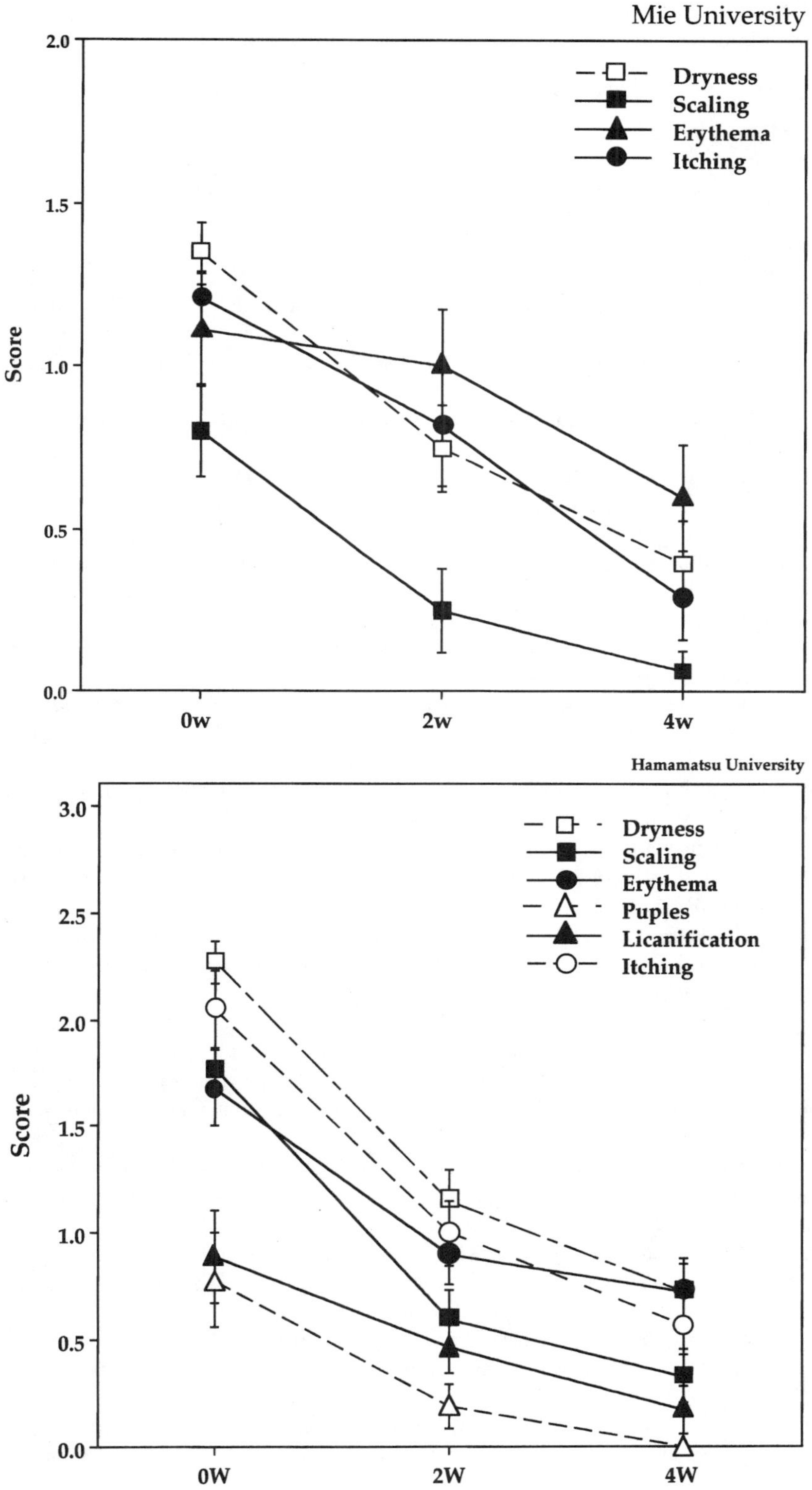

FIGURE 40 Clinical effects of 8% pseudo-ceramide cream on dry forearm skin of atopic dermatitis patients as demonstrated by clinical scores at (A) Mie University and (B) Hamamatsu University.

ideal care. Several clinical trials using pseudo-ceramide-containing cream have demonstrated that the use of pseudo-ceramide was very effective in preventing and restoring dry skin conditions.

REFERENCES

1. Jacobi, O.T. About the mechanisms of moisture regulation in the horny layer of the skin. *Proc. Sci. Sect. Goods Assoc.* 31, 22–24 (1959).
2. Imokawa, G. and Hattori, M. A possible function of structural lipid in the water-holding properties of the stratum corneum. *J. Invest. Dermatol.* 84, 282–284 (1985).
3. Imokawa, G. Stratum corneum moisturizing effect and intercellular lipids. *Fragrance J.* 15, 35–41, (1987).
4. Imokawa, G. *Intercellular Lipids of the Stratum Corneum.* Gendai Hifukagaku Taikei, Nakayama Publish Corporation, pp 43–53 (1990).
5. Imokawa, G. Properties and function of the stratum corneum lipids and its measurement. *Rinshouhifuka* 44, 583–588 (1990).
6. Imokawa, G., Akasaki, S., Minematsu, Y., and Kawai, M. Importance of intercellular lipids in water-retention properties of the stratum corneum: induction and recovery study of surfactant dry skin. *Arch. Dermatol. Res.* 281, 45–51 (1989).
7. Imokawa, G., Akasaki, S., Kuno, O., Zama, M., Kawai, M., Minematsu, Y., Hattori, M., Yoshizuka, N., Kawamata, A., Yano, S., and Takaishi, N. Function of lipids on human skin. *J. Dis. Sci. Tech.* 10, 617–641 (1989).
8. Imokawa, G., Kuno, H., and Kawai, M. Stratum corneum lipids serve as a bound-water modulator. *J. Invest. Dermatol.* 96, 845–851 (1991).
9. Imokawa, G. Water and the stratum corneum. *Bioengineering of Skin. In Vitro and in Vivo Models,* ed. by Elsner, P., Berardesca, E., Maibach, H.I. CRC Press, Boca Raton, FL, Volume 1, Chapter 3 pp 23–47 (1993).
10. Imokawa, G., Akasaki, S., Hattori, M., and Yoshizuka, N. Selective recovery of deranged water-holding properties by stratum corneum lipids. *J. Invest. Dermatol.* 87, 758–761 (1986).
11. Akasaki, S., Minematsu, Y., Yoshizuka, N., and Imokawa, G., The role of intercellular lipids in the water-holding properties of the stratum corneum: recovery effect on experimentally induced dry skin. *Jpn. J. Dermatol.* 98, 40–51 (1988).
12. Jokura, T., Ishikawa, Y., Tokuda, H., and Imokawa, G. Molecular analysis of elastic properties of the stratum corneum by solid-state ^{13}C-nuclear magnetic resonance spectroscopy. *J. Invest. Dermatol.*, 104, 806–812 (1995).
13. Akimoto, K., Yoshikawa, N., Higaki, Y., Kawashima, M., and Imokawa, G. Quantitative analysis of stratum corneum lipids in xerosis and asteatotic eczema. *J. Dermatol. (Tokyo)* 20, 1–6 (1993).
14. Imokawa, G. Atopic dermatitis and abnormality in sphingolipid metabolisms. *Lipid* 7, 428–423 (1996).
15. Imokawa, G. and Kawashima, M. Atopic dermatitis and the stratum corneum lipids. *Tokyo Tanabe Q.* 42, 41–52 (1997).
16. Imokawa, G., Abe, A., Kumi, J., Higaki, Y., Kawashima, M., and Hidano, A. Decreased level of ceramides in stratum corneum of atopic dermatitis: an etiologic factor in atopic dry skin? *J. Invest. Dermatol.* 96, 523–526 (1991).
17. Imokawa, G., Akasaki, S., Zama, M., Minematsu, Y., Kawamata, A., Yano, Y., and Takaishi, N. Selective recovery of deranged water-holding properties in the stratum corneum by synthesized pseudo-ceramide derivatives. *Proc. Jpn. Soc. Invest. Dermatol.* 12, 126–127 (1988).
18. Imokawa, G., Akasaki, S., Kawamata, A., Yano, S., and Takaishi, N. Water-retaining function in the stratum corneum and its recovery properties by synthetic pseudo-ceramides. *J. Soc. Cosmet. Chem.* 40, 273–285 (1989).
19. Imokawa, G. Function of epidermal sphingolipids and their application. *Fragrance J.* 4, 26–34 (1990).
20. Imokawa, G. Structure and function of intercellular lipids in the stratum corneum. *Yukagaku* 44, 751–766 (1995).
21. Imokawa, G. Moisturizers used in dermatology fields. *J. Clin. Dermatol.* 56, 87–96 (1998).

24 The Influence of Fatty Acids and Fatty Alcohols on Skin Permeability

Bruce J. Aungst

CONTENTS

24.1 INTRODUCTION

Long chain, saturated fatty acids and fatty alcohols are commonly used in pharmaceutical, cosmetic, or other formulations applied to the skin. Shorter chain and unsaturated fatty acids and fatty alcohols have been shown to have the potential for influencing the permeability of skin. The effects of fatty acids on skin permeability depend upon the composition of the substances applied to the skin, but in many cases these effects have been very significant. Because of their effects on skin barrier function, fatty acids and fatty alcohols have been utilized, at least experimentally, in topical and transdermal formulations specifically to modulate the permeation of drugs into or through the skin. This chapter reviews the characteristics of fatty acid and fatty alcohol effects on skin.

24.2 STRUCTURAL AND PHYSICAL CHEMICAL PROPERTIES

Fatty acids and fatty alcohols are comprised of a terminal carboxylate or alcohol group on an aliphatic hydrocarbon chain, as depicted by the general structures given below.

$CH_3(CH_2)_nCOOH$ Fatty acids

$CH_3(CH_2)_nOH$ Fatty alcohols

0-8493-7520-7/00/$0.00+$.50

The fatty acids and fatty alcohols primarily discussed in this chapter have n = 6 to 18. Fatty acids and fatty alcohols with one or more unsaturated carbon–carbon bonds have also been commonly used in skin permeation studies. The position of unsaturated groups along the hydrocarbon chain can vary. Also, the positioning around unsaturated bonds can be in the *cis* or *trans* configuration. Some structures to be discussed have additional acyl, hydroxyl, or other groups branching from the chain. Again, the position of these substituents can vary along the hydrocarbon chain. Structures and nomenclature for some of the fatty acids discussed in this chapter and in the references cited herein are given in Table 1. Fatty alcohols follow essentially the same nomenclature. Fatty acid esters, oils, glycerides, and other similar agents are discussed elsewhere in this book, as are the essential fatty acids.

Fatty acids occur in large amounts as components of lipids, but in animal and plant lipids, fatty acids are predominantly found in esterified forms. Small amounts of free fatty acids are found in sebum and epidermal tissue. The most abundant fatty acids in animals and plants have chain lengths of 14 to 22 carbons, and those with 16 or 18 carbons predominate. Unsaturated fatty acids are also common in nature. Most unsaturated fatty acids are found in the *cis* configuration.

Physical chemical properties that influence pharmaceutical applications are water solubility and melting point. Fatty acids and fatty alcohols are generally water insoluble. They are soluble in alcohol, ether, and chlorinated solvents. Melting points of saturated fatty acids and fatty alcohols increase as carbon chain length increases. For example, melting points of lauric acid, myristic acid, palmitic acid, and stearic acid are, respectively, 44, 54, 63, and 70°C. Unsaturated fatty acids have lower melting points than saturated fatty acids of the same chain length. Melting points of 18:0, 18:1, 18:2, and 18:3 fatty acids are 70, 13, –5, and –11°C, respectively. Fatty acids and fatty alcohols can be considered polar because, even though they contain a long hydrocarbon chain, they have a terminal carboxylate or hydroxyl group. Although insoluble in water, they can be spread on the water surface to form a stable monolayer. Fatty acids were shown to have very high partition coefficients ($>10^3$) from water into plasma membranes.[2]

24.3 USES AS EXCIPIENTS

Several fatty acids and fatty alcohols are commonly used as excipients in pharmaceutical and cosmetic preparations. Stearic acid is widely used in topical, as well as oral, pharmaceutical preparations, in addition to cosmetic, skin care, and shaving preparations. In topical preparations, stearic acid has emulsifying and solubilizing properties. Stearic acid is often partially neutralized with cationic excipients in the preparation of creams. This partially neutralized form results in a creamy base when mixed with 5 to 15 times its weight of aqueous liquid. Stearic acid concentrations in topical ointments and creams can range from approximately 1 to 20%. Palmitic acid, myristic acid, lauric acid, and oleic acid can also be found in various consumer products. Oleic acid is used in some eye makeup products and hair care products. Palmitic acid is utilized in eye shadows, skin cleansers, and skin moisturizers, as is myristic acid. Lauric acid can be found in some shampoos, moisturizing skin care preparations, and deodorants.

Another pair of commonly used excipients in topical products is cetyl alcohol, $CH_3(CH_2)_{14}CH_2OH$, and stearyl alcohol, $CH_3(CH_2)_{16}CH_2OH$. Cetyl alcohol gives emollient, water absorptive, and emulsifying properties to lotions, creams, and ointments. The emollient properties are thought to be due to absorption and retention of cetyl alcohol by the epidermis, where it lubricates and softens the skin. Cetyl and stearyl alcohols can also be used to improve the texture of topical formulations, increase their consistency, and enhance their stability. Cetosteryl alcohol, which is comprised of a mixture of fatty alcohols, mainly stearyl and cetyl alcohols with small amounts of other fatty alcohols, is another common excipient. It is used as an emulsifying agent and stiffening agent in cosmetics and topical pharmaceuticals.

TABLE 1
Nomenclature, Chemical Formulas, and Occurrence of Some Fatty Acids

Shorthand Name	Name	Other Names	Formula	Occurrence
6:0	Hexanoic	Caproic	$CH_3(CH_2)_4COOH$	Butter, palm oil, coconut oil
8:0	Octanoic	Caprylic	$CH_3(CH_2)_6COOH$	Butter, palm oil, coconut oil
10:0	Decanoic	Capric	$CH_3(CH_2)_8COOH$	Butter, whale oil, coconut oil
11:0	Undecanoic		$CH_3(CH_2)_9COOH$	
12:0	Lauric	Dodecanoic	$CH_3(CH_2)_{10}COOH$	Seed oils of Lauraceae
14:0	Myristic	Tetradecanoic	$CH_3(CH_2)_{12}COOH$	Widespread
16:0	Palmitic	Hexadecanoic	$CH_3(CH_2)_{14}COOH$	Widespread
18:0	Stearic	Octadecanoic	$CH_3(CH_2)_{16}COOH$	Widespread
20:0	Eicosanoic	Arachic	$CH_3(CH_2)_{18}COOH$	Seed oils, fish oils
12:1	Lauroleic	*cis*-9-Dodecenoic	$CH_3CH_2CH = CH(CH_2)_7COOH$	Butter
12:1		*cis*-5-Dodecenoic	$CH_3(CH_2)_5CH = CH(CH_2)_3COOH$	Fish oils
14:1	Myristoleic	*cis*-9-Tetradecenoic	$CH_3(CH_2)_3CH = CH(CH_2)_7COOH$	Widespread
16:1	Palmitoleic	*cis*-9-Hexadecenoic	$CH_3(CH_2)_5CH = CH(CH_2)_7COOH$	Widespread
18:1	Oleic	*cis*-9-Octadecenoic	$CH_3(CH_2)_7CH = CH(CH_2)_7COOH$	Widespread
18:1	Elaidic	*trans*-9-Octadecenoic	$CH_3(CH_2)_7CH = CH(CH_2)_7COOH$	Widespread
18:1	Vaccenic	*cis*-11-Octadecenoic	$CH_3(CH_2)_5CH = CH(CH_2)_9COOH$	Widespread
18:2	Linoleic	*cis*-9,*cis*-12-Octadecadienoic	$CH_3(CH_2)_4CH = CHCH_2CH = CH(CH_2)_7COOH$	Widespread
18:3	Linolenic	*cis*-9,*cis*-12,*cis*-15-Octadecatrienoic	$CH_3CH_2CH = CHCH_2CH = CHCH_2CH = CH(CH_2)_7COOH$	Widespread
	Isostearic	16-Methylheptadecanoic	$(CH_3)_2CH(CH_2)_{14}COOH$	Wool fat, ox fat
	Ricinoleic	12-Hydroxy-*cis*-9-octadecenoic	$CH_3(CH_2)_5CHOHCH_2CH = CH(CH_2)_7COOH$	Castor oil

Source: Adapted from Davenport, J.B. and Johnson, A.R., *Biochemistry and Methodology of Lipids,* Wiley-Interscience, New York, 1971, 1.

TABLE 2
Examples of the Effects of Fatty Acids Enhancing the Skin Permeation of Various Drugs

Permeant	Fatty Acid	Vehicle	Skin Source	Enhancement Ratio	Ref.
Acyclovir	1%, 5% Oleic acid	Propylene glycol	Human	9–166	3
p-Aminobenzoic acid	0.16 *M* Oleic acid	Propylene glycol	Human	16	4
	0.16 *M* Lauric acid	Propylene glycol	Human	3.5	4
Dihydroergotamine	6% Oleic acid	Propylene glycol	Rabbit	207	5
5-Fluorouracil	5% Oleic acid	Propylene glycol	Human	8	6
	5% Oleic acid	Propylene glycol	Hairless mouse	33	6
Hydrocortisone	5% Oleic acid	Propylene glycol	Human	84	7
Indomethacin	0.15 *M* Oleic acid	Propylene glycol	Rat	29	8
Ketoprofen	10% Oleic acid	Propylene glycol	Rat	13	9
	10% Lauric acid	Propylene glycol	Rat	46	9
Leuprolide	2% Lauric acid	Ethanol/water	Nude mouse	675	10
Mannitol	5% Oleic acid	Propylene glycol	Human	84	7
Progesterone	5% Oleic acid	Propylene glycol	Human	8	7
Testosterone	0.5 *M* Lauric acid	Propylene glycol	Human	5	11

24.4 PERMEATION ENHANCEMENT

As described in the previous section, some fatty acids and fatty alcohols are commonly used as inert ingredients in various products applied to the skin. Fatty acids and fatty alcohols may also have utility for improving the effectiveness of topically applied drugs and for transdermal systemic drug delivery, because numerous studies have shown that they can increase skin permeability to drugs. The effects of fatty acids on drug permeation through or into skin have been described in many publications. The effects of fatty alcohols have also been investigated, although less extensively. Many of these studies involve measuring diffusion rates of a drug of interest across excised skin specimens *in vitro*. In these studies fatty acids and fatty alcohols typically increase drug diffusion rates across the excised skin membranes. The effectiveness of increasing skin permeability can be expressed by calculating the ratio of diffusion rates or permeability coefficients in the presence and absence of the permeation enhancer, producing a value referred to as the enhancement ratio. Table 2 provides examples of drugs whose *in vitro* skin permeability was increased by a fatty acid. These selected examples utilize oleic acid and lauric acid, which are among the most effective and most commonly employed skin permeation enhancers. As this table shows, permeation of these drugs through skin can be increased up to several orders of magnitude in the presence of these fatty acids.

The skin permeation enhancement ratio is influenced by the fatty acid employed, the concentration used, the composition of the vehicle, the skin source studied, and the characteristics of the drug under investigation. The enhancement effect is often greatest for compounds that normally penetrate skin poorly. For example, the drugs in Table 2 subject to greatest permeation enhancement are acyclovir and dihydroergotamine, which are poorly lipophilic, and the peptide leuprolide. The variability of skin permeation from compound to compound depends upon the routes of permeation and the mechanisms of permeation enhancement, which are discussed subsequently.

Skin permeation and permeation enhancement studies using animal skin may not produce the same results as with human skin. For example, using a control vehicle, the permeability coefficients of 5-fluorouracil through human abdominal skin and hairless mouse skin were similar, but with a vehicle containing 5% oleic acid mouse skin showed an exaggerated permeability enhancement relative to human skin.[6] Hairless guinea pig skin was shown to be either more sensitive or less sensitive to permeation enhancement than human skin, depending on the formulation used.[12]

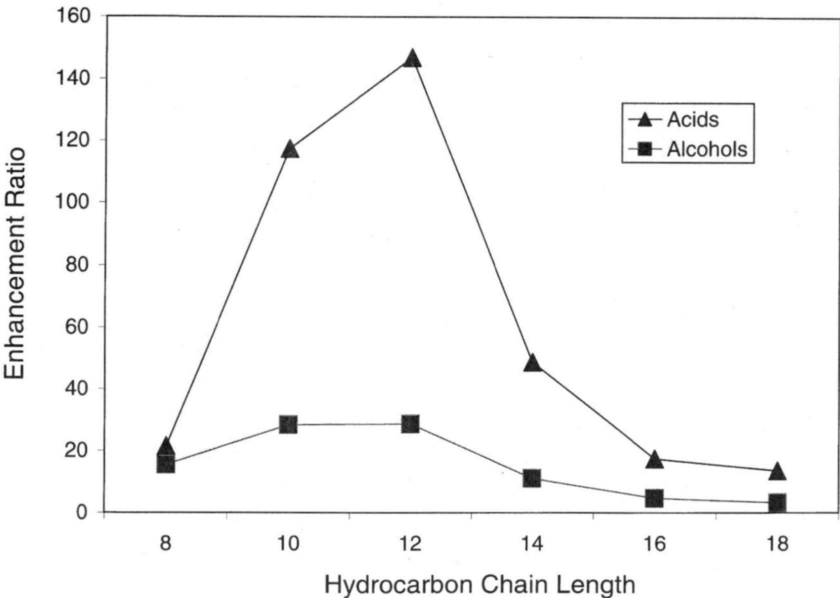

FIGURE 1 Influence of hydrocarbon chain length of saturated fatty acids and alcohols on the human skin permeation enhancement of naloxone using propylene glycol vehicles.

Therefore, caution should be exercised when extrapolating skin permeation results from animals to humans.

24.4.1 Structure/Function Relationships

The skin permeation enhancing effects of fatty acids and fatty alcohols are greatly influenced by the hydrocarbon chain length and degree of unsaturation. Several years ago our laboratory described how fatty acid and fatty alcohol structure influenced skin permeation enhancement using naloxone as the permeant.[13] We were interested in delivering naloxone transdermally at that time, and we realized that for transdermal delivery to be feasible, permeation enhancement would be required. The enhancement ratios for saturated fatty acids and fatty alcohols varied with hydrocarbon chain length. These relationships are depicted in Figure 1. Maximum permeation enhancement was observed for fatty acids of 9 to 12 carbon atoms and for fatty alcohols of 10 to 12 carbons. Tanojo et al.[4] observed a similar parabolic relationship between saturated fatty acid chain length and enhancement of *p*-aminobenzoic acid skin permeation. Permeation of molsidomine through rat skin *in vivo* also showed maximum enhancement by lauric acid when compared with other saturated fatty acids of varying chain length.[14]

Another structure vs. function relationship that has consistently been observed is that unsaturated, long chain fatty acids, C18 in particular, are more effective enhancers than are saturated fatty acids with the same number of carbon atoms. Again using our work with naloxone as an example, in the presence of stearic acid (18:0) the enhancement ratio was 14, oleic acid (18:1) had a ratio of 22, and linoleic acid (18:2) had an enhancement ratio of 64.[13] Further increases in the number of double bonds did not provide greater permeation enhancement. In a study of the effects of monounsaturated fatty acids of varying chain length, in which indomethacin permeation through excised rat skin was measured, the extent of enhancement was oleic acid ≈ palmitoleic acid > myristoleic.[15] However, these three fatty acids had similar enhancement ratios for the permeation of salicylic acid through human skin.[16] The effects of position of the double bond and conformation around the double bond (*cis* vs. *trans*) have also been the subjects of a number of investigations.[16,17]

TABLE 3
Human Skin Permeation Enhancement Ratios for Naloxone Using Various Vehicles Containing 10% Lauric Acid or 10% Lauryl Alcohol

Vehicle	Enhancement Ratio	
	Lauric Acid	Lauryl Alcohol
Propylene glycol	147	29
Isopropanol	10	1.7
PEG 400	26	6.8
Mineral oil	14	8.5
Isopropyl myristate	2.6	Not determined

Note: The enhancement ratio represents the ratio of drug flux from each vehicle in the presence and absence of the enhancer.

Source: Adapted from Aungst, B. J. et al., *Int. J. Pharm.*, 33, 225, 1986.

In the results illustrated in Figure 1, saturated fatty acids were more effective than saturated fatty alcohols of the same chain length. In other investigations, fatty acids and analogous fatty alcohols have had similar effects. Lauric acid and lauryl alcohol enhanced molsidomine permeation through rat skin approximately equally.[14] Oleyl alcohol had slightly greater effects than oleic acid on acyclovir permeation of human skin,[3] and similarly, oleyl alcohol had greater effects than oleic acid on metronidazole human skin penetration.[18]

Other fatty acid structures that have been examined as skin permeation enhancers include branched compounds. Isostearic acid, depicted in Table 1, is one example. Other fatty acids studied had branching at positions closer to the carboxylate, and some had tertiary branching. Some of these more unusual fatty acids were as effective or even more effective as skin permeation enhancers than the straight chain, saturated fatty acid with the same number of carbon atoms.[17]

24.4.2 Influence of Vehicle Composition

The skin permeation enhancing effects of fatty acids and fatty alcohols are highly dependent upon the composition of the vehicle in which they are delivered. As Table 2 shows, many investigators have utilized propylene glycol as the solvent or vehicle. Several studies have compared the permeation enhancement of fatty acids using propylene glycol vs. other vehicles and have shown propylene glycol to provide maximum permeation enhancing effects. A comparison of the effects of lauric acid and lauryl alcohol on naloxone human skin permeation using various vehicles is given in Table 3. In that report lauric acid was at least fivefold more effective when delivered using propylene glycol than with other solvents evaluated. Interestingly, studies have shown that fatty acid vehicles producing maximum skin permeation enhancing effects usually contain a fatty acid concentration <20%. Increasing the concentration of the enhancer results in lower skin permeation. The results of Nomura et al.[19] illustrate this. Indomethacin was incorporated into propylene glycol/stearyl alcohol vehicles containing various concentrations of oleic acid, and these were applied to rat skin. Plasma indomethacin AUC was determined. Indomethacin absorption was increased sixfold using 5% oleic acid, but the increase was only fourfold with 10% oleic acid and threefold with 30% oleic acid. Vehicles containing 50 and 60% oleic acid were similar to the control vehicle not containing oleic acid.

One effect fatty acids and fatty alcohols have is to increase skin permeation of the vehicle. Oleic acid was shown to increase the absorption of propylene glycol, and the greatest extent of propylene glycol absorption was with vehicles containing 5 to 10% oleic acid.[19] Polyethylene glycol 200 and glycerin were more poorly absorbed than propylene glycol, either in the presence or absence of oleic acid.[19] Penetration of the solvent into the skin can alter the skin partitioning behavior of the co-delivered fatty acid or fatty alcohol enhancer or of the drug.[20] Propylene glycol itself can have skin permeation enhancing effects.[7] So there may be synergism involved in the combination of fatty acids or fatty alcohols and propylene glycol.

24.4.3 Mechanisms of Enhancing Permeation

The stratum corneum provides the rate-limiting barrier to skin permeation. The stratum corneum is comprised of layers of flattened, dead cells, whose microscopic appearance has been likened to bricks and mortar. The cells of the stratum corneum lack recognizable organelles, but contain keratinized protein filaments. The intercellular spaces, the mortar in the brick and mortar representation, are filled with lipids. The major components of stratum corneum intercellular lipids are triglycerides, free fatty acids, ceramides, and free sterols.[21] The lipids contained in the stratum corneum have fatty acid groups primarily of 16 and 18 carbon chains, and they are primarily saturated, although some C18 groups contain one or two unsaturated positions. The intercellular lipids appear to be further organized into bilayers, with interdigitation of hydrocarbon chains forming a tight barrier to diffusion through the intercellular spaces.[22] The routes available for drug permeation through the stratum corneum are through the protein-packed keratinocytes, along a tortuous pathway around the keratinocytes through the intercellular lipids, or through the appendages. The appendages, the hair follicles, sweat glands, and sebaceous glands are generally thought to contribute little to skin permeation.

It has been proposed that skin permeation-enhancing effects generally occur via three mechanisms: (1) disruption of the barrier properties of stratum corneum lipids, (2) disruption of cellular proteins, and (3) increased partitioning from the applied vehicle into skin.[20] There is strong evidence indicating that fatty acids alter skin permeability by disrupting the packed structure of intercellular lipids. This evidence has been obtained using various physical techniques which in some way are indicative of the structure of stratum corneum lipids, including Fourier transform infrared spectroscopy (FTIR),[23] differential scanning calorimetry (DSC),[24,26] and fluorescence spectroscopy.[27] FTIR analysis of oleic acid-treated stratum corneum indicated increased motional freedom of the lipid hydrocarbon chains,[25] an effect also referred to as increased lipid fluidity. DSC measures the heat flow associated with phase transitions, and the temperatures at which certain phase transitions occur reflect the structural order of that material. DSC of treated and control stratum corneum indicated that oleic acid treatment was associated with a less ordered, more heterogeneous state of stratum corneum lipids.[25] Furthermore, there were very good correlations between the FTIR or DSC measurements of stratum corneum lipid changes and the increases in permeability to salicylic acid[25] or piroxicam.[26] In contrast to oleic acid, stearic acid treatment did not affect FTIR or DSC profiles, and it did not significantly alter permeability. Fluorescence spectroscopy involves incorporating minute quantities of a lipophilic, fluorescent probe into the membrane structure and then using fluorescence to monitor the structural organization of the membrane lipids. Fluorescence spectroscopy also showed that oleic acid treatment of stratum corneum alters the packing order of intercellular lipids, and the magnitude of those changes also was correlated with increases in permeability to benzoic acid.[27]

The aforementioned influence of fatty acid and fatty alcohol structure on skin permeation-enhancing effects is consistent with a mechanism of disruption of intercellular lipid order. In various studies, maximum skin permeation enhancement has been seen with 10:0 and 12:0 fatty acids and fatty alcohols and with unsaturated C18 hydrocarbons. The hydrocarbon chains of stratum corneum lipids primarily have chain lengths of 16 or more carbons and are mostly saturated. These long, saturated hydrocarbon chains pack tightly together to form bilayer structures. Unsaturated hydrocarbons such as oleic acid may disrupt the packed structure of intercellular lipids because of the incorporation of its kinked structure, the kink arising from *cis* double bonds. Studies with model lipid membranes indicate that packed lipid structures comprised of long, saturated hydrocarbon chains are disrupted by the incorporation of shorter, saturated hydrocarbons. So it can be reasoned that the effects of 10:0 and 12:0 hydrocarbons on stratum corneum lipids are through a similar disruption of intercellular lipid structure.

It has also been proposed that some fatty acids such as oleic acid can incorporate into the stratum corneum lipids heterogeneously, as a separate phase or in pools, creating defects in the barrier structure.[26,28] Water or solvent may then associate within these barrier defects. This proposed mechanism could explain why fatty acids most significantly increased the skin permeabilities of ionized compounds. Thermal analysis supported the proposal for unsaturated fatty acids forming separate domains within the intercellular lipids, but there was no evidence for this mechanism for medium chain, saturated fatty acids.[4]

Some investigators have suggested that oleic acid can cause extraction of lipids from the skin. This could create a void in the membrane allowing the permeation of drugs or solvents. Oleic acid in an ethanol vehicle applied to human stratum corneum led to FTIR and DSC changes suggestive of lipid extraction, in addition to increased disorder of lipid hydrocarbon chains.[29] However, other investigators have found no evidence for lipid extraction following oleic acid treatment.

Another possible mechanism for increasing skin permeation could be to alter the packed intracellular proteins and increase diffusion through the keratinocytes. Solvents such as DMSO and some surfactants probably increase skin permeability, at least partly, via this mechanism. The various studies having evaluated fatty acid effects on intracellular proteins and intercellular lipids have concluded that fatty acids affect the lipids and do not affect stratum corneum proteins. In one study[8] there was evidence that oleic acid, applied in propylene glycol, induced a conformational change in keratinized proteins. However, propylene glycol alone also caused a similar conformational change.

The third general mechanism for increasing skin permeation is to increase the partitioning of the permeant from the vehicle into the skin. One way for fatty acids to increase skin partitioning is through an acid-base ion pairing mechanism. Transport of cationic compounds across an isopropyl myristate membrane was enhanced by the presence of fatty acids within the membrane.[30] For some compounds, there was a close association between the amounts of drug and fatty acid permeating skin, suggesting that they permeate together. This was the case with thiamine disulfide and lauric acid permeation of rat skin.[31] Skin penetration of the vehicle is also an important factor, in that the vehicle can increase skin permeation of solutes via a solvent drag mechanism. There have been studies in which solute and solvent appeared to permeate into skin simultaneously. For example, molsidomine skin permeation using propylene glycol vehicles containing varying concentrations of oleic acid was correlated with the skin permeation of propylene glycol.[32] As mentioned previously, fatty acids can increase skin permeation of the solvent used as the vehicle. This can enhance the skin permeation of dissolved solutes by solvent drag, or in some cases the solvent might have separate barrier disrupting properties.

24.5 SAFETY

Fatty acids can be damaging to skin. Rabbits treated with 10% oleic acid in propylene glycol for 18 h developed exfoliation of the stratum corneum, although shorter times of exposure were less damaging.[33] A rabbit irritation test was performed using topical treatment of various fatty acids in propylene glycol for 6 h, and in that report lauric and oleic acids had low-to-moderate irritation potential, using erythema and edema as end points.[17] Of particular interest from that study was the suggestion that it may be possible to identify fatty acids with effective skin permeation-enhancing properties which affect skin without apparently damaging it. In an irritation test in nude mice using aqueous vehicles, 10% oleic acid caused severe irritation, but 10% oleyl alcohol produced no discernible histological changes,[34] suggesting that fatty alcohols might be a safer alternative to fatty acids. Oleic acid was also evaluated in guinea pigs, with 5% producing significant epidermal damage, but 1% having relatively little effect.[35] Various fatty acids have been examined in humans using laser Doppler velocimetry (LDV), which is an alternative to visual scoring of irritation.[36] Fatty acids were applied for 3 h under occlusion, using 0.16 *M* concentrations in propylene glycol. Saturated fatty acids of 6 to 12 carbons produced no indication of irritation by LDV. Oleic acid resulted in an elevated LDV score and visible erythema and edema.

A consequence of enhanced skin permeability and/or toxicity with fatty acids is increased transdermal water loss (TEWL). TEWL was slightly elevated in humans dosed with 0.16 *M* lauric acid in propylene glycol for 3 hours, and propylene glycol alone also slightly elevated TEWL.[36] Oleic acid and other unsaturated fatty acids caused much greater increases in TEWL under the same conditions. Similar results were observed using human keratinocyte cultures, referred to as a human skin equivalent, as the membrane. Lauric acid caused a slight increase in TEWL and had no effect on LDV, whereas oleic acid had much more significant effects on both end points.[37] Elevations in TEWL were also seen in humans treated with pure oleic acid or with lauric acid applied in acetone.[38] Water permeability through human stratum corneum has been correlated with physical changes of stratum corneum, measured using FTIR, similar to those associated with fatty acid treatments.[39] The intercellular lipids have an important function in maintaining the barrier to water permeation through skin and for holding water in skin, and removal of intercellular lipids produced chapped and scaly skin.[40]

24.6 CONCLUSIONS

Fatty acids and fatty alcohols clearly can change the properties of the intercellular lipids of the stratum corneum. Medium chain, saturated hydrocarbons or longer chain, unsaturated hydrocarbons are most effective. At the extreme, skin permeability to drugs can be increased tremendously, and this result may be desired for improving transdermal or topical drug delivery. But those changes induced in the skin may result in water loss and dry and possibly irritated skin. There are presently no pharmaceutical products on the market in which the most effective fatty acids are used specifically for their skin penetration enhancing effects. Most of the literature on the mechanisms of skin permeation enhancement and toxicity of fatty acids has dealt with oleic acid and lauric acid. It may be possible to identify other fatty acids or fatty alcohols which only moderately affect skin permeability and which may be more acceptable for everyday use. These could then be more useful for enhancing transdermal or topical drug delivery or in topical formulations for other uses.

REFERENCES

1. Davenport, J. B. and Johnson, A. R., The nomenclature and classification of lipids, in *Biochemistry and Methodology of Lipids*, Johnson, A. R. and Davenport, J. B., Eds., Wiley-Interscience, New York, 1971, 1.
2. Pjura, W. J., Kleinfeld, A. M. and Karnovsky, M. J., Partition of fatty acids and fluorescent fatty acids into membranes, *Biochemistry*, 23, 2039, 1984.
3. Cooper, E. R., Merritt, E. W. and Smith, R. L., Effect of fatty acids and alcohols on the penetration of acyclovir across human skin *in vitro*, *J. Pharm. Sci.*, 74, 688, 1985.
4. Tanojo, H., Bouwstra, J. A., Junginger, H. E. and Bodde, H. E., *In vitro* human skin barrier modulation by fatty acids: skin permeation and thermal analysis studies, *Pharm. Res.*, 14, 42, 1997.
5. Niazy, E. M., Influence of oleic acid and other permeation promoters on transdermal delivery of dihydroergotamine through rabbit skin, *Int. J. Pharm.*, 67, 97, 1991.

6. Bond, J. R. and Barry, B. W., Hairless mouse skin is limited as a model for assessing the effects of penetration enhancers in human skin, *J. Invest. Dermatol.*, 90, 810, 1988.
7. Barry, B. W. and Bennett, S. L., Effect of penetration enhancers on the permeation of mannitol, hydrocortisone and progesterone through human skin, *J. Pharm. Pharmacol.,* 39, 535, 1987.
8. Takeuchi, Y., Yasukawa, H., Yamaoka, Y., Kato, Y., Morimoto, Y., Fukumori, Y. and Fukuda, T., Effects of fatty acids, fatty amines and propylene glycol on rat stratum corneum lipids and proteins *in vitro* measured by Fourier transform infrared/attenuated total reflection (F-IR/ATR) spectroscopy, *Chem. Pharm. Bull.,* 40, 1887, 1992.
9. Kim, C. K., Kim, J.-J., Chi, S.-C. and Shim, C.-K., Effect of fatty acids and urea on the penetration of ketoprofen through rat skin, *Int. J. Pharm.,* 99, 109, 1993.
10. Lu, M. F., Lee, D. and Rao, G. S., Percutaneous absorption enhancement of leuprolide, *Pharm. Res.,* 9, 1575, 1992.
11. Aungst, B. J., Blake, J. A. and Hussain, M. A., Contributions of drug solubilization, partitioning, barrier disruption, and solvent permeation to the enhancement of skin permeation of various compounds with fatty acids and amines, *Pharm. Res.,* 7, 712, 1990.
12. Aungst, B. J., Blake, J. A., Rogers, N. J. and Hussain, M. A., Transdermal oxymorphone formulation development and methods for evaluating flux and lag times for two skin permeation-enhancing vehicles, *J. Pharm. Sci.,* 79, 1072, 1990.
13. Aungst, B. J., Rogers, N. J. and Shefter, E., Enhancement of naloxone penetration through human skin *in vitro* using fatty acids, fatty alcohols, surfactants, sulfoxides and amides, *Int. J. Pharm.,* 33, 225, 1986.
14. Yamada, M. and Uda, Y., Enhancement of percutaneous absorption of molsidomine, *Chem. Pharm. Bull.,* 35, 3390, 1987.
15. Morimoto, K., Tojima, H., Haruta, T., Suzuki, M. and Kakemi, M., Enhancing effects of unsaturated fatty acids with various structures on the permeation of indomethacin through rat skin, *J. Pharm. Pharmacol.,* 48, 1133, 1996.
16. Cooper, E. R., Increased skin permeability for lipophilic molecules, *J. Pharm. Sci.,* 73, 1153, 1984.
17. Aungst, B. J., Structure/effect studies of fatty acid isomers as skin penetration enhancers and skin irritants, *Pharm. Res.,* 6, 244, 1989.
18. Hoelgaard, A., Mollgaard, B. and Baker, E., Vehicle effect on topical drug delivery. IV. Effect of N-methylpyrrolidone and polar lipids on percutaneous drug transport, *Int. J. Pharm.,* 43, 233, 1988.
19. Nomura, H., Kaiho, F., Sugimoto, Y., Miyashita, Y., Dohi, M. and Kato, Y., Percutaneous absorption of indomethacin from mixtures of fatty alcohol and propylene glycol (FAPG bases) through rat skin: effects of oleic acid added to FAPG base, *Chem. Pharm. Bull.,* 38, 1421, 1990.
20. Goodman, M. and Barry, B. W., Lipid-protein-partitioning (LPP) theory of skin enhancer activity: finite dose technique, *Int. J. Pharm.,* 57, 29, 1989.
21. Elias, P. M., Structure and function of the stratum corneum permeability barrier, *Drug Develop. Res.,* 13, 97, 1988.
22. Downing, D. T., Lipid and protein structures in the permeability barrier of mammalian epidermis, *J. Lipid Res.,* 33, 301, 1992.
23. Ongpipattanakul, B., Burnette, R. R., Potts, R. O. and Francoeur, M. L., Evidence that oleic acid exists in a separate phase within stratum corneum lipids, *Pharm. Res.*, 8, 350, 1991.
24. Takeuchi, Y., Yasukawa, H., Yamaoka, Y., Takahashi, N., Tamura, C., Morimoto, Y., Fukushima, S. and Vasavada, R. C., Effects of oleic acid/propylene glycol on rat abdominal stratum corneum: lipid extraction and appearance of propylene glycol in the dermis measured by Fourier transform infrared/attenuated total reflectance (FT-IR/ATR) spectroscopy, *Chem. Pharm. Bull.,* 41, 1434, 1993.
25. Golden, G. M., McKie, J. E. and Potts, R. O., Role of stratum corneum lipid fluidity in transdermal drug flux, *J. Pharm. Sci.,* 76, 25, 1987.
26. Francoeur, M. L., Golden, G. M. and Potts, R. O., Oleic acid: its effects on stratum corneum in relation to (trans)dermal drug delivery, *Pharm. Res.*, 7, 621, 1990.
27. Garrison, M. D., Doh, L. M., Potts, R. O. and Abraham, W., Effect of oleic acid on human epidermis: fluorescence spectroscopic investigation, *J. Contr. Rel.,* 31, 263, 1994.
28. Walker, M. and Hadgraft, J., Oleic acid — a membrane 'fluidizer' or fluid within the membrane?, *Int. J. Pharm.,* 71, R1, 1991.

29. Clancy, M. J., Corish, J. and Corrigan, O. I., A comparison of the effects of electrical current and penetration enhancers on the properties of human skin using spectroscopic (FTIR) and calorimetric (DSC) methods, *Int. J. Pharm.,* 105, 47, 1994.
30. Green, P. G., Hadgraft, J. and Ridout, G., Enhanced *in vitro* skin permeation of cationic drugs, *Pharm. Res.,* 6, 628, 1989.
31. Komata, Y., Kaneko, A. and Fujie, T., Accumulation of lauric acid in skin as an enhancer for the percutaneous absorption of thiamine disulfide, *Biol. Pharm. Bull.,* 18, 791, 1995.
32. Yamada, M., Uda, Y. and Tanigawara, Y., Mechanism of enhancement of percutaneous absorption of molsidomine by oleic acid, *Chem. Pharm. Bull.*, 35, 3399, 1987.
33. Hsu, L.-R., Tsai, Y.-H. and Huang, Y.-B., The effect of pretreatment by penetration enhancers on the *in vivo* percutaneous absorption of piroxicam from its gel form in rabbits, *Int. J. Pharm.,* 71, 193, 1991.
34. Lashmar, U. T., Hadgraft, J. and Thomas, N., Topical application of penetration enhancers to the skin of nude mice: a histopathological study, *J. Pharm. Pharmacol.*, 41, 118, 1989.
35. Meshulam, Y., Kadar, T., Wengier, A., Dachir, S. and Levy, A., Transdermal penetration of physostigmine: effects of oleic acid enhancer, *Drug Develop. Res.,* 28, 510, 1993.
36. Tanojo, H., Boelsma, E., Junginger, H. E., Ponec, M. and Bodde, H. E., *In vivo* human skin barrier modulation by topical application of fatty acids, *Skin Pharmacol. Appl. Skin Physiol.,* 11, 87, 1998.
37. Boelsma, E., Tanojo, H., Bodde, H. E. and Ponec, M., An *in vivo-in vitro* study of the use of a human skin equivalent for irritancy screening of fatty acids, *Toxicol. In Vitro*, 11, 365, 1997.
38. Green, P. G., Guy, R. H. and Hadgraft, J., *In vitro* and *in vivo* enhancement of skin permeation with oleic and lauric acids, *Int. J. Pharm.,* 48, 103, 1988.
39. Potts, R. O. and Francoeur, M. L., Lipid biophysics of water loss through the skin, *Proc. Natl. Acad. Sci. U.S.A.,* 87, 3871, 1990.
40. Imokawa, G. and Hattori, M., A possible function of structural lipids in the water-holding properties of the stratum corneum, *J. Invest. Dermatol.*, 84, 282, 1985.

25 Essential Fatty Acids

Lesley E. Rhodes

CONTENTS

25.1 INTRODUCTION

Burr and Burr reported in 1929 on "a new deficiency disease produced by the rigid exclusion of fat from the diet."[1] Rodents fed a fat-free diet showed reduced growth and reproductive failure, accompanied by two prominent changes in the skin: increased scaliness and impaired barrier function, evident as increased water consumption without increase in urine output.[1,2] The reversal of the features of deficiency by administration of linoleic acid led to the concept of essential fatty acids (EFA) that cannot be synthesized by the higher animals.[2] Similarities between the clinical features of EFA deficiency and atopic dermatitis led Hansen in 1937 to discover low blood levels of unsaturated fat in atopic children,[3] and he later reported that EFA-deficient infants developed an eczematous rash which responded to linoleic acid supplements.[4] Several early studies examined a range of dietary oil supplements in atopic dermatitis,[5-8] with generally reported benefit.

There are now recognized to be two families of EFA, the n-6 and the n-3 fatty acids, derived from linoleic acid and α-linolenic acid, respectively. Whereas attention previously focused on the effects of EFA deficiency on the skin, principally the lack of linoleic acid and its metabolites, interest has shifted to the physiological changes in the skin induced by altered EFA status. The n-6 fatty acids are more abundant and more active in the skin than n-3 fatty acids, but the essential role of the latter in neurological development is established,[9] and there is growing recognition of their function in skin as modulators of inflammation and the immune response. The EFA influence skin physiology and pathology via their effects on skin barrier function, eicosanoid production, membrane

0-8493-7520-7/00/$0.00+$.50

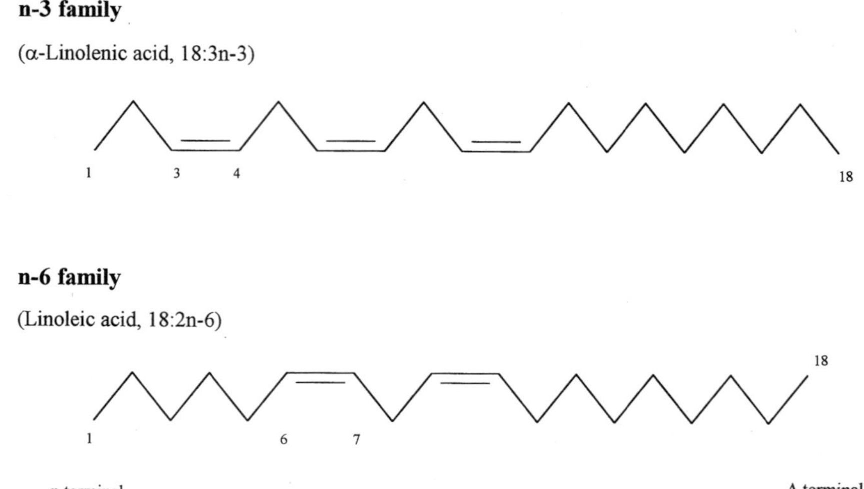

FIGURE 1 Chemical structure of α-linolenic (n-3 fatty acid) and linoleic acids (n-6 fatty acid).

fluidity, and cell signaling and have recently been recognized to alter expression of genes for cell growth and several enzymes.[10]

25.2 CLASSIFICATION AND NOMENCLATURE

Three major families of unsaturated fatty acids are seen in warm-blooded animals, i.e., the n-9, monounsaturated fatty acids, and the n-6 and n-3, both polyunsaturated fatty acids (PUFA). However, only the n-6 and n-3 families, derived from linoleic and α-linolenic acids, respectively, are EFA. These must be obtained from the diet since mammals lack the desaturase enzymes necessary for the insertion of a double bond in the n-6 and n-3 positions of the fatty acid carbon chain.

Fatty acid nomenclature is as follows. The first number denotes the number of carbon atoms in the acyl chain, and the second number refers to the number of unsaturated (double) bonds. This is followed by a symbol n or ω and a number which denotes the number of carbon atoms from the methyl terminal of the molecule to the first double bond. Hence, linoleic acid is 18:2n-6, while the more unsaturated α-linolenic acid is denoted as 18:3n-3 (Figure 1). These fatty acids must be metabolized to their longer chain derivatives before carrying out many of their activities.

25.3 DIETARY SOURCES

Linoleic and α-linolenic acids are mainly obtained from PUFA-rich vegetable oils. Linoleic acid is found in high concentrations in several oils including safflower, corn, and soybean, while α-linolenic acid is found in linseed, canola, and soya bean.[11] While most of the n-6 requirement is obtained from dietary linoleic acid, small amounts of its longer chain metabolite arachidonic acid (AA) may be ingested from food of animal origin, particularly meat, liver, and egg yolk. In contrast, the longer chain n-3 fatty acids eicosapentaenoic acid (EPA) and docosahexaenoic acid (DHA) are found mainly in oily fish and marine animals.

25.4 ESSENTIAL FATTY ACID CONTENT OF SKIN

The EFA are found predominantly within the epidermal phospholipids (e.g., phosphatidylinositol, phosphatidylcholine, phosphatidylethanolamine), with the pattern of incorporation varying between

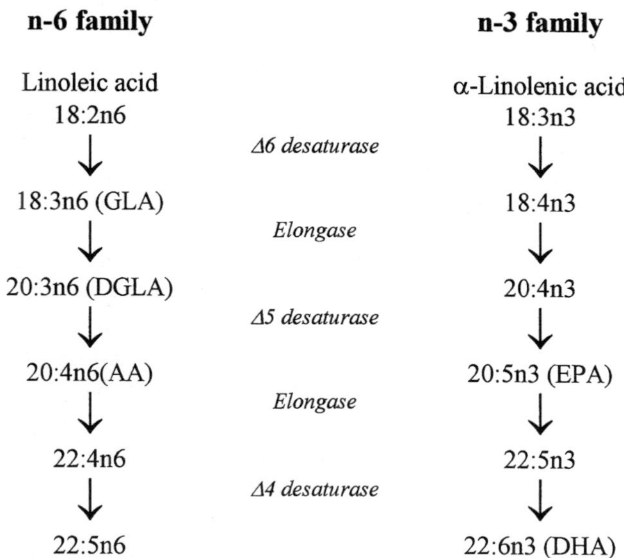

FIGURE 2 Metabolic conversion of linoleic acid and α-linolenic acid to longer chain, more unsaturated fatty acids.

fatty acids. They are also present in small amounts in cholesterol and, importantly, are found linked with ceramides in the granular layer and stratum corneum, where they play a critical role in barrier function. The most abundant EFA in the skin are linoleic acid and its metabolite AA, comprising approximately 12 and 3.5%, respectively, of human epidermal fatty acids.[12]

25.5 METABOLISM OF ESSENTIAL FATTY ACIDS

The metabolism of linoleic and α-linolenic acids involves an alternating sequence of desaturation and elongation to produce longer chain, more unsaturated fatty acids, including AA (20:4n-6), derived from linoleic acid, and EPA (20:5n-3) and DHA (22:6n-3), from α-linolenic acid (Figure 2). The desaturations and elongations all take place near the carboxy terminal (Δ) of the chain, allowing the methyl terminal to preserve its relationship to the first double bond. Hence, in mammals there is no interconversion between the n-3 and n-6 fatty acids. Fatty acids of the n-3, n-6, and n-9 families compete for the same enzymes, and there is preferential desaturation in the order α-linolenic acid > linoleic acid > oleic acid. Thus, the ratio of 20:3n-9 (an oleic acid metabolite) to 20:4n-6, known as the triene-tetraene ratio, is used to assess for deficiency of n-6 and n-3 fatty acids, indicated by a ratio of >0.2. The initial step in the metabolism of linoleic acid and α-linolenic acid to the longer chain fatty acids is the rate-limiting Δ6-desaturase, whose activity is altered by several hormonal and dietary factors.[13]

EFA metabolism is presented in several extensive reviews.[9,14,15] Much of the information concerning EFA physiology and biochemistry has been derived from work in hepatocytes and may be of limited relevance to epidermis, since a major role of the liver is to convert dietary lipids into energy stores. Meanwhile, keratinocytes are involved in the fatty acid metabolism required both for normal cellular processes and the specialized role in the permeability barrier. Unlike the liver, the epidermis does not possess the capacity to desaturate at the Δ5 or Δ6 position,[16] and, therefore, the skin relies on a supply of AA from the circulation, in addition to systemic linoleic acid and α-linolenic acid. There is evidence for a distinct fatty acid binding protein in keratinocyte plasma membranes which is involved in EFA uptake into the skin and also recycling of free fatty acids from the stratum corneum.[17] The transport mechanism in epidermis differs from that in hepatocytes since there is preferential uptake of linoleic acid over oleic acid, which may function to ensure adequate capture of linoleic acid for barrier lipid synthesis.[17]

25.6 FUNCTIONS OF ESSENTIAL FATTY ACIDS IN THE SKIN

25.6.1 Cutaneous Barrier Function

A major role of the skin is to provide an effective barrier against excessive water loss. Increased transepidermal water loss (TEWL), together with scaling and epidermal hyperplasia, are early features of EFA deficiency. It appears that the hyperplasia is at least partly driven by the barrier defect.[18] While administration of linoleic acid restores barrier function and reduces the scaling and epidermal hyperproliferation,[19,20] AA reduces the hyperproliferation, but does not improve barrier function.[21] There is now good evidence that the impaired epidermal barrier is due to the loss of unusual linoleate-containing ceramides from the stratum corneum.

The structure of the permeability barrier is ascribed to sheets of stacked lipid bilayers (lamellae) surrounding the corneocytes in the stratum corneum. These lamellae are rich in ceramides (sphingolipids), in which linoleic acid is the most abundant unsaturated fatty acid.[22] The presence of lamellar bodies, from which the lipid lamellae are derived, is closely associated with the presence of water barrier function, and abnormal lamellar body function is seen in linoleic acid deficiency.[23,24] If young animals are raised on n-6 fatty acid-deficient diets, the lack of linoleic acid results in decreased formation of linoleic acid-rich ceramides.[21]

Evidence suggests that linoleic acid-linked acylglucosylceramides, present in the upper layer of the viable epidermis, are essential for the formation of lamellar granules and for the subsequent assembly of their contents into lamellae.[25,26] In linoleic acid deficiency, the fatty acid is replaced in the ceramide molecule by oleic acid, causing conformational changes which result in the inability to form normal lamellae associated with loss of epidermal barrier.[27] Extrusion of the lamellar granule contents into the stratum corneum is accompanied by removal of the glucose from acylglucosylceramides, resulting in the formation of linoleic acid-linked acylceramides, which are abundant in the lipid lamellae of the stratum corneum.[28] There is evidence that the linoleyl moiety of the acylceramide is further metabolized by lipoxygenase before the barrier function is exhibited,[29] and it is likely that the oxidated metabolite of linoleic acid involved is 13-hydroxyoctadecadienoic acid (13-HODE).[15] 13-HODE also reverses epidermal hyperproliferation, possibly by inhibiting protein kinase C activity.[15]

25.6.2 Production of Eicosanoids

EFA are the precursors of the eicosanoids, namely, prostaglandins, leukotrienes, and hydroxy fatty acids. These important extracellular mediators have critical roles in the inflammatory process and the regulation of cell proliferation and may be involved in epidermal carcinogenesis.[15] Arachidonic acid (AA) is converted into a range of potent mediators (Figure 3), and, in many respects, the n-3 metabolites can be regarded as partial agonists of the n-6 eicosanoids, often producing similar, but less intense reactions.[14]

The EFA stored in the phospholipids of cell membranes are released by phospholipases and then undergo oxidative transformation by the cyclooxygenase (COX) pathway to prostanoids and by the lipoxygenase pathway to hydroxy fatty acids and leukotrienes. The metabolism to prostanoids is catalyzed by two isoenzymes of COX, a constitutive and an inducible form. The main products of COX metabolism of AA are prostaglandin E_2 (PGE_2), $PGF_{2\alpha}$, and PGD_2. In addition, AA is converted via 15-lipoxygenase to 15-hydroxyeicosatetraenoic acid (15-HETE); by 12-lipoxygenase to 12-HETE; and by the 5-lipoxygenase pathway to leukotriene B_4 (LTB_4), LTC_4, and LTD_4.[15] While many of the oxidative metabolites of AA have potent pro-inflammatory actions, including leukocyte chemoattraction by LTB_4 and 12-HETE and vasodilatation by PGE_2, others such as

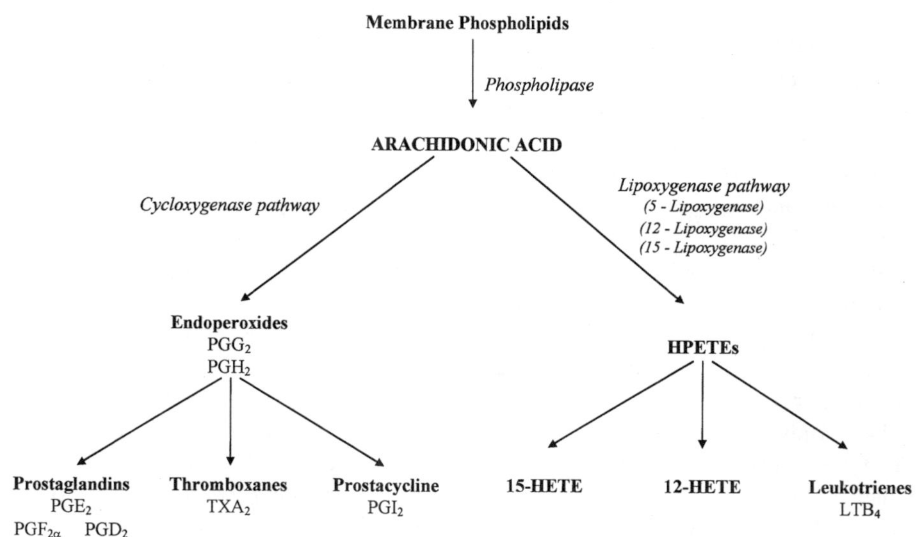

FIGURE 3 Metabolism of AA via the cycloxygenase and lipoxygenase pathways.

15-HETE have anti-inflammatory potential. The parent n-6 fatty acid linoleic acid can also be metabolized directly by COX and lipoxygenase to 9-HODE and 13-HODE,[30] respectively.

The fatty acids of the n-6 series and n-3 series compete with each other for metabolism by COX and lipoxygenase to eicosanoids. While AA is converted to potent inflammatory mediators, namely, PG of the 2 series and lipoxygenase metabolites LTB_4 and 12-HETE, EPA is metabolized to the less inflammatory PG of the 3 series and LTB_5.[14,31] Moreover, a rise in dietary γ-linolenic acid (GLA, 18:3n-6) causes increased production of dihommogammalinolenic acid (DGLA, 20:3n-6), which while being a precursor of AA in the liver and other tissues, also competes with AA for metabolism. Conversion of DGLA by COX and lipoxygenase results in the production of the anti-inflammatory PG of the 1 series,[32] containing one double bond, and 15-hydroxyeicosatrienoic acid (15-HETrE), a potent lipoxygenase inhibitor.[33]

Dietary fatty acid modification has been found to have a profound influence on epidermal fatty acid composition and subsequent eicosanoid production.[34-36] Human supplementation studies with n-3 fatty acids taken as Maxepa® (Seven Seas, Hull, U.K.; 18% EPA, 12% DHA) 10 g daily for 3 months resulted in an increase in epidermal n-3 fatty acids from <2 to >24% of total fatty acids, with a consequent increase in the n-3 to n-6 ratio.[35] Subsequently, this dietary regime was shown to result in a 70% reduction in suction blister fluid PGE_2 levels, and this was associated with a reduced erythemal (sunburn) response to UVB challenge.[36] In guinea pigs, dietary evening primrose oil (EPO) supplements, which are rich in GLA, caused a significant rise in epidermal DGLA content, accompanied by increased generation of PGE_1 and 15-HETrE.[37,38]

25.6.3 Modulation of Cell Signaling

Membrane fluidity is dependent on lipid content, with fluidity generally increasing with the level of unsaturation.[39] Dunham et al. recently showed that in keratinocytes *in vitro* the plasma membrane viscosity ranges over a biologically large factor of 2 depending on the fatty acid profile of the growth media, with the highest viscosity seen in EFA-deficient cells.[40] Since cell membrane-associated proteins are very sensitive to changes in their lipid environment,[41] lipid composition has an important influence on many physiological processes including enzyme and receptor function.

Many extracellular signals act by inducing hydrolysis of cell membrane phospholipids, resulting in the liberation of second messengers, including diacylglycerol (DAG), inositol phosphates, PG, and protein kinase C. Activation of phospholipase C causes degradation of phosphatidyl-inositol 4,5-biphosphate (PIP_2) to inositol triphosphate (IP_3) and DAG. The DAG activates protein kinases, which in turn activate a range of cellular proteins by phosphorylation,[42] while IP_3 acts synergistically to activate cells by increasing ionic calcium. Stimulation of phospholipase A_2 by cell surface signals leads to the release of AA, which is available for eicosanoid synthesis, and free AA may also result from the hydrolysis of DAG. AA can act as a second messenger by activating protein kinase C,[43] which regulates epidermal proliferation, and may also be an important regulator of intracellular calcium concentration.[44]

It is evident from the previous information that modification of EFA content can potentially influence many vital cell-signaling functions. Recent studies have demonstrated that the PUFA content of phospholipids can affect activity of protein kinase C[45] and phospholipase C.[46] EFA of the n-6 and n-3 families also influence cytokine production.[47,48] While dietary n-3 fatty acid supplementation results in reduced production of interleukin (IL)-1 and tumor necrosis factor (TNF)-α by peripheral blood monocytes,[49,50] AA and DGLA reduce synthesis of IL-2 by a PG-independent mechanism.[51] Changes in EFA status also affect the activity of several membrane-associated enzymes.[52-54] Reduced adenyl cyclase activity occurred in EFA-deficient animals,[55] while in animals supplemented with n-6 or n-3 fatty acids increased adenyl cyclase activity was seen in cardiac membranes.[56,57] However, the opposite effect has been reported in other membranes, possibly reflecting differences in initial fatty acid composition.[58]

25.7 ESSENTIAL FATTY ACIDS IN CLINICAL DERMATOLOGY

25.7.1 Atopic Dermatitis

A series of studies over many years have suggested the existence of an abnormal EFA pattern in the tissues of subjects with atopic dermatitis.[3,59,60] The plasma levels of linoleic and α-linolenic acids are normal, and hence there is no evidence of dietary deficiency of EFA. However, low plasma levels of linoleic acid metabolites, i.e., GLA, DGLA, and AA, and also α-linolenic metabolites, EPA and DHA, are reported and are interpreted to be consistent with defective functioning of Δ6-desaturase, which converts LA to GLA.[59,61] Similar findings have been reported in the peripheral blood monocytes in atopic asthma and allergic rhinitis sufferers,[62] and in umbilical cord blood in infants at risk of atopy, where the biochemical abnormality is proportional to the IgE level.[63] Atopic women are also reported to have low levels of GLA, DGLA, and AA in breast milk.[64] However, a recent study showed no difference in the plasma PGE_1 and PGE_2 levels between adults with atopic dermatitis and healthy control subjects, making it unlikely that Δ6-desaturase deficiency is the basic metabolic defect in atopic dermatitis.[65] Abnormalities of lamellar body ultrastructure,[66] altered sphingomyelin metabolism,[67] and reduced levels of ceramide 1[68] are also observed in patients with atopic dermatitis, raising the possibility that a defect in barrier function may account for the dry skin of eczema.[69]

Several clinical trials of n-6 EFA supplementation in atopic dermatitis were performed in the 1980s, usually with the GLA-rich EPO (Epogam®, Scotia Pharmaceuticals, Guildford, U.K.).[70-74] Dietary EPO raises the DGLA/AA concentration ratio, resulting in increased generation of anti-inflammatory and immunomodulatory eicosanoids. Most of these studies were reported to show some clinical improvement of atopic dermatitis following supplementation, particularly with respect to itching. In 1989, the manufacturer's research institute performed a meta-analysis of published and unpublished EPO supplementation studies.[75] This showed a significant clinical benefit in both adults and children, and a correlation between clinical improvement and rise in plasma EFA. Two recent double-blind studies, however, are at odds with these findings. A placebo-controlled trial of EPO alone and of combined EPO and fish oil showed no benefit of either treatment in adult and childhood atopic dermatitis,[76] while EPO in atopic children showed no advantage over sunflower oil.[77] Similarly, a study of EPO in chronic hand dermatitis showed equal improvement in active and control groups,[78] in keeping with a high placebo response rate in dermatitis.

Dietary supplementation studies with n-3 fatty acids alone have generally not been promising in atopic dermatitis. An initial double-blind study reported a subjective improvement on fish oil compared with the control olive oil, but no objective improvement on physician assessment.[79] A further double-blind study using EPA with saturated fatty acids as the control showed equal improvement with both supplements, and the benefit was attributed to increased clinician guidance,[80] while a multicenter study showed a similar improvement in clinical score in subjects taking fish oil or corn oil.[81] The latter results might possibly reflect a beneficial effect of both EFA-containing oils, but more likely imply a placebo effect and illustrate the problems posed both in selection of a suitable control and the interpretation of such studies.

25.7.2 Psoriasis

Disturbances in lipid metabolism occur in the skin in psoriasis. Increased phospholipase A_2 activity is seen in lesional and nonlesional skin, while phospholipase C activity is elevated in lesional skin.[82,83] Increased elongase activity is also observed in psoriatic epidermis. A local increase in AA occurs, and this appears to be preferentially metabolized by the lipoxygenases, resulting in a marked increase in 12-HETE and LTB_4, while there is a relative or absolute reduction in metabolism by the COX pathway.[84] Leukotriene B_4 is a very potent chemoattractant, and topical application causes epidermal hyperproliferation in addition to neutrophil microabscesses.[85] A defective, transmembranous cell-signaling system is also suggested by elevation of both IP_3 and DAG in the psoriatic plaque.[86]

Epidemiological studies reveal a very low prevalence of psoriasis in Greenland Eskimos.[87] Eskimos have high tissue levels of the n-3 fatty acids EPA and DHA, attributable to their high consumption of marine lipids.[88] In contrast, psoriatic plaques contain elevated levels of the n-6 fatty acid AA and its metabolites LTB_4 and 12-HETE. Dietary n-3 supplements result in suppression of these levels due to substitution by less active eicosanoids, including LTB_5 which is a less potent neutrophil chemoattractant and stimulator of keratinocyte proliferation than LTB_4.[89,90] These findings have led to several clinical studies of n-3 (EPA + DHA) fatty acid supplementation in psoriasis with conflicting results. While most of these studies have reported a mild-moderate improvement in the clinical features of psoriasis,[89-92] an 8-week study using olive oil as a control showed no benefit.[93] A more recent multicenter double-blind study showed no advantage of 4 months of treatment with fish oil over control (corn) oil.[94]

It has been suggested that this therapeutic approach may be too simplistic.[95] There might be a genetic difference in EFA metabolism in Eskimos, since they are also noted to have high DGLA levels accompanied by low AA levels, consistent with a lack of the enzyme Δ5-desaturase.[95,96] When Eskimos change from their traditional marine diet to a westernized diet, tissue levels of EPA and DHA fall, but the AA level remains low relative to DGLA. Since DGLA is converted to PGE_1, which has anti-inflammatory properties, it is conceivable that the low prevalence of psoriasis in this population might be partly attributable to the higher DGLA levels.[95] Hence, double-blind studies have recently been performed of combined EPO and n-3 fatty acid supplements (Efamol Marine®, Scotia Pharmaceuticals, Guildford, U.K.) in psoriasis, but no improvement was seen.[97,98]

25.7.3 Acne Vulgaris and Other Disorders

Low levels of linoleic acid are found in the sebum of acne sufferers,[99] and the levels appear to be inversely related to sebum secretion rate.[100] It has been hypothesized that this local EFA deficiency may lead to the follicular hyperkeratosis and occlusion of acne and that an increased supply of linoleate might possibly ameliorate the condition.[101] Recently, digital image analysis has revealed that topical application of linoleic acid over a 1-month period reduces the size of microcomedones.[102] Decreased levels of linoleic acid may also contribute to acne inflammation by failing to inhibit phagocytosis and reactive oxygen species generation by neutrophils.[103]

The effects of EFA on wound healing are variable: some studies report no effect, while others report a beneficial[104] or a detrimental[105] influence. In animal experiments, dietary GLA reduced ionizing radiation-induced adverse skin effects when given over the time course of expression of the damage, raising the possibility of increased therapeutic gain for patients undergoing radiotherapy.[106]

25.7.4 Photodermatology

Dietary n-3 fatty acid (EPA + DHA) supplements reduce the sunburn response in humans.[35,107] In addition, an open study of subjects with the photosensitivity disorder polymorphic light eruption (PLE) showed an increased threshold for provocation of rash after supplementation.[36] These changes were accompanied by incorporation of EPA and DHA into epidermal lipids, reduced levels of PGE_2 in UVB-exposed and unexposed skin, and an increased level of epidermal lipid peroxidation.[35,36] The mechanisms of these photoprotective properties are likely to include reduction in the inflammatory response due to a shift in the balance from the synthesis of n-6 eicosanoids toward the less active n-3 products. There is evidence for a major role of prostaglandins in the sunburn response, and it has been speculated that leukotrienes might also be involved.[15,108] Prostaglandins are elevated in suction blister fluid from UV-exposed human skin,[35,109,110] and nonsteroidal anti-inflammatory drugs reduce both PG levels and erythema.[111,112] It is also speculated that the unstable, highly unsaturated n-3 fatty acids might act as a free-radical buffer, protecting other structures from attack.[35,113,114]

Studies in hairless mice show a significant suppression of UV-induced skin cancers during oral n-3 fatty acid supplementation.[115] UV-induced carcinogenesis is augmented by high levels of PUFA,[116,117] but it is now evident that there is a need to distinguish between long chain n-6 fatty acids, which promote, and n-3 fatty acids, which inhibit, photocarcinogenesis.[115,118] These effects appear to act at the promotion stage of carcinogenesis and are analogous to the respective promoting and inhibiting activities of n-6 and n-3 fatty acids in models of colon and breast cancer.[119] The protective effect of n-3 fatty acid supplementation in photocarcinogenesis may be attributable to suppression of PGE_2[120-122] and modulation of UV-induced immune suppression.[123-125] Since the same wavelengths of UV radiation are implicated in sunburn and photocarcinogenesis,[126] it is speculated that long-term dietary n-3 fatty acid supplements might provide a safe[127] approach to protect against skin cancers in humans.[128] A case-control study of males with NMSC showed an inverse relationship between skin cancer risk and dietary fish intake,[129] and, clearly, this area needs exploration in further human intervention studies.

25.8 CONJUGATED LINOLEIC ACID

Recently, there has also been much interest in the anticarcinogenic properties of conjugated linoleic acid (CLA, C18:2), derivatives of linoleic acid found particularly in cooked meats and processed dairy products.[130,131] The isomeric products differ from linoleic acid in the position and configuration of the double bonds, and it is suspected that the *cis* 9, *trans* 11 isomer is the most biologically active. These linoleic acid derivatives are incorporated into keratinocyte phospholipids in the same distribution as linoleic acid, where they result in decreased AA content and PGE_2 synthesis.[132] Studies of CLA administration in mouse carcinogenesis models give evidence of inhibition of both the initiation and promotion stages of chemically induced skin cancer.[133,134] Potential mechanisms include modulation of eicosanoid synthesis, signal transduction, and oxidative stress.[131,132]

25.9 ESSENTIAL FATTY ACID STATUS IN THE MODULATION OF CUTANEOUS RESPONSES

It is clear from the previous information that alterations in dietary lipid intake can profoundly affect epidermal fatty acid composition and consequently influence many physiological and pathological processes in the skin. While deficiency of linoleic acid results in loss of water barrier and hyperproliferation, an altered balance of n-3 and n-6 EFA may affect many processes including inflammatory and immune responses, cell proliferation, and carcinogenesis. There is evidence that many of the effects are mediated by alterations in eicosanoid production, and an increased understanding is developing of the influence exerted by phospholipid-PUFA via modulation of signal transduction.

The treatment of eczema and psoriasis with n-3 or n-6 fatty acids remains controversial. The etiology of these disorders is still poorly understood, and EFA supplementation is addressing one potential factor. In addition, since AA is metabolized to both pro-inflammatory and anti-inflammatory metabolites, more selective inhibition may be needed. However, a general advantage of fatty acid supplementation is its safety compared with the pharmacological approach. Moreover, EFA may be incorporated into epidermal phospholipids via both the dietary and topical routes.[135] The frequent finding of a laboratory-documented anti-inflammatory effect with only minimal clinical benefit suggests that larger doses of EFA may be needed for a more effective monotherapy or that their role may lie as an adjunctive therapy to improve the therapeutic gain of other treatments. Further research is needed into the roles of individual n-3 and n-6 fatty acids, their optimal balance in the skin, and the effect of their manipulation on skin inflammation and carcinogenesis.

25.10 ACKNOWLEDGMENT

With gratitude to Michael Dean for assistance with preparation of this manuscript and to Linda Fenton for secretarial support.

REFERENCES

1. Burr, G. O., Burr, M. M., A new deficiency disease produced by the rigid exclusion of fat from the diet, *J Biol Chem,* 82, 345, 1929.
2. Burr, G. O., Burr, M. M., On the nature and role of the essential fatty acids in nutrition, *J Biol Chem,* 86, 587, 1930.
3. Hansen, A. E., Serum lipids in eczema and other pathological conditions, *Am J Dis Child,* 59, 933, 1937.
4. Hansen, A. E., Haggard, M. E., Boelsche, A. N., Adam, D. J. D., Wiese, M. F., Essential fatty acids in infant nutrition III. Clinical manifestations of linoleic acid deficiency, *J Nutr,* 66, 565, 1958.
5. Hansen, A. E., Serum lipid changes and therapeutic effects of various oils in infantile eczema, *Proc Soc Exp Biol Med,* 31, 160, 1933.
6. Cornbleet, T., Use of maize oil (unsaturated fatty acids) in the treatment of eczema, *Arch Dermatol Syph,* 31, 224, 1935.
7. Ginsberg, G. E., Bernstein, C. Jr., Effects of oils containing unsaturated fatty acids on patients with dermatitis, *Arch Dermatol Syph,* 36, 1033, 1937.
8. Hansen, A. E., Knott, E. M., Weise, H. F., Shaperman, E., McQuarie, I., Eczema and essential fatty acids, *Am J Dis Child*, 73, 1, 1947.
9. Innis, S. M., Essential fatty acids in growth and development, *Prog Lipid Res,* 30, 39, 1991.
10. Clarke, S. D., Jump, D. B., Regulation of gene transcription by polyunsaturated fatty acids, *Prog Lipid Res*, 32, 132, 1993.
11. Innis, S. M., Essential dietary lipids, *Present Knowledge in Nutrition,* 7th ed., Ziegler, E. E., Filer Jr., L. J., ILSI Press, Washington, D.C., 1994, 58.
12. O'Farrell, S., Dietary Polyunsaturated Fatty Acids and Oxidation Damage to Heart, Skeletal Muscle and Skin, Ph.D. Thesis, University of Liverpool, 1994.
13. Brenner, R. R., Hormonal control of fatty acid desaturation, *Biochem Soc Trans*, 18, 773, 1990.
14. Lands, W. E. M., Biochemistry and physiology of n-3 fatty acids, *FASEB J,* 6, 2530, 1992.
15. Ziboh, V. A., Essential fatty acids/eicosanoid biosynthesis in the skin: biological significance, *Soc Exp Biol Med*, 205(1), 1, 1994.

16. Chapkin, R. S., Ziboh, V. A., Inability of skin enzyme preparations to biosynthesise arachidonic acid from linoleic acid, *Biochem Biophys Res Commun,* 124, 784, 1984.
17. Schurer, N. Y., Stremmel, W., Grundmann, J.-U., Schliep, V., Kleinert, H., Bass, N. M., Williams, M. L., Evidence for a novel keratinocyte fatty acid uptake mechanism with preference for linoleic acid: comparison of oleic and linoleic acid uptake by cultured human keratinocytes, fibroblasts and a human hepatoma cell line, *Biochim. Biophys.* Acta, 1211, 51, 1994.
18. Proksch, E., Feingold, K. R., Mao-Quiang, M., Elias, P. M., Barrier function regulates epidermal DNA synthesis, *J Clin Invest,* 87, 1668, 1991.
19. Prottey, C., Hartop, P. J., Press, M., Correction of the cutaneous manifestations of essential fatty acid deficiency in man by application of sunflower-seed oil to the skin, *J Invest Dermatol,* 64, 228, 1975.
20. Hartop, P. J., Prottey, C., Changes in transepidermal water loss and the composition of epidermal lecithin after applications of pure fatty triglycerides to the skin of essential fatty acid-deficient rats, *Br J Dermatol*, 95, 255, 1976.
21. Hansen, H. S., Jensen, B., Essential function of linoleic acid esterified in acylglucosyl ceramide and acylceramide in maintaining the epidermal water permeability barrier: evidence from feeding studies with oleate, linoleate, arachidonate, columbinate and alpha-linoleate, *Biochim Biophys Acta,* 834, 357, 1985.
22. Abraham, W., Wertz, P. W., Downing, D. T., Linoleate-rich acylglucosyl ceramides of pig epidermis: structure determination by proton magnetic resonance, *J Lipid Res,* 26, 761, 1985.
23. Landmann, L., The epidermal permeability barrier, *Anat Embryol,* 178, 1, 1975.
24. Wertz, P. W., Swartzendruber, C., Abraham, W., Maddison, K. C., Downing, D. T., Essential fatty acids and epidermal integrity, *Arch Dermatol*, 123, 1381, 1987.
25. Wertz, P. W., Downing, D. T., Glycolipids in mammalian epidermis, structure and function in the water barrier, *Science*, 217, 1261, 1982.
26. Hou, S. Y. E., Mitra, A. K., White, S. H., Membrane structures in normal and essential fatty acid deficient stratum corneum: characterisation by ruthenium tetroxide staining and X-ray diffraction, *J Invest Dermatol,* 96, 215, 1991.
27. Elias, P. M., Brown, B. E., The mammalian cutaneous permeability barrier: defective barrier function in essential fatty acid deficiency correlates with the abnormal intercellular lipid deposition, *Lab Invest*, 39, 574, 1978.
28. Wertz, P. W., Miethke, M. C., Long, S. A., The composition of ceramides from human stratum corneum and from comedones, *J Invest Dermatol,* 84, 410, 1985.
29. Nugteren, D. H., Christ-Hazelhof, E., van der Beek, A., Houtsmuller, U. M. T., Metabolism of linoleic acid and other essential fatty acids in the epidermis of the rat, *Biochim. Biophy. Acta*, 834, 429, 1985.
30. Nugteren, D. H., Kivits, G. A. A., Conversion of linoleic acid and arachidonic acid by skin epidermal lipoxygenases, *Biochimica et Biophysica Acta*, 921, 135, 1987.
31. Lee, T. H., Hoover, R. L., Williams, J. D., Sperling, R. I., Ravalese III, J., Spur, B. W., Robinson, D. R., Corey, E. J., Lewis, R. A., Austen, K. F., Effect of dietary enrichment with eicosapentaenoic and docasahexaenoic acids on *in vitro* neutrophil and monocyte leukotriene generation and neutrophil function, *N Engl J Med,* 312, 1217, 1985.
32. Kirtland, S. J., Prostaglandin E_1: a review, *Prostaglandins Leukotrienes and Essential Fatty Acids,* 32, 165, 1988.
33. Miller, C. C., Ziboh, V. A., Jones, A. D., Guinea pig epidermis synthesis of 15-hydroxy-8,11,13-eicosatrienoic acid (15 OH 20:3n-6) from dihomogammalinolenic acid: a potent lipoxygenase inhibitor derived from evening primrose oil, *J Invest Dermatol*, 88, 507, 1987.
34. Ziboh, V. A., Cohen, K. A., Ellis, C. N., Miller, C., Hamilton, T. A., Kragballe, K., Hydrick, C. R., Voorhees, J. J., Effects of dietary supplementation of fish oil on neutrophil and epidermal fatty acids, *Arch Dermatol,* 122, 1277, 1986.
35. Rhodes, L. E., O'Farrell, S., Jackson, M. J., Friedmann, P. S., Dietary fish-oil supplementation in humans reduces UVB-erythemal sensitivity but increases epidermal lipid peroxidation, *J Invest Dermatol,* 103, 151, 1994.
36. Rhodes, L. E., Durham, B. H., Fraser, W. D., Friedmann, P. S., Dietary fish oil reduces basal and ultraviolet B-generated PGE_2 levels in skin and increases the threshold to provocation of polymorphic light eruption, *J Invest Dermatol,* 105, 532, 1995.

37. Chapkin, R. S., Ziboh, V. A., McCullough, J. L., Dietary influences of evening primrose oil and fish oil on the skin of essential fatty acid deficient guinea pigs, *J Nutr,* 117, 1360, 1987.
38. McCreedy, C., Wong, T., Ziboh, V. A., Generation of prostaglandins of the E_1 series from dihommogammalinolenic acid by guinea pig epidermal preparations, *J Invest Dermatol,* 88, 506, 1987.
39. Stubbs, C. D., Smith, A. D., The modification of mammalian cell membrane polyunsaturated fatty acid composition in relation to membrane fluidity and function, *Biochim Biophys Acta,* 779, 89, 1984.
40. Dunham, W. R., Klein, S. B., Rhodes, L. M., Marcelo, C. L., Oleic acid and linoleic acid are the major determinants of changes in keratinocyte plasma membrane viscosity, *J Invest Dermatol*, 107, 332, 1996.
41. Yeagle, P. L., Lipid regulation of cell membrane structure and function, *FASEB J,* 3, 1833, 1989.
42. Nishizuka, Y., The molecular heterogeneity of protein kinase C and its implications for cellular regulation, *Nature,* 334, 661, 1988.
43. Murakami, K., Routtenberg, A., Direct activation of purified protein kinase (by unsaturated fatty acids toleate and arachidonate) in the absence of phospholipids and calcium, *FEBS Lett,* 192, 189, 1986.
44. Chaudry, A., Rubin, R. P., Mediators of Ca^{2+} dependent secretion, *Environ Health Perspect,* 84, 35, 1990.
45. Lo, H. H., Bartek, G. A., Fischer, S. M., *In vitro* activation of mouse skin protein kinase C by fatty acids and their hydroxylated metabolites, *Lipids,* 29, 547, 1994.
46. Estes, K. C., Rose, B. T., Speck, J. J., Nutter, M. L., Reitz, R. C., Effects of omega 3 fatty acids on receptor tyrosine kinase and PLC activities in EMT6 cells, *J Lipid Mediat Cell Signal,* 17, 81, 1997.
47. Grimble, R. F., Tappia, P. S., Modulatory influence of unsaturated fatty acids on the biology of tumour necrosis factor-α, *Biochem Soc Trans,* 23, 282, 1995.
48. Blok, W. L., Deslypere, J. P., Demacker, P. N., van der Ven Jongekrijg, J., Hectors, M. P., van der Meer, J. W., Katan, M. B., Pro and anti-inflammatory cytokines in healthy volunteers fed various doses of fish oil for 1 year, *Eur J Clin Invest,* 27, 1003, 1997.
49. Endres, S., Ghorbani, R., Kelley, V. E., Georgilis, K., Lonnemann, G., van der Meer, J. W. M., Cannon, J. G., Rogers, T. S., Klempner, M. S., Weber, P. C., Schaefer, E. J., Wolff, S. M., Dinarello, C. A., The effect of dietary supplementation with n-3 polyunsaturated fatty acids on the synthesis of interleukin-1 and tumour necrosis factor by mononuclear cells, *N Engl J Med,* 320, 265, 1989.
50. Calder, P. C., n-3 polyunsaturated fatty acids and cytokine production in health and disease, *Ann Nutr Metab,* 41, 203, 1997.
51. Santoli, D., Zurier, R. B., Prostaglandin E precursor fatty acids inhibit human IL-2 production by a prostaglandin E-independent mechanism, *J Immunol,* 143, 1303, 1989.
52. Engelhard, V. H., Esko, J. D., Storm, D. R., Glaser, M., Modification of adenyl cyclase activity in LM cells by manipulation of the membrane lipid composition *in vivo*, *Proc Natl Acad Sci,* 73, 4482, 1976.
53. Momchilova, A., Petkova, D., Mechev, I., Sensitivity of 5′ nuleotidase and phospholipase A_2 towards liver plasma membrane modifications, *Int J Biochem,* 17, 787, 1985.
54. Murphy, M. G., Dietary fatty acids and membrane protein function, *J Nutr Biochem,* 1, 68, 1990.
55. Alam, S. Q., Alam, B. S., Ren, Y. F., Adenyl cyclase activity, membrane fluidity and fatty acid composition of rat heart in essential fatty acid deficiency, *J Mol Cell Cardiol,* 19, 465, 1987.
56. Hamm, M. W., Shei, G. J., Dietary lipid, adenyl cyclase activity and β adrenergic binding in rat heart, *FASEB J*, 2, 639, 1988.
57. McMurchie, E. J., Patten, G. S., McLennan, P. L., The influence of dietary lipid supplementation on cardiac beta-adrenergic receptor adenyl cyclase activity in the marmoset monkey, *Biochim Biophys Acta*, 937, 347, 1988.
58. Wright, S., Essential fatty acids and the skin, *Br J Dermatol,* 125, 503, 1991.
59. Manku, M. S., Horrobin, D. F., Morse, N. L., Wright, S., Burton, J. L., Essential fatty acids in the plasma phospholipids of patients with atopic eczema, *Br J Dermatol*, 110, 643, 1984.
60. Oliwiecki, S., Burton, J. L., Elles, K., Horrobin, D. F., Level of essential and other fatty acids in plasma and red cell phospholipids from normal controls and patients with atopic eczema, *Acta Derm Venereol* (*Stockh.*)*,* 71, 224, 1991.
61. Manku, M. S., Horrobin, D. F., Morse, N., Kyte, V., Jenkins, K., Reduced levels of prostaglandin precursors in the blood of atopic patients: defective delta-6-desaturase function as a biochemical basis for atopy, *Prostaglandins Leukotrienes Medicine*, 9, 615, 1982.

62. Rocklin, R. E., Thistle, L., Gallant, L., Altered arachidonic acid content in polymorphonuclear and mononuclear cells from patients with allergic rhinitis and/or asthma, *Lipids,* 21, 17, 1986.
63. Strannegard, I.-L., Svennerholm, L., Strannegard, O., Essential fatty acids in serum lecithin of children with atopic dermatitis and in umbilical cord serum of infants with high or low IgE levels, *Int Arch Allergy Appl Immunol*, 82, 422, 1987.
64. Wright, S., Bolton, C. H., Breast milk fatty acid composition in mothers of children with atopic eczema, *Br J Nutr,* 62, 693, 1989.
65. Leonhardt, A., Krauss, M., Gieler, U., Schweer, H., Happle, R., Seyberth, H. W., *In vivo* formation of prostaglandin E_1 and prostaglandin E_2 in atopic dermatitis, *Br J Dermatol,* 136, 337, 1997.
66. Werner, Y., Lindberg, M., Forslind, B., Membrane-coating granules in dry non-eczematous skin of patients with atopic dermatitis, *Acta Derm Venereol (Stockh.),* 67, 385, 1987.
67. Murata, Y., Ogata, J., Higaki, Y., Kawashima, M., Yada, Y., Higuchi, K., Tsuchiya, T., Kawaminami, S., Imokawa, G., Abnormal expression of sphingomyelin acylase in atopic dermatitis: an etiologic factor for ceramide deficiency?, *J Invest Dermatol,* 106, 1242, 1996.
68. Imokaura, G., Abe, A., Jin, K., Kawashima, M., Hidano, A., Decreased level of ceramides in stratum corneum of atopic dermatitis: an etiological factor in atopic dry skin, *J Invest Dermatol,* 96, 523, 1991.
69. Melnik, B. C., Hollmann, J., Plewig, G., Decreased stratum corneum ceramides in atopic individuals-pathobiochemical factor in xerosis, *Br J Dermatol,* 119, 547, 1988.
70. Lovell, C. R., Burton, J. L., Horrobin, D. F., Treatment of atopic eczema with evening primrose oil, *Lancet,* 1, 278, 1981.
71. Wright, S., Burton, J. L., Evening primrose seed oil improves atopic eczema, *Lancet,* ii, 1120, 1982.
72. Bamford, J. T. M., Gibson, R. W., Renier, C. M., Atopic eczema unresponsive to evening primrose oil (linoleic and°–linolenic acids), *J Am Acad Dermatol*, 13, 959, 1985.
73. Schalin-Karrila, M., Mattila, L., Jansen, C. T., Uottila, P., Evening primrose oil in the treatment of atopic eczema: effect on clinical status, plasma phospholipid fatty acids and circulating blood prostaglandins, *Br J Dermatol,* 117, 11, 1987.
74. Bordoni, A., Biagi, P. L., Masi, M., Ricci, G., Fanelli, C., Patrizi, A., Ceccoline, E., Evening primrose oil (efamol) in the treatment of children with atopic eczema, *Drugs Exp. Clin Res*, 14, 291, 1988.
75. Morse, P. F., Horrobin, D. F., Manku, M. S., Stewart, J. C. M., Allen, R., Littlewood, S., Wright, S., Burton, J., Gould, D. J., Holt, P. J., Jansen, C. T., Mattila, L.M, Meigel, W., Dettke, Th., Wexler, D., Guenther, L., Bordoni, A., Patrizi, A., Meta-analysis of placebo-controlled studies of the efficacy of Epogam in the treatment of atopic eczema. Relationship between plasma essential fatty acid changes and clinical response, *Br J Dermatol*, 121, 75, 1989.
76. Berth-Jones, J., Graham-Brown, R. A. C., Placebo-controlled trial of essential fatty acid supplementation in atopic dermatitis, *Lancet,* 341, 1557, 1993.
77. Hederos, C.-A., Berg, A., Epogam evening primrose oil treatment in atopic dermatitis and asthma, *Arch Dis Child*, 75, 494, 1996.
78. Whitaker, D. K., Cilliers, J., de Beer, C., Evening primrose oil (Epogam) in the treatment of chronic hand dermatitis: disappointing therapeutic results, *Dermatology,* 193, 115, 1996.
79. Bjørneboe, A., Søyland, E., Bjørneboe, G-E. A., Rajka, G., Drevon, C. A., Effect of dietary supplementation with eicosapentaenoic acid in the treatment of atopic dermatitis, *Br J Dermatol,* 117, 463, 1987.
80. Kunz, B., Ring, J., Braun-Falco, O., Eicosapentaenoic acid (EPA) treatment in atopic eczema: a prospective double-blind trial, *J Allergy Clin Immunol,* 83, 196, 1987.
81. Søyland, E., Funk, J., Rajka, G., Sandberg, M., Thune, P., Rustad, L., Helland, S., Middelfart, K., Odu, S., Falk, E. S., Solvoll, K., Bjørneboe, G.-E. A., Drevon, C. A., Dietary supplementation with very-long chain n-3 fatty acids in patients with atopic dermatitis. A double-blind, multicentre study, *Br J Dermatol,* 130, 757, 1994.
82. Forster, S., Ilderton, E., Norris, J. F. B., Characterisation and activity of phospholipase A_2 in normal human epidermis and in lesion free epidermis of patients with psoriasis or eczema, *Br J Dermatol,* 112, 135, 1985.
83. Fisher, G. J., Talwar, H. S., Baldassare, J. J., Increased phospholipase C-catalysed hydrolysis of phosphatidylinositol-4, 5-bisphosphate and 1, 2-sn-diacylglycerol content in psoriatic involved compared to uninvolved and normal epidermis, *J Invest Dermatol,* 95, 428, 1990.
84. Horrobin, D. F., Essential fatty acids in clinical dermatology, *J Am Acad Dermatol*, 20, 1045, 1989.

85. Bauer, F. W., Van de Kerkhof, P. C. M., Maassen-De Good, R. M., Epidermal hyperproliferation following the induction of microabscesses by leukotriene B4, *Br J Dermatol,* 114, 409, 1986.
86. Burton, J. L., Dietary fatty acids and inflammatory skin disease, *Lancet,* i, 27,1989.
87. Kromann, N., Green, A., Epidemiological studies in the Upernavik district, Greenland, *Acta Med Scand*, 208, 401, 1980.
88. Bang, H., Dyerberg, J., Horne, N., The composition of food consumed by Greenland eskimos, *Acta Med Scand,* 200, 69, 1976.
89. Maurice, P. D. L., Allen, B. R., Barkley, A. S. J., Cockbill, S. R., Stammers, J., Bather, P. C., The effects of dietary supplementation with fish oil in patients with psoriasis, *Br J Dermatol,* 117, 599, 1987.
90. Kragballe, K., Fogh, K., A low-fat diet supplemented with dietary fish oil (Max-EPA) results in improvement of psoriasis and in formation of leukotriene B_5, *Acta Derm Venereol (Stockh.),* 69, 23, 1989.
91. Bittiner, S. B., Tucker, W. F. G., Cartwright, I., Bleehen, S. S., A double-blind, randomised, placebo-controlled trial of fish oil in psoriasis, *Lancet,* i, 378, 1988.
92. Allen, B. R., Fish oil in combination with other therapies in the treatment of psoriasis, *World Rev Nutr Diet,* 66, 436, 1991.
93. Bjørneboe, A., Klemeyer Smith, A., Gunn Elin, A. A., Bjørneboe, P. O., Thune, P. O., Drevon, C. A., Effect of dietary supplementation with n-3 fatty acids on clinical manifestations of psoriasis, *Br J Dermatol,* 118, 77, 1988.
94. Søyland, E., Funk, J., Rajka, G., Sandberg, M., Thune, P., Rustad, L., Helland, S., Middelfart, K., Odu, S., Falk, E. S., Solvoll, K., Bjørneboe, G.-E. A., Drevon, C. A., Effect of dietary supplementation with very-long chain n-3 fatty acids in patients with psoriasis, *N Engl J Med,* 328, 1812, 1993.
95. Horrobin, D. F., Low prevalences of coronary heart disease (CHD), psoriasis, asthma and rheumatoid arthritis in Eskimos: are they caused by high dietary intake of eicosapentaenoic acid (EPA), a genetic variation of essential fatty acid (EFA) metabolism or a combination of both?, *Med. Hypotheses*, 22, 421, 1987.
96. Gibson, R. A., Sinclair, A. J., Are Eskimos obligate carnivores?, *Lancet,* 1, 1100, 1981.
97. Veale, D. J., Torley, H. I., Richards, I. M., O'Dowd, A., Fitzsimons, C., Belch, J. J. F., Sturrock, R. D., A double-blind placebo controlled trial of efamol marine on skin and joint symptoms of psoriatic arthritis, *Br J Rheumatol*, 33, 954, 1994.
98. Oliwiecki, S., Burton, J. L., Evening primrose oil and marine oil in the treatment of psoriasis, *Clin Exp Dermatol*, 19, 127, 1994.
99. Morello, A. M., Downing, D. T., Strauss, J. S., Octadecadienoic acids in the skin surface lipids of acne patients and normal subjects, *J Invest Dermatol,* 66, 319, 1976.
100. Stewart, M. E., Wertz, P. W., Granek, M. O., Downing, D. T., Relationship between sebum secretion rates and the concentration of linoleate in sebum and epidermal lipids, *Clin Res,* 33, 684, 1985.
101. Downing, D. T., Stewart, M. E., Wertz, P. W., Strauss, J. S., Essential fatty acids and acne, *J Am Acad Dermatol*, 14, 221, 1986.
102. Letawe, C., Boone, M., Pierard, G. E., Digital image analysis of the effect of topically applied linoleic acid on acne microcomedones, *Clin Exp Dermatol,* 23, 56, 1998.
103. Akamatsu, H., Komura, J., Miyachi, Y., Asada, Y., Niwa, Y., Suppressive effects of linoleic acid on neutrophil oxygen metabolism and phagocytosis, *J Invest Dermatol,* 95, 271, 1990.
104. Moreno-Gimenez, J. C., Bueno, J., Navas, J., Camacho, F., Treatment of skin ulcer using oil of mosqueta rose, *Med Cutanea Ibero Lat Am,* 18, 63, 1990.
105. Albina, J. E., Gladden, P., Walsh, W. R., Detrimental effects of an omega-3 fatty acid-enriched diet on wound healing, *J Parenter Enteral Nutr,* 17, 519, 1993.
106. Hopewell, J. W., van den Aardweg, G. J., Morris, G. M., Rezvani, M., Robbins, M. E., Ross, G. A., Whitehouse, E. M., Scott, C. A., Horrobin, D. F., Amelioration of both early and late radiation-induced damage to pig skin by essential fatty acids, *Int J Rad Oncol, Biol, Physics,* 30, 1119, 1994.
107. Orengo, I. F., Black, H. S., Wolf, J. E. Jr., Influence of fish oil supplementation on the minimal erythema dose in humans, *Arch Dermatol Res,* 284, 219, 1992.
108. Rhodes, L. E., Mechanisms of UVB Induced Erythema, M.D. Thesis, University of Liverpool, 1995.
109. Black, A. G., Greaves, M. W., Hensby, C. N., Plummer, N. A., Increased prostaglandins E_2 and $F_{2\alpha}$ in human skin at 6 and 24 H after ultraviolet B irradiation, *Br J Clin Pharmacol,* 5, 431, 1978.

110. Gilchrest, B. A., Soter, N. A., Stoff, J. S., Mihm, M. C., The human sunburn reaction. Histologic and biochemical studies, *J Am Acad Dermatol,* 5, 411, 1981.
111. Black, A. K., Greaves, M. W., Hensby, C. N., Plummer, N. A., Warin, A. P., The effects of indomethacin on arachidonic acid and prostaglandins E_2 and $F_{2\alpha}$ levels in human skin 24 H after UVB and UVC irradiation, *Br J Clin Pharmacol,* 6, 261, 1978.
112. Farr, P. M., Diffey, B. L., A quantitative study on the effect of topical indomethacin on cutaneous erythema induced by UVB and UVC radiation, *Br J Dermatol,* 115, 453, 1986.
113. van den Berg, J. J. M., de Fouw, N. J., Kuypers, F. A., Roelofsen, B., Houtsmuller, U. M. T., Op den Kamp, J. A. F., Increased n-3 polyunsaturated fatty acid content of red blood cells from fish oil-fed rabbits increases *in vitro* lipid peroxidation, but decreases haemolysis, *Free Rad Biol Med,* 11, 393, 1991.
114. Budowski, P., The omega-3 fatty acid peroxidation paradox, *Redox Rep,* 21, 75, 1996.
115. Oregno, I. F., Black, H. S., Kettler, A. H., Wolf, J. E., Influence of dietary menhaden oil upon carcinogenesis and various cutaneous responses to ultraviolet radiation, *Photochem Photobiol,* 49, 71, 1989.
116. Reeve, V. E., Matheson, M. J., Greenoak, G. E., Canfield, P. J., Boehm-Wilcox, C., Gallagher, C. H., Effects of dietary lipid on UV light carcinogenesis in the hairless mouse, *Photochem Photobiol,* 48, 689, 1988.
117. Reeve, V. E., Bosnic, M., Boehm-Wilcox, C., Dependence of photocarcinogenesis and photoimmunosuppression in the hairless mouse on dietary polyunsaturated fat, *Cancer Lett,* 108, 271, 1996.
118. Black, H. S., Thornby, J. I., Gergius, J., Lenger, W., Influence of dietary omega-6, -3 fatty acid sources on the initiation and promotion stages of photocarcinogenesis, *Photochem Photobiol,* 56, 195, 1992.
119. Weisburger, J. H., Dietary fat and risk of chronic disease: mechanistic insights from experimental studies, *J Am Diet Assoc,* 7, 16, 1997.
120. Henderson, C. D., Black, H. S., Wolf, J. E., Influence of omega-3 and omega-6 fatty acid sources on prostaglandin levels in mice, *Lipids,* 24, 502, 1989.
121. Haedersdal, M., Poulsen, T., Wulf, H. C., Effects of systemic indomethacin on photocarcinogenesis in hairless mice, *J Cancer Res Clin Oncol,* 121, 257, 1995.
122. Reeve, V. E., Matheson, M. J., Bosnic, M., Boehm-Wilcox, C., The protective effect of indomethacin on photocarcinogenesis in hairless mice, *Cancer Lett,* 95, 213, 1995.
123. Chung, H. T., Burnham, D. R., Robertson, B., Roberts, L. K., Daynes, R. A., Involvement of prostaglandins in the immune alterations caused by the exposure of mice to ultraviolet radiation, *J Immunol,* 137, 2478, 1986.
124. Fischer, M. A., Black, H. S., Modification of membrane composition, eicosanoid metabolism, and immunoresponsiveness by dietary omega-3 and omega-6 fatty acid sources, modulators of ultraviolet-carcinogenesis, *Photochem Photobiol,* 54, 381, 1991.
125. Black, H. S., Diet and skin cancer, in *Nutritional Oncology,* Heber, D., Blackburn, G. L., Go, V. L. W., Eds., Academic Press, San Diego, CA, 1999, 405.
126. de Gruijl, F. R., Sterenborg, H. J. C. M., Forbes, P. D., Davies, R. E., Cole, C., Kelfkens, G., van Weelden, H., Slaper, H., van der Leun, J. C., Wavelength dependence of skin cancer induction by ultraviolet irradiation of albino hairless mice, *Cancer Res,* 53, 53, 1993.
127. Saynor, R., Gillott, T., Changes in blood lipids and fibrinogen with a note on safety in a long term study on the effects of n-3 fatty acids in subjects receiving fish oil supplements and followed for seven years, *Lipids,* 27, 533, 1992.
128. Rhodes, L. E., Topical and systemic approaches for protection against solar radiation-induced skin damage, *Clin Dermatol,* 16, 75, 1998.
129. Kune, G. A., Bannerman, S., Field, B., Watson, L. F., Cleland, H., Merenstein, D., Vitetta, L., Diet, alcohol, smoking, serum β-carotene, and vitamin A in male nonmelanocytic skin cancer patients and controls, *Nutr Cancer,* 18, 237, 1992.
130. Ip, C., Scimeca, J. A., Thompson, H. J., Conjugated linoleic acid: a powerful anticarcinogen from animal fat sources, *Cancer,* 74, 1050, 1994.
131. Belury, M. A., Conjugated dienoic linoleate: a polyunsaturated fatty acid with unique chemoprotective properties, *Nutr Rev,* 53, 83, 1995.
132. Liu, K.-L., Belury, M. A., Conjugated linoleic acid reduces arachidonic acid content and PGE_2 synthesis in murine keratinocytes, *Cancer Lett,* 74, 1050, 1998.

133. Ha, Y. L., Grimm, N. K., Pariza, M. W., Anticarcinogens from fried ground beef: heat altered derivatives of linoleic acid, *Carcinogenesis,* 8, 1881, 1987.
134. Belury, M. A., Nickel, K. P., Bird, C. E., Wu, Y., Dietary conjugated linoleic acid modulation of phorbol ester skin tumor promotion, *Nutr Cancer,* 26, 149, 1996.
135. Prottey, C., Essential fatty acids and the skin, *Br J Dermatol*, 94, 579, 1976.

26 Sphingolipids: From Chemistry to Possible Biologic Influence on the Skin

Hisashi Wakita

CONTENTS

26.1 CHEMISTRY OF SPHINGOLIPIDS: OVERVIEW

Over 300 types of sphingolipids are synthesized in various mammalian cell types. Structurally, sphingolipids are composed of a long-chain aliphatic 2-amino-1,3-diol (sphingoid base), an attached amide-linked fatty acyl′chain varying in length from 16 to 24 carbon atoms, and a polar head group at the 1-position (Figure 1). The diversity of sphingolipids originates from a variety of head groups: ceramide has a hydroxyl at the 1-position, sphingomyelin has phosphorylcholine head groups, and glycosphingolipids contain carbohydrate head groups. Glycosphingolipids are further classified according to the sequence of sugars and the chemical bonds which link them together: cerebrosides have a single glucose or galactose, other neutral lipids such as latotosyl-ceramide and trihexosides have higher order glycose units, and acidic glycosphingolipids contain one or more sialic acid residues (gangliosides) or sulfate monoester groups (sulfatides). For every sphingolipid there is a corresponding lysosphingolipid, which has the identical polar head group at the 1-position, but lacks the amide-linked fatty acyl group at the 2-position. For example, deacylation of ceramide produces sphingosine, a representative of free long-chain bases (FLCBs). Sphingosine can be further converted to highly biologically active metabolites such as sphingosine-1-phosphate via sphingosine kinase-catalyzed phosphorylation at the 1-position,[1] and *N,N*-dimethylsphingosine via amino-dimethylation.[2]

0-8493-7520-7/00/$0.00+$.50

Basic Structure of Sphingolipid

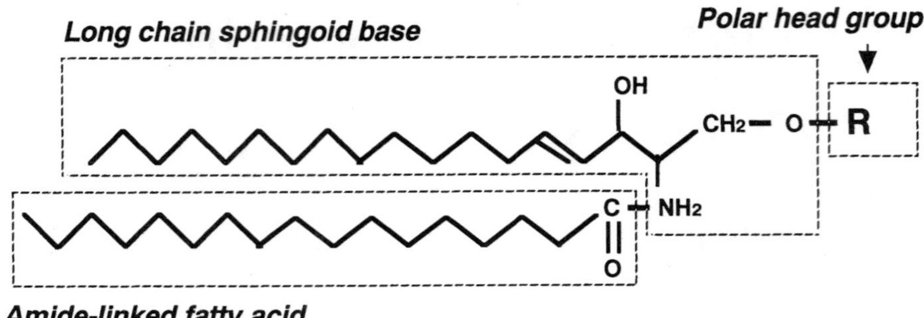

R	Sphingolipid
Hydrogen	Ceramide
Phosphorylcholine	Sphingomyelin
Single sugar	Cerebroside
Sugar chains with sialic acid	Ganglioside
Sugar chains with sulfate	Sulfatide

FIGURE 1 Structural formulas of sphingolipids.

26.2 CHEMISTRY OF SPHINGOLIPIDS IN THE SKIN

Epidermal sphingolipids play important roles in cell construction, growth, and differentiation of keratinocytes and in cohesion, desquamation, and a permeability barrier formation of the stratum corneum. To better understand these functions, the structure and composition of the epidermal sphingolipids have been elucidated.[3] Sphingolipid composition generally changes dramatically during differentiation, development, and oncogenic transformation. In the epidermis, the amount of sphingolipid such as FLCBs, ceramides, glucosylceramides, and gangliosides is increased with keratinocyte differentiation, especially with transition from the granular layer to the stratum corneum. In contrast, almost complete disappearance of glycerophospholipids is observed during this process.[4] Therefore, the stratum corneum is one of the richest tissues containing sphingolipids, and, in fact, various biologic functions of sphingolipids on the body surface have been revealed.

26.2.1 Free Long-Chain Bases

The major FLCBs in the stratum corneum of human skin include both dihydrosphingosines (sphinganines) and sphingosines (sphingenines) with 18 to 20 carbons, in addition to some phytosphingosines (hydroxysphinganines).[5-7] Moreover, an FLCB with three hydroxyl groups and one double bond (6-hydroxysphingosine) was specifically identified in the stratum corneum of the human skin.[6,7] Although the biological significance of such a variety of FLCB molecular species remains unknown, the relative percentage of each molecular species shows site-related differences in normal skin and differs between normal and pathologic skin conditions.[6] Compared with the stratum corneum of normal lower legs, molar percentages of FLCB having 18 carbons and those with 20 carbons were higher and lower, respectively, in normal plantar epidermis. Psoriatic scales and hyperkeratotic stratum corneum from the clavus and plantar keratoderma contain increased levels of FLCB with 18 carbons and decreased levels of FLCB with 20 carbons, possibly reflecting the abnormal keratinization in hyperkeratotic skin conditions.

26.2.2 Glycosphingolipids

Although glucosylceramides are the predominant epidermal glycosphingolipids,[8] various classes of glycosphingolipids such as acylglucosylceramides and gangliosides have been identified in epidermis and cultured keratinocytes.

26.2.2.1 Epidermosides

One group of sphingolipids characteristic to epidermis is acylglucosylceramides (AGCs). Hamanaka et al. reported that human epidermal AGCs consisted of *N*-(*O*-linoleoyl)-ω-hydroxy fatty acyl sphingosyl glucose and *N*-(*O*-linoleoyl)-ω-hydroxy fatty acyl phytosphingosyl glucose and named the epidermal AGCs "Epidermosides."[9] The main role of epidermosides in the stratum corneum is thought to be participation in the formation of the epidermal permeability barrier in conjunction with other lipids including (acyl)ceramide, cholesterol, and free fatty acids.

26.2.2.2 Gangliosides

The existence of trace amounts of gangliosides in epidermis had been reported already by Gray and Yardley in 1975.[8] However, they could not identify the individual compounds. Paller et al. demonstrated that the total ganglioside content of the epidermis was about 1 μg of lipid-bound sialic acid per milligram of dry weight and compromised 0.1% of the total epidermal lipids.[10] They determined that GM3 was the predominant ganglioside of the epidermis followed by GM2 and GD3, and polysialylated gangliosides such as GT1b were also presented in trace amounts.

Not only biochemical analysis, but immunohistochemical staining with antibodies against gangliosides has similarly revealed the existence and distribution of gangliosides in epidermis. Nakakuma et al. showed that epidermal keratinocytes reacted with an anti-GM3 monoclonal antibody, but not an anti-GD3 mAb.[11] Expression of GM3, predominantly in the stratum corneum, was reported by Paller et al.[12] In contrast, Hersey et al. detected GD2 in the basal and spinous layers of the epidermis, whereas neither GM3 nor GD3 was detected in normal skin.[13] However, the epidermis adjacent to naevi and primary melanoma strongly expressed GD3.[13]

One of the biologically important gangliosides in epidermis is 9-*O*-acetyl-GD3. The ganglioside was initially thought to be a surface marker for basal cell carcinoma of the skin because of the presence of the ganglioside in basal cell carcinoma, but not in normal epidermis.[10,14] However, 9-*O*-acetyl-GD3 was identified as CDw60 antigen,[15] which is expressed on a subset of lymphocytes such as activated human B lymphocytes[16] and Th2-type CD8+ T (Tc2) cells,[17] and has been implicated in the control of cellular proliferation. CDw60 antigen was also expressed in activated epidermal keratinocytes in psoriasis vulgaris. Moreover, T cell lines obtained from lesional skin of psoriasis vulgaris up-regulated CDw60 expression in cultured normal keratinocytes via IL-13.[18] This finding suggests the role of 9-*O*-acetyl-GD3 in the pathogenesis of psoriasis vulgaris. Furthermore, alterations in the amount and composition of individual gangliosides on neoplastic and activated keratinocytes may lead to novel therapeutic interventions.

26.3 POSSIBLE INFLUENCE OF SPHINGOLIPIDS ON THE SKIN

Few reports have investigated the therapeutic and cosmetic applications of sphingolipids on skin, except for ceramides, which can be used for treatment of dry skin such as atopic dermatitis. However, various *in vitro* studies have demonstrated the biological effects of sphingolipids on differentiation and proliferation of keratinocytes, which are the predominant cell type in epidermis. Therefore, it is possible in the future that sphingolipids might be utilized as an ingredient in topical medicine or cosmetics. In this chapter, the biological effects of sphingolipids on cultured keratinocytes are mainly discussed.

26.3.1 Free Long-Chain Bases

The discovery that sphingosine inhibited protein kinase C (PKC) activity spurred interest in sphingolipids as modulators of cell function.[19] In epidermis, it was initially speculated that free sphingosine liberated from ceramides in the stratum corneum may provide a feedback mechanism for regulating the differentiation process. Based on this hypothesis, we investigated the direct biologic action of sphingosine on a transformed human keratinocyte cell line and reported the proliferation-promoting effects of sphingosine on the cells.[20] However, the effects of sphingosine on cultured, normal human keratinocytes remain to be elucidated. In contrast, some studies have examined the biological effects of topical application of sphingosine on the skin. Arnold et al. assessed the effects of sphingosine following tape stripping, which is a potential PKC activator, on the level of induction of ornithine decarboxylase (ODC), and found that application of 0.1 *M* sphingosine resulted in a decrease in ODC activity of approximately 50%.[21] Gupta et al. demonstrated that sphingosine inhibited 12-*0*-tetradecanoylphorbol-13-acetate (TPA)-induced inflammation, hyperplasia, induction of ODC activity and ODC mRNA, and activation of PKC in mouse skin.[22] Their data are compatible with the hypothesis that PKC is a major mediator of the phorbol ester response and that PKC inhibitors may have therapeutic potential in the treatment of inflammatory skin diseases such as psoriasis.

In epidermis, however, unusually large concentrations of free sphingosines are found in the stratum corneum, where free sphingosines make up about 0.5% of the total lipids.[23] Therefore, it is doubtful that temporary release of a small amount of sphingosine could have any important effect on keratinocytes.[7] In addition, FLCBs in epidermis are "detoxified" by forming a complex with cholesterol sulfate,[24] possibly because of the highly cytotoxic nature of FLCBs. However, at the very surface of the skin, cholesterol sulfate disappears during desquamation and released FLCB might play a physiological role at this site. In fact, Bibel et al. have demonstrated a role for sphingosine in the stratum corneum as a cutaneous antimicrobial barrier.[25-27] Their *in vitro* examination of the antimicrobial activity of stratum corneum phospholipids and sphingolipids showed that only the FLCBs were effective against *Staphylococcus aureus*, *Streptococcus pyogenes*, *Micrococcus luteus*, *Propionibacterium acnes*, *Brevibacterium epidermidis*, *Pseudomonas aeruginosa*, and *Candida albicans*. Of note is that antimicrobial activity was duplicated *in vivo* by topical application and microbial challenge, suggesting the usage of FLCB as a topical applicant for antimicrobial regimen.[26,27]

26.3.2 Glycosphingolipids

Glycosphingolipids in cellular membranes generally play two major functional roles: as mediators of cell–cell and cell-substratum interaction and as modulators of transmembrane signaling.[28] In epidermis, however, the main role of sphingolipids, especially ceramides, has been thought to function as an extracellular barrier in the stratum corneum, the nonliving epidermal layer. Since the barrier function of sphingolipids is discussed in further detail in other sections, we have focused mainly on the biological effects of sphingolipids on the viable cell layers.

26.3.2.1 Epidermosides

In addition to participation in epidermal permeability barrier formation, epidermosides are likely associated with autoregulation of epidermal differentiation. Uchida et al. showed that chemically synthesized analogs of epidermosides enhanced keratin synthesis in cultured human keratinocytes and induced the morphological changes such as enlargement and flattening, which are compatible with the morphology of differentiated keratinocytes.[29] The results suggest that AGC, which appears as a consequence of terminal differentiation of keratinocytes, supports the differentiation process. Since the amounts of acylceramide, a breakdown product of AGC, are decreased in the stratum corneum of psoriasis vulgaris,[30] which shows an altered pattern of differentiation,[31] AGC might be a potential topical medicine in the future.

26.3.2.2 Gangliosides

Direct pharmacological effects of gangliosides on cultured keratinocytes have been vigorously investigated. Suppressive effects of gangliosides on keratinocyte proliferation were initially reported by Paller et al.[32] They showed that (1) ganglioside GM3, which is the predominant ganglioside of keratinocyte membranes, inhibited the growth of cultured normal human keratinocytes without modulating keratinocyte differentiation; (2) GD3, 9-*0*-acetyl-GD3, and GD1b also inhibited keratinocyte proliferation; and (3) GM1, GD1a, and sialic acid had little effect. They suggest that hematoside (GM3) and "b" pathway gangliosides (GD3, GD1b), generated by the preferential activation of sialyltransferase II vs. *N*-acetylgalactosaminyltransferase, may be involved in control of keratinocyte growth but not of differentiation. It was subsequently demonstrated that highly sialylated gangliosides, GT1b and GQ1b could promote keratinocyte differentiation.[33,34] However, the pattern of differentiation induced by GT1b and GQ1b seems to be distinct. Paller et al. showed that ganglioside GT1b induced both early (desmosome formation and keratin 1 expression) and late (involucrin expression and cornified envelope formation) phase differentiation markers,[33] whereas Seishima et al. reported that GQ1b, a tetrasialoganglioside containing two disialosyl residues, induced cornified envelope formation and enhancement of transglutaminase activity, which are characteristic steps in the late phase of terminal differentiation in cultured keratinocytes, while GT1b was much less effective.[34] Both reports suggest that GT1b preferentially promotes the initial phase of keratinocyte differentiation, whereas GQ1b predominantly accelerates the late phase of differentiation. These observations suggest that the mechanisms which mediate the differentiation induced by these gangliosides are different, since GT1b could not cause a shift in intracellular free calcium or alter PKC activity,[33] while GQ1b induces a increase in intracellular free calcium and activates PKC[34] via the activation of phospholipase D.[35] Since the transition from the epidermal spinous to granular cell layer is mainly dependent on PKC activation,[36] it is highly likely that the biologic effects of GQ1b on keratinocyte differentiation are mediated by activation of PKC. In contrast, the differentiation modulating effects of GT1b seem to be mainly dependent on its action on the cell–cell and cell–extracellular matrix interaction of keratinocytes. We recently observed that GT1b enhanced the cell surface expression of E-cadherin, which is the major homotypic cell–cell adhesion molecule on keratinocytes and which plays a crucial role in stratification.[37] In addition, the ganglioside GT1b prevents attachment of keratinocytes to fibronectin,[38] which has the ability to inhibit the suspension-induced differentiation of keratinocytes.[39] Therefore, GT1b might promote differentiation by up-regulating cell–cell interaction and down-regulating cell–extracellular matrix interaction, which accelerate the stratification of keratinocytes.

Gangliosides also modulate the biological functions of cutaneous residential cells other than keratinocytes, which might be pathophysiologically relevant. For example, gangliosides GM2, GM3, and GD1a augmented anti-IgE-induced mediator release from human skin mast cells,[40] suggesting that gangliosides optimize IgE-receptor-ligand interaction and that alterations in cellular gangliosides could thus induce enhanced releasability, as observed in atopics.

26.3.3 Acidic Phospholipid Autacoid

Much attention has recently focused on lyso-formed phospholipids, including both glycerophospholipids such as lysophosphatidic acid (LPA) and lysosphingolipids such as sphingosine-1-phosphate (S-1-P) and sphingosylphosphorylcholine (SPC) (Figure 2), since they elicit diverse cellular

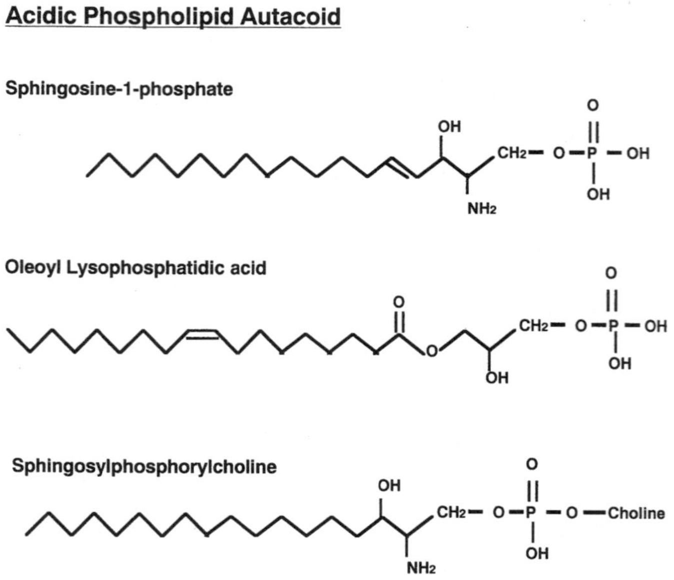

Acidic Phospholipid Autacoid

Sphingosine-1-phosphate

Oleoyl Lysophosphatidic acid

Sphingosylphosphorylcholine

FIGURE 2 Structure of acidic phospholipid autacoid.

effects that range from mitogenesis to the prevention of programmed cell death via the interaction of specific cell surface receptors.[41-43] Therefore, these active lipids are termed the "acidic phospholipid autacoid (APA) family of lipid mediators."[44,45] Since the main source of APA is platelets and APA is released from activated platelets[46,47] a role for APA lipids in the wound healing process has been speculated. In fact, the topical application of SPC has been reported to accelerate cutaneous wound healing in the diabetic mouse.[48,49] SPC is a potent mitogen of cultured keratinocytes,[49] in addition to dermal fibroblasts.[48] LPA is also mitogenic for keratinocytes via the induction of TGF (transforming growth factor)-α.[50] In addition, LPA induces both the active and latent forms of TGF-β in cultured keratinocytes and increases involucrin synthesis in differentiation-committed keratinocytes.[50] The effects of LPA on TGF-α and TGF-β production by keratinocytes likely have *in vivo* relevance, as concluded from rodent studies involving topical LPA treatment.[50] Although, the biologic effects of S-1-P on keratinocytes remain to be reported, S-1-P promotes the morphogenesis of endothelial cells via induction of cadherin-mediated cell–cell interaction[42] and we othat S-1-P could enhance the E-cadherin-mediated cell–cell interaction of keratinocytes. Since E-cadherin is crucial for normal epidermal tissue morphogenesis,[51] S-1-P released from platelets might also modulate reepithelization in healing of cutaneous wound.

In conclusion, this chapter discusses the composition of sphingolipids in epidermis and their possible influences on the skin in the context of recent findings regarding the direct action of sphingolipids on cultured keratinocytes. Although it is commonly thought that sphingolipids are rather cytotoxic because of their detergent-like characteristics, we hopefully await their successful application on the skin as therapeutic agents in the treatment of various cutaneous and other human disorders.

REFERENCES

1. Stoffel, W., Heimann, G., and Hellenbroich, B., Sphingosine kinase in blood platelets, *Hoppe-Seylers Z. Physiol. Chem.*, 354, 562, 1973.
2. Igarashi, Y., and Hakomori, S., Enzymatic synthesis of N,N-dimethyl-sphingosine: demonstration of the sphingosine: N-methyltransferase in mouse brain, *Biochem. Biophys. Res. Commun.*, 164, 1411, 1989.
3. Wertz, P.W., Epidermal lipids, Semin. Dermatol., 11, 106, 1992.

4. Yardley, H.J., and Summerly, R., Lipid composition and metabolism in normal and diseased epidermis, *Pharmacol. Ther.*, 13, 357, 1981.
5. Wertz, P.W., and Downing, D.T., Free sphingosine in human epidermis, *J. Invest. Dermatol.*, 94, 159, 1990.
6. Wakita, H., Nishimura, K., and Takigawa, M., Composition of free long-chain (sphingoid) bases in stratum corneum of normal and pathologic human skin conditions, *J. Invest. Dermatol.*, 99, 617, 1992.
7. Stewart, M.E., and Downing, D.T., Free sphingosines of human skin include 6-hydroxysphingosine and unusually long-chain dihydrosphingosines, *J. Invest. Dermatol.*, 105, 613, 1995.
8. Gray, G.M., and Yardley, H.J., Lipid compositions of cells isolated from pig, human, and rat epidermis, *J. Lipid Res.*, 16, 434, 1975.
9. Hamanaka, S., Asagami, C., Suzuki, M., Inagaki, F., and Suzuki, A., Structure determination of glucosyl beta 1-N-(omega-O-linoleoyl)-acylsphingosines of human epidermis, *J. Biochem.*, 105, 684, 1989.
10. Paller, A.S., Arnsmeier, S.L, Robinson, J.K., and Bremer, E.G., Alteration in keratinocyte ganglioside content in basal cell carcinomas, *J. Invest. Dermatol.*, 98, 226, 1992.
11. Nakakuma, H., Horikawa, K., Kawaguchi, T., Hidaka, M., Nagakura, S., Hirai, S., Kageshita, T., Ono, T., Kagimoto, T., and Iwamori, M., Common phenotypic expression of gangliosides GM3 and GD3 in normal human tissues and neoplastic skin lesions, *Jpn. J. Clin. Oncol.*, 22, 308, 1992.
12. Paller, A.S., Siegel, J.N., Spalding, D.E., and Bremer, E.G., Absence of a stratum corneum antigen in disorders of epidermal cell proliferation: detection with an anti-ganglioside GM3 antibody, *J. Invest. Dermatol.*, 92, 240, 1989.
13. Hersey, P., Jamal, O., Henderson, C., Zardawi, I., and D'Alessandro, G., Expression of the gangliosides GM3, GD3 and GD2 in tissue sections of normal skin, naevi, primary and metastatic melanoma, *Int. J. Cancer*, 41, 336, 1988.
14. Heidenheim, M., Hansen, E.R., and Baadsgaard, O., CDW60, which identifies the acetylated form of GD3 gangliosides, is strongly expressed in human basal cell carcinoma, *Br. J. Dermatol.*, 133, 392, 1995.
15. Kniep, B., Flegel, W.A., Northoff, H., and Rieber, E.P., CDw60 glycolipid antigens of human leukocytes: structural characterization and cellular distribution, *Blood*, 82, 1776, 1993.
16. Vater, M., Kniep, B., Gross, H.J., Claus, C., Dippold, W., and Schwartz-Albiez, R., The 9-O-acetylated disialosyl carbohydrate sequence of CDw60 is a marker on activated human B lymphocytes, *Immunol. Lett.*, 59, 151, 1997.
17. Rieber, E.P., and Rank, G., CDw60: a marker for human CD8+ T helper cells, *J. Exp. Med.*, 179, 1385, 1994.
18. Skov, L., Chan, L.S., Fox, D.A., Larsen, J.K., Voorhees, J.J., Cooper, K.D., and Baadsgaard, O., Lesional psoriatic T cells contain the capacity to induce a T cell activation molecule CDw60 on normal keratinocytes, *Am. J. Pathol.*, 150, 675, 1997.
19. Hannun, Y.A., Loomis, C.R., Merrill, A.H. Jr., and Bell, R.M., Sphingosine inhibition of protein kinase C activity and of phorbol dibutyrate binding *in vitro* and in human platelets, *J. Biol. Chem.*, 261, 12604, 1986.
20. Wakita, H., Tokura, Y., Yagi, H., Nishimura, K., Furukawa, F., and Takigawa, M. Keratinocyte differentiation is induced by cell-permeant ceramides and its proliferation is promoted by sphingosine, *Arch. Dermatol. Res.*, 286, 350, 1994.
21. Arnold, W.P., Glade, C.P., Mier, P.D., and van de Kerkhof, P.C., Effects of sphingosine, isoquinoline and tannic acid on the human tape-stripping model and the psoriatic lesion, *Skin Pharmacol.*, 6, 193, 1993.
22. Gupta, A.K., Fisher, G.J., Elder, J.T., Nickoloff, B.J., and Voorhees, J.J., Sphingosine inhibits phorbol ester-induced inflammation, ornithine decarboxylase activity, and activation of protein kinase C in mouse skin, *J. Invest. Dermatol.,* 91, 486–491, 1988.
23. Wertz, P.W., and Downing, D.T., Free sphingosines in porcine epidermis, *Biochim. Biophys. Acta*, 1002, 213, 1989.
24. Downing, D.T., Dose, R.W., and Abraham, W., Interaction between sphingosine and cholesteryl sulfate in epidermal lipids, *J. Lipid Res.*, 34, 563, 1993.
25. Bibel, D.J., Aly, R., and Shinefield, H.R., Antimicrobial activity of sphingosines, *J. Invest. Dermatol.*, 98, 269, 1992.

26. Bibel, D.J., Aly, R., Shah, S., and Shinefield, H.R., Sphingosines: antimicrobial barriers of the skin, *Acta Derm. Venereol.*, 73, 407, 1993.
27. Bibel, D.J., Aly, R., and Shinefield, H.R., Topical sphingolipids in antisepsis and antifungal therapy, *Clin. Exp. Dermatol.*, 20, 395, 1995.
28. Hakomori, S., Sphingolipid-dependent protein kinases, *Adv. Pharmacol.*, 36, 155, 1996.
29. Uchida, Y., Hamanaka, S., Matsuda, K., Mimura, K., and Otsuka, F., Effect of a chemically-synthesized acylglucosylceramide, epidermoside, on normal human keratinocyte differentiation, *J. Dermatol. Sci.*, 12, 64, 1996.
30. Motta, S., Monti, M., Sesana, S., Mellesi, L., Ghidoni, R., and Caputo, R., Abnormality of water barrier function in psoriasis. Role of ceramide fractions, *Arch. Dermatol.*, 130, 452, 1994.
31. Ortonne, J.P., Aetiology and pathogenesis of psoriasis, *Br. J. Dermatol.*, 135, Suppl. 49, 1, 1996.
32. Paller, A.S., Arnsmeier, S.L., Alvarez-Franco, M., and Bremer, E.G., Ganglioside GM3 inhibits the proliferation of cultured keratinocytes, *J. Invest. Dermatol.*, 100, 841, 1993.
33. Paller, A.S., Arnsmeier, S.L., Fisher, G.J., and Yu, Q.C., Ganglioside GT1b induces keratinocyte differentiation without activating protein kinase C, *Exp. Cell Res.*, 217, 118, 1995.
34. Seishima, M., Takagi, H., Okano, Y., Mori, S., and Nozawa, Y., Ganglioside-induced terminal differentiation of human keratinocytes: early biochemical events in signal transduction, *Arch. Dermatol. Res.*, 285, 397, 1993.
35. Seishima, M., Aoyama, Y., Mori, S., and Nozawa, Y., Involvement of phospholipase D in ganglioside GQ1b-induced biphasic diacylglycerol production in human keratinocytes, *J. Invest. Dermatol.*, 104, 835, 1995.
36. Dlugosz, A.A., and Yuspa, S.H., Coordinate changes in gene expression which mark the spinous to granular cell transition in epidermis are regulated by protein kinase C, *J. Cell Biol.*, 120, 217, 1993.
37. Lewis, J.E., Jensen, P.J., and Wheelock, M.J., Cadherin function is required for human keratinocytes to assemble desmosomes and stratify in response to calcium, *J. Invest. Dermatol.*, 102, 870, 1994.
38. Paller, A.S., Arnsmeier, S.L., Chen, J.D., and Woodley, D.T., Ganglioside GT1b inhibits keratinocyte adhesion and migration on a fibronectin matrix, *J. Invest. Dermatol.*, 105, 237, 1995.
39. Watt, F.M., Kubler, M.D., Hotchin, N.A., Nicholson, L.J., and Adams, J.C., Regulation of keratinocyte terminal differentiation by integrin-extracellular matrix interactions, *J. Cell Sci.*, 106, 175, 1993.
40. Zuberbier, T., Pfrommer, C., Beinholzl, J., Hartmann, K., Ricklinkat, J., and Czarnetzki, B.M., Gangliosides enhance IgE receptor-dependent histamine and LTC4 release from human mast cells, *Biochim. Biophys. Acta*, 1269, 79, 1995.
41 Spiegel, S., and Merrill, A.H. Jr., Sphingolipid metabolism and cell growth regulation, *FASEB J.*, 10, 1388, 1996.
42. Lee, M.J., Van Brocklyn, J.R., Thangada, S., Liu, C.H., Hand, A.R., Menzeleev, R., Spiegel, S., and Hla, T., Sphingosine-1-phosphate as a ligand for the G protein-coupled receptor EDG-1, *Science*, 279, 1552, 1998.
43. Igarashi, Y., Sphingosine-1-phosphate as an intercellular signaling molecule, *Ann. N.Y. Acad. Sci.*, 845, 19, 1998.
44. Tokumura, A., A family of phospholipid autacoids: occurrence, metabolism and bioactions, *Prog. Lipid Res.*, 34, 151, 1995.
45. Liliom, K., Fischer, D.J., Virag, T., Sun, G., Miller, D.D., Tseng, J.L., Desiderio, D.M., Seidel, M.C., Erickson, J.R., and Tigyi, G., Identification of a novel growth factor-like lipid, 1-O-cis-alk-1'-enyl-2-lyso-sn-glycero-3-phosphate (alkenyl-GP) that is present in commercial sphingolipid preparations, *J. Biol. Chem.*, 273, 13461, 1998.
46. Yatomi, Y., Igarashi, Y., Yang, L., Hisano, N., Qi, R., Asazuma, N., Satoh, K., Ozaki Y., and Kume, S., Sphingosine 1-phosphate, a bioactive sphingolipid abundantly stored in platelets, is a normal constituent of human plasma and serum, *J. Biochem.*, 121, 969, 1997.
47. Alexander, J.S., Patton, W.F., Christman, B.W., Cuiper, L.L., and Haselton, F.R., Platelet-derived lysophosphatidic acid decreases endothelial permeability *in vitro*, *Am. J. Physiol.*, 274, H115, 1998.
48. Sun, L., Xu, L., Henry, F.A., Spiegel, S., and Nielsen, T.B., A new wound healing agent — sphingosylphosphorylcholine, *J. Invest. Dermatol.*, 106, 232, 1996.
49. Wakita, H., Matsushita, K., Nishimura, K., Tokura, Y., Furukawa, F., and Takigawa, M., Sphingosylphosphorylcholine stimulates proliferation and upregulates cell surface-associated plasminogen activator activity in cultured human keratinocytes, *J. Invest. Dermatol.*, 110, 253, 1998.

50. Piazza, G.A., Ritter, J.L., and Baracka, C.A., Lysophosphatidic acid induction of transforming growth factors alpha and beta: modulation of proliferation and differentiation in cultured human keratinocytes and mouse skin, *Exp. Cell Res.*, 216, 51, 1995.
51. Wheelock, M.J., and Jensen, P.J., Regulation of keratinocyte intercellular junction organization and epidermal morphogenesis by E-cadherin, *J. Cell Biol.*, 117, 415, 1992.

27 Critical and Optimal Molar Ratios of Key Lipids

Carl Thornfeldt

CONTENTS

27.1 BACKGROUND

It is now generally accepted that the functional cutaneous permeability barrier resides within the stratum corneum intercellular multilamellar sheets consisting predominantly of ceramides and cholesterol, as well as essential and nonessential free fatty acids. The importance of these three key stratum corneum lipid species to the integrity of the cutaneous permeability barrier is demonstrated by their synthetic activity being regulated by alterations in stratum corneum barrier structure. When such alterations occur, not all epidermal lipids are synthesized in parallel. Cholesterol and free fatty acids are synthesized immediately after barrier disruption, while ceramide synthesis begins about 2 h later in the recovering of barrier homeostasis.[1-4]

Barrier function not only regulates lipid synthesis, but also epidermal DNA synthesis, thereby providing an additional pool of lipid biosynthetic enzymes and precursor substrates.[4] The stimulation of epidermal lipid and DNA synthesis was observed in both acute and chronic murine models of barrier disruption, indicating the crucial roles for both lipid and DNA synthesis for the maintenance of permeability barrier homeostasis.[5,6]

With the proliferation of skin care products and cosmeceuticals, distinction between the functionality of pure moisturizers and barrier-repairing moisturizers should be made. This information will assist health care providers and skin care professionals in selecting the products which improve stratum corneum barrier function, our first line of defense. Optimizing skin health in this manner should diminish the adverse impact of environmental insults and may be prophylaxis against certain mucocutaneous diseases.

Moisturizers are defined as compositions which increase the stratum corneum water content, also known as hydration. Skin conductance measurement is among the most accurate methods of assaying the water content. While high water content determined by high skin conductance measurements indicates a high degree of moisturization, it does not indicate excellent barrier function. Mucous membranes, for example, are moist with an extremely high water content, but have poor barrier function.[7,8] Substances which induce and/or accelerate barrier repair are all

0-8493-7520-7/00/$0.00+$.50

TABLE 1
Comparison of Hydration

Composition Applied (Mole Ratios)	Mean Conductance (Siemens)
None (measurement taken prior to treatment with test formulation)	−1.9
LacHydrin V	237.7
Avon ANEW	624.4
Vehicle plus additives shown below (vehicle is proylene glycol/ethanol, 7:3, additive totaling 2 to 3% by weight of formulation)	
CH/AC (2:1)	126.9
CH/Cer/LA/PA (3:1:1:1)	122.4
CH/AC/PA (4:1:2:5)	130.4
50% CH/AC (2:1) with 25% Pet, 25% Gly	383.2

Note: AC, acylceramide; Cer, bovine ceramide; CH, cholesterol; LA, linoleic acid; PA, palmitic acid; SA, stearic acid; Pet, petrolatum; Gly, glycerin.

effective moisturizers, but all pure moisturizers do not improve barrier function. While all pure moisturizers will temporarily decrease visible scaling and roughness, most further disrupt the integrity or do not allow normal repair of the stratum corneum barrier.

Barrier-repairing moisturizers increase hydration due to efficacy of the three physiologic lipids, but especially ceramides which are known potent humectants.[8,9] Studies have demonstrated that many of the individual lipids and lipid combinations known for their hydrating properties actually impede rather than facilitate barrier repair when applied to damaged skin. Therefore, these formulations will be expected to worsen the lesions of mucocutaneous diseases because an acute or chronically damaged epidermal barrier responds differently than either normal skin or merely dry, rough skin when epidermal lipids are applied.

An assessment of the moisturizing capability of several key physiologic lipid compositions including critical and optimal molar ratios compared to marketed products was undertaken in Table 1.[9] The test procedure was as follows. Twelve female humans aged 18 to 55, in two panels of six each, were pretreated for one week by washing their forearms daily with Ivory Soap®. Following the pretreatment, the test formulations were applied to three sites on the volar side of each forearm. Skin conductance was measured prior to application of the formulations to establish a baseline and again at 4 h after application of the formulations. Measurements were taken using a SKINCON 200 MT probe. The mean values are shown in Table 1.

Table 1 shows that all of these tested formulations serve as effective moisturizing agents, with the greatest benefit from the noncommercial formulation consisting of key physiologic lipids with added petrolatum and glycerin. Comparing Table 1 data with Test Series 2 of Table 2 demonstrates the lack of correlation between excellent moisturization and improving barrier repair. The four compositions containing the key physiologic lipid dramatically accelerate repair of the disrupted barrier, while the most hydrating commercially available moisturizers do not accelerate normal barrier repair.[9]

Scaling and roughness of the skin are a manifestation of an abnormally desquamating stratum corneum, but often these conditions do not correlate with the abnormal function of the stratum corneum barrier as with ichthyosus vulgaris. Conversely, people afflicted with the atopic diathesis with intermittent flares of dermatitis have areas of normal appearing nonlesional skin without scale, yet the stratum corneum barrier function is compromised.

Stratum corneum thickness also does not correlate with barrier function. Palms and soles that appear normal have the thickest stratum corneum and a high water content, but relatively poor barrier function.[4,6]

27.2 CRITICAL AND OPTIMAL RATIOS

Ceramide, cholesterol, and free fatty acids account for about 40, 25, and 20%, respectively, by weight of the stratum corneum lipids. Cholesterol has a molecular weight of 387. The molecular weight of the multiple ceramides was averaged at 875. Free fatty acids were averaged at a molecular weight of 285. Thus, a normally functioning stratum corneum barrier has an approximately equimolar critical physiologic lipid ratio of ceramide 1/cholesterol 1/free fatty acid 1. This was confirmed clinically by screening normal young adults who did not suffer from nor have a family history of any chronic cutaneous diseases (unpublished).

A variable amount of the ceramides exists as acylceramides, uniquely human ceramides with omega esterified fatty acids such as ceramide 1 linoleate. The most effective barrier-repairing ceramides are acylceramides linked to linoleic, palmitic, or stearic fatty acids. Acylceramides usually function as two physiologic lipids because stratum corneum lipases release the fatty acid moiety from the ceramide backbone.[5,8,13]

Utilizing pharmacologic inhibitors of their rate-limiting enzymes, each of the three key lipids has been shown to be required for barrier homeostasis. These rate-limiting synthetic enzymes include 3-hydroxy-3-methyl-glutaryl coenzyme A reductase for cholesterol, serine palmitoyl transferase for ceramides, and acetyl Co A carboxylase for fatty acids. Co-applications of the distal products of each enzyme with the inhibitor normalized repair kinetics, indicating that the barrier abnormality could be attributed to synthetic enzyme inhibition.[1-4] Deletion or diminution of any of these three key lipids results in delayed recovery, further disruption, and/or abnormal homeostasis of the intact stratum corneum barrier due to a deficiency of one of the three crucial components of the physiologic barrier lipid complex.

The importance of this critical equimolar lipid ratio for normal stratum corneum barrier function was further substantiated when topical application of this physiologic lipid composition to disrupted young murine and human skin allowed normal barrier recovery, as in Table 2.[10-12] Moreover, many pure moisturizers further disrupt the stratum corneum barrier and/or prevent its recovery by perturbing this critical equimolar ratio of the three key physiologic lipids as in Tables 1 and 2. Additional evidence for the importance of this critical ratio is that co-application of two rate-limiting enzyme inhibitors of cholesterol and ceramides decreases the lipid quantity but maintains the critical molar lipid ratio and thus normal barrier function.[14]

The discovery of this critical equimolar ratio for normal stratum corneum barrier function stimulated the search for compositions which would accelerate repair of a compromised barrier known as the optimal molar ratio. There are multiple prophylactic and therapeutic applications for topical products containing these optimal ratios of the three key physiologic lipids because multiple diseases and disorders of the skin and mucous membrane are associated with, caused by, or result in a compromised stratum corneum barrier. Barrier disruption not only contributes significantly to the morphology of the cutaneous lesions, but also may activate certain mucocutaneous conditions such as the Koebner phenomenon, psoriasis and other papulosquamous diseases, and atopic and irritant dermatoses.

Mucocutaneous conditions characterized by a compromised stratum corneum permeability barrier include the following:

1. Premature infants under 33 weeks gestational age
2. Atopic and seborrheic dermatitis and other genetically predisposed dermatitides
3. Eczematous dermatitis induced by environmental or occupational insults, specifically allergic and irritant contact, eczema craquelé, photoallergic, phototoxic, phytophotodermatitis, radiation, and stasis dermatitis

4. Ulcers and erosions due to cutaneous trauma, including chemical or thermal burns or vascular compromise or ischemia including venous, arterial, arterial, or embolic or diabetic ulcers
5. Ichthyoses
6. Epidermolysis bullosa
7. Psoriasis, lichen planus, and other papulosquamous diseases
8. Cutaneous changes of intrinsic aging and/or photoaging
9. Mechanical friction blistering
10. Atrophy due to corticosteroids and actinic damage[9]

Other clinical uses for these optimal ratio key lipid compositions include the following:

1. Prevent cutaneous occupationally and environmentally induced irritant and allergic reactions
2. Minimize barrier disruption by other known or potential therapeutic products
3. Prevent activation, minimize severity and distribution, and prolong remission of genetically predisposed mucocutaneous disorders
4. Enhance the therapeutic activity of other known pharmacologically active agents

These optimal molar ratio physiologic lipid compositions, by accelerating barrier recovery, decrease epidermal DNA synthesis, thus ameliorating hyperproliferation. These compositions also diminish inflammation by inhibiting stratum corneum biological response modifiers released to induce repair of a disrupted barrier and protect the organism. Significantly impeding release of these modifiers by inducing or maintaining normal barrier function may prolong or induce complete remission, prevent recurrences, and/or minimize the severity and distribution of lesions of mucocutanateous diseases.

The impact upon stratum corneum barrier integrity and recovery of compositions comprising various ratios of the three key physiologic lipids was assessed. To rapidly assess many compositions of different molar ratios, mice were used as the *in vivo* subjects. However, to ensure these data predicted the potential utility in humans known to have thicker stratum corneum, a very stringent environment was created by dissolving only 1.5% lipids in a vehicle consisting of 70% propylene glycol/30% ethanol. This active vehicle is commonly used in many therapeutic products as a penetration enhancer. Later human trials confirmed the relative potency of barrier-repairing activity by these lipid compositions.[9]

Hairless mice, aged 8 to 12 weeks, were treated by repeated application of absolute acetone to one flank to perturb the cutaneous barrier. The rate of transepidermal water loss (TEWL) was then measured periodically by use of an electrolytic water analyzer (Meeco, Inc., Warrington, PA). As soon as the TEWL rates exceeded 2.0 g/m^2/h, test formulations were applied topically to the barrier-perturbed areas, over an area of 5 cm^2. The formulations consisted of either a lipid or lipid combination dissolved in a vehicle consisting of a mixture of propylene glycol and ethanol at a volume/volume ratio of 7:3 or the vehicle alone. Each test formulation was applied to 10 to 12 mice. Further measurements of TEWL were then taken at 45 min, 4 h, and 8 h after application of the test formulations. The values from these measurements were compared with the values obtained just before the test formulations were applied to determine the degree of barrier recovery. The degrees of recovery for each lipid or lipid combination can be compared with the values obtained with the vehicle alone to determine what effect can be attributed to the inclusion of the lipid or lipid combination.[9]

In Table 2, the values listed in the second, third, and fifth columns represent the TEWL at 45 min, 4 h, and 8 h, respectively, after application of each test formulation. The values are expressed as percentages of the TEWL value immediately before the test formulations were applied. Percentages below 100 indicate improved recovery of barrier function. Recovery attributable to the lipid(s) is seen only when the percentages fall below those obtained for the vehicle alone. Percentages above 100 indicate further deterioration of barrier function attributable to the test formulation rather than recovery. Although not shown in the table, applications of these test formulations resulted in 0% TEWL or full recovery of the barrier integrity 30 to 36 h after application compared to normal recovery at 72 h.

These topically applied key physiologic lipid compositions traverse the stratum corneum and enter into the nucleated cell layers. The lipids are incorporated into lamellar bodies and then secreted into the intercellular spaces at the superficial junction of the stratum granulosum, forming the multiple lipid lamella between the cornified keratinocytes. Because of this metabolic processing, these lipids have the greatest impact on barrier recovery beginning at about 2 h. The inhibition of stratum granulosum lamellar body secretion with monensin prevents the beneficial effects of these key molar ratio lipid mixtures.[4-6]

The barrier-repairing activity of these key lipid compositions is not simply due to passive blockade of evaporation due to an occlusive film type quality, as with petrolatum.[15] Effects of petrolatum do not need active lamellar body secretion and thus are not inhibited by monensin. Furthermore, petrolatum induces earlier barrier repair than the key lipid mixtures. Contrarily, the molar ratio lipid mixtures are accelerating the normal epidermal repair process. Glycerin accelerates barrier repair, but later than optimal molar lipid ratio compositions as seen in Table 2.

Logically, the application of each of the key physiologic lipids individually or combined with another key lipid in a two-component system should normalize or accelerate barrier recovery when applied to damaged skin, but this does not occur as seen in Table 2, Test Series 1. When cholesterol, free fatty acids, ceramides, or even acylceramides are applied alone to compromised skin, they inhibit rather than improve barrier repair. Any two-component system of the three key lipids also inhibits repair. The exception is when cholesterol and acylceramide are mixed, as this composition accelerates barrier repair. Compositions with all three key lipids in critical molar ratios allow normal barrier recovery. Optimal molar ratio lipid compositions accelerate barrier recovery to varying degrees. Barrier recovery after 2 to 4 h was enhanced by these compositions, even if it had been delayed during the first hour after the application of the optimal lipid ratio compositions.[9]

The most effective compositions in accelerating barrier recovery after acute disruption in Table 2 are the optimal molar ratio key lipid combinations with the greatest statistical significance ($p < 0.0001$). Furthermore, these optimal compositions are expected to be the most effective prophylactic and therapeutic agents for mucocutaneous disorders. The optimal compositions include the following:

1. Two-component combinations include cholesterol and acylceramide. Ratios within the range of 1.5:1 to 3.5:1 are most effective, with a particularly effective molar ratio being cholesterol 2/acylceramide 1.
2. Three-component combinations include cholesterol, acylceramides, or ceramides and one or more fatty acids preferably with 16 to 18 carbon atom lengths, but especially linoleic, palmitic, and stearic acid. The most effective molar ratios include cholesterol 1.5-2/acylceramide 1/free fatty acids 3, cholesterol 4/ceramide 1/palmitic acid 2.5, and cholesterol 2/ceramide 1/stearic acid 3.
3. Four-component combinations include cholesterol, ceramide, essential fatty acid, and nonessential or bulk fatty acid. The essential fatty acid is linoleic acid, and the preferred nonessential fatty acids are those of 16 to 18 carbon atom lengths, especially palmitic and stearic acids. The most effective molar ratio compositions include cholesterol 2/ceramide 1/stearic or palmitic acid 1/linoleic acid 1. This ratio is the most effective when stearic acid is the nonessential fatty acid. Other effective combinations include cholesterol 2/ceramide 1/linoleic acid 1/bulk fatty acid 1, 2:2:1:1, 1:1:1:2, and 1:1:1:3.[9]

TABLE 2
Barrier Function Recovery: Transepidermal Water Loss at Various Intervals Expressed as Percent of Transepidermal Water Loss at 0 Hours (Maximal Level)

Composition Applied (Mole Ratios of Active Ingradients)	n	TEWL at 0.75 Hours (as % of TEWL at 0 Hours)	TEWL at 4 Hours (as % of TEWL at 0 Hours)	P Value[a]	TEWL at 8 Hours (as % of TEWL at 0 Hours)
Test Series 1					
Vehicle alone (propylene glycol/ethanol, 7:3)	25	87 ± 3.8	67.5 ± 3.8	—	52.1 ± 4.9
Vehicle plus (additive weight at 1.5% by weight)					
Cer	5	—	113.8 ± 11.7	<0.001	—
AC	10	—	93.5 ± 4.4	<0.001	—
CH	35	—	69.5 ± 2.8	NS	—
PA	10	—	67.3 ± 5.8	NS	—
SA	10	—	69.1 ± 4.1	NS	—
Pet (25%)	23	49.2 + 3.8	50.0 ± 3.4	<0.01	—
Pet (2%)	10	59.0 ± 6.3	—	—	—
Gly (30%)	10	93.2 ± 6.2	66.7 ± 9.0	NS	33.7 ± 5.4
Gly (10%)	10	—	33.0 ± 6.5	<0.0001	16.8 ± 4.3
CH/Cer (1:1)	14	—	91.7 ± 5.4	<0.001	—
CH/LA (1:1)	10	—	88.0 ± 2.3	<0.0001	—
Ch/Cer/:LA (1:1:1)	10	—	66.0 ± 4.6	NS	—
CH/Cer/PA (1:1:1)	11	—	66.8 ± 4.2	NS	—
CH/Cer/SA (1:1:1)	11	—	67.4 ± 2.7	NS	—
CH/AC (0.25:1)	11	—	50.2 ± 3.1	<0.01	—
CH/AC (0.67:1)	10	—	23.6 ± 2.8	<0.0001	—
CH/AC (1.33:1)	10	—	26.9 ± 1.3	<0.0001	—
CH/AC (1.5:1)	11	—	18.4 ± 1.0	<0.0001	—
CH/AC (2:1)	11	102.3 ± 5.8	17.4 ± 2.1	<0.0001	11.0 ± 1.1
CH/AC (2.5:1)	11	—	24.5 ± 3.2	<0.0001	—
CH/AC (3:1)	11	—	22.1 ± 4.0	<0.0001	—
CH/AC (3.5:1)	10	—	20.3 ± 1.2	<0.0001	—
CH/AC (4.6:1)	10	—	47.0 ± 3.4	<0.01	—
50% CH/AC (2:1) 25% Pet 25% Gly	9	40.2 ± 4.2	17.9 ± 3.0	<0.0001	7.0 ± 1.2
CH/AC/PA (1:1:2.5)	11	—	26.8 ± 3.1	<0.0001	—
Avon ANEW	9	—	71.9 ± 4.6	NS	—
LacHydrin	11	63.3 ± 6.1	63.8 ± 5.9	NS	—
Test Series 2					
Vehicle alone (propylene glycol/ethanol, 7:3)	25	—	67.5 ± 3.8	—	—
Vehicle plus (additives totaling 1.5% by weight):					
CH/Cer/La/PA (1:1:1:1)	11	—	60.7 ± 4.2	NS	—
CH/Cer/LA/PA (2:1:1:1)	11	—	37.4 ± 2.0	<0.0001	—
CH/Cer/LA/PA (3:1:1:1)	12	—	28.0 ± 2.0	<.0001	—
CH/Cer/LA/PA (4:1:1:1)	12	—	49.5 ± 3.5	<0.01	—

TABLE 2 (continued)
Barrier Function Recovery: Transepidermal Water Loss at Various Intervals Expressed as Percent of Transepidermal Water Loss at 0 Hours (Maximal Level)

Composition Applied (Mole Ratios of Active Ingradients)	n	TEWL at 0.75 Hours (as % of TEWL at 0 Hours)	TEWL at 4 Hours (as % of TEWL at 0 Hours)	P Value[a]	TEWL at 8 Hours (as % of TEWL at 0 Hours)
CH/Cer/LA/PA (5:1:1:1)	12	—	56.6 ± 3.6	<0.05	—
CH/Cer/LA/PA (5.5:1:1:1)	12	—	61.5 ± 3.5	NS	—
CH/Cer/LA/PA (1:1:1:1.5)	11	—	58.6 ± 3.9	<0.1	—
CH/Cer/LA/PA (3:1:1:2)	11	—	46.0 ± 5.6	<0.01	—
CH/Cer/LA/PA (3:1:1:3)	21	—	32.0 ± 2.3	<0.0001	—
CH/Cer/LA/PA (3:1:1:3.5)	11	—	56.0 ± 4.7	<0.1	—
CH/Cer/LA/PA (3:1:1:4)	12	—	69.7 ± 4.9	NS	—
CH/Cer/LA/PA (3:1:1:2)	12	—	50.2 ± 4.3	<0.01	—

Note: AC = acylceramide; Cer, bovine ceramide; CH, cholesterol; LA, linoleic acid; PA, palmitic acid; SA, stearic acid; Pet, petrolatum; Gly, glycerin.

[a] NS: difference not statistically significant, i.e., $p > 0.1$.

To correlate this murine data with human clinical situations, two different formulations comprising optimal molar ratios of lipids that accelerated barrier recovery with $p < 0.0001$ were tested in three groups of human patients. The following results were obtained.

Topical Formulation A was prepared as a creamy emulsion. The key lipid mole ratio was cholesterol 3/ceramide 1/linoleic acid 1. Five health care workers whose daily routine involved frequent changing of gloves and hand washing and who all suffered from noninflammatory, scaly, intermittently pruritic hands as a result experienced only minimal relief by commercial moisturizing lotions and partial relief by occlusive greases. Application of Formula A three times daily by each worker completely relieved the scaling and symptoms within an average of 6 days. Continued use of the product every other day effectively maintained normal skin despite the workers' continued exposure to the same environmental insults.

Three people with a history of atopic dermatitis but suffering from marked xerosis most prominently on the distal extremities, failed many commercially available moisturizing products. The use of occlusive hydrocarbon mixtures such as petrolatum produced pruritus. Formulation A applied two to four times daily produced complete resolution of scaling without inducing pruritis within 3 to 4 days. Daily application for maintenance prevented recurrence.

Topical Formulation B was also prepared as a creamy emulsion with a lipid molar ratio of cholesterol 3/ceramide 1/linoleic acid 1/palmitic acid 1. Four middle-aged women, all outdoor agriculture workers and all of whom had scaly, leathery-textured, finely wrinkled facial skin, experienced only poor response to a variety of moisturizing lotions. Each of the women applied Topical Formulation B twice daily, and the scaling was cleared within 1 week in all cases. After 4 weeks of twice daily applications, the skin of all four women exhibited a noticeable improvement in skin suppleness.[9]

These previously mentioned experiments indicate that compositions with critical and optimal ratios of the three key physiologic lipids would be expected to effectively produce prophylactic and therapeutic benefits to mucocutaneous membranes. Thus, dermatologists, cosmetic surgeons, and skin care professionals should recommend such products. Moreover, these experiments indicate that *in vivo* mouse models with approriately stringent vehicles are useful for designing human products that impact the stratum corneum barrier.

27.3 ENDOGENOUS VARIABILITY OF PHYSIOLOGIC LIPIDS

There exist significant differences in the physiologic lipid composition and quantity over different anatomic regions. For example, the proportion of ceramides and cholesterol is much higher in palm and sole stratum corneum than on the extensor surfaces of the extremities, abdomen, and face. Adjusting for the 2% lipid weight at the palms and soles, the absolute amounts of ceramides and cholesterol in the intercellular spaces are significantly lower than the other three anatomic sites. Thus, there is an inverse relationship between lipid weight percentage and the permeability properties of any particular mucocutaneous membrane.[4,6,7,16]

A sphingolipid gradient exists in the stratum corneum with ceramide accounting for 98% of the epidermal surface sphingolipid species in keratinizing membranes. Precursor species are dominant in the epidermal basal layer. Less well-keratinized membranes such as the palate and fixed gingiva have 77 and 73%, respectively, of the sphingolipid converted into ceramides. Nonkeratinized buccal and the floor of the mouth membranes have 5 to 6% of sphingolipids converted to ceramide. Phospholipids, glycolipids, cholesterol, and fatty acids were the dominant lipid species by weight in the buccal and mouth floor mucosa.7

Similar epidermal gradients exist for cholesterol and free fatty acids with the precursors dominating in the basal strata resulting in different mole ratios of the key lipids at different levels within the stratum corneum. The ratio of free fatty acid/cholesterol decreases from 1.6 to 1.2 between tape strip levels 3 and 5, while free fatty acid/ceramide ratio decreases from 0.8 to 0.66 at these same levels.[17]

Chronologically aged mice (<18 months) and humans (>75 years) have morphologically compromised stratum corneum barrier with reduced total lipids and decreased numbers of intercellular lipid lamellae. These changes are manifested by a delay in barrier recovery, but have no impact upon the normal permeability function. These aged mice also display a global decrease in synthesis of the three key lipids, but it is especially pronounced with cholesterol synthesis.[18-20] Therefore, in contrast to younger animals, topical application of cholesterol alone and the critical equimolar ratio of the three key lipids both accelerate repair of a compromised barrier. Applying an optimal molar ratio composition of cholesterol 3/ceramide 1/linoleic acid 1/palmitic acid 1 significantly accelerated barrier repair beyond that of either the critical equimolar lipid composition or by cholesterol alone. Ultrastructure supported these effects by demonstrating increased lipid lamellar units in the stratum corneum intercellular spaces after application of this optimal lipid composition.[21]

In aged human skin, the same 3:1:1:1 optimal lipid ratio with cholesterol dominance increased barrier repair by 30% at 6 h over the optimal equimolar ratio.[21] Total lipid levels in this population were decreased about 30%, but the ratios of the three key physiological lipids remained constant, maintaining the structural integrity of the lipid bilayers and thus preserving normal barrier function. However, the increased susceptibility of the stratum corneum barrier to damage, the delay in barrier repair after injury, and the increased permeability to certain compounds are due primarily to the age-related decline in ceramide 1 linoleate and acylceramide, cholesterol, and free fatty acid levels.[18-20,22,23]

Systemic homeostasis generally has little influence on cutaneous lipid synthesis. Although dramatic changes in thyroid hormone, testosterone, and estrogen modulate epidermal lipid synthesis, these hormones do not regulate daily cutaneous lipid synthesis.[23] In contrast, recent female sex hormones have been shown to influence cutaneous thickness, keratinocyte proliferation, and ceramide synthesis.[24-25]

27.4 EXOGENOUS VARIABILITY OF PHYSIOLOGIC LIPIDS

In addition to the decline in the mass quantity of the different ceramide species, the relative proportion of ceramide 1 linoleate (acylceramide) was decreased in winter. This compound is also reduced in atopic dermatitis and xerosis and within acne follicles. This acylceramide functions in maintaining stratum corneum flexibility and bilayer fluidity, as previously observed only for glycerol.[13,20,26-29]

Low ambient temperature and decreasing skin surface temperature diminishes epidermal lipid synthesis capacity, inhibits barrier repair, and masks a compromised permeability barrier.[28,30,31] This reduction in total lipid quantity and function accounts for the increased incidence of wintertime xerosis and itch even though the permeability layer is not compromised. Other documented seasonal changes include increased levels of both palmitic and palmitoleic fatty acids in the summer.[20,32,33]

Another clinical condition characterized by a significant reduction in lipid content and compromised stratum corneum barrier results from topical corticosteroid application. These drugs induce mucocutaneous atrophy by: (1) decreasing the number of layers of cornified keratinocytes due to antiproliferative effect and (2) decreasing the numbers of intercellular lipid lamellae, seen with ultrastructure microscopy.[34,35]

The stratum corneum permeability barrier is disrupted by solvents such as acetone or petroleum ether which remove different lipid species and by mechanical methods such as tape stripping. Both mechanical and solvent disruption is reversed by application of a composition containing the three key barrier lipids in an optimal molar ratio. Barrier disruption with different detergents resulted in an unpredictable variable response. The detergent disruption by either *N*-laurosarcosine or dodecylbenzensulfuric was repaired in an accelerated manner following an application of an optimal molar ratio consisting of cholesterol 4.3/ceramide 2.3/palmitic acid 1.0/linoleic acid 1.08. When the barrier was disrupted with either of two other detergents, sodium dodecyl sulfate and ammonium lauryl sulphosuccinate, this same optimal lipid mixture did not even effectively repair the compromised stratum corneum barrier.[36]

The fact that these critical and optimal molar ratios are physiologically processed suggests that mixtures of the three key lipid precursors may also positively impact barrier repair. Utilizing a mixture of triglyceride and glycosylceramide/sphingomyelin replacing fatty acids and ceramides, respectively, combined with cholesterol significantly accelerated barrier repair.[10,11] A naturally occurring mixture comprising predominantly precursors in addition to very small amounts of the three key lipids accelerated barrier repair and increased hydration.[35] The large amount of epidermal hydrolase activity in the upper epidermis appears to catabolize the complex lipid precursors into mature key physiologic lipids.[38-40]

27.5 SUMMARY

The preceding review shows the importance of not only the presence of the three key lipid species — cholesterol, ceramide, and free fatty acids — for normal stratum corneum barrier function, but also the importance of the interrelationships of the quantities of these lipids, i.e., molar ratios. The data indicate the critical molar ratio for normal stratum corneum permeability barrier function is an equimolar ratio of cholesterol 1/ceramide 1/essential free fatty acid 1/bulk fatty acid 1. When the barrier is compromised in response to cutaneous injury at a specific anatomic site or environmental insults such as seasons and chronological age, critical molar ratio lipid compositions allow normal recovery of permeability barrier function. The majority of people are afflicted by multiple environmental insults, chronological aging, or have overt predisposition to mucocutaneous diseases characterized by a compromised stratum corneum barrier. Formulations containing optimal molar ratios of the three key physiologic lipids and those with naturally occurring lipid complexes of precursor barrier lipids accelerate repair of a compromised permeability barrier except when induced by certain detergents. These optimal lipid compositions are expected to have great utility in preventing and treating mucocutaneous diseases and conditions as well as improving "wellness" of these epithelial membranes.

REFERENCES

1. Holleran WM, Mao-Qiang M, Gao WN, Menon GK, Elias PM, Feingold KR, Sphingolipids are required for mammalian barrier function: inhibition of sphingolipid synthesis delays barrier recovery after acute perturbation. *J Clin Invest* 88: 1338–1345. 1991.
2. Feingold KR, Mao-Qiang M, Menon GK, Cho SS, Brown BE, Elias PM. Cholesterol synthesis is required for cutaneous barrier function in mice. *J Clin Invest* 86:1738–1745. 1990.
3. Mao-Qiang M. Elias PM, Feingold KR. Fatty acids are required for epidermal permeability barrier function. *J Clin Invest* 92: 791–798. 1993.
4. Elias PM, Feingold KR. Lipids and the epidermal water barrier: metabolism, regulation, and pathophysiology. *Sem Dermatol* 11: 176–182. 1992.
5. Feingold KR. The regulation and role of epidermal lipid syntheses. *Adv Lipid Res* 24: 57–59. 1991.
6. Elias PM. Dynamics of the epidermal barrier: new implications for percutaneous drug delivery, topical therapeutics, and disease pathogenesis. *Prog Dermatol.* 2: 1–8. 1992.
7. Law S, Wertz PW, Swartzenderuber DC, Squier CA. Regional variation in content, composition and organization of porcine epithelial barrier lipids revealed by thin-layer chromatography and transmission electron microscopy. *Arch Oral Biol.* 4(12):1085–1091. 1995.
8. Imokawa G, Hattori M. A possible function of structural lipid in the water holding properties of the stratum corneum. *J Invest Dermatol* 84: 282–284. 1985.
9. Thornfeldt CR, Elias PM, Feingold KR. Lipids for Epidermal Moisturization and Repair of Barrier Function. US Patent No. 5,693,899; July 1, 1997.
10. Mao-Qiang M, Feingold KR, Elias PM. Exogenous lipids influence permeability barrier recovery in acetone treated murine skin. *Arch Dermatol* 129: 729–738. 1993.
11. Mao-Qiang M, Thornfeldt CR, Feingold KR, Elias PM. Optimization of physiological lipid mixtures for barrier repair. *J Invest Dermatol* 106: 1096–1101. 1996.
12. Mao-Qiang M, Brown BE, Wu-Pong S et al. Exogenous non-physiologic vs. physiologic lipids: divergent mechanisms for correction of permeability barrier dysfunction. *Arch Dermatol* 131: 809–816. 1995.
13. Oldroyd J, Critchley P, Tiddy G, Turner J, Rawlings A. Specialized role for ceramide one in the stratum corneum water barrier. *J Invest Dermatol* 102: 525. 1994.
14. Mao-Quiang M, Feingold KR, Elias PM. Inhibition of cholesterol and sphingoloid synthese causes paradoxial effects on permeability barrier homeostatis. *J Invest Dermatol* 101: 185–190. 1993.
15. Ghadially RG, Halkier-Sorensen L, Elias PM. The effects of petrolatum on stratum corneum structure and function. *J Am Acad Dermatol* 26: 387–396. 1992.
16. Lampe MA, Burlingame AL, Whiney J, Williams ML, Brown BE, Roitman E, Elias PM. Human stratum corneum lipids: characterization and regional variations. *J Lipid Res* 24: 120–150. 1983.
17. Bonte F, Saunois A. Pinguet P, Meybeck A. Existence of a lipid gradient in the upper stratum corneum and its possible biological significance. *Arch Dermatol Res* 289: 78–82. 1997.
18. Ghadially R, Brown BE, Sequeira-Martin SM et al. The aged epidemial permeability barrier: structural, functional, and lipid biochemical abnormalities in humans and a senescent murine model. *J Clin Invest* 95: 2281–2290. 1995.
19. Ghadially R, Brown BE, Hanley K et al. Decreased epidermal lipid synthesis accounts for altered barrier functions in aged mice. *J Invest Dermatol* 106: 1064–1069. 1996.
20. Rogers J, Harding C, Mayo A, Banks J, Rawlings A. Stratum corneum lipids: the effect of ageing and the seasons. *Arch Dermatol Res* 288: 765–770. 1996.
21. Zettersten EM, Ghadially R, Feingold KR, Crumrine D, Elias PM. Optimal ratios of topical stratum corneum lipids improve barrier recovery in chronologically aged skin. *J Am Acad Dermatol* 37: 403–408. 1997.
22. Grove GL, Kligman AM. Age-associated change in human epidermal cell renewal. *J Gerontol* 38: 137–142. 1983.
23. Shuster S, Black MM, McVitie E. Influences of age and sex on skin thickness, skin collagen and density. *Br J Dermatol* 93: 639–643. 1975.
24. Brincat M, Moniz CF, Studd JWW, Darby AJ, Magos A, Cooper D. Sex hormones and skin collagen content in postmenopausal women. *Br Med J* 287: 1337–1338. 1983.

25. Urano R, Sakabe K, Kawashima I, Ohkido M, Seiki K. Effects of estrogen and progesterone on induction and proliferation of normal human keratinocytes. *J Dermatol Sci* 4: 141. 1992.
26. Yumamoto A, Serizawa M, Ito M, Sato Y. Stratum corneum lipid abnormalities in atopic dermatitis. *Arch Dermatol Res* 283: 219–223. 1991.
27. Wertz PW, Miethke MC, Long SA, Strauss JS, Downing DT. The composition of the ceramides from human stratum corneum and from comedones. *J Invest Dermatol* 84: 410–412. 1985.
28. Abe T, Mayazumi J, Kikuchi N, Arai S. Seasonal variations in skin temperature, skin pH, evaporative water loss and skin surface lipid values on human skin. *Chem Pharm Bull* 38: 387–392. 1989.
29. Rawlings A, Hope J, Watkinson A, Harding C, Egelrud T. The biological effect of glycerol. *J Invest Dermatol* 100: 526. 1993.
30. Halkier-Sorensen L, Menon GK, Elias PM, Thestrup-Pedersen K, Feingold KR. Cutaneous barrier function after cold exposure in hairless mice: a model to demonstrate how cold interferes with barrier homeostasis among workers in the fish-processing industry. *Br J Dermatol* 132: 391–401. 1995.
31. Grubaeur G, Feingold KR, Harris RM, Elias PM. Lipid content and lipid type as determinants of the epidermal permeability barrier. *J Lipid Res* 30: 89–96. 1989.
32. Akimoto K, Yoshikawa N, Higaki Y, Kawashima M, Imokawa G. Quantitative analysis of stratum corneum lipids in xerosis and asteatotic eczema. *J Dermatol* 20: 1–6. 1993.
33. Rawlings A, Hope J, Rogers J, Watkinson A, Scott I. Abnormalities in stratum corneum structure, lipid composition, and desmosome degradation in soap induced winter xerosis. *J Soc Cosmet Chem* 45: 203–220. 1994.
34. Sheu H-M, Lee JY-Y, Chai C-Y, Kuo K-W. Depletion of stratum corneum intercellular lipid lamellae and barrier function abnormalities after long-term topical corticosteroids. *Br J Dermatol* 136: 884–890. 1997.
35. Malkinson FD. Studies of the percutaneous absorption of C^{14} labelled steroids by use of the gas-flow cell. *J Invest Dermatol* 31: 19–28. 1958.
36. Yang L, Ma-Qiang M, Taljebini M, Elias PM, Feingold KR. Topical stratum corneum lipids accelerate barrier repair after tape stripping, solvent treatment and some but not all types of detergent treatment. *Br J Dermatol* 133: 679–685. 1995.
37. Mao-Qiang M, Thornfeldt CR, Feingold KR, Wang F, Elias PM. A natural lipid mixture improves barrier function and hydration in human and murine skin. *J Soc Cosmet Chem* 47: 157–166. 1997.
38. Bowser P, Gray M. Sphingomyelinase in pig and human epidermis. *J Invest Dermatol* 74: 331–335. 1978.
39. Freinkel R, Traczyk T. The phospholipases A of epidermis. *J Invest Dermatol* 70: 169–173. 1980.
40. Freinkel R, Traczyk T. Acid hydrolases of the epidermis: subcellular localization and relationship to cornification. *J Invest Dermatol* 78: 441–446. 1983.

28 Effect of Moisturizing Products on the Structure of Lipids in the Outer Stratum Corneum of Humans

Ronald R. Warner and Ying Liu Boissy

CONTENTS

28.1 INTRODUCTION

The lipids in the stratum corneum (SC) constitute the primary barrier of the skin,[1-5] forming a protective sheath that shields the skin from desiccation and external assault.[6] These barrier lipids exist in the SC intercellular space as highly organized lamellar bilayers, readily visualized by the marriage of transmission electron microscopy (TEM) with RuO_4 staining.[7,8] The lamellar

0-8493-7520-7/00/$0.00+$.50

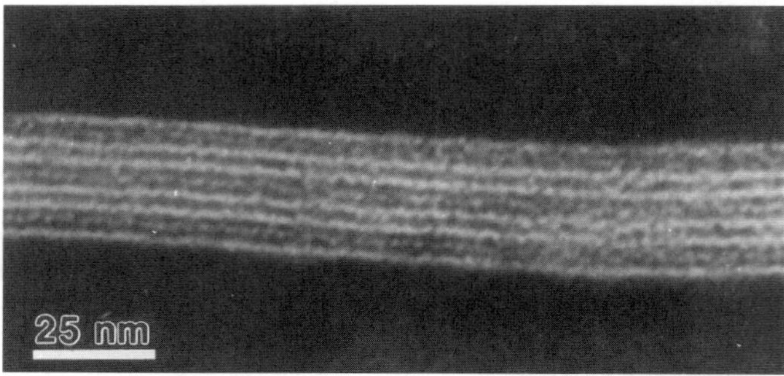

FIGURE 1 Normal structure of the lipid lamellae in the intercellular space. Shown are three Landmann units separating the darkly staining corneocytes above and below this intercellular space. Bar = 25 nm.

organization consists of a unique pattern of alternating electron-lucent and electron-dense lamellae forming repeating structures[7-10] often referred to as Landmann units.[10] This lipid structure appears to be the same throughout most of the SC, with variability occurring primarily in the number of Landmann units (typically two or three) that bridge the intercellular space.[8,10-12] However, more diverse structures have been described in the outer SC,[11-14] perhaps reflecting environmental impact[12,14] or inherent differences in lipid composition.[15-18] This chapter focuses on the lipid structure of the *outer* SC in humans. We present a modified TEM technique to investigate this structure. We attempt to organize and understand the variability in lipid structure we observe in the outer SC. We further explore the alterations (repair) of the lipid structure in the outer SC due to the application of moisturizing products.

28.1.1 Inner Stratum Corneum Lipids

The Landmann-unit structure of intercellular lipid lamellae is illustrated in Figure 1. A plausible molecular model has been published that accounts for the electron-lucent and electron-dense lamellar structure of the Landmann unit.[10] The Landmann-unit structure is consistently found throughout nearly all of the normal SC. It is known that these lipid lamellae are not constant structures. At least in the inner and middle SC they are known to be altered by age[19] and disease,[8,11,20-22] to be altered with experimental solvent treatment[23-25] and topical inhibitor treatment,[26,27] to reform relatively quickly following solvent extraction,[5,24] and to be repaired rapidly with appropriate exogenous lipid treatment.[28,29] Thus, they appear to be somewhat dynamic in nature.

28.1.2 Outer Stratum Corneum Lipids

In contrast to the more extensive studies of the intercellular lipid lamellae in the inner and middle SC, there are few studies of the lipid structure in the outer SC. It has been reported that the outer SC can have a substantial increase in the number of intercellular lamellae, increasing from the normal 2 or 3 Landmann units to numbers in excess of 100 bilayers.[13] It has been reported that for normal skin with little or no visible dryness, the outer SC intercellular space is filled with an amorphous material, whereas in soap-treated skin with pronounced visible dryness, the outer SC intercellular space is filled with numerous disorganized lamellae.[14] A separate study using human skin *in vitro* also found disordered lipid lamellae in the outer SC following soap use, less disruption following use of a soap/glycerin/oil bar, and normal lamellae following use of an isethionate bar.[12]

To the extent that lipids are involved in corneocyte cohesion and desquamation,[30-33] the lipid structure in this outer layer is presumably very important for proper desquamation. However, due to its fate of being at the surface, the outer SC is also likely to be the most susceptible to environmental insult and consumer products such as surfactants and solvents.[5,12,28] There may be a functional correlation between the lipid structure of the outer SC and skin dryness.

If consumer products like soaps and surfactants can damage this outer SC lipid structure, moisturizers might aid its repair. It is increasingly clear that moisturizing ingredients like petrolatum can enter into the upper layers of the SC, affect SC lipid structure, and accelerate repair.[34] Conversely, it was recently shown that some commercial moisturizers actually interfere with skin barrier recovery following barrier disruption with acetone.[35] Although moisturizer use typically results in improvements in skin condition, little is known about *how* moisturizers improve skin condition. There would appear to be a continuum of moisturizer action, from the purely cosmetic effect of "hiding" visible skin dryness to a functional effect in which a moisturizer may actively abet the biological repair process.[36] Evidence suggests that one mechanism of moisturizer action is to aid in the digestion of desmosomes that are abnormally retained in the outer SC.[37,38] Another mechanism, however, may involve the SC lipids. Moisturizers contain lipids, and lipids play a very important role in skin barrier properties,[39,40] so it is reasonable to assume that moisturizers interact in some way with the lipids in the skin's SC to improve the skin barrier and thereby enhance skin water content.[34,35,39-41]

In this chapter we will investigate alterations in the lipid structure of the outer SC induced by moisturizing ingredients and commercial moisturizing products. As a preface to this investigation, we will examine the normal variability in lipid structure of the outer SC and how it is affected by age, level of visible dryness, and soap use.

28.2 TAPE STRIP PROTOCOL

Similar to a previously reported procedure,[14] we sampled the outer SC with a tape strip using Scotch Magic Tape 810 (3M). Using gentle pressure, the tape was applied to the skin surface — in the studies reported here, the lower leg — and carefully removed after approximately 30 seconds. Under stereo-microscope observation, regions of the tape having large clusters of skin flakes were cut out and placed in 0.25% RuO_4 in a 0.1 *M* cacodylate buffer for 1 h at 4°C, rinsed briefly in 0.1 *M* cacodylate buffer, and then dehydrated through a graded acetone series prior to Epon embedding and overnight polymerization at 65°C. Thin sections were obtained on an ultramicrotome, counterstained with uranyl acetate and lead citrate, and analyzed in a Philips CM12 at 100 KeV. It is known that the lipid structure of the SC improves as a function of depth into the SC; by the third tape strip, lipid structure has normalized to the typical Landmann pattern.[14] In our study, only one tape strip was taken, and whenever possible, micrographs were obtained only from the outermost three to four corneocytes (adjacent to the tape). Similarly, to minimize possible artifacts resulting from the mechanical process of tape stripping or from previously uplifted scale, micrographs were only taken (whenever possible) from intercellular regions that were closely apposed, thus minimizing potential problems of physical trauma or ready access of tape adhesive or bulk moisturizing lotion. Since our assessments of lipid structure are qualitative and subjective, we were blinded to treatment identity during sample analysis.

Although we feel this tape-stripping approach is a very useful procedure, it does have some limitations. Limitations are inherent with RuO_4 staining due to its poor penetration and high reactivity, as discussed previously.[22] With our tape-stripping approach, these staining limitations are superimposed on problems of representative sampling. In our experience only limited areas are available that meet our analysis criteria for TEM inspection, and variation in lipid structure does exist within a single tape strip. Nevertheless, this variation is relatively small in the context of the large variations in lipid structure that are encountered in the outer SC, as will be seen. In particular, in our experience, the outer SC lipid structure of an individual's skin is constant over large areas, such that a person's lipid structure is very similar over the entire lower leg and similar for both legs, which is critical for paired studies and valid conclusions. Nevertheless, the variation that does exist limits the ability to detect small changes in lipid structure; in particular, it has been difficult to observe improvements in lipid structure due to the use of moisturizing products when the skin was in good condition initially.

Another limitation is the labor-intensive nature of TEM investigations; the number of samples that can be analyzed in a reasonable time is small. In the studies we will present, "n," the number of samples per treatment that we analyzed, is variable, but is no smaller than n = 3, except for mineral oil (n = 1).

28.3 NORMAL LIPID STRUCTURE IN THE OUTER STRATUM CORNEUM

Our intent for this study was to observe the lipid structure of the outer SC in a population of people engaged in their normal, personal skin care habits. Accordingly, in this study of normal lipid structure we selected female participants at random without advance knowledge of their normal skin care and without any pretreatment protocol. Prior to tape stripping, their skin was graded by an expert grader using a 0 to 6 scale developed for skin dryness, 0 being no dryness.[42] The ages of the individuals investigated ranged from 22 to 52.

28.3.1 Young Skin

The lipids of young skin (individuals in their early 20s) with little or no visible dryness typically have a good Landmann unit structure even at the surface of the SC, as shown in Figure 2a. Youthful skin in good condition is invariably associated with closely apposed corneocytes and narrow intercellular spaces. In contrast, young individuals with dry skin do not have Landmann units in their outer SC. A great variety of intercellular lipid morphologies is observed in different individuals with poor skin grade, including fibrous, mesh, and amorphous structures. Usually the intercellular spaces are considerably widened. An example of the latter is shown in Figure 2b, in which the intercellular spaces are filled with amorphous material having a variety of textures.

28.3.2 Old Skin

We typically did not observe intercellular lipids with a Landmann unit structure in the outer SC in individuals over 40 years of age, regardless of skin condition. On this basis we define "old skin" to be skin from a person greater than age 40. An example of lipid structure from an "old" person with good skin condition is shown in Figure 3a. It is common to find lamellae, but these lamellae are seldom present as fully formed Landmann units. Often lamellae are present at the periphery of corneocytes, separated by a central band of nonlamellar amorphous/fibrous material as shown in Figure 3a. Other intercellular spaces are simply filled with this nonlamellar material (not shown). As with more youthful skin, the intercellular spaces are nevertheless typically closely apposed. In older individuals with dry skin, the intercellular spaces can become spectacularly abnormal. Very widened intercellular spaces are common. A great diversity of structures can be observed, although amorphous material is quite common. An example is shown in Figure 3b; the outermost intercellular space appears to consist of a two-phase system, with the noncontinuous phase being membrane bound. Vesicles are apparent. The intercellular spaces are widened. There is no organized lamellar structure.

28.4 THE EFFECT OF HARSH SOAP

Protocols that employ controlled soap washing on the lower leg, such as a daily use of soap for 2 weeks, result in worsening of visual skin (dryness) grade and distinctive alterations in the lipid structure of the outer SC. We observe a soap-induced formation of two distinct intercellular structures. In one form, intercellular spaces appear "invaded" by heavily staining globules of a variety of sizes, as shown in Figure 4a. A more frequently observed response to soap use is the formation of profuse disorganized lamellae within widened intercellular spaces, as illustrated by Figure 4b and as seen previously.[14] In this latter figure, although localized domains of ordered

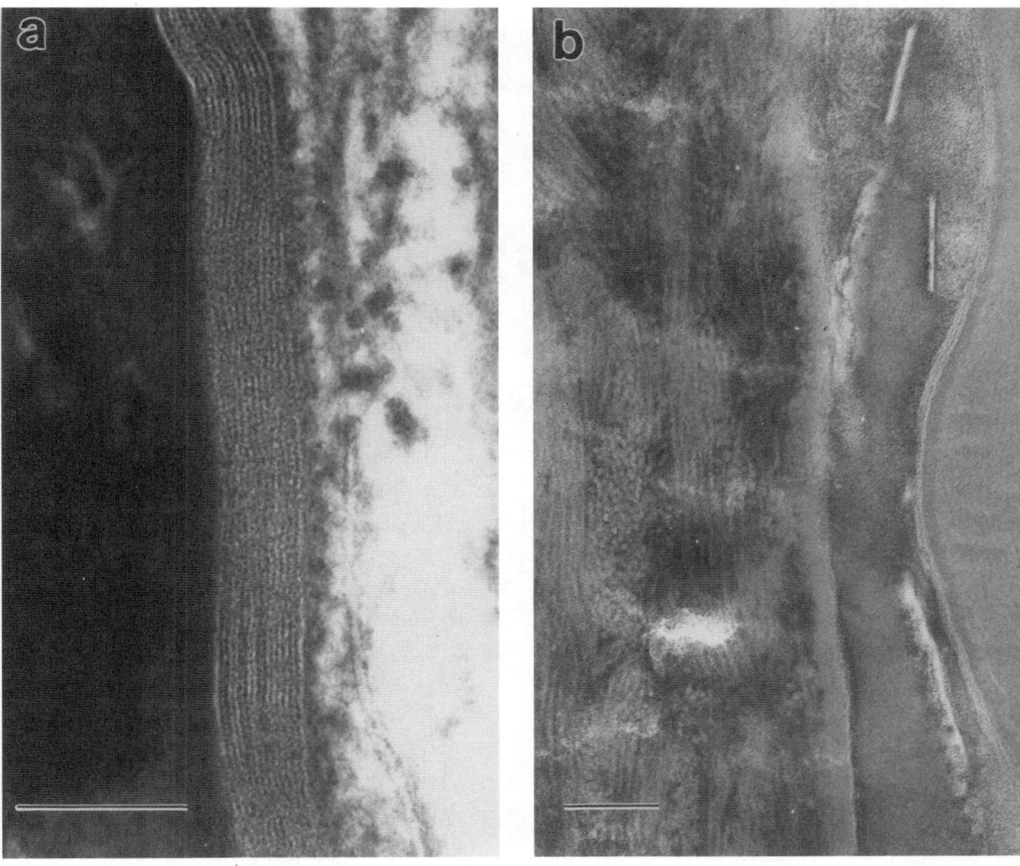

FIGURE 2 (a) Landmann units from the outer SC of a person 24 years old, skin grade 0.5. (b) A mixture of amorphous materials with different textures in the intercellular space of the outer SC from a person 28 years old, skin grade 5.0. Bar = 100 nm.

lamellae exist (over short dimensions), the lamellae are visualized as single electron-dense and electron-lucent lines with no evidence of the distinct substructure of the Landmann unit.

28.5 THE EFFECT OF MOISTURIZING PRODUCTS

We have shown that the lipid structure of the outer SC varies as a function of age and dry skin condition. We have shown that the use of soap alters this lipid structure. Can the use of a skin moisturizer improve this lipid structure? Do moisturizing ingredients penetrate into the SC? Can a skin moisturizer convert the lipid structure of aged skin back to the Landmann unit structure of youth? To answer such questions we investigated the effect of neat moisturizing ingredients, reduced concentration (formulated) moisturizing ingredients, and fully formulated commercial products on the lipid structure of the outer SC of the leg following 2 or 3 weeks of product use. For its comparative value, we will show results on the moisturizing ingredients primarily using matched studies done with a single person, a 42-year-old male. Mineral oil, petrolatum formulated at 10% in an oil-in-water emulsion vehicle containing high levels of humectants, and SEFA (sucrose esters of fatty acids), formulated at 2 and 10% in the same vehicle, were applied at 3 mg/cm^2 on the lower leg twice a day for 2 weeks. Neat petrolatum and neat SEFA were applied ad-lib twice a day for 2 weeks. Final product application was 12 h before tape stripping. The individual used a synthetic bar for daily personal cleansing.

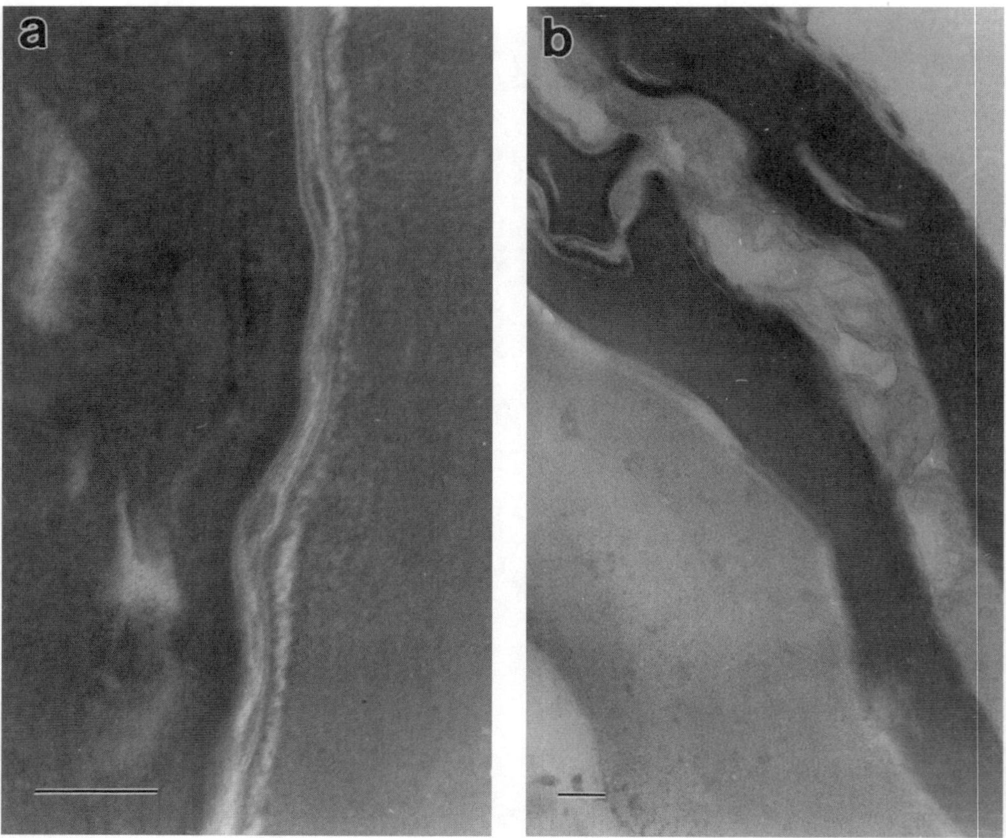

FIGURE 3 (a) Lipid structure in the intercellular space from a person 45 years old, skin grade 1.0. The corneocytes are closely apposed and lamellae are frequent, but these lamellae appear somewhat disorganized and do not form Landmann units. The core of the intercellular space is filled with nonlamellar material that is amorphous and fibrous with interspersed granular deposits. (b) Lipid structure from a person 49 years old, skin grade 3.5. The outermost intercellular space contains vesicular structures and membrane-bound phases. Inner intercellular spaces appear to contain largely amorphous material. Bar = 100 nm.

28.5.1 Mineral Oil

The control, nontreated site is shown in Figure 5a, and the mineral-oil-treated site is shown in Figure 5b (same magnification). In the control skin, the outermost layers contain amorphous material and darkly staining globules. Lamellar structures can be found in lower layers, but the lamellae do not appear to form Landmann units. Following use of mineral oil, the intercellular space is relatively uniformly filled with a smooth-appearing amorphous material, presumably the mineral oil (Figure 5b). Intercellular spaces were occasionally focally dilated. There seemed to be little effect of the mineral oil other than as a "spacer" separating corneocytes.

28.5.2 Petrolatum

28.5.2.1 Neat Petrolatum

As shown in Figure 6a, neat petrolatum forms lamellar-like "streamers" in the intercellular space, as seen previously.[34] The streamers appear to be suspended in a nonstaining or empty intercellular medium (water?). In other areas, petrolatum forms a more continuous amorphous phase, also seen previously.[34] Petrolatum also forms intercellular structures intermediate between these two appearances (data not shown).

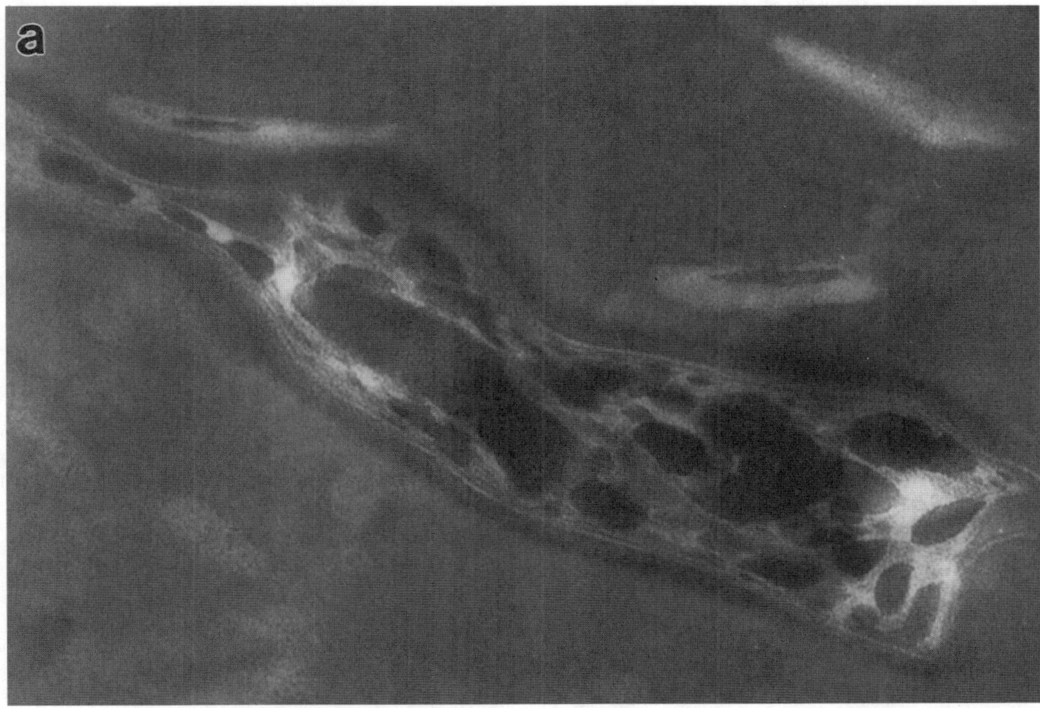

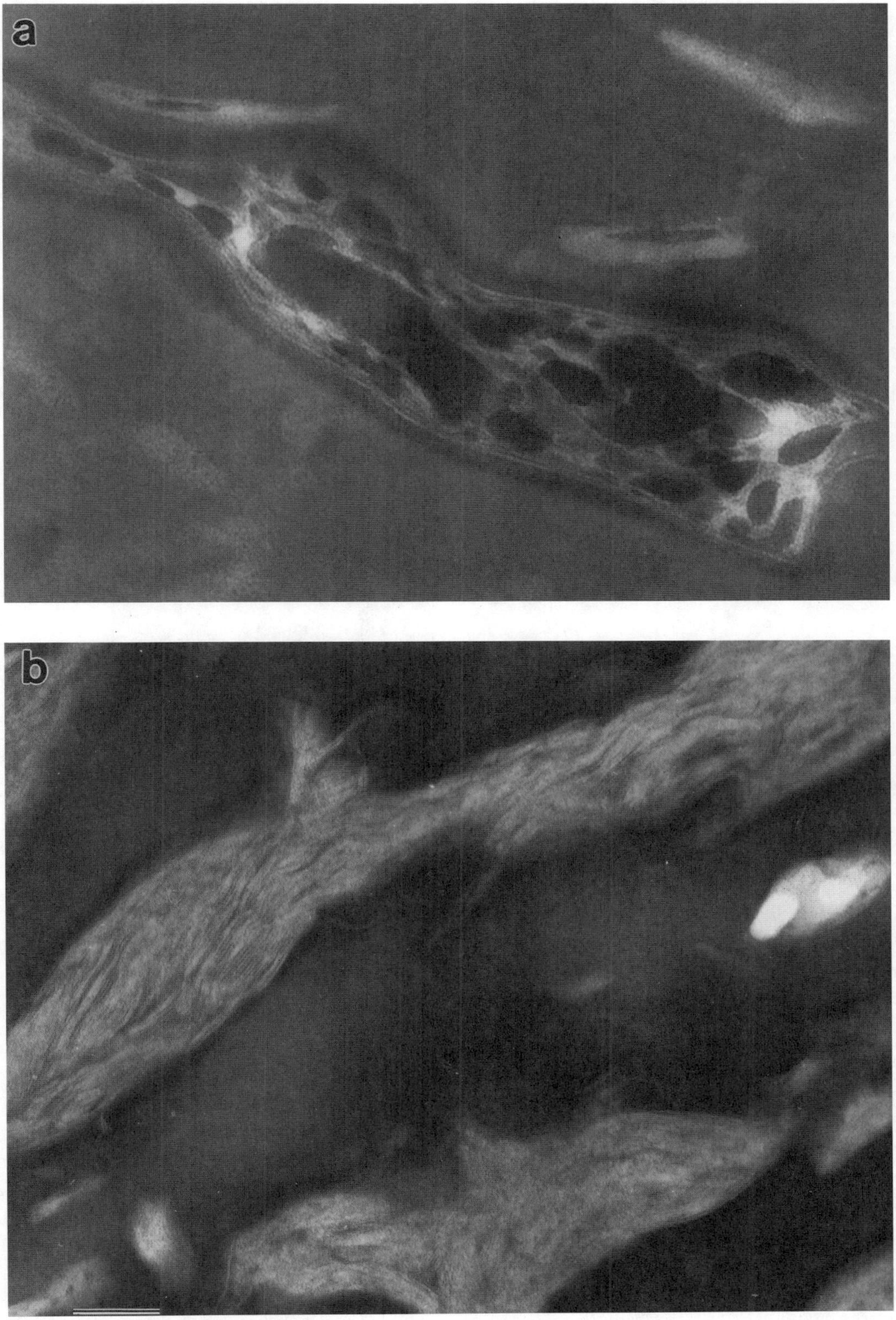

FIGURE 4 (a) Soap treatment frequently results in the formation of many darkly staining globular bodies in an amorphous matrix. (b) The signature pattern of soap use is the presence of widened intercellular spaces that are filled with numerous disorganized lamellae without a Landmann pattern. Bar = 100 nm.

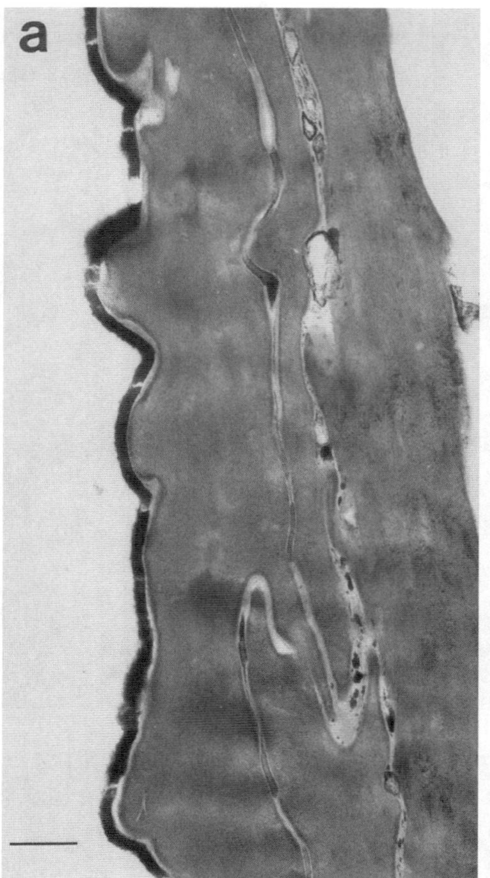

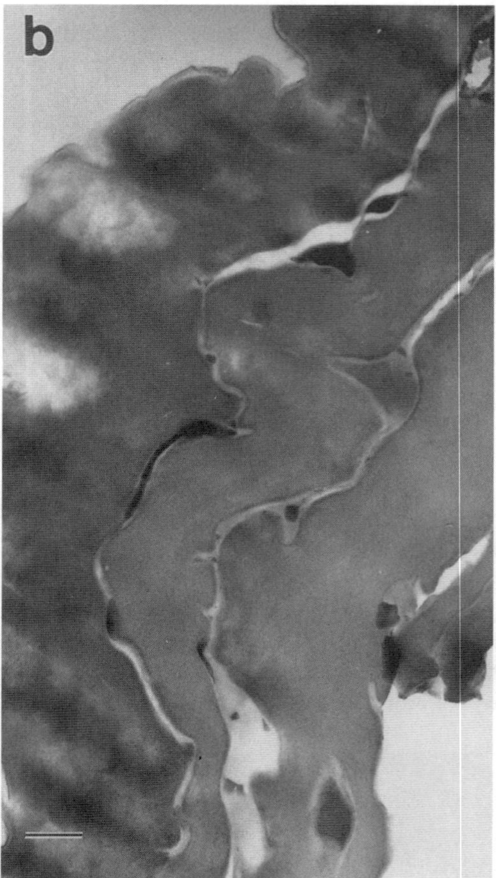

FIGURE 5 (a) Control, nontreated site from a 42-year-old male. The outermost (right) layers contain darkly staining globules in an amorphous matrix. Lamellae are present in deeper corneocyte layers, but Landmann units are rare. (b) Treatment with mineral oil results in the formation of large amorphous phases containing some darkly staining material. Bar = 200 nm.

In other studies, similar streamer and amorphous structures were observed in a young female with dry skin following the previously mentioned treatment protocol, although the amorphous phase was less prominent. In contrast, it was the streamer phase that was less obvious in older individuals treated with 2 mg/cm^2 twice a day for 3 weeks.

28.5.2.2 Formulated Petrolatum

The "streamer" phase observed with neat petrolatum (Figure 6a) is not seen. Amorphous material is common (data not shown). Reasonable lamellae are occasionally encountered, as shown in Figure 6b. Often these lamellae are separated by a thin stretch of amorphous material, as shown in the center of Figure 6b. In general, treatment with formulated petrolatum resulted in an appearance of the intercellular lipids which was much improved over that of neat petrolatum or mineral oil. The corneocytes were more closely apposed, and Landmann units were more common.

28.5.3 Sucrose Esters of Fatty Acids (SEFA)

SEFA, CAS No. 93571-82-5, was obtained from the Procter & Gamble Co., Cincinnati, OH.

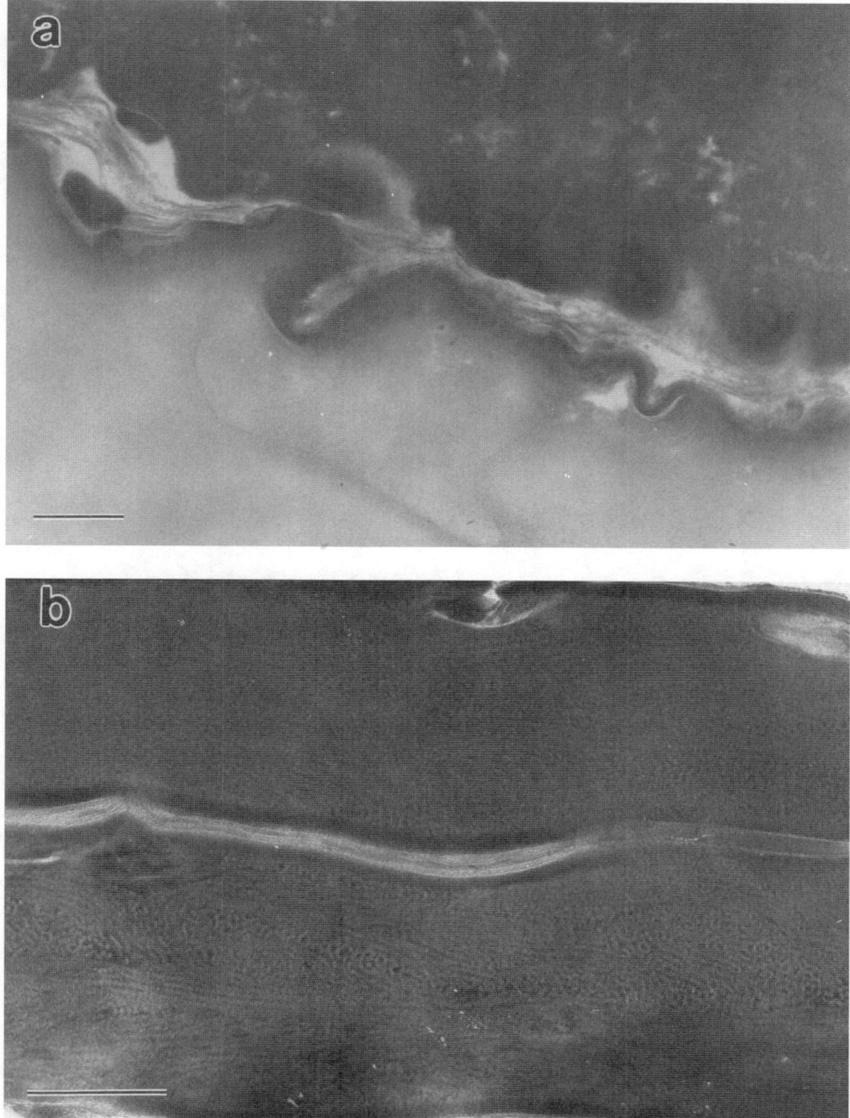

FIGURE 6 (a) Neat petrolatum site from a 42-year-old male. Flocculent/fibrous material existing as "streamers" or bands is present within an otherwise empty-appearing intercellular space. (b) Formulated (10%) petrolatum site. Lamellae, occasionally forming Landmann units, are sometimes separated by a thin layer of more darkly staining amorphous material. Bar = 200 nm.

28.5.3.1 Neat Sucrose Esters of Fatty Acids

SEFA use results in a very characteristic appearance of the intercellular space, shown in Figure 7a, which we describe as the "SEFA look." The corneocytes are relatively closely apposed; single Landmann units are present at corneocyte margins, and the slightly expanded intervening space is "plugged" with an amorphous material, presumably SEFA. Unlike the previous products, multiple Landmann units are occasionally present, although the multiple units are usually present in short regions within the SEFA "plug," as shown in Figure 7b. Very similar results were obtained in a young female with dry skin.

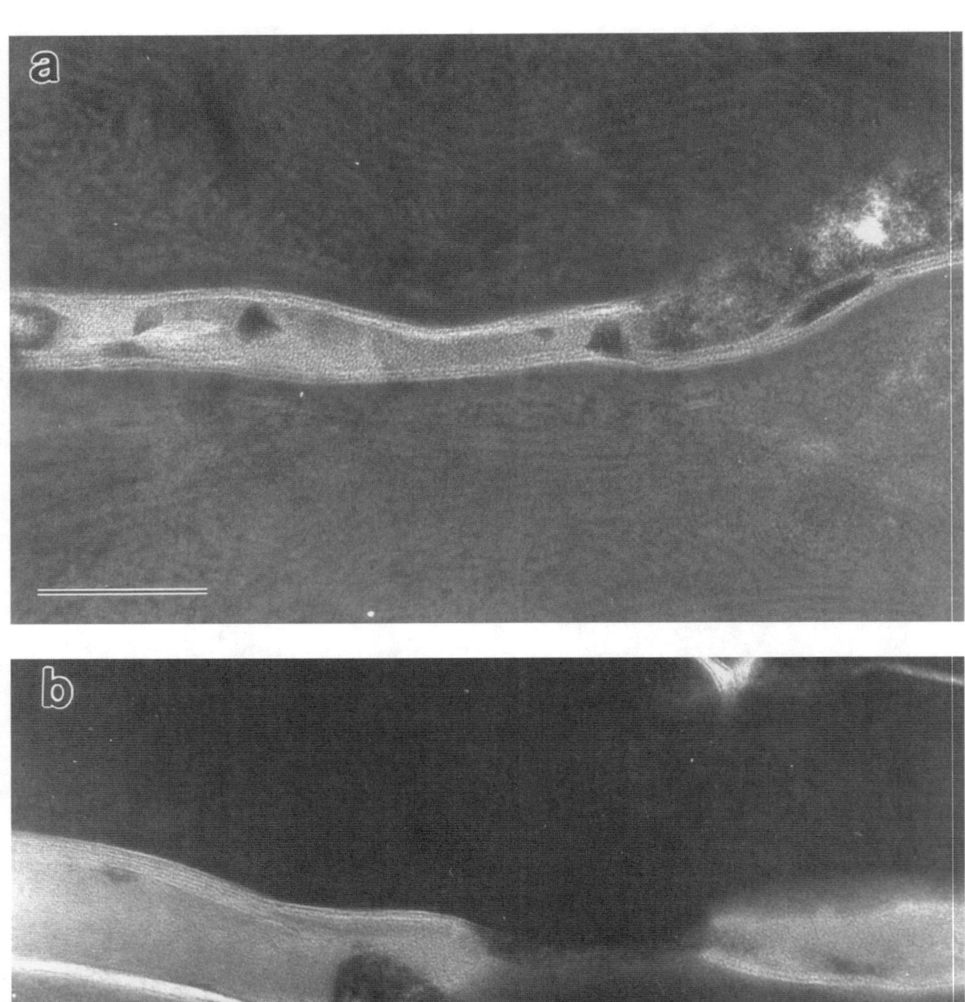

FIGURE 7 Neat SEFA site from a 42-year-old male. (a) Corneocytes are closely apposed, with well-formed lamellae at the corneocyte surface. Between the lamellae is a relatively uniform layer of an amorphous material. This pattern is referred to as the "SEFA look." (b) Occasionally, multiple Landmann units are present in the intercellular space. The length of the double Landmann units is always relatively short. Bar = 100 nm.

28.5.3.2 Formulated Sucrose Esters of Fatty Acids

The structure of the lipids in the intercellular space is overwhelmingly the SEFA look for both the 2 and 10% formulations, as shown in Figure 8a. With the 10% formulation, extra Landmann units within the SEFA phase are occasionally seen, as shown in Figure 8b.

In a separate clinical study, 2 mg/cm^2 of 2 or 10% SEFA in a humectant vehicle was applied to the lower leg twice a day for 3 weeks. The control, nontreated site of a 52-year-old female panelist, shown in Figure 9a, is characterized by numerous disorganized lamellae which are characteristic of

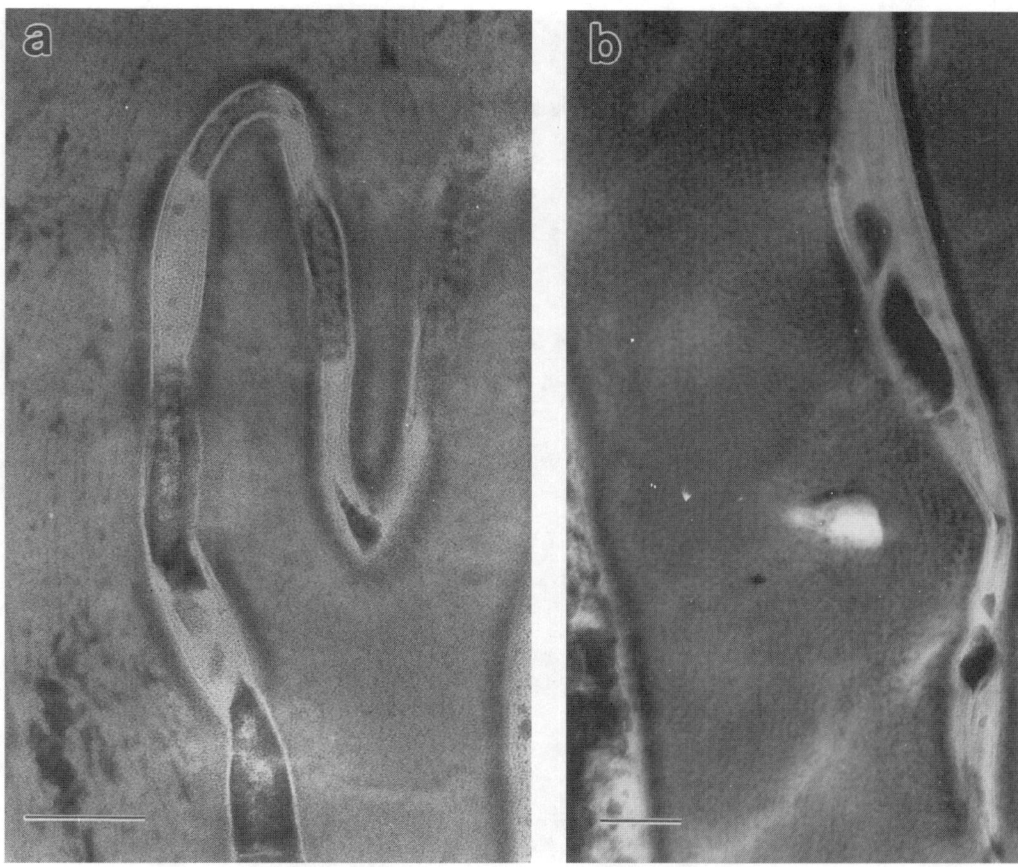

FIGURE 8 (a) Formulated (2%) SEFA site from a 42-year-old male. The characteristic SEFA look. (b) Formulated (10%) SEFA site. In addition to the SEFA look, an extra Landmann unit is present within the amorphous material. This extra Landmann unit is slightly separated from the peripheral lamella, which is common. Bar = 100 nm.

soap use; numerous darkly staining globular deposits were also common (data not shown). The humectant vehicle alone resulted in substantial improvement in lipid structure, but Landmann units were not common, and many intercellular spaces contained indistinct or amorphous material (data not shown). The vehicle did not produce the SEFA look. Following 2% SEFA treatment, the SEFA look was commonly observed (Figure 9b), but so too were Landmann units, unusual for a person of this age. Following the 10% SEFA treatment, the SEFA look was less common and the Landmann units more common (Figure 9c).

28.5.4 Product Comparisons from Clinical Studies

28.5.4.1 Neat Petrolatum vs. Neat Sucrose Esters of Fatty Acids vs. Market-Leading Moisturizing Lotion

Products were applied at 2 mg/cm^2 to the lower leg twice a day for 3 weeks. Typical results are presented from a 52-year-old female panelist. Petrolatum use results in an intercellular space containing diverse intercellular structures, including darkly staining globular material, amorphous regions, and some lamellae, but few Landmann units, as shown in Figure 10a. SEFA substantially improves the intercellular structures, as shown in Figure 10b, including the occasional formation of multiple Landmann units characteristic of younger skin (insert, Figure 10b). In striking contrast,

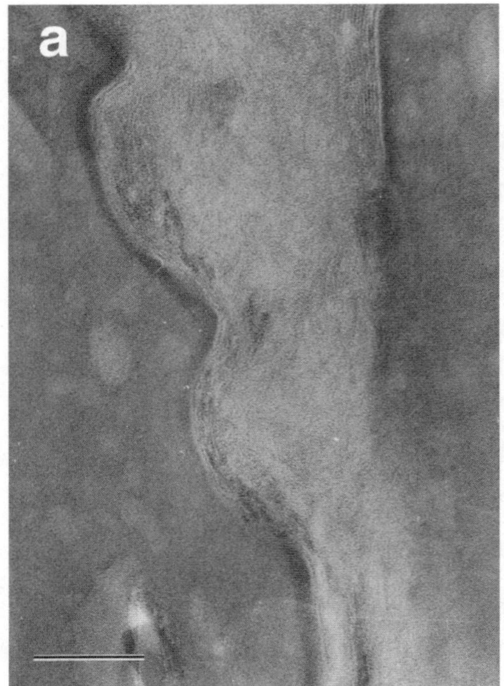

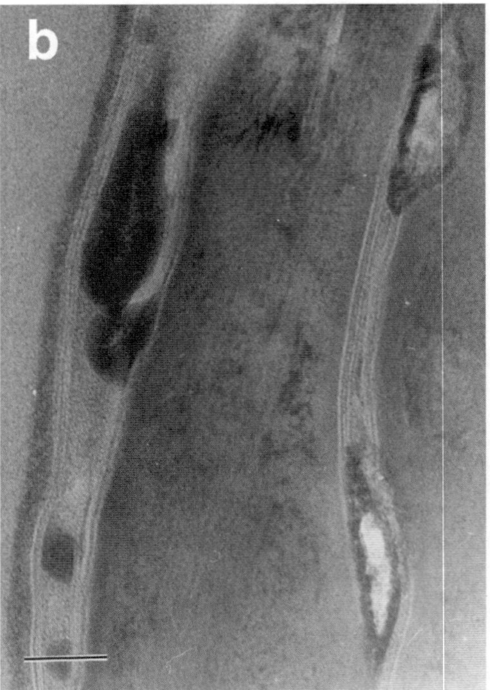

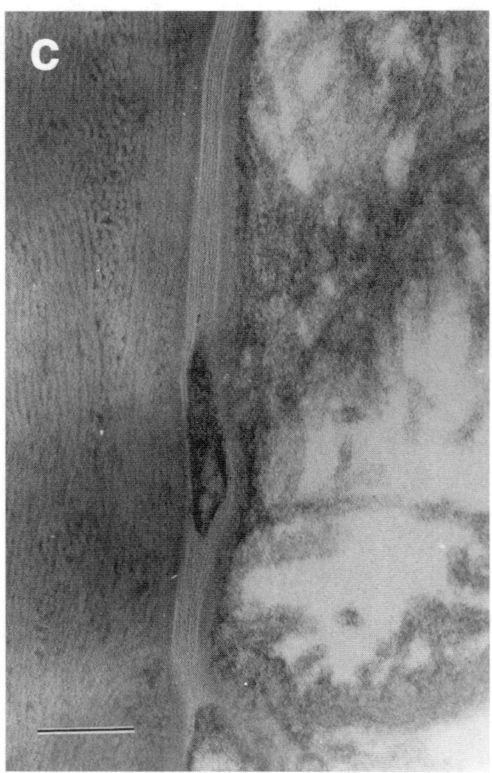

FIGURE 9 (a) Control, nontreated site from a 52-year-old female. The characteristic lipid structure resulting from soap use ("winter xerosis"[14]) is evident — compare with Figure 4b. (b) Use of formulated (2%) SEFA results in the SEFA look, as well as Landmann units. (c) With use of formulated (10%) SEFA, Landmann units are commonly observed. Bar = 100 nm.

a market-leading moisturizing lotion produces diverse and unusual structures, including mixtures of amorphous and fibrous material (Figure 11a); phase-separated amorphous lipids (not shown); and frequent, bizarre vesicular structures (Figure 11b). Landmann units were rarely observed. Of some note, in our (blinded) TEM studies on the improvement of lipid ultrastructure, we always rated neat SEFA as performing better than neat petrolatum, which was better than the lotion. However, by expert visual grading in this particular study, the reverse was true, with lotion better than neat petrolatum better than neat SEFA. This discrepancy further supports the notion that moisturizer action can be separated into two components: (1) a predominantly cosmetic or physical effect that does physical things like hiding visible skin dryness or diminishing brittleness, and (2) a functional effect in which a moisturizer aids biological repair.[36] These results show that the cosmetic and functional effects of moisturizers or moisturizing ingredients need not both be operational in treated skin and, further, suggest that they need not be acting in parallel.

28.5.4.2 Moisturizing Body Wash vs. Synthetic Bar + Moisturizing Lotion

In a clinical study, body wash treatment at 10 μl/cm² and lotion treatment at 1 μl/cm² were applied to the lower leg of female panelists once a day for 25 days. Good repair of the lipids in the intercellular space was routinely obtained with a moisturizing body wash that contains petrolatum, as illustrated by a particularly dramatic improvement in Figure 12. The "no treatment" (water only) site of a 28-year-old panelist, shown in Figure 12a, is characterized by intercellular spaces filled with amorphous material. The effect of the moisturizing body wash is shown in Figure 12b. The majority of the intercellular space is filled with Landmann units, although amorphous material was occasionally found in some regions. The effect of a mild synthetic bar followed by application of a market-leading moisturizing lotion is shown in Figure 12c. This bar/lotion treatment results in a clear improvement from the no-treatment control, but many regions are still dilated with amorphous material. Although lamellae are present, Landmann units are relatively rare.

A more typical response for these treatments is shown in Figure 13 from a separate clinical study that used the same treatment regimen, but for only 14 days. The 48-year-old panelist had a moderate amount of skin dryness, and the "no treatment" control region exhibited an intercellular lipid structure similar to that of Figure 3a (a good lipid structure for that age). In this case the moisturizing body wash results in no dramatic change in intercellular lipid structure, shown in Figure 13a, although there was significant improvement in the visual skin grade. In contrast, use of the synthetic bar followed by the moisturizing lotion degrades the lipid ultrastructure, as shown in Figure 13b. The intercellular spaces contain amorphous and "fuzzy" material and prominent disorganized, undulating lamellae. Nevertheless, the visual skin grade was dramatically improved, again illustrating a separation between cosmetic and functional effects.[36]

28.6 CONCLUSIONS

An improved understanding of the structure of the SC barrier is of interest for many reasons such as the improvement of percutaneous penetration and (particularly for this chapter) the optimization of topical therapy for the treatment of damaged skin. We have shown that the lipid structure of the outer SC is quite variable. Typically, the intercellular spaces in the outer SC are considerably widened and filled with nonlamellar material. These data are consistent with earlier TEM studies[13,14] and with an infrared spectroscopy study that found less structured lipids and greater amounts of lipid in the outer SC.[16]

Contrary to an earlier report that lipids have an amorphous structure in the outer SC of normal skin (with good visual skin grade),[14] we instead find an enormous variation in this lipid structure among individuals. Attempting to make sense of this variation, we believe we can generalize and conclude that the outer SC lipid structure is a function of age and skin condition (visual dryness grade). In particular, we find that lipids in young skin with good skin grade typically have a good

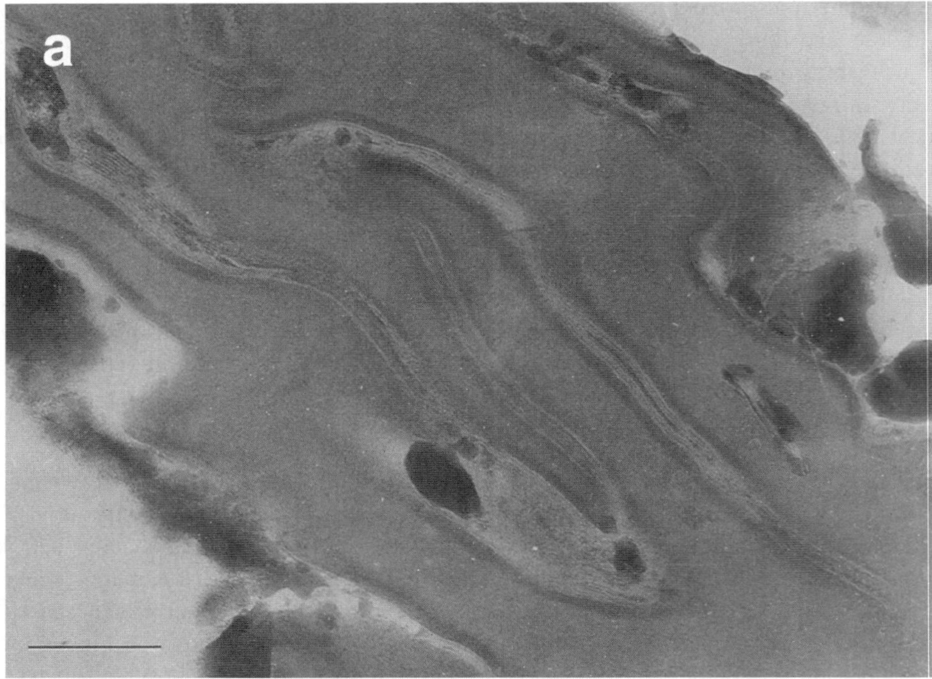

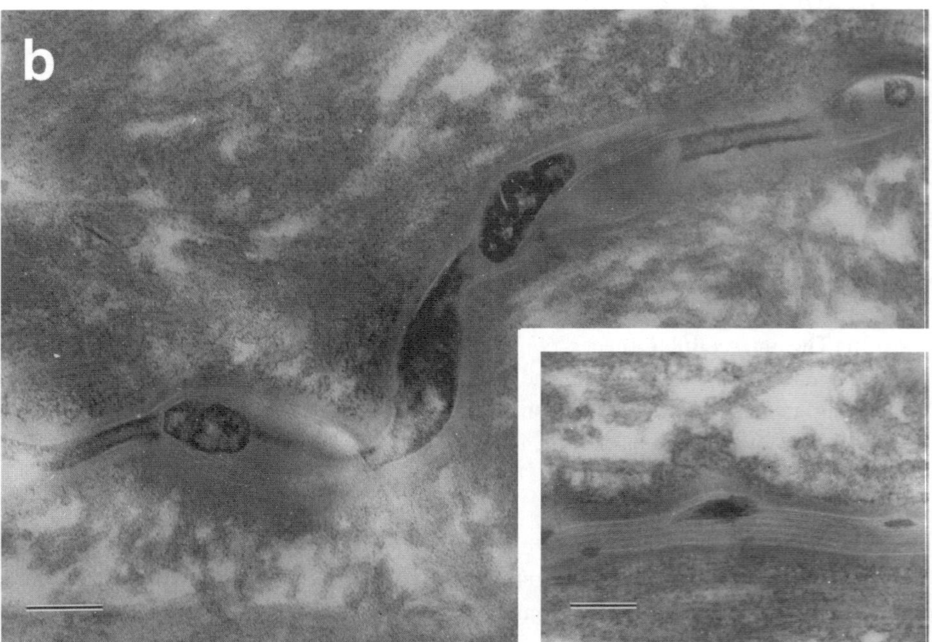

FIGURE 10 Neat petrolatum-treated site from a (different) 52-year-old female. (a) A great variety of intercellular structures are present, but the "streamer" phase typical of petrolatum (Figure 6a) was not seen. Amorphous regions and expanded intercellular regions containing many darkly staining globular regions are very common, as are lamellae without a Landmann pattern. Landmann units were rare. (b) Neat SEFA-treated site. The SEFA look is evident. The dark, spindle-shaped structures near the center of the micrograph are presumably desmosomes undergoing degradation. In many areas with the SEFA look, multiple, short-length Landmann units are common in the intercellular space, as shown. Normal, well-formed Landmann units are relatively common, as shown in the insert. Bar = 100 nm.

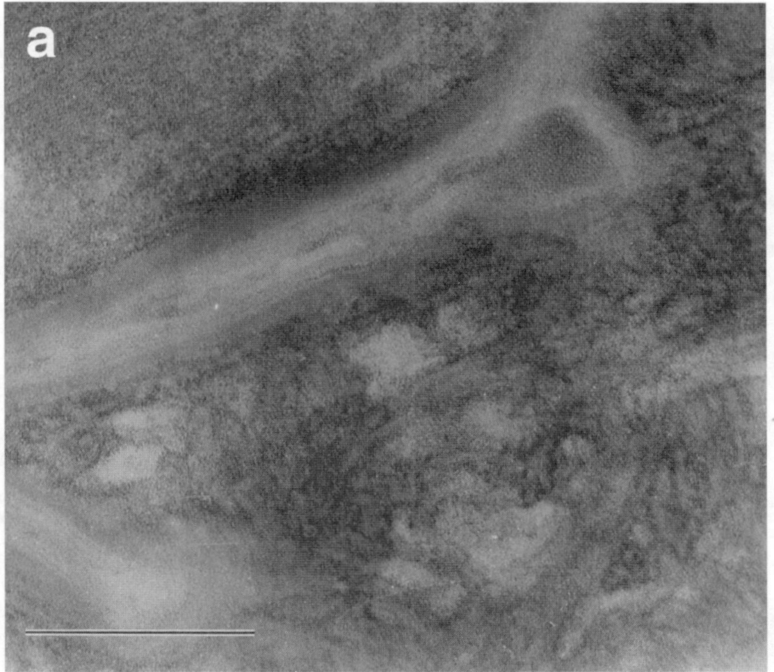

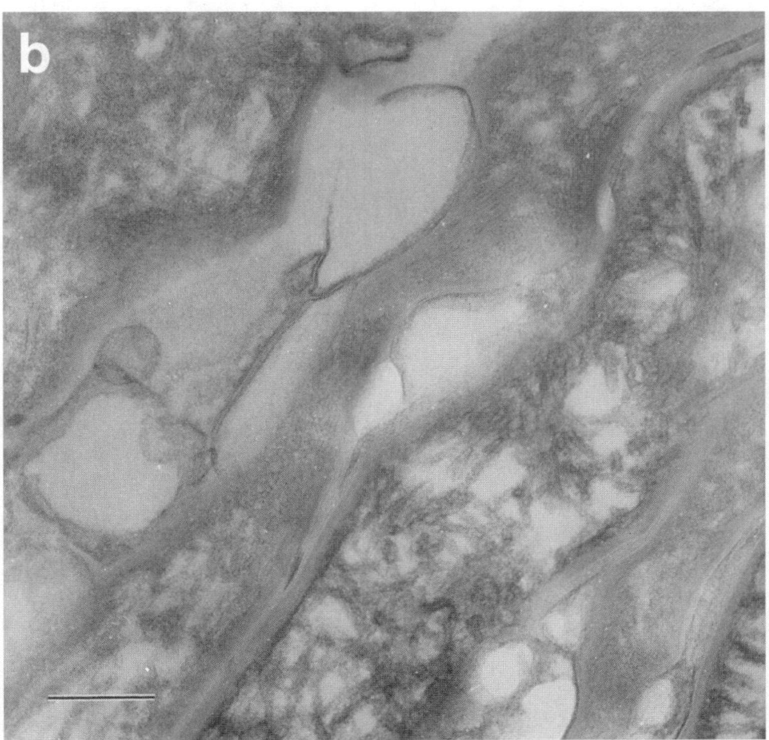

FIGURE 11 Site of market-leading moisturizing lotion from the 52-year-old female of Figure 10. The structure of the intercellular space is unusual. (a) Many areas contain amorphous and fibrous material in the intercellular space. (b) Other areas contain vesicles, membrane-bound compartments, and a mesh-like material. Bar = 200 nm.

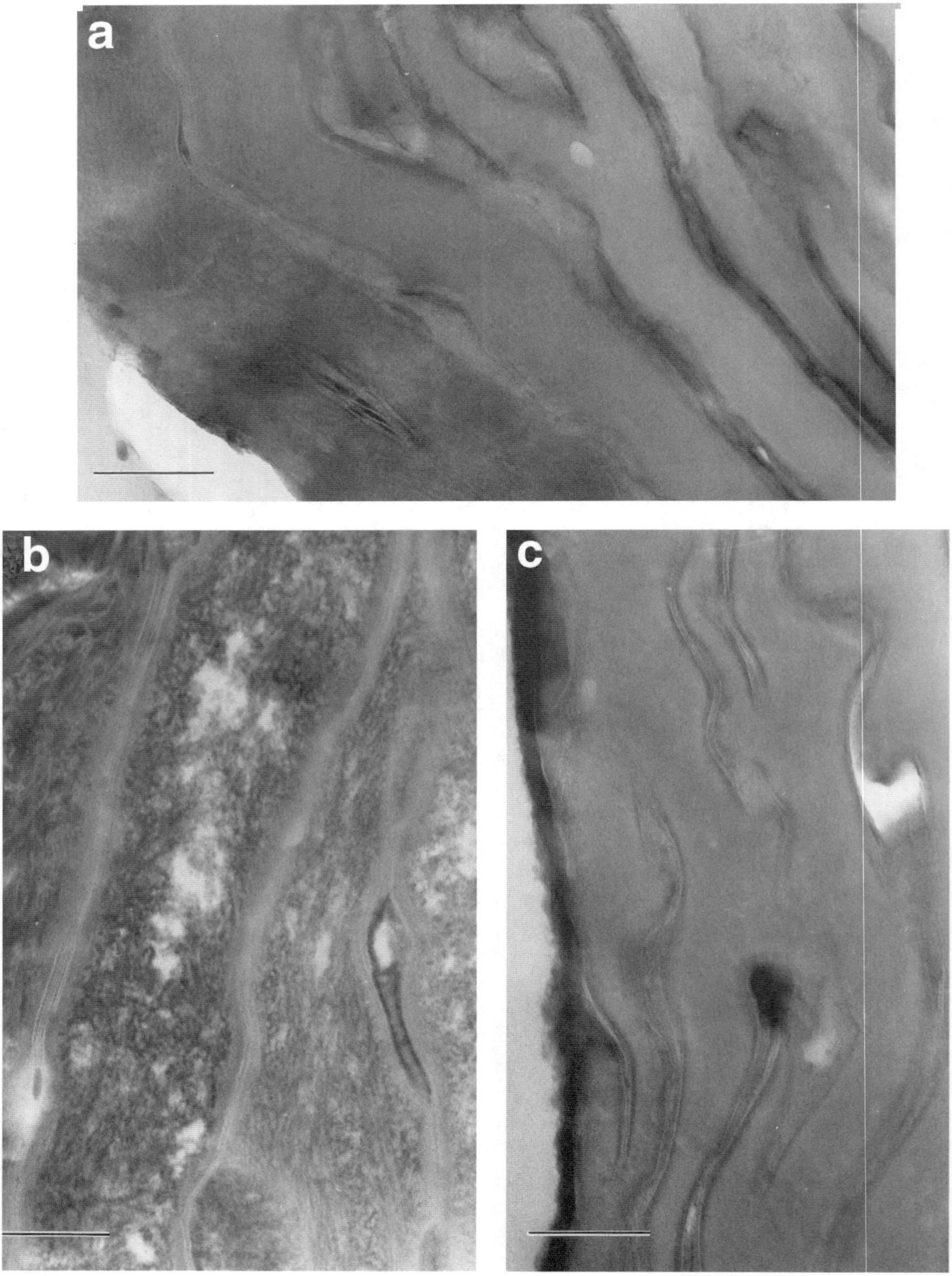

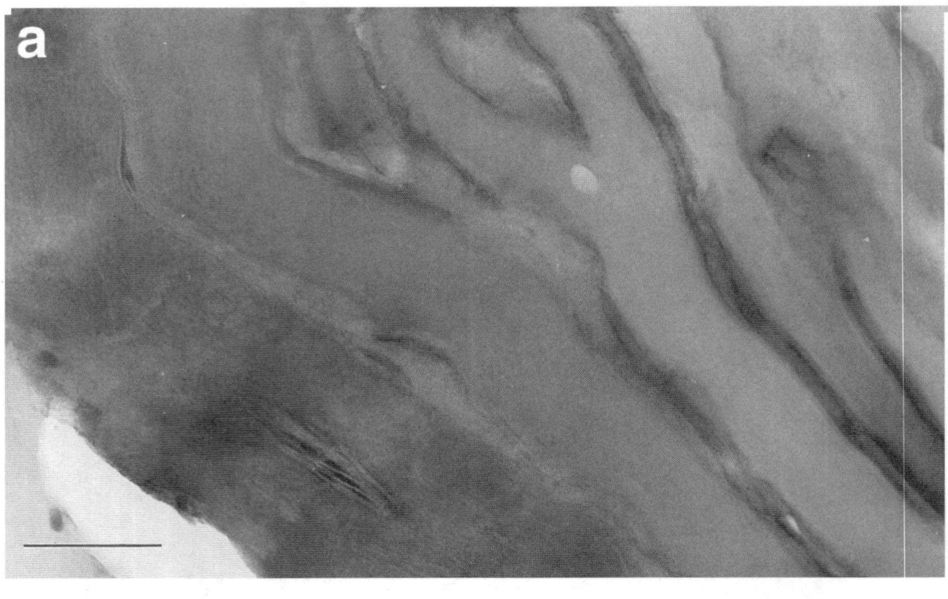

b

c

FIGURE 12 (a) Control, nontreated site from a 28-year-old female. The intercellular spaces are completely filled with amorphous material. Lamellar structures are rare. (b) Site of application of a commercial moisturizing body wash containing petrolatum. Lamellae are common, as are Landmann units. (c) Site of application of a mild synthetic bar followed by a market-leading moisturizing lotion. Lamellae are present, but few have the Landmann unit structure. Amorphous material is still common. Bar = 200 nm.

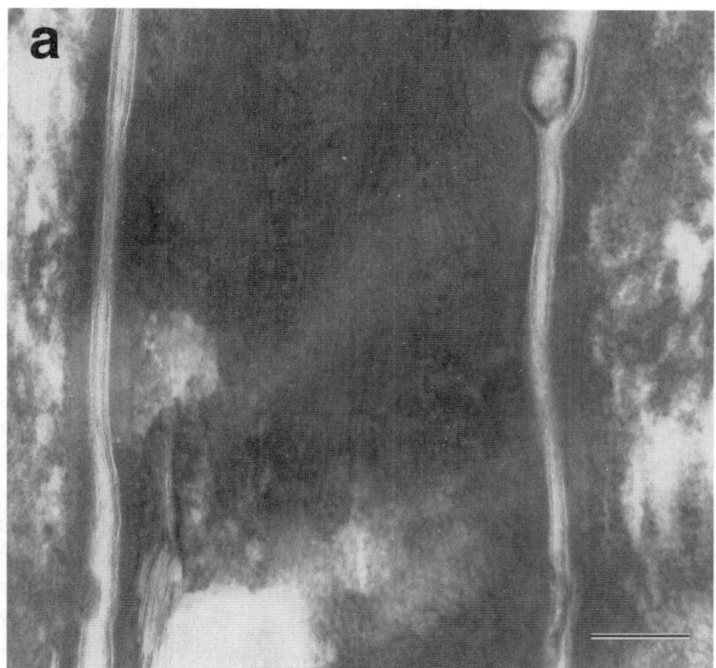

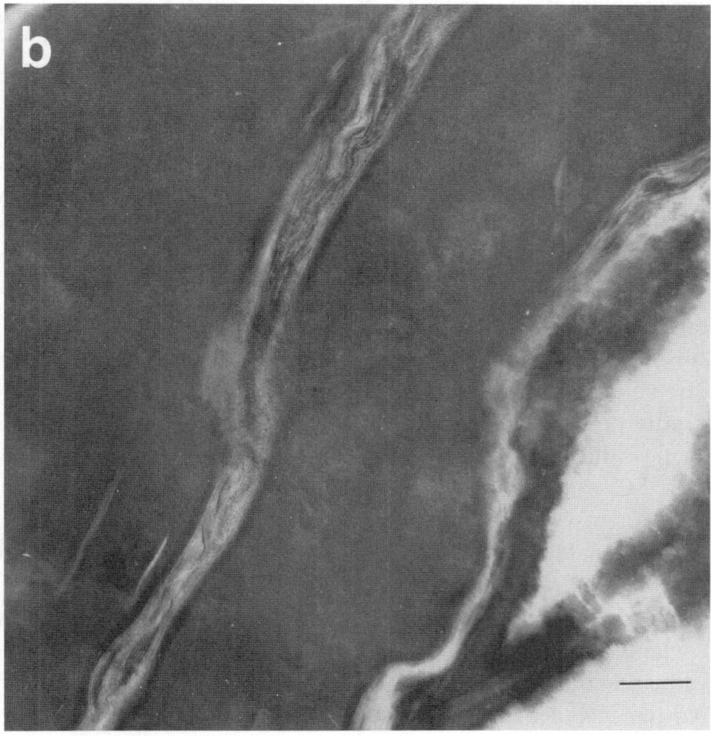

FIGURE 13 Tape strips from a 48-year-old female. (a) Site of application of a commercial moisturizing body wash containing petrolatum. The appearance is typical of a person over age 40 with good skin condition. The corneocytes are closely apposed and lamellae are frequent, but the lamellae appear somewhat disorganized and amorphous/fibrous material is present between lamellae. Nevertheless, Landmann units are easy to find, as shown in the left intercellular space. (b) Site of application of a mild synthetic bar followed by a market-leading moisturizing lotion. The intercellular spaces contain amorphous and fibrous material as well as prominent wavy lamellae without a Landmann pattern. Bar = 100 nm.

Landmann unit structure even at the surface of the SC. This ideal Landmann unit structure is typically not seen in individuals over the age of 40 regardless of dry skin level. We also find that a Landmann unit structure in the outer SC tends to be inversely correlated with skin dryness.

The lipid structure of the SC of older individuals is known to be altered from that of youth, with the older SC having fewer lipid lamellae and more open intercellular clefts.[19] This paucity of lamellae is likely due to a decrease in SC lipid synthesis resulting in a decreased SC lipid content.[41] Whereas these observations were made on individuals of advanced age, 80 years old, we see changes in lipid structure of the outer SC at a much earlier age, 40 years old, far from the "aged" designation. Data in the literature support skin being old at 40. Stratum corneum lipids change with age, with sharp decreases occurring by age 45 and a nearly constant SC lipid profile afterward.[43] Total SC ceramides appear to undergo a sharp drop in concentration at age 40.[44] A challenge to skin moisturizers is to reverse this age-related decline in the SC lipid barrier.

We observed a correlation between dry skin condition and lipid structure in the outer SC. Although there was generally a good correlation between our assessment of changes in SC lipid structure and independent assessment of changes in skin visual grade, nevertheless there were striking outliers that indicated the lipid structure was not the major factor determining dry appearance. A good example was the neat petrolatum/SEFA/lotion comparison mentioned earlier, in which neat SEFA produced a large improvement in lipid structure but got a poor skin grade, whereas the commercial lotion made the lipid structure worse but got high visual marks. We surmise that desmosomal breakdown rather than lipid structure is the more important determinant of visual grade. However, a healthy skin may ultimately rely more on the integrity of the lipid barrier than on the state of degradation of desmosomes in the outer SC layers.

We believe the discrepancies we have seen between visual grade and lipid structure are a result of commercial products being formulated to achieve visual improvement rather than skin health. Improvement in visual appearance need not mean that there is an improvement in the overall functional health of the skin, only that it looks better. Relying on this visual method for evaluating cosmetic product efficacy can yield commercially successful products that do not necessarily benefit skin health. In fact, some investigators have recently presented the stunning discovery that commercial moisturizing lotions may impede barrier recovery after experimental barrier perturbation.[35,45] A cosmetic product should ideally address not only visual skin problems, but also address the underlying biological causes to achieve healthy skin; there is a clear need for evaluation tools for skin health beyond visual grades.

We observed distinctive changes in the outer SC lipid structure with use of different products from soap to oil. Some of these lipid structures were sufficiently unique that they could be used to successfully identify product use (and to some degree, panelist age/skin condition). Based on appearances, we believe that moisturizing products enter the intercellular space of the SC and become a part of the SC, as was shown for petrolatum.[34] The mechanism by which the entry of moisturizing material improves skin barrier lipids is uncertain. We consider it unlikely that any of the products we studied could directly and physically participate in the formation of Landmann units. Of some note, we observed that petrolatum and SEFA were not as effective in reforming Landmann units when applied neat as when applied as a formulated product. Since the moisturizing body wash only contains petrolatum and polymers as moisturizing ingredients, this would suggest that the quantity of petrolatum or the form of its delivery is important for promoting the necessary conditions for lipid repair. For SEFA in formulated product, it may be that the combination of humectants and some occlusivity promotes internal conditions needed for the intrinsic formation of Landmann units. However, the inability of a market-leading moisturizer to reform Landmann units implies that the choices of ingredients for the formulated product is important to reform the ideal lipid structure.[46,47]

We do not pretend to fully understand the lipid structure of the outer SC in this initial extended investigation of this region. The variability is confusing, the number of observations small, and our survey large. Our conclusions are predicated on certain key observations and assumptions. We observed the ideal Landmann unit lipid structure in young individuals with no skin dryness, the absence of this structure in individuals with a high level of dryness, and the reappearance of Landmann units with treatment by moisturizing products. We assume, therefore, that this Landmann unit structure is the ideal lipid structure for the outer SC. In a system undergoing desquamation that may involve lipids,[30-33] this is an important assumption and one that should be tested further, particularly on young individuals with no skin dryness. We have further assumed that this ideal Landmann unit structure in the outer SC is important to skin health and a parameter by which moisturizers should be judged. This assumption, too, warrants further challenges.

In summary, from our microscopy study, moisturizers appear to enter into the SC and affect lipid structure. The lipid structure appears to be a function of the visual skin dryness grade, but is not the primary factor affecting the visual grade. Formulated products do a better job at helping to restore normal Landmann unit lipid structure than do the neat oils themselves. In our experience most of the moisturizing materials and products that we investigated to date are effective at reversing the abnormal lipid structures of soap use (winter xerosis)[14] back to a "status quo," but far fewer materials are able to substantially reform Landmann units, particularly in individuals over 40. Is there hope that moisturizers might restore the ideal Landmann unit lipid structure common in the healthy skin of youth? We believe the promise is there, as shown for older individuals in Figures 9 and 10.

28.7 ACKNOWLEDGMENTS

The authors wish to acknowledge the helpful suggestions of Connie Comstock, Keith Ertel, Robert Date, and Bruce Semple of Procter & Gamble in the writing of this manuscript.

REFERENCES

1. Berenson, G. S., Burch, G. E., Studies of diffusion of water through dead human skin: the effect of different environmental states and of chemical alterations of the epidermis, *Am. J. Trop. Med.*, 31, 842, 1951.
2. Onken, H. D., Moyer, C. A., The water barrier in human epidermis, *Archiv. Dermatol.*, 87, 584, 1963.
3. Elias, P. M., Lipids and the epidermal permeability barrier, *Arch. Dermatol. Res.*, 270, 95, 1981.
4. Elias, P. M., Cooper, E. R., Korc, A., Brown, B. E., Percutaneous transport in relation to stratum corneum structure and lipid composition, *J. Invest. Dermatol.*, 76, 297, 1981.
5. Grubauer, G., Feingold, K. R., Harris, R. M., Elias, P.M., Lipid content and lipid type as determinants of the epidermal permeability barrier. *J. Lipid Res.*, 30, 89, 1989.
6. Elias, P. M., Epidermal lipids, membranes, and keratinization, *Int. J. Dermatol.*, 20, 1, 1981.
7. Madison, K. C., Swartzendruber, D. C., Wertz, P. W., Downing, D. T., Presence of intact intercellular lipid lamellae in the upper layers of the stratum corneum, *J. Invest. Dermatol.*, 88, 714, 1987.
8. Hou, S. Y. E., Mitra, A. K., White, S. H., Menon, G. K., Ghadially, R., Elias, P. M., Membrane structures in normal and essential fatty acid-deficient stratum corneum: characterization by ruthenium tetroxide staining and X-ray diffraction, *J. Invest. Dermatol.*, 96, 215, 1991.
9. Landmann, L., Epidermal permeability barrier: transformation of lamellar granule disks into intercellular sheets by a membrane fusion process, *J. Invest. Dermatol.*, 87, 202, 1986.
10. Swartzendruber, D. C., Wertz, P. W., Kitko, D. J., Madison, K. C., Downing, D. T., Molecular models of the intercellular lipid lamellae in mammalian stratum corneum, *J. Invest. Dermatol.*, 92, 251, 1989.
11. Fartasch, M., Epidermal barrier in disorders of the skin, *Microsc. Res. Tech.*, 38, 361, 1997.
12. Misra, M., Ananthapadmanabhan, K. P., Hoyberg, K., Gursky, R. P., Prowell, S., Aronson, M., Correlation between surfactant-induced ultrastructural changes in epidermis and transepidermal water loss, *J. Soc. Cosmet. Chem.*, 48, 219, 1997.
13. Fartasch, M., Bassukas, I. D., Diepgen, T. L., Structural relationship between epidermal lipid lamellae, lamellar bodies and desmosomes in human epidermis: an ultrastructural study, *Br. J. Dermatol.*, 128, 1, 1993.

14. Rawlings, A., Watkinson, A., Rogers, J., Mayo, A.-M., Hope, J., Scott, I. R., Abnormalities in stratum corneum structure, lipid composition, and desmosome degradation in soap-induced winter xerosis, *J. Soc. Cosmet. Chem.*, 45, 203, 1994.
15. Elias, P. M., Menon, G. K., Grayson, S., Brown, B. E., Membrane structural alterations in murine stratum corneum: relationship to the localization of polar lipids and phospholipases, *J. Invest. Dermatol.*, 91, 3, 1988.
16. Bommannan, D., Potts, R. O., Guy, R. H., Examination of stratum corneum barrier function *in vivo* by infrared specstroscopy, *J. Invest. Dermatol.*, 95, 403, 1990.
17. Bonté, F., Saunois, A., Pinguet, P., Meybeck, A., Existence of a lipid gradient in the upper stratum corneum and its possible biological significance, *Arch. Dermatol. Res.*, 289, 78, 1997.
18. Long, S. A., Wertz, P. W., Strauss, J. S., Downing, D. T., Human stratum corneum polar lipids and desquamation, *Arch. Dermatol. Res.*, 277, 284, 1985.
19. Ghadially, R., Brown, B. E., Sequeira-Martin, S. M., Feingold, K. R., Elias, P. M., The aged epidermal permeability barrier, *J. Clin. Invest.*, 95, 2281, 1995.
20. Ghadially, R., Williams, M. L., Hou, S. Y. E., Elias, P. M., Membrane structural abnormalities in the stratum corneum of the autosomal recessive ichthyoses, *J. Invest. Dermatol.*, 99, 755, 1992.
21. Ghadially, R., Reed, J. T., Elias, P. M., Stratum corneum structure and function correlates with phenotype in psoriasis, *J. Invest. Dermatol.*, 107, 558, 1996.
22. Menon, G., Ghadially, R., Morphology of lipid alterations in the epidermis: a review, *Microsc. Res. Tech.,* 37, 180, 1997.
23. Imokawa, G., Kuno, H., Kawai, M., Stratum corneum lipids serve as a bound-water modulator, *J. Invest. Dermatol.*, 96, 845, 1991.
24. Menon, G. K., Feingold, K. R., Elias, P. M., Lamellar body secretory response to barrier disruption, *J. Invest. Dermatol.*, 98, 278, 1992.
25. Fartasch, M., Ultrastructure of the epidermal barrier after irritation, *Microsc. Res. Tech.,* 37, 193, 1997.
26. Menon, G. K., Feingold, K. R., Mao-Qiang, M., Schaude, M., Elias, P.M., Structural basis for the barrier abnormality following inhibition of HMG CoA reductase in murine epidermis, *J. Invest. Dermatol.*, 98, 209, 1992.
27. Mao-Qiang, M., Brown, B. E., Wu-Pong, S., Feingold, K. R., Elias, P. M., Exogenous nonphysiologic vs. physiologic lipids, *Arch. Dermatol.*, 131, 809, 1995.
28. Imokawa, G., Akasaki, S., Minematsu, Y., Kawai, M., Importance of intercellular lipids in water-retention properties of the stratum corneum: induction and recovery study of surfactant dry skin, *Arch. Dermatol. Res.*, 281, 45, 1989.
29. Man, M.-Q., Feingold, K. R., Elias, P. M., Exogenous lipids influence permeability barrier recovery in acetone-treated murine skin, *Arch. Dermatol.,* 129, 728, 1993.
30. Elias, P. M., Epidermal lipids, barrier function, and desquamation, *J. Invest. Dermatol.*, 80, 44s, 1983.
31. Chapman, S. J., Walsh, A., Jackson, S. M., Friedmann, P. S., Lipids, proteins and corneocyte adhesion, *Arch. Dermatol. Res.*, 283, 167, 1991.
32. Rawlings, A. V., Scott, I. R., Harding, C. R., Bowser, P.A., Stratum corneum moisturization at the molecular level, *J. Invest. Dermatol.,* 103, 731, 1994.
33. Sato, J., Denda, M., Nakanishi, J., Nomura, J., Koyama, J., Cholesterol sulfate inhibits proteases that are involved in desquamation of stratum corneum, *J. Invest. Dermatol.*, 111, 189, 1998.
34. Ghadially, R., Halkier-Sorensen, L., Elias, P. M., Effects of petrolatum on stratum corneum structure and function, *J. Am. Acad. Dermatol.*, 26, 387, 1992.
35. Halkier-Sorensen, L., Occupational skin diseases, *Contact Dermatitis*, 35 (Suppl. 1), 89, 1996.
36. Prall, J. K., Theiler, R. F., Bowser, P. A., Walsh, M., The effectiveness of cosmetic products in alleviating a range of skin dryness conditions as determined by clinical and instrumental techniques, *Int. J. Cosmet. Sci.*, 8, 159, 1986.
37. Rawlings, A., Harding, C., Watkinson, A., Banks, J., Ackerman, C., Sabin, R., The effect of glycerol and humidity on desmosome degradation in stratum corneum, *Arch. Dermatol. Res.*, 287, 457, 1995.
38. Fartasch, M., Teal, J., Menon, G. K., Mode of action of glycolic acid on human stratum corneum: ultrastructural and functional evaluation of the epidermal barrier, *Arch. Dermatol. Res.*, 289, 404, 1997.
39. Elias, P. M., Menon, G. K., Structural and lipid biochemical correlates of the epidermal permeability barrier, in *Advances in Lipid Research*, Vol. 24, Elias, P. M., Havel, R. J., Small, D. M., Eds, Academic Press, New York, 1991, 1.

40. Jass, H. E., Elias, P. M., The living stratum corneum: implications for cosmetic formulation, *Cosm. Toiletries*, 106, 47, 1991.
41. Ghadially, R., Brown, B. E., Hanley, K., Reed, J. T., Feingold, K. R., Elias, P. M., Decreased epidermal lipid synthesis accounts for altered barrier function in aged mice, *J. Invest. Dermatol.*, 106, 1064, 1996.
42. Lukacovic, M. F., Dunlap, F. E., Michaels, S. E., Visscher, M. O., Watson, D. D., Forearm wash test to evaluate the clinical mildness of cleansing products, *J. Soc. Cosmet. Chem.*, 39, 355, 1988.
43. Imokawa, G., Abe, A., Jin, K., Higaki, Y., Kawashima, M., Hidano, A., Decreased level of ceramides in stratum corneum of atopic dermatitis: an etiologic factor in atopic dry skin?, *J. Invest. Dermatol.*, 96, 523, 1991.
44. Saint Léger, D., François, A. M., Lévêque, J. L., Stoudemayer, T. J., Grove, G. L., Kligman, A. M., Age-associated changes in stratum corneum lipids and their relation to dryness, *Dermatologica*, 177, 159, 1988.
45. Mortz, C. G., Andersen, K. E., Halkier-Sorensen, L., Occupational skin diseases, *Contact Dermatitis*, 36, 297, 1997.
46. Man, M.-Q., Feingold, K. R., Elias, P. M., Exogenous lipids influence permeability barrier recovery in acetone-treated murine skin, *Arch. Dermatol.*, 129, 728, 1993.
47. Summers, R. S., Summers, B., Chandar, P., Feinberg, C., Gursky, R., Rawlings, A. V., The effect of lipids, with and without humectant, on skin xerosis, *J. Soc. Cosmet. Chem.*, 47, 27, 1996.

Part 5

Evaluation and Safety

29 Study Design

David Salter

CONTENTS

29.1 INTRODUCTION

Harmlessness is important, but hardly enough to convince someone to buy and use a product. Hence, claims of efficacy are made for cosmetics and toiletries. The validity of such claims needs to be assured by their being subject to objective review from inside and outside the industry, a matter which is being addressed by legislation at many different levels. However, despite the increasing interest in efficacy, the concept itself has still not been authoritatively defined. Hence, consumer protection in respect of efficacy remains far less developed than is the case for safety. While there is no agreement on exactly what we are discussing, there is unlikely to be agreement on the quality and quantity of efficacy present in a particular case. To move forward, a working definition should presumably relate to fitness for purpose, where "purpose" is the explicit performance claim or claims if any, and "fitness" is validated according to some procedure which is not just legally, but also scientifically and ethically defensible. This breadth of validity is essential to convey the proper professionalism of the cosmetic and toiletries industry toward the consumers of its products and can only be achieved by following adequate principles of study design, analysis, and reporting.

There are also increasing legal pressures to follow such principles. For the more than 370 million consumers in the Member States of the European Union, the law now defines a cosmetic product in very broad terms:

> A 'cosmetic product' shall mean any substance or preparation intended to be placed in contact with the various external parts of the human body (epidermis, hair system, nails, lips and external genital organs) or with the teeth and the mucous membranes of the oral cavity with a view exclusively or mainly to cleaning them, perfuming them, changing their appearance and/or correcting body odours and/or protecting them or keeping them in good condition. (Sixth Amendment to the Cosmetics Directive[1])

Furthermore, for this broad range of products, the amended Article 7a, paragraph 1(g) requires the European cosmetic manufacturer or initial importer to hold available *"proof of the effect claimed for the cosmetic product, where justified by the nature of the effect or product."*[1]

Compliance with these provisions has been required since January 1, 1997.[1] However, the task remains difficult because it is not yet clear what exactly triggers the requirement of proof of efficacy

0-8493-7520-7/00/$0.00+$.50

or what constitutes sufficient proof of efficacy once that proof is required. We only know that much depends upon *"the nature of the effect or product."*

Presumably the categories of effect or product for which proof of claim is required will be identified over the progress of time at least on a case-by-case basis, according to the significance of the anticipated or claimed biological effect. This may limit the instances in which such efficacy will have to be proved in detail. Everyone is against the proliferation of new and burdensome standards, so it seems helpful to widely discuss and agree to some firmly grounded criteria defining exactly what *is* necessary, or else this will remain a matter of arbitrary opinion.

Some may believe that the data already held by manufacturers and initial importers are sufficient to satisfy the requirements of the Sixth Amendment quoted previously. While not necessarily doubting it, it would be interesting to know how such a conclusion could presently be arrived at, since the criteria to be met do not seem to be widely known either within the industry or by the consumers wanting to buy the best products. This is a less than ideal situation which should be rectified as soon as possible for everyone's benefit.

Of course, some products, for example, sunscreens, already have widely debated and agreed standards of proof of cosmetic efficacy, which may well be sufficient. In the case of other cosmetics, for example, moisturizers and antiwrinkle products, agreeing on a basis for establishing their claims of efficacy might also be considered desirable. The enhanced consumer confidence would surely be in the best interests of both the consumers and the cosmetics industry, provided always that the proofs of efficacy are relevant, reliable, and practical for everyone. Nevertheless, no procedural guidelines have yet been officially sanctioned, and the various guidelines that have been proposed by unofficial groups have been viewed as not adequately flexible, that is, not sufficiently adaptable to the needs of product manufacturers and testing organizations both large and small.

Yet whatever the continuing debate may bring, it can be expected that most of those interested in cosmetics will wish to encourage efficacy study methodologies which simultaneously (1) ensure an adequate level of quality based on accepted principles of good scientific investigation; (2) are broad and flexible so that detailed procedure can be adapted to suit local needs and conditions; and (3) are relevant to the needs of producers, regulatory authorities, and consumers.

Furthermore, the scientific literature and personal experience in this field tend to encourage the belief that much the same basic set of procedural considerations arises in all contexts if proof of efficacy is to meet generally accepted standards of valid scientific investigation.[2,3]

Putting all this together, one can arrive at a generic yet flexible basic set of procedural considerations for valid study design, analysis, and reporting. What follows here has been successfully piloted in several European countries and commercial organizations, resulting in practical and flexible guidelines which have already appeared in English, German, and French[4-6] and are presently being translated into other languages.

29.2 OBJECTIVE(S)

Define and set a clear statement of *the product and/or physiological claim to be made* (e.g., "the water content of the stratum corneum on the forearm averages 12% *in vivo*") or *the hypothesis to be tested* (e.g., "product A is more effective than product B in producing lasting moisturization"). Studies to test hypotheses which are clearly defined in advance are likely to derive more reliable conclusions than studies which merely explore a large dataset with the aim of discovering apparent relationships retrospectively.

29.3 LEVEL OF SOPHISTICATION

Consider and state clearly *how good an answer is required* to satisfy the objective(s), in the view of those commissioning the study. Studies can be simple and yet entirely adequate so long as no claim to significant innovation in physiological understanding, product, or marketing concept depends upon them. If a significant innovation is claimed, then the study can reasonably be required to be more carefully planned and conducted.

Because the concept of levels of study sophistication can be helpful, three such levels are proposed here, as follows:

RESEARCH — Work publishable as an advance in a peer-reviewed scientific journal; a new claim for radical improvement, qualitative or quantitative, in physiological understanding or in product action.

STANDARD — Work conducted according to current procedures, publishable as a record in a peer-reviewed scientific journal or as news in a trade journal, quantitatively but not qualitatively extending knowledge of physiology or product action, and which could be used to support an existing product claim.

GUIDANCE — A largely or entirely routine study conducted for purposes of performance confirmation, formulation, or re-formulation guidance, and unlikely to be published.

29.4 STUDY DESIGN AND PROTOCOL

Before the study begins, a written protocol should be prepared. This fact and this sequence are not trivial. All studies on which claim support may be based (i.e., Research, Standard, and usually Guidance) should be conducted according to a protocol which addresses *at least* the questions in the following checklist (based on Reference 3 and Table I of Reference 7, which are recommended for direct consultation). If investigators record in the protocol their views on only some of these issues, an unnecessary risk of errors of omission may arise, adding to the inevitable risk of errors of commission. Hence, this is considered a minimum list, but of course each topic need not be discussed at length.

- What are the objectives of the work?
- What information is required to achieve the objectives?
- What function or structure is to be investigated?
- Which measurable variables could serve for description, comparison, support, or rejection of the claim or hypothesis?
- What are the most relevant variables to be assessed, and why?
- Is each chosen variable a *direct* measure of the quantity or quantities of interest? If not, how indirect is it, and what factors can influence the connecting relationship?
- To what extent can the variables chosen for measurement be influenced by the variable factors in the experiment and especially any factors not controlled in the experimental context (i.e., potential "confounding variables")?
- What is the expected time course of the variables chosen, i.e., are the variables expected to develop linearly or in some other way (for example, a cyclical dependence upon time of day or time of year)?
- At what time point(s) should the measurements be performed, and why?
- What is known about the ranges of the variables to be measured in relation to the expected phenomena or structure being studied, including inter- and intra-individual variation and dependence upon
  - Anatomical site
  - Sex
  - Age
  - Environmental conditions
  - Time of day and proximity of mealtimes
  - Time of year
  - Number and duration of previous measurements

- Is the study sample sufficiently representative of the group from which it is drawn (the study population), and is this group itself sufficiently representative of the wider population to which the results might apply (the target population)?
- Is the measuring area so much smaller than the area of the skin site that extra measurements need to be taken to estimate the intra-site variability?
- Are measurements with the equipment reproducible, and is the accuracy acceptable relative to the variables being measured and their expected range?
- What are the measuring standards and calibration procedures?
- In view of the available information on the dependence on environmental conditions, is there a need to conduct the measurements in a controlled environment?
- Is it necessary to precondition the individuals before testing, and if so, how should this be done? (Factors to consider here could include, for example, the procedure, if any, for cleaning the site to be tested and the procedure, if any, for product sample application, including amount and mode of application.)
- How many measurements need be taken in order to detect a result meaningful in physiological or consumer terms at an acceptable level of statistical significance? N.b. It is strongly recommended that a sufficiently experienced statistician be consulted to answer and document this question, since the necessary sample size will depend upon
  - The anticipated or known response of the controls
  - The anticipated response of the test group
  - The statistical significance level or Type I error rate α (usually $\alpha = 0.05$)
  - The statistical power (1 minus the Type II error rate β, where usually $\beta = 0.1$)
- If this adequate sample size is not used in the study, then an explicit justification should be provided for the number actually used.
- Are there restrictions upon conducting the measurements involved in the study?
- How will the overall design of the study take account of all the considerations above?
- What is the evidence that the principal investigator and any assistants have both the educational background and enough practical experience to conduct the investigation to the required standard of quality?

A Research study may wish to follow the guidelines recommended for Good Clinical Practice (GCP) studies on medicinal products,[8] especially if the cosmetic products involved contain ingredients which may show a high degree of physiological activity (i.e., so-called "actives"). However, following the GCP guidelines requires direction by a medically qualified person, and this is not at present mandatory or even necessarily appropriate unless the treatment of illness is involved.

29.5 CONTENT AND FORMAT OF PROTOCOL AND SUPPORTING DOCUMENTS

Depending on the nature of the cosmetic and the level of study concerned, the following headings may be found useful as a checklist of points to consider in the protocol and supporting documents.

1. Background
2. Specific Objective(s) and Relevance of the Study
3. Methods of Measurement to be Used
   3.1 Rationale for Choice of Method(s), including Relevance to Meet Objective(s)
   3.2 Rationale for Type(s) of Measurement Scale Used (i.e., Nominal, Ordinal, Interval, or Ratio)
   3.3 Anticipated Relationship Between Instrumental Measures and Self-Assessment Scores

3.4 Rationale for Wording and Design of Questionnaire(s), if Used for Claim Support
3.5 Calibration and Control Procedures
3.6 Standard Operating Procedures and/or Literature Precedents

4. Design Rationale and Statistics
   4.1 Statistical Design, Experimental Layout, Randomization, and Blinding
   4.2 Rationale for the Number of Measurements Required
   4.3 Treatment Site(s), Measurement Procedure, Time(s), and Duration(s)
   4.4 Type(s) of Statistical Analysis to Be Used
   4.5 Possible Combination of Data Subgroups (e.g., from Different Geographical Locations)
   4.6 Intended Use and Influence of Interim Analyses of Data
5. Test Preparations and Control Procedures
   5.1 Background
   5.2 Composition/Formulation(s)
   5.3 Origin and Preparation
   5.4 Packaging
   5.5 Analytical
   5.6 Labelling
   5.7 Coding
   5.8 Usage
   5.9 Procedure for the Return and Analysis of Unused Materials
6. Panellist Selection
   6.1 Inclusion Criteria
   6.2 Exclusion Criteria
   6.3 Prohibitions and Restrictions
   6.4 Withdrawal from the Study
   6.5 Dismissal from the Study
   6.6 Consequences of Missing Assessments
7. Safety and Ethical Procedures for Panellist Protection
   7.1 Safety Clearance Requirements
   7.2 Ethical Review Requirements
   7.3 Foreseeable Effects of the Treatments
   7.4 Action in the Event of Unexpected Effects
   7.5 Emergency Procedures
   7.6 Compliance with Safety Regulations and Special Precautions
   7.7 Insurance
   7.8 Informed Consent
   7.9 Confidentiality and Data Protection
   7.10 The Form and Timing of Recompense for Panellists
8. Logistics and Administration
   8.1 Study Schedule
   8.2 Data Handling, Validation, Security, and Archiving
   8.3 Responsibilities of Principal Investigator and Assistants
   8.4 Procedure for Dealing with Protocol Amendments
9. Auditing Procedures
   9.1 Stages of Review of Protocol
   9.2 Monitoring of Study Progress and Quality Assurance
   9.3 Auditing Procedures for Data
10. Record of Authorizations and Approvals
11. Plan for Reporting and Publishing

29.6 ANALYSIS AND INTERPRETATION OF RESULTS

The danger of reading too much (or too little) into the results of the study can be reduced by avoidance of common errors of data analysis.[9-14] Such errors might invalidate the conclusions if these were subjected to close scrutiny.[14] Lack of attention to proper controls, believing proof of association to be proof of causation, the possible need for data transformations, forgetting the preferability of confidence intervals to p-values, and the analysis of multiple or repeated measurements are all common sources of error.

It is therefore recommended that References 2, 3, and 7 to 14 should be consulted as representing internationally recognized standards of product research on human beings. Research and Standard studies should be planned to avoid the dangers outlined in these and similar publications. Furthermore, all studies should take care to avoid the dangers of overinterpretation, which may apply particularly to cosmetic product efficacy investigations.[14,15]

REFERENCES

1. The Council of the European Communities, Council Directive 93/35/EEC of 14 June 1993 amending for the sixth time Directive 76/768/EEC on the approximation of the laws of the Member States relating to cosmetic products, *Official Journal of the European Communities*, No L 151, 32–36, 1993.
2. Salter, D. C., Ethics of human testing, *International Journal of Cosmetic Science,* 12, 165–173, 1990.
3. Fowkes, F. G. R., Fulton, P. M., Critical appraisal of published research: introductory guidelines, *British Medical Journal*, 302, 1136–1140, 1991.
4. Salter, D. C., Non-invasive cosmetic efficacy testing in human volunteers: some general principles, *Skin Research and Technology*, 2, 59–63, 1996.
5. Salter, D. C., Wolf, F., Nicht-invasive Wirksamkeitsprüfungen von Kosmetika an Probanden: einige allgemeine Prinzipien, *Parfümerie und Kosmetik*, 78, 24–27, 1997.
6. Salter, D. C., Leneveu-Duchemin, M.-L., Evaluation non invasive sur humain de l'efficacité des produits cosmétiques, *Parfums Cosmétiques Actualités*, 136, 67–69, 1997.
7. Serup, J., Bioengineering and the skin: from standard error to standard operating procedure, *Acta Dermato-Venereologica (Stockholm),* Suppl. 185, 5–8, 1994.
8. CPMP Working Party on Efficacy of Medicinal Products, EEC Note for Guidance: Good Clinical Practice for trials on medicinal products in the European Community, *Phamacology & Toxicology*, 67, 361–372, 1990.
9. Altman, D. G., Gore, S. M., Gardner, M. J., Pocock, S. J., Statistical guidelines for contributors to medical journals, *British Medical Journal,* 286, 1489–1493, 1983.
10. Bland, J. M., Altman, D. G., Calculating correlation coefficients with repeated observations: Part 1 — correlation within subjects, *British Medical Journal*, 310, 446, 1995.
11. Bland, J. M., Altman, D. G., Calculating correlation coefficients with repeated observations: Part 2 — correlation between subjects, *British Medical Journal,* 310, 633, 1995.
12. Gardner, M. J., Altman, D. G., Confidence intervals rather than P-values: estimation rather than hypothesis testing, *British Medical Journal*, 292, 746–750, 1986.
13. Gardner, M. J., Machin, D., Campbell, M. J., Use of checklists in assessing the statistical content of medical studies, *British Medical Journal*, 292, 810–812, 1986.
14. Skrabanek, P., The epidemiology of errors, *The Lancet*, 342, 1502, 1993.
15. Grove, G. L., Design of studies to measure skin care product performance, *Bioengineering and the Skin*, 3, 359–373, 1987.

30 Safety Assessment

Monica Tammela

CONTENTS

30.1 INTRODUCTION

Skin moisturizers are used by a majority of the population in different degrees. Skin moisturizers, in addition to their beneficial effect on the skin, must be devoid of any other deleterious effect on human health. They must not cause damage to human health under normal or reasonably foreseeable conditions of use.

In most cases, skin moisturizers are considered as cosmetic/hygienic products and must comply with the legislation for these products. The manufacturer of the products is responsible for the safety of each product. However, in addition, the legislation in many countries may restrict the use of certain ingredients, mainly preservatives, colors, and UV-filters.

Certain skin moisturizers, however, may be considered as medicinal products and are then covered by special documentation and registration requirements.

The main part of the safety assessment of finished products could be based, in principle, on data from the different ingredients used. The many thousands of different products on the market are all derived from a smaller number of ingredients. The toxicological profiles are also adequately

0-8493-7520-7/00/$0.00+$.50

studied on separate substances. To avoid costly duplication of studies and unjustifiable use of animals, toxicity testing in this area must be concentrated on the different ingredients and particularly those of most concern. For example, the listing of coloring agents, preservatives, and UV-filters within EU and the Cosmetic Ingredient Review within the U.S. is important.

30.2 TOXICOLOGICAL REQUIREMENTS ON INGREDIENTS

To assure that an ingredient does not pose a risk for human health, all possible toxicological endpoints must be considered. That includes possible acute and chronic effects both locally and systemically. The exact information and studies needed depend on the compound and its properties. As a guidance to the toxicological properties to be considered, annex 1 in the Notes of guidance from the SCC could be used.[1] In this guidance the first part of the lists (Sections 30.2.1 to 30.2.9) constitutes items necessary for all compounds. Depending on the properties and outcome of this first part, additional points (Sections 30.2.10 to 30.2.11) might be necessary. Considerable oral intake or skin absorption are examples of circumstances where these additional points are necessary.

It is important to remember that as our knowledge about the effects of different substances on the human body increases, ingredients already in use might need reevaluation.

30.2.1 Acute Toxicity

Acute toxicity is necessary to evaluate the amounts that do or, in many cases, do not affect the living organism at a single exposure. It can be necessary for assessment of accidental exposure. However, mostly it is helpful to choose the levels in subsequent toxicological examinations. For new substances it should be performed only for the need in other legal requirements, for example, due to chemicals legislation and/or worker protection. No exact figures are required, and ranges or intervals might be enough. Both oral and dermal routes might be adequate, but in most cases the oral route is used. Acute toxicity is of minor importance for most ingredients in skin moisturizers, but can be important for additives with special effects.

30.2.2 Skin Absorption

As skin moisturizers are applied to the minor or major outer parts of the human body, the skin absorption of ingredients is important to estimate the systemic exposure. If skin absorption studies are lacking, 100% absorption could be assumed in the safety evaluation.

30.2.3 Skin Irritation

Possible irritative effects of the substance on the skin must be assessed. Preliminary knowledge, can in this case, can be derived from experiences of other substances with similar structure. If any hesitation exists, studies must be performed.

30.2.4 Mucous Membrane Irritation

Since most of the products intentionally or unintentionally can come in contact with different mucous membranes, local deleterious effects must be considered.

30.2.5 Skin Sensitization

Predictive tests on the potential of the compound to cause skin sensitization are essential. The introduction of new potent sensitizers must be avoided. So far only animal tests are sufficiently reliable to predict a low sensitizing potential, although alternatives can exclude potent sensitizers.

30.2.6 Sub-Chronic Toxicity

To substantiate the safety of the substance for the population exposed, a subchronic study must be performed. The study should be designed to obtain a no-adverse-effect level. A 90- or 28-day study in rats is usually used.

30.2.7 Mutagenicity

To exclude substances with mutagenic effects, as a minimum, the mutagenicity should be assessed in three different systems with and without metabolizing medium.

30.2.8 Phototoxicity and Photomutagenicity

Most of the toxicological studies mentioned previously are needed also for other uses of the substance. However, different types of investigations involving light sources also are, in many cases, a special requirement for use in cosmetic products. This is important for UV-light absorbing substances.

30.2.9 Human Data

For many substances used in cosmetics, humans might have been exposed earlier intentionally or unintentionally. All data from these experiences are useful in the safety evaluation both for substances and later for the products.

30.2.10 Toxicokinetics

If there is a systemic exposure of the substance it is important to examine the disposition, metabolism, and excretion of the substance.

30.2.11 Teratogenicity and Reproduction Toxicity

The risk of different reproduction disorders must be evaluated if there is a considerable systemic exposure, as moisturizers are extensively used within the population.

30.2.12 Additional Genotoxicity and Carcinogenicity

Depending on the outcome of previous testing on mutagenicity and systemic exposure, complete carcinogenicity or at least additional genotoxicity testing is necessary to exclude these risks.

30.3 SOURCES OF TOXICOLOGICAL INFORMATION

First, a request about toxicological information to the raw material supplier should be made. In addition, data from usual toxicological sources, databases, and literature are supplementary. As toxicological studies substantiating safety of a substance are prepared within companies and not usually published, different attempts have been made to make them more avaible. In the U.S. the Cosmetic Ingredient Review reports on the safety of different ingredients.[2] Within EU, reports from the Scientific Committee on Cosmetics and Non-Food Products (former Scientific Committee on Cosmetology) are available for some ingredients.

If sufficient toxicological information is not to be found, studies must be conducted.

30.4 METHODS

For the toxicity studies needed, internationally accepted methods as those reported within EU[3] or in accordance with the OECD Guidelines for testing of chemicals are recommended. Tests for assessing photomutagenicity, photoirritationcy, photosensitization, and skin absoprtion have not been included so far in the previously mentioned guidelines. Some guidance to these types of tests could be found in the document from the SCC.[1]

New studies have to be conducted according to Good Laboratory Practice (GLP). However, old studies should not automatically be invalidated if they do not comply with guidelines or GLP requirements. Due to ethical reasons other testing procedures based on scientifically justified models and procedures can be accepted.

30.5 DIFFERENT TYPES OF INGREDIENTS

As reviewed in this book, skin moisturizers contain a long variety of ingredients that have beneficial effects on the skin. So far some types of ingredients have been of the most toxicological concern. Preservatives and perfumes are two types of ingredients which need special toxicological attention. Colors and UV-filters are two other types of ingredients for which special requirements have been made. Within EU compounds used as preservatives, UV-filter and colors require an evaluation by authorities prior to their use in cosmetic products. Their documentation and safety are evaluated by the Scientific Committee on Cosmetics and Non-Food Products before they are permitted and placed on the lists of the Cosmetics Directive.[4] Within the fragrance industry, self-regulatory work is increasing the safety of the substances used as they comply with the IFRA Code of Practice.[5]

30.6 SAFETY EVALUATION OF PRODUCTS

In general the safety evaluation of the finished product can be obtained by ascertaining the toxicity profile of the different ingredients. But it is important to evaluate each different toxicological end point and to examine the documentation to see if it is adequate for the assessment.

Important factors to consider in calculating the exposure are, for example, concentration of ingredients in the product, quantity, frequency and area of skin contact, and the nature of consumers.

For some of the effects the concentration in the products is most important, e.g., the local tolerance on the skin and eye. For some of the other effects it is necessary to estimate the presumed use by a normal or perhaps an eager user and the total amounts are more adequate. The European cosmetics industry has estimated the exposure levels to be 0.8 g/day of face cream, 1 to 2 g/day of general cream, and 8 to 16 g/day of body lotion for a female user.[6] It is also important to predict the use of the special product and the expectations from the single user. Groups of users with especially sensitive skin are important to take into account.

It is also necessary to look at the product as a composition. Possible interactions and potentiations of effects between the different ingredients locally or systemically must be considered. The possibility of altered penetration due to the composition and the possible effect on toxicity must be evaluated. For skin moisturizers a lot of experience is gathered for previous compositions and products on the market. For local effects such experience may be reliable, but one has to pay special attention to systemic toxicity which is difficult to discover during use by consumers.

30.7 ADDITIONAL TOXICOLOGICAL ASPECTS

Apart from the strictly regulated types of ingredients, colors, preservatives, and UV-filters, the main part can be used under the manufacturers responsibility. From the past we can get important toxicological aspects that ought to be noticed. In some cases toxicological problems have been discovered among constituents such as emulsifiers and emollients.

30.7.1 Contaminants

In the manufacturing process of ingredients a lot of different chemicals are used. The residue levels of these starting materials must be controlled, not only to have a high quality raw material, but also in relation to their toxicological profile. In the past, the residue level of dioxane used in the manufacturing process for ethoxylated substances was considered as a health hazard, as dioxane was shown to be carcinogenic in mice. It is important also to state that the specification of the ingredient during the toxicological testing and evaluation to make the results relevant for the ingredient when used in a cosmetic product.

30.7.2 Formation of New Substances

Under certain circumstances, formation of new substances can be seen during manufacturing, storage, or use. Formation of different nitrosamines were found in products with dialkanolamines together with some nitrosating agents. 2-Bromo-2-nitropropane-1,3-diol and 5-bromo-5-nitro-1,3-dioxane are two, but not the only, examples of such substances. This formation of nitrosamines is important to avoid or reduce, as many different nitrosamines are shown to be carcinogenic in animals.

REFERENCES

1. Notes of guidance for testing of cosmetic ingredients for their safety evaluation (Second revision) Scientific Committee on Cosmetology. European Commission, Directorate General DG XXIV Consumer Policy and Consumer Health Protection. http://dg3.eudra.org/dgiii3/docs.htm.
2. Cosmetics Ingredients Review. http://www.ctfa-cir.org.
3. Commission Directive 87/302/EEC (Annex Part B: Methods for the determination of toxicity) and Annex to Commission Directive 92/69/EEC.
4. Council Directive (76/768/EEC) on the approximation of laws of the Member States relating to cosmetic products O.J. L262 27.09.76 (amended).
5. IFRA Code of Practice. IFRA General Secretary, 8 Rue Charles Humbert, CH-1205 GENEVA.
6. ECETOC Technical Report No 58. Assessment of Non-Occupational Exposure to Chemicals. Brussels, 1994.

31 Human *In Vivo* Skin Irritancy Testing

Ebba Bárány

CONTENTS

31.1 INTRODUCTION

In the toxicological safety assessment of topical preparations, tests to predict skin irritation are regularly included. There are several ways to perform irritancy tests, with both *in vitro* and *in vivo* methods described, the latter both in animals and humans. Assessing the skin irritancy potential of topicals in humans has a great advantage to other tests, in that extrapolation from other species or *in vitro* models to man is not necessary. In this way, criticism of the relevance to man does not arise. Moreover, subjective effects on the skin may also be evaluated. Animal testing is a controversial issue, and using animals for testing of finished cosmetic products will also be banned within the EU shortly.[1] Therefore, this chapter will only discuss human *in vivo* tests for skin irritation from moisturizers. The general requirements for studies involving human volunteers are touched upon, the different test methods to assess the irritancy potential are reviewed, and the ways of evaluation are described. In the last part of the chapter the clinical relevance is commented.

Skin irritation is a complex biological event, commonly described by the observed clinical response (erythema, edema, scaling) to stimuli, both chemical and physical, that produces inflammation at the

0-8493-7520-7/00/$0.00+$.50

contact site.[2] Multiple external and internal factors influence the clinical appearance of irritant contact dermatitis. Elicitation of an irritant reaction occurs after single or repeated exposures. There may be skin barrier perturbation with subsequent increase in transepidermal water loss (TEWL) and stimulation of cytokine production.[3] Hereby, an inflammatory skin reaction is promoted. Direct damage to the keratinocytes is also possible, inducing release of mediators of inflammation. However, in subacute or nonvisible conditions of irritation, inflammation can be absent or minimal, but the skin barrier can still be disrupted.[3] Moreover, subjective irritation without visible signs, e.g., stinging or itching, may also occur.[4] There does not seem to be a direct correlation between subjective and objective irritation.[4,5]

31.2 WHEN IS TESTING REQUIRED?

The objective of irritancy testing is to establish the clinical safety of all topical preparations. Data on the preclinical and clinical safety of a pharmaceutical moisturizer are to be reviewed during the new drug application process. In the EU, a cosmetic moisturizer must be safe under normal conditions of use and foreseeable misuse.[1] Guidelines for the safety assessment were issued by the Scientific Committee on Cosmetology of the Commission of the European Union in 1997.[6] The FDA requires manufacturers to adequately substantiate cosmetic product safety, which can be done by already available data on ingredients or similar formulations, or by performing additional toxicological tests.[7]

In order to substantiate the safety of a topical preparation after application to the skin, a stepwise approach of predictive tests can be used (Figure 1). In general, safety substantiation can be derived from knowledge of the inherent properties of the ingredients, making it unnecessary to test the final product. This is often the case for cosmetic moisturizers. Still, in some cases, testing of the final product may be justified. One example is when the combination of ingredients in the vehicle results in considerably greater skin penetration than expected from their individual effects. Another reason can be when interaction between ingredients may result in the formation of new, potentially irritating substances. Guidelines for the assessment of skin compatibility of cosmetic finished products in humans were recently published by the European Cosmetic, Toiletries and Perfumery Association, COLIPA.[8] Postmarketing control such as monitoring of complaints data is also important.

31.3 GENERAL REQUIREMENTS AND PREPARATIONS

31.3.1 Good Laboratory Practice and Good Clinical Practice

Good Laboratory Practice (GLP)[9] and Good Clinical Practice (GCP)[10] set the standard for the organization and circumstances under which studies are planned, conducted, monitored, recorded, and reported. These guidelines are intended to promote the quality and validity of test data.

31.3.2 Ethical Requirements

All human studies must be conducted in accordance with the Declaration of Helsinki (1964) and subsequent revisions.[11, 12] If appropriate, an ethical review committee shall approve the study.

31.3.3 Informed Consent

The participants must give their informed consent before entering a study, which is done by signing a consent agreement form. An example of such a form can be found in the COLIPA guidelines by Walker et al.[8] It is important to specify that the participant may discontinue the study at any time without further explanation.

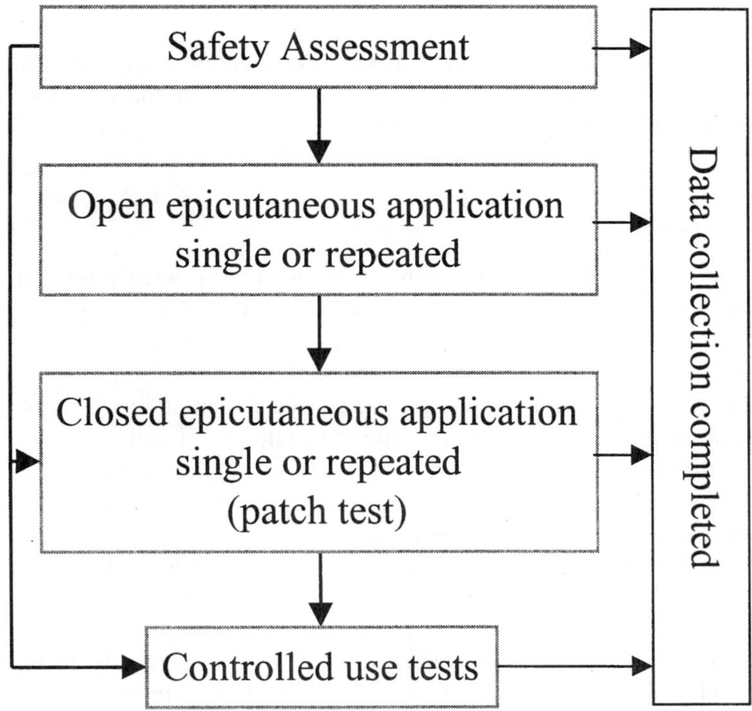

FIGURE 1 A stepwise approach is useful in order to substantiate the safety of a topical preparation.

31.3.4 Safety Assessment

Before a study can commence, a thorough safety review is needed to conclude that the study will involve no significant risk to the volunteers. This includes the elimination of severe skin irritants through consideration of the structure activity relations (SARs)[13] and structure property relations (SPRs), physicochemical properties, and data obtained from *in vitro* corrosion tests.[6] Moreover, available toxicological data on the ingredients or on products similar in composition to the product being evaluated should be considered.

31.3.5 Participants

The susceptibility of the subjects to skin irritation may be influenced by many different factors, which are important in considering in the selection. Examples of such factors are age, race, sex, test site, and preexisting dermatitis.[3] External factors to consider are, e.g., environmental conditions.[14]

31.4 TEST STRATEGIES

There are several human tests to predict the skin irritation potential of different formulations. Most are rank methods and include reference materials. Many consist of exaggerated and/or prolonged exposure, aiming to compare the inherent properties of the test products. Use tests are performed to investigate the acceptability of a formulation under realistic conditions of use. Moisturizers are usually tested undiluted in all tests due to their relatively low potential for skin irritation.

31.4.1 Open Test

In an open test, the formulation is applied to the skin without occlusion. The repeated open application test (ROAT) consists of application of the moisturizer to the same test site twice daily for 7 days.[15] This is a way to mimic everyday exposure. The study design may be suitable for new formulations where the irritation potential is unknown.

31.4.2 Patch Tests

Application under occlusion by using the patch testing technique is widely used for the assessment of irritation. This procedure enhances, by use of occlusion, the effect of the test products on the skin. Three types of prognostic patch tests are generally practiced: single closed patch test evolving from the diagnostic tests, cumulative irritancy patch test,[16] and repeated insult patch test.[17] The single closed patch test is commonly used as a screening test for acute skin irritation potential. Often both positive (e.g., sodium lauryl sulfate, SLS) and negative controls (well-tolerated marketed products, water, or petrolatum) are included as comparisons. Patches with the undiluted product are applied for 24 to 48 h to the arm or back of 10 to 20 test subjects, the patches are then removed, and the irritation is assessed 0.5 to 1 and/or 24 h later.[2] Recently, a 4-h patch test has been developed and characterized.[18,19] However, the OECD has recently evaluated and turned down a proposal for a new guideline for "Acute Dermal Irritation Study in Human Volunteers" based on the 4-h patch test.

Cumulative irritancy tests exist in many varieties,[20,21] but are basically 10 to 21 consecutive patches applied and read at 24-h intervals. Twenty-five test subjects are recommended for biostatistical significance.[22] The number of patches may be estimated using the IT50 method (time to produce irritation in 50% of subjects after 24 h exposure) of Kligman and Wooding.[16] Repeated insult patch test is used to predict the irritancy from low-level irritants and the sensitizing ability of test substances or formulas. It consists of a number of induction exposures, originally 15, and when testing for sensitizing ability, a challenge application 2 weeks later. Larger groups of test subjects are involved, normally 50 to 100.

The chamber scarification test was developed to investigate and compare cosmetic ingredients and consumer products intended for repeated use on normal and diseased skin.[23] It is a predictive test, which amplifies irritant reactions to products by scarification of the test area prior to the first application. The investigated materials are then applied in closed patch tests daily for 3 days, and the sites are read each day. A high reproducibility of the reactions have been shown.[24] The scarification procedure can be likened to a worst case scenario, indicating what might happen under unusually provocative circumstances.[14]

31.4.3 Controlled Use Test

In a controlled use test, the participants use the product for a defined period of time, usually up to 4 weeks,[25] under realistic conditions of use. Subjective irritation is important to consider when assessing the irritation potential of a product. Controlled use testing can supplement a safety assessment with data on possible stinging, itching, or burning sensations experienced.

31.5 EVALUATION OF TEST REACTIONS

31.5.1 Clinical Assessment

A ROAT is considered positive when dermatitis appears.[15] In patch tests, treatment and control sites are examined for signs of irritation, and responses are scored at, for example, 1 and 24 to 96 h after patch removal. The reactions should be scored throughout the test by the same experienced assessor. Visual assessment can then be both sensitive and reproducible.[26] A scoring scale for

TABLE 1
Example of Scoring Scale for Skin Irritation[27]

Score	Erythema	Dryness
0	No reaction	No reaction
½	Minimal or doubtful	Dry without scaling
1	Slight redness, spotty, and diffuse	Fine/mild scaling
2	Moderate, uniform redness	Moderate scaling
3	Strong, uniform redness	Severe scaling with large flakes
4	Fiery redness	—

different aspects of skin irritation is shown in Table 1.[27] Edema is graded separately as absence (–) or presence (+).[27] The clinical appearance of acute and cumulative irritation may differ. Therefore, two different standard clinical scoring schemes can be used, as suggested by the Standardization Group of the European Society of Contact Dermatitis, ESCD.[28]

31.5.2 Bioengineering Methods

Exposure to chemicals may induce invisible but functional skin changes. Biophysical methods can be used to evaluate different aspects of an irritant reaction and to supplement the visual evaluation. Changes in TEWL are a sensitive measure of skin barrier damage.[29-31] Techniques that are supposed to reflect skin hydration, e.g., impedance[32] and capacitance,[33] also detect subtle skin damage. The skin capacitance has also been reported to correlate with the clinical appearance of scaling.[34,35]

Moreover, inflammatory changes can be evaluated. The microvascular blood flow can be measured using an optical technique such as the laser Doppler flowmeter.[36] Colorimetry measures the skin color and can be used to quantify erythema in the irritant response.[37]

The development of noninvasive measuring techniques have increased the ability to distinguish between the irritation potentials of different products. All instrumental evaluations are to be made following an acclimatization period in an environmentally conditioned room (e.g., controlled temperature, relative humidity).[31,36] Other important aspects are removal of the test product when appropriate before measurements, since, for example, remains of occlusive substances give false reduction in TEWL measurements. There are several textbooks providing further information in the field of bioengineering methods.[38,39]

31.5.3 Subjective Evaluation

Subjective evaluation can be accomplished by questionnaires completed by the study participants. One drawback of controlled use tests is the lack of objective criteria in evaluation of the test subjects experiences, thus limiting the information gathered in respect to quality and quantity of the sensations. A possible way to overcome this is by use of the visual analog scale (VAS). Another option is using the scoring system introduced by the ESCD (Table 2).[28]

31.6 IRRITATING SUBSTANCES IN MOISTURIZERS

Moisturizers may contain substances with the potential for skin irritation, yet they are required for the structure or function of the product (Table 3). For instance, moisturizers require the presence of emulsifiers to stabilize the emulsion. Emulsifiers are potential irritants, but unexpectedly some have been shown not to amplify the irritation in already damaged skin, but rather to decrease TEWL.[40] Other included irritants are often used at a tolerable level, and furthermore the preparation can be formulated to diminish these effects. Substances included for the moisturizing effect, e.g.,

TABLE 2
Subjective Scoring System of Irritant Reactions During or After Exposure[28]

Score	Quality	Description
0	Negative	No burning/stinging sensation
1	Weak	Weak burning/stinging
2	Moderate	Moderate burning/stinging
3	Strong	Strong burning/stinging

TABLE 3
Examples of Substance with Potential for Skin Irritation Found in Moisturizers

Substance (test concentration)	Test strategy	Result	Ref.
PEG stearates (5%)	48-h patch test	Increased TEWL	40
Stearethes (5%)			
Wool wax alcohol (30%)	48-h patch test	Erythema	41
Benzalkonium chloride (7.5 to 10%)	4-h patch test	Clinical irritation	19
Lactic acid (undiluted)	4-h patch test	Clinical irritation	19
Oleic acid	3- or 24-h occlusive application		
Oleic acid (25%)	21-day cumulative irritation test	Increased laser Doppler value and skin permeability	43
		Clinical irritation	14
Propylene Glycol (100%)	48-h patch test	Erythema	42

wool wax alcohols[41] or propylene glycol,[42] may cause skin irritation in some cases. In a 4-h patch test, undiluted lactic acid caused more positive reactions than 20% sodium lauryl sulfate,[19] which is a well-known model irritant.[28] Fatty acids, naturally occurring in the skin such as oleic acid, may also be offending agents.[14,43] Certain preservatives, e.g., benzalkonium chloride, are irritants.[19] However, the effects of the substances mentioned previously, when applied in occluded patch tests, are certainly different than in a moisturizer during normal use conditions.

Ingredients which have been reported to induce subjective irritation include lactic acid, propylene glycol,[44] and salicylic acid.[45]

31.7 CLINICAL RELEVANCE OF TESTING

There are many predictive tests developed in order to evaluate the skin irritation potential of individual chemicals or formulations. Most are relative methods, ranking the irritation potential compared to known reference materials. Therefore, the choice of standard reference materials is important to consider. Also, the method of application, occlusive or open, single or repeated, as well as the anatomical site used, must be related to the data collected. A single exposure is a relatively quick and cheap way of ranking the irritancy of products and reflects the inherent properties. On the other hand, it may not reflect an in-use situation appropriately, as extrapolation to these conditions are not well characterized.[46] Moreover, stay-on products of the skin care type generally reveal no significant adverse effects even after contact times of 24 h.[8] The response is generally sporadic and rapidly declining erythema, of the same magnitude as from water. Therefore, repeated applications may be necessary to assess the range of possible effects, if the formula is new and without reference data from related products. Controlled use testing provides additional information. The exaggerated exposure of a patch test on the arm or back of healthy volunteers is quite different from using the same product on, for example, facial skin or diseased skin. The former demonstrates the inherent irritant properties, while the latter focus on the acceptability of the formulation.

31.8 CONCLUSION

There are to date no definite guidelines on how human tests should be performed for the safety assessment of moisturizers. Therefore, the approach to assessment of irritancy can be flexible to avoid unnecessary human tests. The method for apprising the skin irritation potential of a moisturizer is determined by the quantity and quality of information available on ingredients and similar formulations. A stepwise procedure is advantageous, first establishing the inherent properties of the formulation. This is done by safety assessment of raw materials and then, if considered necessary, open test and/or occluded patch test. The characteristics during use situations are then established.

REFERENCES

1. EC, D. 9. Amending for the 6th time Directive 76/768/EEC on the approximation of the laws of the member states relating to cosmetic products. *Off J European Communities* L151, (1993).
2. Weltfriend, S., Bason, M., Lammintausta, K., Maibach, H. I. *Irritant dermatitis (Irritation)*. In *Dermatotoxicology* (5th ed). Edited by Marzulli F. N. and Maibach H. I. Taylor & Francis, Washington. (1996) pp 87.
3. Berardesca, E., Distante, F. *Mechanisms of skin irritation.* In *Irritant Dermatitis New Clinical and Experimental Aspects. Current Problems in Dermatology,* 23, Edited by Elsner P. and Maibach H. I. Karger, Basel. (1995) pp 1.
4. Frosch, P., Kligman, A. M. A method for appraising the stinging capacity of topically applied substances. *J Soc Cosmet Chem* 28, 197(1977).
5. Basketter, D. A., Griffiths, H. A. A study of the relationship between susceptibility to skin stinging and skin irritation. *Contact Dermatitis* 29, 185(1993).
6. Scientific Committee on Cosmetology. 2 rev, EUROPEAN COMMISSION, Brussels. (1997).
7. 40 *Fed. Reg.* (1975).
8. Walker, A. P., Basketter, D. A., Baverel, M., Diemsbeck, W., Matthies, W., Mougin, D., Paye, M., Röthlisberger, R., Dupois, J. Test guidelines for assessment of skin compatibility of cosmetic finished products in man. *Food Chem. Toxicol.* 34, 651(1996).
9. OECD, E. D. Environment monograph no. 45. OECD, Paris. (1992).
10. ICH. GCP: Consolidated guidelines. ICH. (1996).
11. World Medical Association. 2, WMA, Ferney Voltaire. (1989).
12. CIOMS/WHO. CIOMS, Geneva. (1993).
13. Basketter, D. A. Chemistry of contact allergens and irritants. *Am J Contact Dermatitis* 9, 119(1998).
14. Kligman, A. M. *Assessment of mild irritants in humans.* In Current Concepts in Cutaneous Toxicology. Edited by Drill L. Academic Press, New York. (1980) pp 69.
15. Hannuksela, M., Salo, H. The repeated open application test (ROAT). *Contact Dermatitis* 14, 221 (1986).
16. Kligman, A. M., Wooding, W. M. A method for the measurement and evaluation of irritants on human skin. *J Invest Dermatol* 49, 78 (1967).
17. Shelanski, H. A., Shelanski, M. V. New technique of patch tests. *Drug Cosmet Ind* 73, 186(1953).
18. Basketter, D. A., Whittle, E., Griffiths, H. A., York, M. The identification and classification of skin irritation hazard by a human patch test. *Food Chem Toxicol* 32, 769(1994).
19. York, M., Griffiths, H. A., Whittle, E., Basketter, D. A. Evaluation of a human patch test for the identification and classification of skin irritation potential. *Contact Dermatitis* 34, 204(1996).

20. Patil, S. M., Patrick, E., Maibach, H. I. *Animal, human, and in vitro test methods for predicting skin irritation.* In *Dermatotoxicology* (5th Ed). Edited by Marzulli F. N. and Maibach H. I. Taylor & Francis, Washington. (1996) pp 411.
21. Jackson, E. M. Prognostic patch testing: the other kind of patch test. *Am J Contact Dermatitis* 9, 237(1998).
22. Jackson, E. M. The biostatistical significance of panel size in patch testing. *Am J Contact Dermatitis* 5, 228(1994).
23. Frosch, P. J., Kligman, A. M. The chamber scarification test for irritancy. *Contact Dermatitis* 2, 314(1976).
24. Andersen, K. E. Reproducibility of the chamber scarification test. *Contact Dermatitis* 34, 181(1996).
25. Jackson, E. M. Irritation and sensitization. In *Safety and Efficacy Testing of Cosmetic Products.* Edited by Waggoner W. C. Marcel Dekker, New York. (1990) pp 23.
26. Basketter, D., Reynolds, F., Rowson, M., Talbot, C., Whittle, E. Visual assessment of human skin irritation: a sensitive and reproducible tool. *Contact Dermatitis* 37, 218(1997).
27. Frosch, P. J., Kligman, A. M. The soap chamber test. *J Am Acad Dermatol* 1, 35(1979).
28. Tupker, R. A., Willis, C., Berardesca, E., Lee, C. H., Fartasch, M., Agner, T., Serup, T. Guidelines on sodium lauryl sulfate (SLS) exposure tests. *Contact Dermatitis* 37, 53(1997).
29. van der Valk, P. G. M., Nater, J. P., Bleumink, E. Skin irritancy of surfactants as assessed by water vapour loss measurements. *J Invest Dermatol* 82, 291(1984).
30. Agner, T., Serup, J. Sodium lauryl sulfate for irritant patch testing — a dose–response study using bioengineering methods for determination of skin irritation. *J Invest Dermatol* 95, 543(1990).
31. Pinnagoda, J., Tupker, R. A., Agner, T., Serup, J. Guidelines for transepidermal water loss (TEWL) measurements. A report from the standardization group of the European society of contact dermatitis. *Contact Dermatitis* 22, 164(1990).
32. Tagami, H. Measurements of electrical conductance and impedance. In *Handbook of Non-Invasive Methods and the Skin.* Edited by Serup J. and Jemec G. B. E. CRC Press, Boca Raton, FL. (1995) pp 159.
33. Courage, W. Hardware and measuring principle: corneometer. In *Bioengineering of the Skin: Water and the Stratum Corneum.* Edited by Elsner P., Berardesca E. and Maibach H. CRC Press, Boca Raton, FL. (1994) pp 171.
34. Wilhelm, K. P., Freitag, G., Wolff, H. H. Surfactant-induced skin irritation and skin repair. *J Am Acad Dermatol* 30, 944(1994).
35. Lodén, M. Barrier recovery and influence of irritant stimuli in skin treated with a moisturizing cream. *Contact Dermatitis* 36, 256(1997).
36. Bircher, A., de Boer, E. M., Agner, T., Wahlberg, J. E., Serup, J. Guidelines for measurements of cutaneous blood flow by laser doppler flowmetry. A report from the standardization group of the European Society of Contact Dermatitis. *Contact Dermatitis* 30, 65(1994).
37. Westerhof, W. CIE Colorimetry. In *Handbook of Non-Invasive Methods and the Skin.* Edited by Serup J. and Jemec G. B. E. CRC Press, Boca Raton, FL. (1995) pp 385.
38. Serup, J., Jemec, G. B. E. *Handbook of Non-Invasive Methods and the Skin.* CRC Press, Boca Raton, FL. (1995).
39. Elsner, P., Berardesca, E., Maibach, H. I. *Bioengineering of the Skin: Water and the Stratum Corneum.* CRC Press, Boca Raton, FL. (1994).
40. Bárány, E., Lindberg, M., Lodén, M. *Int J Pharm* In press.
41. Kligman, A. M. The myth of lanolin allergy. *Contact Dermatitis* 39, 103(1998).
42. Cosmetic Ingredient Review, CIR. Final report on the safety assessment of propylene glycol and polypropylene glycols (PPG-9, -12, -15, -17, -20, -26, -30, -34). *J Am Coll Toxicol* 13 (1994).
43. Tanojo, H., Boelsma, E., Junginger, H. E., Ponec, M., Bodde, H. E. *In vivo* human skin permeability enhancement by oleic adic: a laser Doppler velocimetry study. *J. Controlled Release* 58, 97(1999).
44. Frosch, P. J., Kligman, A. M. A method for appraising the stinging capacity of topically applied substances. *J Soc Cosmet Chem* 28, 197(1977).
45. Toro, J. R., Engasser, P. G., Maibach, H. I. Cosmetic reactions. In *Dermatotoxicology* (5th Ed). Edited by Marzulli F. N. and Maibach H. I. Taylor & Francis, Washington. (1996) pp 607.
46. Basketter, D., Gilpin, G., Kuhn, M., Lawrence, D., Reynolds, F., Whittle, E. Patch test vs. use test in skin irritation risk assessment. *Contact Dermatitis* 39, 252(1998).

32 Non-Invasive Methods for Testing the Stratum Corneum Barrier

Ludger Kolbe

CONTENTS

32.1 INTRODUCTION

Moisturizers are marketed as products that combat the signs of dry skin by delivering moisture to the skin. They are appreciated by the consumer for making the skin smooth and pliable. Since the discovery of Blank,[1] that water had a plasticizing effect on the stratum corneum, the main goal of formulators was to develop moisturizers that deliver more moisture. However, enhancement of hydration, softness, and smoothness are short-lived effects, lasting only for hours. Therefore, moisturizers need to be reapplied frequently. In short-term, *in vivo* studies the improvement of skin mechanics or plasticity[2] and hydration parameters[3] have been analyzed following a single application of a moisturizer.

The traditional view of moisturizers is that they increase the moisture content of the skin by forming an occlusive, hydrophobic film on the surface of the stratum corneum, thereby trapping moisture in the underlying tissue. However, restoration of barrier function after disruption can be accelerated by the application of lipids such as free fatty acids, cholesterol, and nonphysiological lipids like the complex hydrocarbon mixture petrolatum.[4] Barrier repair can be measured within an hour after barrier disruption and leads to normalization of barrier function within hours to days, depending on the initial insult.

0-8493-7520-7/00/$0.00+$.50

TABLE 1
Selection of Tests for the Investigation of Skin Barrier Function

	Ref.
Tests involving chemical probes	
Ammonium hydroxide blister test	29
Chloroform:methanol burning test	29
Dimethyl sulfoxide (DMSO) test	20
Erythema after sodium lauryl sulfate provocation assay	25
Lactic acid sting test	29
Nicotinate test	29
Repetitive irritation test	16
Sodium hydroxide erosion assay	10
Bioengineering methods to measure skin responses to chemical probes	
Chromametry	29
Evaporimetry	29
Hydration measurements with various electrical devices	29
Laser Doppler imaging	29

Consumers use moisturizers frequently, especially women who use them often on a twice daily basis for years or even decades. Therefore, it is appropriate to ask for the consequences of this life-long treatment on the barrier function of the skin. Fortunately, we do not see adverse reactions after long-term use of moisturizers. Individuals identifying themselves as having sensitive skin will change their cosmetics as soon as they perceive itching, tingling, or other adverse effects. However, there are positive consequences of moisturizers on barrier properties which are evident only after long-term use, i.e., twice daily applications for several weeks. Such an improvement of barrier function occurs even in normal skin,[5] but skin conditions with impaired barrier function, such as winter xerosis, represent an excellent model for studying barrier improvement by moisturizers. Moisturizers are well known for relieving the symptoms of dry, scaly, and itchy skin. The efficacy of moisturizers for the treatment of dry skin of the lower leg is usually assessed by the regression method,[6] estimating the time course for reduction of scaliness and reappearance after treatment. However, this method gives little information on barrier properties.

Experience has taught us that products that are equivalent in removing scales may have different effects on the integrity of the horny layer.

The stratum corneum is not only a barrier preventing excessive diffusional water loss, it is also a mechanical and permeability barrier reducing the absorption of substances from the environment. All these barrier properties can be tested in order to gain a complete picture of the state of the horny layer.

32.2 TECHNIQUES

Over the years a panel of methods has been published for testing different properties of the stratum corneum barrier (Table 1). The combination of tests employing the application of chemical probes to the skin and the measurement of skin responses with new bioengineering read-out systems allows the measurement of changes in barrier properties with high sensitivity and reliability. A subjective selection of skin barrier tests will be discussed further in this chapter.

32.2.1 Transepidermal Water Loss

Measurement of the transepidermal water loss (TEWL) is the standard method to determine stratum corneum barrier status. A disturbed skin barrier is characterized by high TEWL.[7] TEWL measurement has been a valuable tool in barrier repair experiments where repair kinetics were followed by TEWL. However, there are some problems with this method when the efficacy of moisturizers is to be evaluated. Some ingredients of moisturizers like petrolatum are shown to be occlusive.[8] Therefore, TEWL readings might reflect the occlusive effect of the cream, rather than an improved, less permeable stratum corneum. Measurements performed shortly after application of the moisturizer may represent surface water loss of residual emulsion water instead of TEWL. The TEWL measurements must be performed in an environmental chamber with constant temperature and humidity after an appropriate rest period in order to minimize the contribution of sweat gland activity.[9]

32.2.2 Sodium Hydroxide Erosion Assay

This assay is a recently published modification of the alkali resistance test.[10] Sodium hydroxide (NaOH) is strongly keratolytic and rapidly introduces structural defects in the horny layer. Burckhardt introduced the alkali resistance test in 1947.[11] His goal was to develop a procedure that would enable the identification of individuals at increased risk of chemical injury to skin. In some European centers the alkali resistance test subsequently became an accepted screening procedure, in the U.S. the test never caught on. Researchers after Burckhardt largely found the alkali resistance test to be unreliable and unreproducible.[12,13] Attempts to improve the method failed,[14] and therefore the alkali resistance test fell into disuse. However, NaOH has been used as an irritant in other tests.[15,16]

Burckhardt's original test involved application of a drop of 0.5 N sodium hydroxide under each of three glass blocks for periods of ten min. The end point was the time required for ten small vesicles and erosions to develop.

In an attempt to strengthen the reliability and sensitivity of Burckhardt's method the procedure was changed substantially and became the erosion assay: 15 μl of 1.0 *M* sodium hydroxide was applied to the test site and covered immediately by a circular plastic disc 1.3 cm in diameter to achieve uniform distribution. After 1 min the solution was wiped off with a facial tissue; the test site was then gently rubbed with a cotton swab soaked in a solution of the pH-indicator nitrazine yellow. Erosions stain deeply blue due to the higher pH of the living epidermis. If no erosions developed after the first minute, fresh solution was reapplied in a series of 1-min intervals. Precautions have been introduced in order to avoid severe alkali necrosis, a occasional adverse effect of the original alkali resistance test, by recommending a less ambiguous end point for the NaOH erosion assay. The appearance of the first erosion(s) was found to be both safer and more reliable than counting multiple erosions as Burckhardt did. The time in minutes required for the development of the first erosion is recorded as erosion time. The usual size of an erosion is about 0.5 mm. Exposed sites were allowed to heal spontaneously without treatment or bandaging.

32.2.3 Dimethyl Sulfoxide (DMSO) Whealing Test

The use of dimethyl sulfoxide (DMSO) in dermatology has a long history.[17,18] In concentrations up to 50%, DMSO is used for topical treatment of amyloidosis,[19] but in concentrations of 90% and higher it is known to induce whealing and a flare reaction. The procedure described here is a modification of that described by Frosch et al.[20] for the identification of individuals with sensitive skin. The DMSO reaction can be assessed clinically or measured with the laser Doppler flowmeter.[21] The recent development of laser Doppler imagers[28] makes it possible to measure the DMSO-induced increase in blood flow with unparalleled accuracy. To elicit the reaction, 15 μl of 90, 95, and 100% DMSO was applied to three adjacent sites and immediately covered with a circular plastic disk,1.3 cm in diameter, spreading the solution evenly over the skin. The disks were removed after 15 min, and the surface was wiped with tissue paper. Five minutes later (approximately the peak response), readings were made clinically according to the following scale: 0 = no reaction; 1 = discrete, follicular wheals; 2 = flat wheals, with partial convergence; 3 = confluent solid wheal.

The DMSO-induced increased blood flow was measured using the moorLDI laser Doppler imager (Moor Instruments Ltd., Devon, U.K.). The instrument scans a low power laser beam in a raster pattern over the skin. Moving blood in the microvasculature causes a Doppler shift, which is processed to build up a color-coded image of cutaneous blood flow. The mean and standard deviation of the blood perfusion units in a region of interest was calculated.

32.2.4 Sodium Lauryl Sulfate (SLS) Irritation

Sodium lauryl sulfate (SLS) is frequently used to induce experimental irritant dermatitis. The reaction is characterized by erythema, increased TWL, and scaliness. Susceptibility to SLS irritation can be used as an assay for the prevention of irritant reaction by moisturizers.[22-24]

A vast number of different protocols for the induction of SLS irritancy can be found in the literature.[25] Concentrations spanning several orders of magnitude have been used for single or multiple applications with exposure times ranging from minutes to days. In order to show the efficacy of moisturizers to prevent SLS irritation low concentrations should be used. With higher concentrations the individual differences between subjects tend to increase. The prevention of irritant dermatitis from a strong insult with high concentrations of SLS is probably beyond the capacity of bland moisturizers and more the domain of barrier creams.

32.3 DATA

32.3.1 Xerotic Leg Skin

32.3.1.1 Erosion Assay

On normal skin NaOH erosions first develop at hair follicles and orifices of sweat gland ducts, usually after 4 to 5 min. They are small and circular in appearance. However, erosions on xerotic leg skin look different; they often develop along cracks in the stratum corneum, revealing the weak spots of xerotic skin. Erosion times are significantly reduced, and on severely dry skin erosions develop within the first minute.

In a small test group of only five subjects, erosion times of the dry skin of the calves were determined before and after 4 weeks of treatment with either Nivea Creme® (Beiersdorf AG, Hamburg, Germany) or a 12% lactic acid lotion (Figure 1). The assay was performed on four adjacent spots per leg. Spot-to-spot variation was on average less than 1 min. In the majority of subjects erosions formed within 2 min. Erosion times on Nivea-treated legs were strongly increased, whereas the opposite legs, treated with the lactic acid lotion, showed only slight improvement. This is not unexpected since alpha-hydroxy acids are known for their keratolytic activity which will weaken the horny layer. The improvement by moisturizers is probably not due to a protective moisturizer film in the outer layers of the stratum corneum, since there was no significant increase of erosion times after only a few applications. Erosion times gradually increase over the treatment period.

32.3.1.2 Dimethyl Sulfoxide Reaction

DMSO readily penetrates the stratum corneum of dry leg skin and induces an inflammatory response, characterized by a strong whealing reaction and increased cutaneous blood flow. Determination of blood perfusion units with a laser Doppler imager showed a dose-dependent response (Figure 2). However, after 6 weeks of treatment with Eucerin® cream (Beiersdorf AG, Hamburg, Germany) the reaction was markedly reduced, only 1 out of 14 subjects responded slightly to 90% DMSO. Laser Doppler imaging is a reliable and sensitive method, and the obtained images can be stored in the computer for further investigation (Figure 3). Nevertheless, a trained examiner will also get good results with clinical grading.

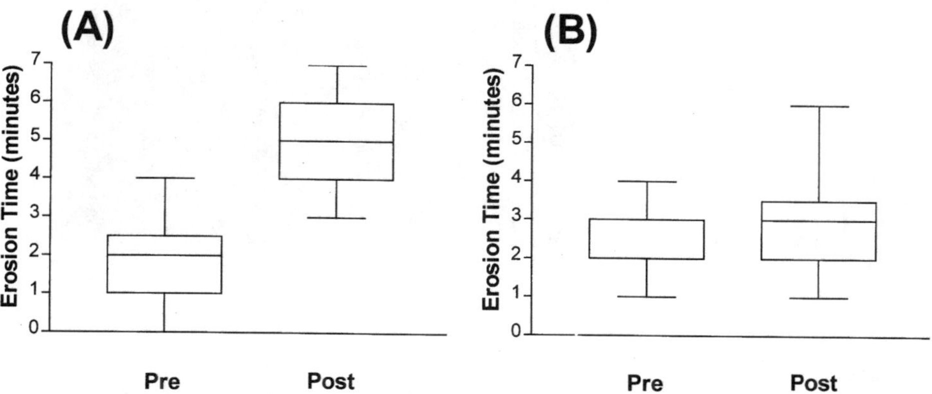

FIGURE 1 Effect of moisturizer treatment on NaOH erosion time of xerotic leg skin. (A) Marked improvement of alkali resistance after treatment with Nivea Creme for 4 weeks (p <0.0001). (B) Slight but significant improvement after treatment with a lotion containing 12% lactic acid (p <0.01). Erosion assays were performed before and after treatment on four adjacent spots per leg. Data are shown as box plots. Statistical analysis was performed with the paired t-test.

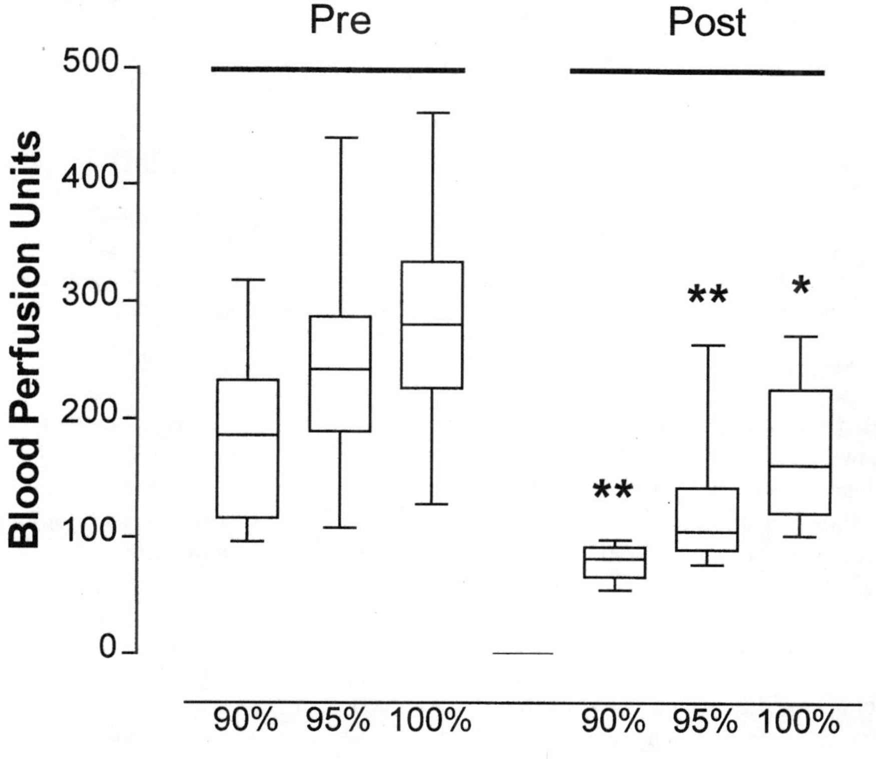

FIGURE 2 DMSO response of xerotic leg skin. (A) Dose-dependent increase of DMSO induced cutaneous blood flow on untreated skin. (B) After twice daily applications of Eucerin cream for 6 weeks, the response was markedly reduced. DMSO-induced blood flow was measured with a laser Doppler imager. Data are expressed as blood perfusion units. Statistical significance was determined using the paired t-test (* p >0.05, ** p <0.01).

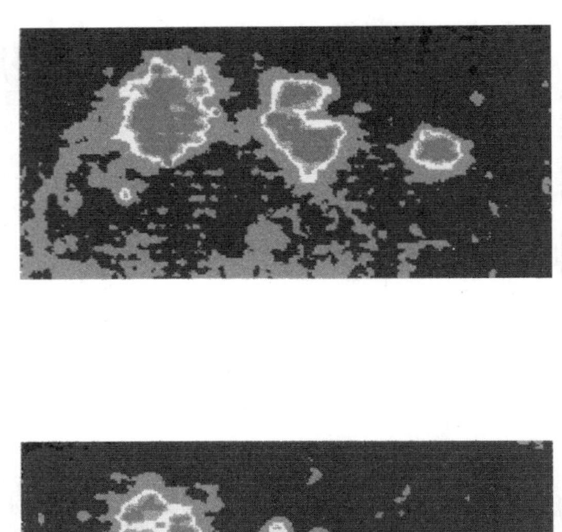

FIGURE 3 The laser Doppler imager generates a pseudo-colored image of blood flow. In this gray scale image the various shades of gray represent regions with increased blood flow. The dark background represents the baseline blood flow. At baseline DMSO evoked a dose-dependent increase in cutaneous blood flow. After six weeks of treatment with Eucerin cream the DMSO response was markedly reduced.

32.3.2 Normal Volar Forearm Skin

At first glance it might seem a bizarre idea to improve a normal skin barrier. Can there be a better barrier than the normal barrier? However, we know there is considerable individual variation. Marie Lodén[5] demonstrated that indeed some moisturizers improve barrier properties of normal skin. Sensitive skin is a multidimensional phenomenon, but at least in part a weak stratum corneum barrier contributes to the problem.[26,27] Moisturizers formulated for individuals with sensitive skin accordingly should be aimed at improving the barrier function.

32.3.2.1 Sodium Lauryl Sulfate Irritation

Susceptibility to SLS irritancy was analyzed before and after treatment with Nivea Creme for 4 weeks. Patches with SLS ranging from 0.025 to 0.1% were applied to the volar forearm of nine subjects for 24 h. At 48 h SLS-induced erythema was measured with the Minolta Chromameter and the laser Doppler imager from Moor Instruments (Figure 4). The laser Doppler imager revealed a significantly lower vascular response to SLS at all concentrations after treatment. There was also a decrease of background blood flow, measured at adjacent unchallenged skin. This probably reflects a subclinical response of the supplying and draining blood vessels in larger areas surrounding the exposure sites, which was also reduced by the moisturizer. No significant differences were found with the Chromameter.

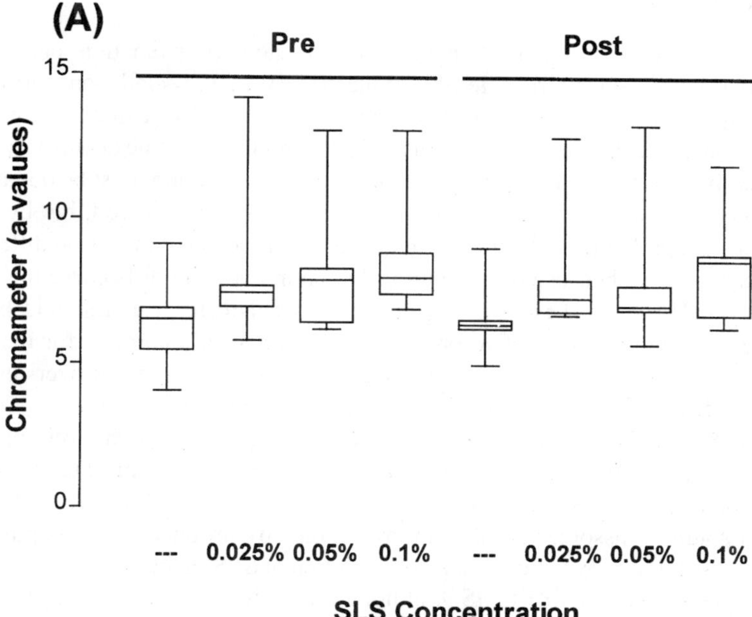

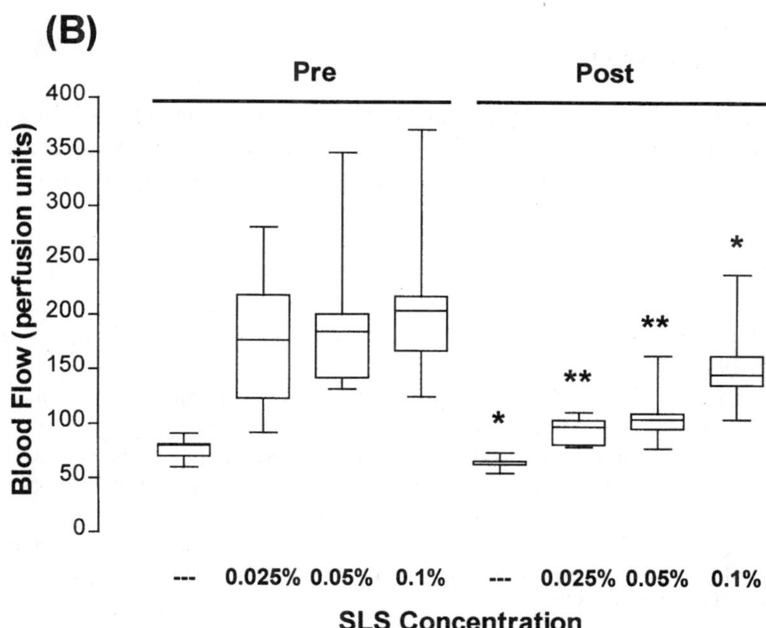

FIGURE 4 SLS irritation and moisturizer treatment. (A) No significant differences in skin color (a-values) were detectable with the Minolta Chromameter. (B) The same sites scanned with the laser Doppler imager showed marked reduction of erythema. Volar forearms were treated with Nivea Creme twice daily for 4 weeks. Statistical significance was determined using the paired t-test ($_{*}\ p > 0.05$, $_{**}\ p < 0.01$).

32.3.2.2 TEWL, Erosion Assay, and Dimethyl Sulfoxide Reaction

In this study no significant reduction of TEWL was detected, but DMSO test and erosion assay demonstrated a significant improvement of barrier function (data not shown).

32.4 CONCLUSION

TEWL measurement is an indispensable method to evaluate barrier function, but improvement of barrier properties is not always reflected by reduced TEWL. Especially on normal skin where TEWL is already low the slight additional reduction after moisturizer treatment might not reach statistical significance. Furthermore, reduction of TEWL might reflect the occlusivity of the product rather than a less permeable horny layer. Hence, additional information must be obtained with other methods. Product occlusivity might interfere with other techniques as well, but by using a set of different methods the problem can be minimized. One can argue that it makes no difference whether a moisturizer is protective because of an improved stratum corneum or because the product forms an occlusive layer. However, these are two different mechanisms which should be investigated separately. The evaluation of protective product layers is a valid approach for the evaluation of barrier creams in short-term studies,[28,29] but in long-term studies with moisturizers improvement of the structural integrity of the horny layer itself should be evaluated.

DMSO, NaOH, and SLS are useful chemical probes because of the different properties of the substances and the different mechanisms by which they induce irritation. Due to its amphiphilic nature DMSO rapidly penetrates the stratum corneum and induces whealing and erythema. The aqueous NaOH solution dissolves the keratin layers, thereby introducing structural defects in the horny layer. The mechanism by which an aqueous solution of SLS induces irritation is still unknown, but SLS penetrates the barrier like DMSO, although at a much slower rate. Tests with these and other chemical probes, when combined, provide valuable information on the barrier properties of the stratum corneum.

32.5 ACKNOWLEDGMENT

I am grateful to Dr. Albert Kligman for all the fruitful discussions on moisturizers and barrier enhancement and his helpful advice. I also thank Tracy Stoudemayer, Managing Director of S.K.I.N. Inc., Conshohocken, PA, where most of the work described in this chapter was done.

REFERENCES

1. Blank, I. H., Factors which influence the water content of the stratum corneum, *J Invest Dermatol*, 18, 433, 1952.
2. Jemec, G. B. E. and Wulf, H. C., The plasticizing effect of moisturisers on human skin *in vivo*: a measure of moisturising potency?, *Skin Res Technol*, 4, 88, 1998.
3. Blichmann, C. W., Serup, J., and Winther, A., Effect of single application of a moisturizer: evaporation of emulsion water, skin surface temperature, electrical conductance, electrical capacitance, and skin surface (emulsion) lipids, *Acta Derm Venereol*, 69, 327, 1989.
4. Man, M.-Q., Brown, B. E., Wu-Pong, S., Feingold, K. R., and Elias, P. M., Exogenous nonphysiologic vs. physiologic lipids: divergent mechanisms for correction of permeability barrier dysfunction, *Arch Dermatol*, 131, 809, 1995.
5. Lodén, M., Urea-containing moisturizers influence barrier properties of normal skin, *Arch Dermatol Res*, 288, 103, 1996.
6. Kligman, A. M., Regression method for assessing the efficacy of moisturizers, *Cosm Toil*, 93, 27, 1978.
7. Shahidullah, M., Raffle, E. J., Rimmer, A. R., and Frain-Bell, W., Transepidermal water loss in patients with dermatitis, *Br J Dermatol*, 81, 722, 1969.
8. Rietschel, R. L., A method to evaluate skin moisturizers *in vivo*, *J Invest Dermatol*, 70, 152, 1978.
9. Pinnagoda, J., Tupker, R. A., Agner, T., and Serup, J., Guidelines for transepidermal water loss (TEWL) measurement, *Contact Dermatitis*, 22, 164, 1990.
10. Kolbe, L., Kligman, A. M., and Stoudemayer, T., The sodium hydroxide erosion assay: a revision of the alkali resistance test, *Arch Dermatol Res*, 290, 382, 1998.

11. Burckhardt, W., Neuere Untersuchungen über die Alkaliempfindlichkeit der Haut, *Dermatologica*, 94, 73, 1947.
12. Björnberg, A., Low alkali resistance and slow alkali neutralization of the eczematous subject, *Dematologica*, 149, 90, 1974.
13. Schnyder, U.W., Gloor, M., and Taugner, M., Über die sozialmedizinische Bedeutung von Alkaliresistenz, Alkalineutralisation und Hautoberflächenlipide bei Neurodermitis atopica und Ichtyosis vulgaris, *Berufsdermatosen*, 25, 101, 1977.
14. Ummenhofer, B., Zur Methodik der Alkaliresistenzprüfung, *Dermatosen*, 28, 104, 1980.
15. Wilhelm, K. P., Pasche, F., Surber, C., and Maibach, H. I., Sodium hydroxide- duced subclinical irritation, *Acta Derm Venereol*, 70, 463, 1990.
16. Frosch, P. J. and Kurte, A., Efficacy of skin barrier creams (IV). The repetitive irritation test (RIT) with a set of 4 standard irritants, *Contact Dermatitis*, 31, 161, 1994.
17. Kligman, A. M., Topical pharmacology and toxicology of dimethyl sulphoxide. Part 1, *JAMA*, 193, 796, 1965.
18. Kligman, A. M., Topical pharmacology and toxicology of dimethyl sulphoxide. Part 2, *JAMA*, 193, 923, 1965.
19. Özkaya-Bayazit, E., Baykal, C., and Kavak, A., Lokale DMSO-Behandlung der makulösen und papulösen Amyloidose, *Hautarzt*, 48, 31, 1997.
20. Frosch, P. J., Duncan, S., and Kligman, A. M., Cutaneous biometrics. I. The response of human skin to dimethyl sulphoxide, *Br J Dermatol*, 102, 263, 1980.
21. Agner, T. and Serup, J., Quantification of the DMSO-response: a test for assessment of sensitive skin, *Clin Exp Dermatol*, 14, 214, 1989.
22. Lodén, M. and Andersson, A.-C., Effect of topically applied lipids on surfactant-irritated skin, *Br J Dermatol*, 134, 215, 1996.
23. Ramsing, D. W. and Agner, T., Preventive and therapeutic effects of a moisturizer, *Acta Derm Venereol (Stockh.)*, 77, 335, 1997.
24. Lodén, M., Barrier recovery and influence of irritant stimuli in skin treated with a moisturizing cream, *Contact Dermatitis*, 36, 256, 1997.
25. Tupker, R. A., Willis, C., Berardesca, E., Lee, C. H., Fartasch, M., Agner, T., and Serup, J., Guidelines on sodium lauryl sulfate (SLS) exposure tests. A report from the Standardization Group of the European Society of Contact Dermatitis. *Contact Dermatitis*, 37, 53, 1997.
26. Draelos, Z. D., Sensitive skin: perception, evaluation, and treatment, *Am J Contact Dermatitis*, 8, 67, 1997.
27. Morizot, F., Le Fur, I., and Tschachler, E., Sensitive skin, definitions, prevalence and possible causes, *Cosm Toil*, 113, 59, 1998.
28. Wigger-Alberti, W. and Elsner, P., Petrolatum prevents irritation in a human cumulative exposure model *in vivo*, *Dermatology*, 194, 247, 1997.
29. Frosch, P. J., Kurte, A., and Pilz, B., Efficacy of skin barrier creams (III). The repetitive irritation test (RIT) in humans, *Contact Dermatitis*, 29, 113, 1993.

33 Sensitizing Substances

Anton C. de Groot

CONTENTS

33.1 SIDE EFFECTS OF SKIN CARE PRODUCTS

Skin care products (moisturizing and cleansing creams, lotions, tonics, etc.) sometimes cause adverse effects in consumers. Such unwanted effects include irritation (subjective [i.e., sensory] and objective), allergic contact dermatitis, photocontact dermatitis, and immediate contact reactions.[1,2] The side effect most frequently seen by dermatologists is allergic contact dermatitis. Usually, such reactions are caused by the fragrances and preservatives present in the products used. Less often, moisturizers such as lanolin and derivatives, humectants such as propylene glycol, emulsifiers such as cocamidopropyl betaine, emollients, and UV filters are the culprit.

In this chapter, these allergens and their role in allergic contact dermatitis from skin care products are discussed. For a full review of side effects of cosmetics, see Reference 1. Other valuable sources of information include References 2 and 3.

33.2 EPIDEMIOLOGY OF CONTACT ALLERGY

There are no studies that have specifically investigated contact allergy to skin care products. However, in investigations on cosmetic allergy (all products), skin care products are always an important category and usually are the most frequent causative products with 30 to 50% of the total number of reactions.[1] In the general population, 2 to 3% are allergic to substances that may be present in skin care products and other cosmetics.[4,5] Of patients seen by dermatologists with eczema and tested for suspected allergic contact dermatitis, some 10% are allergic to cosmetic products.[1-4]

0-8493-7520-7/00/$0.00+$.50

33.3 THE ALLERGENS

33.3.1 Fragrances

Fragrances are not only used in cosmetics specifically designed for their smell (perfumes, after-shaves, deodorants, etc.); virtually all cosmetics and toiletries are scented. In addition, many other products including household products, occupational products, paper and paper products, and topical drugs contain fragrances. As a consequence, virtually everybody is in daily contact with fragrance materials.[6,7] In the general population, 1% is allergic to fragrances;[5] in eczema patients seen by dermatologists, the prevalence is between 6 to 14%.[6,8] Fragrances are the most frequent sensitizers in cosmetic products including skin care products. Over 100 fragrance materials have been identified as allergens.[6] Most reactions are caused by the eight fragrances in the perfume mix, which is used by dermatologists to detect fragrance sensitivity: α-amylcinnamic aldehyde, cinnamic alcohol, cinnamal (cinnamic aldehyde), eugenol, geraniol, hydroxycitronellal, isoeugenol, and oak moss absolute. Of these, oak moss, isoeugenol, and cinnamal are the main sensitisers. Most of these fragrance-sensitive patients are aware that the use of scented products may cause skin problems.[9] Indeed, one or more of the ingredients of the mix are present in nearly all deodorants, popular prestige perfumes, natural ingredient based cosmetics, and perfumes used in the formulation of other cosmetics such as skin care products.[8] Other fragrances which sensitize more than occasionally include benzyl salicylate, citral, coumarin,[10] dihydrocoumarin, hydroabietyl alcohol, jasmine absolute/synthetic, lilial, methyl salicylate, narcissus absolute, sandalwood oil, spearmint oil, and ylang-ylang oil.[6,11,12] For a full review of side effects to fragrances, see Reference 6. A recent book on beneficial and adverse reactions to fragrances also provides valuable information.[7] Other relevant reviews include References 12 and 13.

33.3.2 Preservatives

Preservatives are chemicals added to food, cosmetics, topical drugs, and industrial products with an aqueous compartment to inhibit the growth of pathogenic and non-pathogenic microorganisms, which may cause degradation of the product or endanger the health of the consumers. After fragrances, preservatives are the most common sensitizers in skin care products. Various review articles on the subject of preservative allergy have been published.[14-19] The main allergens are methyl(chloro)isothiazolinone (Kathon® CG), methyldibromo glutaronitrile (in the preservative system Euxyl® K 400), and the formaldehyde donors. The parabens have, incorrectly, a bad reputation of being notorious sensitizers.

- *Methylisothiazolinone + methylchloroisothiazolinone* (Kathon CG) until recently was a major cause of cosmetic allergy in most European countries[17] and the U.S.[20] Currently, the preservative system is mainly used in rinse-off products at low concentrations, which infrequently leads to induction or elicitation of contact allergy.[21] As a consequence, prevalence rates in Europe are decreasing.
- *Methyldibromo glutaronitrile* (synonym: 1,2-dibromo-2,4-dicyanobutane) is the allergen in the preservative system Euxyl® K 400, which also contains (the non-sensitizing) phenoxyethanol. It was thought to be a suitable alternative to methyl(chloro)isothiazolinone, but unfortunately Euxyl K 400 soon proved to be a frequent cause of contact allergy to cosmetics in Europe[18,19] and the U.S.[22] and, in the Netherlands, to moistened toilet tissues. It is currently the most important cosmetic preservative allergen.
- *Formaldehyde donors* are preservatives that, in the presence of water, release formaldehyde. These include quaternium-15; imidazolidinyl urea; diazolidinyl urea, 2-bromo-2-nitropropane-1,3-diol; and DMDM hydantoin. Contact allergy to formaldehyde donors may be due either to the preservative itself or to formaldehyde sensitivity.[14,15] Quaternium-15 and

diazolidinyl urea allergy are important in the U.S.,[20] and less so in Europe. Imidazolidinyl urea and 2-bromo-2-nitropropane-1,3-diol sensitize occasionally.
- The *paraben esters* (methyl, ethyl, propyl, butyl) are the most widely used preservatives in cosmetic products. With many dermatologists, the parabens have a bad reputation as notorious sensitizers. However, most cases of paraben sensitivity are caused by topical drugs applied to leg ulcers or used on eczematous skin. At the usual concentration of 0.1 to 0.3% in cosmetics, parabens rarely cause adverse reactions. Moreover, sensitized individuals may be able to tolerate products containing it, a phenomenon which has been called the paraben paradox.[16,23]

In Table 1, preservatives that have caused cosmetic allergy are tabulated. Their risk of causing contact allergy is rated as "low," "intermediate," or "high." It should be appreciated that this is a very superficial, personal, and tentative assessment. The sensitizing *potential* of various allergens can only be calculated or reliably estimated when quantitative exposure data are known; for the cosmetic preservatives, these are largely lacking. The assessment pertains to their use in products intended to stay on the skin. Rinse-off products very infrequently cause cosmetic dermatitis because of the immediate dilution of potential allergens under use conditions and the short skin contact time. Even strong allergens such as formaldehyde, methyl(chloro)isothiazolinone, and methyldibromo glutaronitrile will rarely cause problems in such products. Preservatives not mentioned in the table are, from an allergological point of view, safe for use in cosmetic products.

33.3.3 Emulsifiers, Surfactants, Emollients, and Humectants

After fragrances and preservatives, the (heterogeneous) group of emulsifiers, surfactants, emollients, and humectants are the third most common cause of cosmetic allergy. In a U.S. study, they constituted 9.2% of allergens identified in 403 patients with proven cosmetic allergy.[24] In a Dutch study in 119 patients suffering from cosmetic-related allergic contact dermatitis, emulsifiers and other base ingredients were the cause in 20%.[25] Most recently, a European study performed in Belgium, the U.K., and Germany identified 475 patients with contact allergy to cosmetic ingredients.[26] In cleansers and skin care products, the three most important causative classes again were fragrances (39%), preservatives (36%), and excipients/emulsifiers (25%).[26] Thus, the latter category certainly is an important source of cosmetic allergens. However, it should be appreciated that, although the list of individual allergens identified is long (Table 2), the majority of reactions are caused by a limited number of emulsifiers: lanolin and its derivatives,[24-26] (formerly) oleamidopropyl dimethylamine,[27] and (currently) cocamidopropyl betaine. All other substances belonging to this group of ingredients sensitize only very occasionally, rarely, or not at all. The risk of sensitization to such ingredients is increased when products containing them are applied to leg ulcers and stasis dermatitis.[28]

33.3.3.1 Lanolin and Lanolin Derivatives

Lanolin and lanolin derivatives are used extensively in cosmetic products as emollients and emulsifiers. Some dermatologists consider the lanolins to be a frequent cause of contact allergy. This is because their (putative, but unproven) allergenic constituents, the wool alcohols, are routinely tested in all patients suspected of allergic contact dermatitis and react positively in up to 3.3% of these patients.[29] However, most cases of allergy are not from the use of cosmetic products, but from the use of topical preparations applied to stasis dermatitis and leg ulcers.[28] In addition, it should be realized that many "positive" patch test reactions (which usually are the basis for the diagnosis of "contact allergy") to wool alcohols[30] and to cetylstearyl alcohol[31] are not reproducible. This may indicate that the currently used test allergens (30% wool alcohols and 20% cetylstearyl alcohol) and possibly also the lanolin derivative Amerchol® L-101 (suggested as an alternative for testing[32])

TABLE 1
Allergenic Cosmetic Preservatives: Risk of Sensitization

Preservative	Risk of Sensitization
Formaldehyde donors	
2-Bromo-2-nitropropane-1,3-diol	Intermediate
Diazolidinyl urea (Germall® II)	High
DMDM hydantoin	Low
Formaldehyde	High
Imidazolidinyl urea (Germall 115)	Intermediate
Quaternium-15 (Dowicil® 200)	High
Isothiazolinones	
Methylisothiazolinone + Methyl(chloro)isothiazolinone (Kathon® CG)	High
Parabens (butyl, ethyl, methyl, propyl paraben)	Low
Phenolics	
4-Chloro-*m*-cresol	Low
Chloroxylenol	Low
Miscellaneous preservatives	
Benzalkonium chloride	Intermediate
Benzethonium chloride	Low
Benzoxonium chloride	Low
Benzyl alcohol	Low
Cetalkonium chloride	Low
Chlorhexidine digluconate	Intermediate
Chloroacetamide	Intermediate
Dichlorophene	Low
Fenticlor	Low
Glutaraldehyde	Intermediate
Hexachlorophene	Low
Mercurials	Intermediate-high
Methyldibromo glutaronitrile (in Euxyl® K 400)	High
Phenoxyethanol	Low
Phenylmercuric acetate	Intermediate
Sodium benzoate	Low
Sorbic acid	Low-intermediate
Thimerosal (merthiolate)	High
Trichlorocarbanilide (triclocarban, TCC)	Low
Triclosan	Low

cause many cases of irritant, false-positive reactions.[30,33] This, in turn, suggests that many patients labelled as "lanolin-allergic" in fact are not! Evidently, patients who are indeed allergic to lanolin (derivatives) may suffer from cosmetic allergy when using products containing these substances. However, the risk of becoming sensitized *from the use of cosmetics* appears to be small,[34] and the prevalence of lanolin allergy in the general population is considered to be very small.[30,33]

33.3.3.2 Propylene Glycol[35-37]

Propylene glycol is widely used in dermatological and non-dermatological topical formulations, including cosmetics, as well as in numerous oral and parenteral medications, hygiene products, and food products. It was reported to be a common cause of cosmetic dermatitis in the U.S.[24] However, in this and earlier studies, high concentrations of propylene glycol used for patch testing (the basis for the diagnosis of "contact allergy") may have induced many cases of false-positive,

TABLE 2
Emulsifiers, Surfactants, Emollients, and Humectants that Have Caused Contact Allergy[1,3]

	Ref.		Ref.
Avocado oil			
Butylene glycol		Methyl glucose sesquistearate	26
Castor oil derivatives	26	Miranol MSA®	
Cetylpyridinium chloride		Myristyl alcohol	48
Cocamide DEA	26	Octyl dodecanol	
Coco-betaine		Oleamide DEA	
Colophony (rosin)	26	Oleth-5	
Cyclomethicone		Oleth-3 phosphate	
DEA-dihydroxypalmityl phosphate		Oleyl alcohol	48
Decyl oleate		Olive oil	
Diethyl sebacate		Paraffinum liquidum	
Diisopropanolamine (DIPA)		PEG-4 dilaurate	
Disodium oleamido sulfosuccinate		PEG-5 lanolate	
Emulgol®		PEG-40 sorbitan lanolate	
Eumulgin®		PEG-32 stearate	
Glycerin		Petrolatum	
Glyceryl diisostearate		Polysorbate 40, 60, 80	49
Glyceryl isostearate		Potassium cocoyl hydrolyzed animal protein	
Glyceryl oleate		PPG-2-ceteareth-9	26
Glyceryl ricinoleate		Ricinoleic acid	
Glyceryl stearate		Sesame oil	
Hydroabietyl alcohol	26	Sodium laureth sulfate	
Hydrogenated castor oil		Sodium lauryl sulfate	
Hydrolyzed animal protein		Sorbitan laurate	26
Isopropyl hydroxypalmityl ether		Sorbitan oleate	26
Isopropyl lanolate	26	Sorbitan sesquioleate	26
Isopropyl myristate		Stearamidoethyl diethylamine	
Isopropyl palmitate		Stearic acid	
Isostearyl alcohol		Stearyl alcohol	48
Jojoba oil		Sulfated castor oil	
Lauramide DEA		TEA-cocoyl hydrolyzed animal protein	
Lauramine oxide		TEA-PEG-3 cocamide sulfate	
Laureth-4	26	TEA-stearate	
Lauryl alcohol	26	Triethanolamine	26
Maleated soybean oil	26	Trilaureth-4 phosphate	
Methyl glucose dioleate		Undecylenamide DEA	

irritant patch test reactions. Consequently, a (significant) number of patients identified as "allergic to propylene glycol" in fact were probably not. Currently, it is generally believed that contact allergy to propylene glycol is uncommon, and the clinical significance has formerly been overestimated. Indeed, in the most recent European study of 475 patients allergic to cosmetics, only 3 reacted to propylene glycol. They all came from one center: in the German and U.K. centers no reactions to propylene glycol were observed at all.[26]

Apart from allergic contact dermatitis, propylene glycol may also cause irritant contact dermatitis, nonimmunological immediate contact reactions (Chapter 35), and subjective (synonym: sensory) irritation. Subjective or sensory irritation, with itching, burning, or stinging sensations, but no signs of inflammation, is a commonly noticed reaction among users of cosmetic products. It is a phenomenon that also occurs in volunteers after application of propylene glycol in different concentrations.[35]

33.3.3.3 Cocamidopropyl Betaine[2,38-40]

Cocamidopropyl betaine is an amphoteric surfactant, which enjoys increasing popularity among cosmetic chemists because of its low potential for irritation of the skin. It is used especially in shampoos and bath products such as bath and shower gels. Most cases of allergy are caused by shampoos. Thus, cocamidopropyl betaine is the exception to the rule that allergic reactions are usually caused by "stay-on" ("leave-on") cosmetic products. However, cocamidopropyl betaine may also be an allergen in other cosmetic products such as skin care products and deodorants and in contact lens fluids.

By its presence in shampoos, cocamidopropyl betaine appears to be an important occupational hazard to hairdressers. Prevalence rates of sensitization range from 3.7 to 5% in these patients and from 1.4 to 3.8% in patients routinely tested for suspected allergic contact dermatitis. Contact allergy to cocamidopropyl betaine is observed especially in patients clinically suspected to suffer from cosmetic-related allergic contact dermatitis and/or dermatitis of the head and neck area.[41]

Depending on its source, cocamidopropyl betaine contains varying amounts of the reactants and intermediates involved in its synthesis. There probably is more than one allergenic component in cocamidopropyl betaine, with dimethylaminopropylamine being the most important one.[42] However, as the amounts of dimethylaminopropylamine found in commercial preparations containing cocamidopropyl betaine are far lower than the concentrations needed to induce contact allergy, this concept may be challenged.[44] Another possible allergenic ingredient is cocamidopropyl dimethylamine.[45]

Thus, cocamidopropyl betaine would appear to be an important cosmetic allergen. Among 475 patients allergic to cosmetic ingredients, 19 (4%) reacted to it.[26] However, cocamidopropyl betaine in the usual and commercially available concentration of 1% in water is a marginal irritant and not all "positive" patch test reactions indicate (relevant) contact allergy to it. As with wool alcohols (lanolin) and propylene glycol, the number of patients actually allergic to cocamidopropyl betaine may be (far) less than the number of positive patch test reactions reported.

33.3.3.4 Oleamidopropyl Dimethylamine

Some ten years ago, the cationic emulsifier oleamidopropyl dimethylamine was responsible for many cases of cosmetic sensitization in the Netherlands by its presence in a baby body lotion.[27] Of 119 patients with proven cosmetic-related allergic contact dermatitis, 13 (11%) were allergic to oleamidopropyl dimethylamine.[25] Especially women who used the product for removing eye makeup became sensitized. They also reacted ("cross-reactions") to a large number of related amide-amine type cationic surfactants, including ricinoleamidopropyl dimethylamine lactate and tallowamidopropyl dimethylamine.[46] After removal of the offending product from the baby body lotion, the clinical problem disappeared.

Later, in Italy, some patients routinely tested with oleamidopropyl dimethylamine had positive reactions, although there are hardly any cosmetic products in Italy containing the surfactant.[47] Many of these patients also reacted to cocamidopropyl betaine, and it was suggested that the allergenic ingredient in oleamidopropyl betaine (and the cross-reacting substances) may, as in cocamidopropyl betaine, have been dimethylaminopropylamine.[47]

33.3.3.5 Miscellaneous Emulsifiers, Surfactants, Emollients, and Humectants

A large number of other emulsifiers, surfactants, emollients, and humectants have been reported as contact allergens. These are summarized in Table 2. Their risk of sensitization can be classsified as "small" or "very small."

33.3.4 MISCELLANEOUS ALLERGENS IN SKIN CARE PRODUCTS

Ultraviolet light filters (UV filters, sunscreens) are used in sunscreens to protect the consumer from harmful UV irradiation from the sun and are increasingly incorporated in some cosmetics, notably facial skin care products, to inhibit UV photodegradation of the product and protect the skin of the user. Not surprisingly, the number of published reports of sunscreen allergy has increased. Both allergic and photoallergic reactions are reported to the main classes of UV-A filters: benzophenones and dibenzoylmethanes. Isopropyl dibenzoylmethane caused so many cases of photocontact allergy that its use was discontinued in 1993. Currently, the main (photo) allergen is benzophenone-3 (oxybenzone). The subject has been reviewed.[50,51]

Antioxidants are added to cosmetics to prevent the deterioration of unsaturated fatty acids and are an occasional cause of cosmetic allergy: BHA (butylated hydroxyanisole), BHT (butylated hydroxytoluene), *t*-butylhydroquinone, di-*t*-butyl-hydroquinone, nordihydroguiaretic acid, gallates (dodecyl, octyl, propyl), and tocopherol (vitamin E).[1-3]

Miscellaneous ingredients of cosmetics which are occasional causes of allergy to cosmetics include colophony (rosin), phenyl salicylate (salol), propolis, and colors. The vitamin E derivative tocopheryl linoleate caused an epidemic of (allergic and irritant) contact dermatitis in Switerland.[52] The depigmenting agent kojic acid is a common allergen in Japan.[53]

REFERENCES

1. De Groot, A. C., Weyland, J. W., Nater, J. P., *Unwanted Effects of Cosmetics and Drugs Used in Dermatology,* Elsevier, Amsterdam, 1994.*
2. De Groot, A. C., Fatal attractiveness: the shady side of cosmetics, *Clinics in Dermatology,* 16, 167, 1998.*
3. De Groot, A. C., White, I. R., Cosmetics and skin care products, in *Textbook of Contact Dermatitis,* 3rd Edition, Rycroft, R., Menné, T., Frosch, P. J., Lepoittevin, J.-P., Eds., Springer-Verlag, Heidelberg, 2000.*
4. De Groot, A. C., Labelling cosmetics with their ingredients, *British Medical Journal,* 300, 1636, 1990.
5. Nielsen, N. H., Menné, T., Allergic contact sensitization in an unselected Danish population, *Acta Dermato-Venereologica,* 72, 456, 1992.
6. De Groot, A. C., Frosch, P. J., Adverse reactions to fragrances. A clinical review, *Contact Dermatitis,* 36, 57, 1997.*
7. De Groot, A. C., Frosch, P. J., Fragrances as a cause of contact dermatitis in cosmetics: clinical aspects and epidemiological data, in *Fragrances. Beneficial and Adverse Effects,* Frosch, P. J., Johansen, J. D., White, I. R., Eds., Springer-Verlag, Berlin, 1998, 66.*
8. Johansen, J. D., Rastogi, S. C., Andersen, K. E., Menné, T., Content and reactivity to product perfumes in fragrance mix positive and negative eczema patients. A study of perfumes used in toiletries and skin-care products, *Contact Dermatitis,* 36, 291, 1997.
9. Johansen, J. D., Andersen, T. F., Veien, N., Avnstorp, C., Andersen, K. E., Menné, T., Patch testing with markers of fragrance contact allergy. Do clinical tests correspond to patients' self-reported problems?, *Acta Dermato-Venereologica,* 77, 149, 1997.
10. Kunkeler, A. C. M., Weijland, J. W., Bruynzeel, D. P., The role of coumarin in patch testing, *Contact Dermatitis,* 39, 327, 1998.
11. Larsen, W., Nakayama, H., Fischer, T., Elsner, P., Frosch, P. J., Burrows, D., Jordan, W., Shaw, S., Wilkinson, J., Marks, J., Jr., Sugawara, M., Nethercott, M., Nethercott, J., A study of new fragrance mixtures, *American Journal of Contact Dermatitis,* 9, 202, 1998.
12. Larsen, W. G., Nethercott, J. R., Fragrances, *Clinics in Dermatology,* 15, 499, 1997.*
13. Scheinman, P. L., Allergic contact dermatitis to fragrances: a review, *American Journal of Contact Dermatitis,* 7, 65, 1996.*
14. Fransway, A. F., The problem of preservation in the 1990s: I. Statement of the problem, solution of the industry, and the current use of formaldehyde and formaldehyde biocides, *American Journal of Contact Dermatitis,* 2, 6, 1991.*

15. Fransway, A. F., Schmitz, N. A., The problem of preservation in the 1990s: II. Formaldehyde and formaldehyde-releasing biocides: incidences of cross-reactivity and the significance of the positive response to formaldehyde, *American Journal of Contact Dermatitis,* 2, 78, 1991.*
16. Fransway, A. F., The problem of preservation in the 1990s: III. Agents with preservative function independent of formaldehyde release, *American Journal of Contact Dermatitis,* 2, 145, 1991.*
17. De Groot, A. C., Methylisothiazolinone/methylchloroisothiazolinone (Kathon CG) allergy: an updated review, *American Journal of Contact Dermatitis,* 1, 151, 1990.*
18. De Groot, A. C., Contact allergens. What's new? Cosmetic dermatitis, *Clinics in Dermatology,* 15, 485, 1997.*
19. De Groot, A. C., van Ginkel, C. J. W., Weyland, J. W., Methyldibromo glutaronitrile (Euxyl K 400): an important "new" allergen in cosmetics, *Journal of the American Academy of Dermatology,* 35, 743, 1996.*
20. Marks, J. G., Jr., Belsito, D. V., DeLeo, V. A., Fowler, J. F., Jr., Fransway, A. F., Maibach, H. I., North American Contact Dermatitis Group patch test results for the detection of delayed-type hypersensitivity to topical allergens, *Journal of the American Academy of Dermatology,* 38, 911, 1998.
21. Frosch, P. J., Hannuksela, M., Andersen, K. E., Wilkinson, J. D., Shaw, S., Lachapelle, J. M., Chloromethylisothiazolinone/methylisothiazolinone (CMI/MI) use test with a shampoo on patch-test-positive subjects, *Contact Dermatitis,* 32, 210, 1995.
22. Jackson, J. M, Fowler, J. F., Methyldibromoglutaronitrile (Euxyl K 400): a new and important sensitiser in the United States? *Journal of the American Academy of Dermatology,* 38, 934, 1998.
23. Fisher, A. A., The parabens: paradoxical preservatives, *Cutis,* 51, 405, 1993.
24. Adams, R. M., Maibach, H. I., A five-year study of cosmetic reactions, *Journal of the American Academy of Dermatology,* 13, 1062, 1985.
25. De Groot, A. C., Bruynzeel, D. P., Bos, J. D., van der Meeren, H. L. M., van Joost, Th., Jagtman, B. A., Weijland, J. W., The allergens in cosmetics, *Archives of Dermatology,* 124, 1525, 1988.
26. Goossens, A., Beck, M. H., McFadden, J. P., Nolting, S., Durupt, G., Ries, G., Adverse cutaneous reactions to cosmetic allergens, *Contact Dermatitis,* 40, 112, 1999.
27. De Groot, A. C., Liem, D. H., Contact allergy to oleamidopropyl dimethylamine, *Contact Dermatitis,* 11, 298, 1984.
28. Wilson, C. I., Cameron, J., Powell, S. M., Cherry, G., Ryan, T. J., High incidence of contact dermatitis in leg ulcer patients — implications for management, *Clinical and Experimental Dermatology,* 16, 250, 1997.
29. Marks, J. G., Jr., Belsito, D. V., DeLeo, V. A., Fowler, J. F., Jr., Fransway, A. F., Maibach, H. I., North American Contact Dermatitis Group patch test results for the detection of delayed-type hypersensitivity to topical allergens, *Journal of the American Academy of Dermatology,* 38, 911, 1998.
30. Nachbar, F., Korting, H. C., Plewig, G., Zur Bedeutung des positiven Epikutantests auf Lanolin, *Dermatosen,* 41, 227, 1993.
31. Von der Werth, J. M., English, J. S. C., Dalziel, K. L., Loss of patch test positivity to cetylsteraryl alcohol, *Contact Dermatit*is, 38, 109, 1998.
32. Matthieu, L., Dockx, P., Discrepancy in patch test results with wool wax alcohols and Amerchol® L-101, *Contact Dermatitis,* 36, 150, 1997.
33. Kligman, A. M., The myth of lanolin allergy, *Contact Dermatitis,* 39, 103, 1998.*
34. Wolf, R., The lanolin paradox, *Dermatology,* 192, 198, 1996.*
35. Funk, J. O., Maibach, H. I., Propylene glycol dermatitis: re-evaluation of an old problem, *Contact Dermatitis,* 31, 236, 1994.*
36. Aberer, W., Fuchs, Th., Peters, K.-P., Propylenglykol: Kutane Nebenwirkungen und Testmethodik, *Dermatosen,* 41, 25, 1993.*
37. Wahlberg, J. E., Propylene glycol: search for a proper and nonirritant patch test preparation, *American Journal of Contact Dermatitis,* 5, 156, 1994.*
38. De Groot, A. C., Cocamidopropyl betaine: a "new" important cosmetic allergen, *Dermatosen,* 45, 60, 1997.*
39. De Groot, A. C., van der Walle, H. B., Weijland, J. W., Contact allergy to cocamidopropyl betaine, *Contact Dermatitis,* 33, 419, 1995.
40. De Groot, A. C., Contact allergens. What's new? Cosmetic dermatitis, *Clinics in Dermatology,* 15, 485, 1997.*

41. Fowler, J. F., Cocamidopropyl betaine: the significance of positive patch test results in twelve patients, *Cutis,* 52, 281, 1993.
42. Pigatto, P. D., Bigardi, A. S., Cusano, F., Contact dermatitis to cocamidopropylbetaine is caused by residual amines: relevance, clinical characteristics, and review of the literature, *American Journal of Contact Dermatitis,* 6, 13–16, 1995.
43. Angelini, G., Rigano, L., Foti, C., Contact allergy to impurities in surfactants: amount, chemical structure and carrier effect in reactions to 3-dimethylaminopropylamine, *Contact Dermatitis,* 34, 248, 1996.
44. Basketter, D. A., Lea, L., Ross, J. S., Does DMAPA play a role in CAPB allergy? in *Book of Abstracts, Jadassohn Centenary Congress*, London, October 9–12, 1996, 44.
45. Fowler, J. F., Jr., Fowler, L. M., Hunter, J. E., Allergy to cocamidopropyl betaine may be due to amidoamine: a patch test and product use test study, *Contact Dermatitis,* 37, 276, 1997.
46. De Groot, A. C., Jagtman, B. A., van der Meeren, H. L. M., Bruynzeel, D. P., Bos, J. D., Den Hengst, C. W., Weijland, J. W., Cross-reaction pattern of the cationic emulsifier oleamidopropyl dimethylamine, *Contact Dermatitis,* 19, 284, 1988.
47. Foti, C., Rigano, L., Vena, G. A., Grandolfo, M., Liguori, G., Angelini, G., Contact allergy to oleamidopropyl dimethylamine and related substances, *Contact Dermatitis,* 33, 132, 1995.
48. Tosti, A., Vincenzi, C., Guerra, L., Andrisano, E., Contact dermatitis from fatty alcohols, *Contact Dermatitis,* 35, 287, 1996.
49. Bergh, M., Magnusson, K., Nilsson, J. L. G., Karlberg, A.-T., Contact allergenic activity of Tween® 80 before and after air exposure, *Contact Dermatitis,* 37, 9, 1997.
50. Funk, J. O., Dromgoole, S. H., Maibach, H. I., Sunscreen intolerance. Contact sensitization, photocontact sensitization, and irritancy of sunscreen agents, *Clinics in Dermatology,* 13, 473, 1995.*
51. Schauder, S., Ippen, H., Contact and photocontact sensitivity to sunscreens: review of a 15-year experience and of the literature, *Contact Dermatitis,* 37, 221, 1995.*
52. Wyss, M., Elsner, P., Homberger, H.-P., Greco, P., Gloor, M., Burg, G., Follikuläres Kontaktekzem auf eine Tocopherol-linoleat-haltige Körpermilch, *Dermatosen,* 45, 25, 1997.*
53. Nakagawa, M., Kawai, K., Kawai, K., Contact allergy to kojic acid in skin care products, *Contact Dermatitis,* 32, 9–13, 1995.

*Reviews. Advised readings.

34 Glycols

Matti Hannuksela

CONTENTS

34.1 PROPYLENE GLYCOL

34.1.1 Properties and Use

Propylene glycol (PG) belongs to dialcohols, diols, some of which are widely used in cosmetics and dermatological formulations. Of the two PGs, 1,2-propanediol is far more often used than 1,3-propanediol. PG and 1,2-propanediol are usually used as synonyms. Its molecular weight is 74.13 and its chemical structure is $CH_2OHCHOHCH_3$. It is an odorless, viscous liquid; is readily miscible with water, acetone, chloroform, and essential oils; and is soluble in ether. Its isotonic concentration is 2% in water, and in higher concentrations it is very hygroscopic.

Taken internally, PG is oxidized to pyruvic and acetic acids. Small internal amounts are harmless. In man, amounts exceeding 5 ml perorally may cause a sensation of drunkenness. When administered intravenously, PG has been shown to have low short- and long-term toxicity.[1] However, intravenous PG, 5 g/kg in 12 h, caused hyperosmolality with an increased osmolal gap, hemolysis, hemoglobinuria, and metabolic acidosis.[2] Acute renal failure has also been attributed to PG, but the mechanism has not been solved.[3] In horses, 6 ml of PG per kilogram of body weight causes severe depression, ataxia, and malodorous breath.[4] In rat, PG has been shown to increase insulin resistance.[5] Ethanol is metabolized partly to diols, and diols are potent inhibitors of basal and insulin-stimulated adipocyte metabolism.[6] These findings may partly explain the link between high plasma diol concentrations in alcohol abusers and their increased susceptibility to noninsulin-dependent diabetes mellitus.[5]

0-8493-7520-7/00/$0.00+$.50

TABLE 1
The Main Effects of Propylene Glycol in Living Organisms

Property/Effect	Consequences, Uses
Hygroscopic	PG in over 2% concentration is hygroscopic and is used widely as a humectant.
Antimicrobic	PG is a preservative in many pharmaceutics and cosmetic products. It is also used as a treatment for pityriasis versicolor and secondary infected dermatitis.
Penetration enhancer	PG is used in many transdermal pharmaceuticals and cosmeceuticals (e.g., antiperspirants) as a penetration enhancer.
Keratolysis	PG can be used in ichthyosis and other hyperkeratotic conditions as a keratolytic agent.
Irritancy	Many people experience itching, burning, tingling, or stinging when using topical preparations containing PG. However, no objective signs of inflammation can be seen. Under occlusion irritation is common.

Topical PG is known to raise serum osmolality in burn patients. In dermatitis patients, PG did not change the electrolyte, lactate, or osmolality results when PG was applied to the skin at a maximum of 6.1 g/kg every 24 h for 5 days.[7]

The main effects of PG for living organisms are listed in Table 1. For its hygroscopic, antiseptic, and solubility properties, PG has become a popular ingredient of dermatological and cosmetic products within the past three decades. It is also used in many oral and parenteral medications, e.g., in antitussive mixtures.

The antimicrobial properties of PG are well known. Vehicles containing more than 5% PG are superior to those with glycerol. When *Candida albicans, Staphylococcus aureus, S. epidermidis, Streptococcus pyogenes A, S. mitis,* and *Eshericia coli* were studied *in vitro*, PG at 30% was able to kill the microorganisms in 20 h.[8] The antimicrobial effect of PG was noticed already at 5%, and at 3 to 9% inhibited the growth of *C. albicans, Trichophyton mentagrophytes, T. rubrum,* and *Pityrosporum orbiculare in vitro.*[9] Pityriasis versicolor can be treated with 50% PG in water.[10] A combination of PG, urea, and lactic acid has been used in the treatment of onychomycosis, but only 2 of 23 patients were totally cured, while 11 improved greatly and 8 to some extent.[11]

Transdermal administration of various drugs has increased greatly in recent years. PG is an important part of the vehicles of most of them. The penetration of corticosteroids is usually greatly enhanced by PG.[12-15] It also enhances the penetration, e.g., of minoxidil,[16] methotrexate,[17] tranilast,[18] yohimbine,[19] diclofenac,[20] and norfloxacin.[21] It also increases the risk of contact sensitization obviously in two ways: (1) by increasing the penetration of the allergen and (2) by irritating the skin especially under occlusion, thus promoting the development of contact hypersensitivity to potential allergens.[22-24]

In cosmetic vehicles PG has been shown to increase the penetration of allantoin[25] but not N-nitrosodiethanolamine, an impurity in many cosmetic products.[26] When applied together with agents causing nonimmunologic contact urticaria (NICU), the NICU reaction is greatly enhanced.[27] On the contrary, pretreatment with PG did not alter the strength of the NICU reaction to benzoic acid.[28]

PG is a mild keratolytic agent and can be used with occlusion for the treatment of ichtyosis.[29] It has also been used together with salicylic acid[30] and as a component of an emollient[31] in hyperkeratosis.

34.1.2 Adverse Effects

34.1.2.1 Irritant Reactions

When applied without occlusion, PG is usually a nonirritant. Subjective sensations such as itching, tingling, burning, or stinging without any signs of inflammation are sometimes reported.[32] Transepidermal water loss was found to increase significantly in atopics, but not in nonatopics when 50% PG in water was applied twice daily for 2.5 days to the back skin.[28] PG itself can rarely cause a NICU reaction.[33]

When applied with occlusion, irritant reactions to PG have been encountered in 12 to 16% of dermatitis.[34,35] The percentage of reactors was 18 to 22% in winter and 5 to 8% in summer, reflecting either a lower penetration rate of PG due to the increase in the thickness of epidermis induced by UV irradiation of the sun or the antiinflammatory effect of UV in summertime or lower ambient water content in winter. When 30% PG in water was tested as an additional test together with standard patch tests (PT), irritant or questionable reactions were found in 10.2% of 1701 patients.[36] Twenty percent PG in petrolatum has been found to be a nonirritant in occlusive PT in healthy volunteers.[37]

34.1.2.2 Delayed Contact Hypersensitivity

PG has been considered to be a weak sensitizer.[38] The evaluation of PT reactions to various concentrations of PG is difficult. While irritant reactions from 100% PG are encountered usually in 10 to 20% (see earlier), the number of allergic and allergic-type PT reactions depends on the concentration of PG and the vehicle. A positive reaction to 2% PG in water was encountered in 2 of 880 (0.2%) dermatological patients subjected for routine patch.[38] Five percent PG in water produced allergic reactions in 27 out of 3364 (0.8%) dermatitis patients.[39]

In the repeated open application test (ROAT), 4 of 12 patients with a positive reaction to 30% or stronger, but not to lower concentrations of PG in water, showed a positive result in ROAT by using a cream with 5% PG.[40] In the same study, all five patients reacting to 1% PG in PT were ROAT positive to the cream with 5% PG. The corresponding number was one of two patients with positive PT results to 10% PG but not to 1% PG.[40] In other investigations with a few patients this result has been confirmed.[33,36,41]

The mechanism of skin contact reactions induced by PG has been evaluated further by making peroral challenge tests. Eight of ten patients reacting to 2% aqueous PG in PT got a widespread exanthema (systemic contact dermatitis) in 3 to 16 h after a peroral challenge with 2 to 15 ml of PG diluted with water.[42] Four of the ten patients reacted to 2 ml, three further patients to 5 ml, and one further patient to 15 ml of PG. Twenty-eight patients reacting to 10 to 100% PG in PT were also subjected for peroral challenge with 5 to 15 ml of PG. Only seven of them reacted. None of the 20 control patients showed any signs of dermatitis from 5 ml of PG, and none of the four controls from 15 ml of PG in peroral.[42]

In their review on PG dermatitis, Funk and Maibach[43] concluded that only combining PT, ROAT, or other use tests, and peroral challenge tests could reliably do the diagnosis of PG allergy. Biopsies taken from positive cutaneous reactions may also be helpful.

34.2 BUTYLENE GLYCOL

34.2.1 Properties and Use

Butylene glycol (BG) usually means 1,3-butanediol, $CH_3CHOHCH_2CH_2OH$, but the term can also be used for 2,3-butanediol. BG, mol wt 90.1, is also a viscous liquid with a distinctive mild odor. It is miscible with water, alcohol, and acetone. It is very hygroscopic like PG. As an antimicrobic agent, BG is approximately as effective as PG,[8,44] but BG is less irritating and a poorer penetration enhancer than PG. All these properties make it more suitable as a hygroscopic and antimicrobial ingredient of cosmetics than PG.

34.2.2 Adverse Effects

34.2.2.1 Irritant Reactions

When patch testing 1701 consecutive eczema patients with 1,3-BG and 2,3-BG at 20% in water, 7.8% showed irritant or questionable reaction to 1,3-BG and 7.0% to 2,3-BG.[36] In that particular study, 30% PG produced irritant or questionable PT reactions in 10.2%. The skin irritation potential of 1,3-BG has been found to be lower than that of PG in other studies, also.[45]

34.2.2.2 Delayed Contact Hypersensitivity

Patients with PT reactions fulfilling the criteria of a positive allergic reaction have been rarely published in the dermatological literature. Sugiura and Hayakawa[45] published five patients with a positive PT reaction from 5% aqueous 1,3-BG. At least three of them had a history of contact dermatitis from cosmetics containing 1,3-BG. One patient was further tested with cosmetics, and she reacted to a foundation cream and 18 hypoirritant cosmetics all containing 1,3-BG. The patient got rid of her dermatitis when avoiding products with 1,3-BG.[45]

Positive (+, ++) PT reaction to 20% 1,3-BG was encountered in 4 of 1701 (0.2%) consecutive eczema patients subjected for routine PT.[36] The corresponding number for 2,3-BG was 5 of 1701 (0.3%). Four patients reacted to both BGs, and three of them reacted also to 30% PG in PTs. ROAT was performed with 20% BG in water in one and with 20% 2,3-BG in two of them. The test was positive in the two cases tested with 2,3-BG, but negative in the particular patient tested with 1,3-BG.[36] The results speak in favor that both 1,3-BG and 2,3-BG are weak irritants and their sensitizing capacity is low.

34.3 HEXYLENE GLYCOL

34.3.1 Properties and Use

Hexylene glycol (HG), $(CH_3)_2COHCH_2CHOHCH_3$, is another diol used in cosmeticals and dermatologicals. It is also known as 2-methyl-2,4-pentanediol and as 2,4-pentanediol, 2-methyl. It is a viscous liquid with the distinctive odor of "an old man." Its mol wt is 118.2. It is very hygroscopic like other glycols mentioned previously. In cosmetics it is used mainly as a defoaming agent, coupling agent, humectant, antimicrobial, or an emulsifier in hair and bath preparations, soaps, eye makeups, and skin care products at 0.1 to 25%. In dermatology it is mainly used as an antimicrobial and a penetration enhancer in topical corticosteroids. Like other glycols it possesses good antimicrobic capacity.[46] The longer the chain is, the more effective antimicrobic agent the diol is.[9] The effect of 10% HG equals approximately that of 30% PG and 30% BG.[8]

34.3.2 Adverse Effects

34.3.2.1 Irritant Reactions

When tested under occlusion, HG is less irritating than PG. The irritation capacity of 50% HG in water equaled approximately that of 30% PG in water.[28] Twice daily applications of 50% HG for 2.5 days on the back skin neither caused any symptoms or signs of irritation nor increased the transepidermal water loss when tested in a group or 11 nonatopic and 8 atopic people.[28] ROAT with 30% HG in water was negative in all four patients showing an irritant PT reaction to the test material.[36]

34.3.2.2 Delayed Contact Hypersensitivity

The risk of contact allergy from HG is obviously approximately the same level as from PG and BG. One positive ROAT result has been published from 50% HG and two from 30% HG in water.[28,36] However, true contact allergy could not be verified in these particular cases.

34.4 CONCLUSIONS

All three glycols dealt with in this chapter are good humectants, and they also possess antimicrobial capacity and are penetration enhancers. They irritate the skin when applied under occlusion but without occlusion, their irritating capacity is very low. Delayed contact allergy can be expected in less than 1% of eczema patients. The verification of contact allergy is still a matter of controversy. Most patients reacting to 1 to 2% PG, BG, or HG in water in ordinary PTs experience eczematous dermatitis when using dermatological or cosmetic preparations containing the corresponding glycol. However, 1 to 2% glycol in water does not pick up all allergic people. It is advisable to use 20% glycol in water for screening. Positive cases are further subjected for PT with dilution series. ROAT and other use tests as well as peroral challenge tests may be used for further confirmation of the diagnosis.

REFERENCES

1. Ruddick, J. A., Toxicology, metabolism, and biochemistry of 1,2-propanediol, *Toxicol. Appl. Pharmacol.,* 21, 102, 1972.
2. van de Wiele, B., Rubinstein, E., Peacock, W., Martin N., Propylene glycol toxicity caused by prolonged infusion of etomidate, *J. Neurosurg. Anesthesiol.,* 7, 259, 1995.
3. Yorgin, P. D., Theodorou, A. A., Al-Uzri, A., Davenport, K., Boyer-Hassen, L. V., Johnson, M. I., Propylene glycol-induced proximal renal tubular cell injury, *Am. J. Kidney Dis.,* 30, 134, 1997.
4. McClanahan, S., Hunter, J., Murphy, M., Valberg, S., Propylene glycol toxicosis in a mare, *Vet. Hum. Toxicol.,* 40, 294, 1998.
5. Xu, D., Dhillon, A. S., Abelmann, A., Croft, K., Peters, T. J., Palmer, T. N., Alcohol-related diols cause acute insulin resistance *in vivo, Metabolism,* 47, 1180, 1998.
6. Lomeo, F., Khokher, M. A., Dandona, P., Ethanol and its novel metabolites inhibit insulin action on adipocytes, *Diabetes,* 37, 912, 1988.
7. Commens, C. A., Topical propylene glycol and hyperosmolality, *Br. J. Dermatol.,* 122, 77, 1990.
8. Kinnunen, T., Koskela, M., Antibacterial and antifungal properties of propylene glycol, hexylene glycol, and 1,3-butylene glycol *in vitro, Acta Derm. Venereol.,* 71, 148, 1991.
9. Faergemann, J., Fredriksson, T., The antimycotic activity *in vitro* of five diols, *Sabouraudia,* 18, 287, 1980.
10. Faergemann, J., Fredriksson, T., Antimycotic activity of propane-1,2-diol (propylene glycol), *Sabouraudia,* 18, 163, 1980.
11. Faergemann, J., Swanbeck, G., Treatment of onychomycosis with a propylene glycol-urea-lactic acid solution, *Mycoses,* 32, 536, 1989.
12. Ponec, M., Penetration of corticosteroids through the skin in relation to the vehicle, *Dermatologica,* 152, Suppl. 1, 37, 1976.
13. Polano, M. K., Ponec, M., Dependence of corticosteroid penetration on the vehicle, *Arch. Dermatol.,* 112, 675, 1976.
14. Kansky, A., The effects of increased penetration of betamethasone dipropionate in a propylene glycol base (Diprolene) for psoriasis, *Int. J. Med. Res.,* 9, 128, 1981.
15. Barry, B. W., Bennett, S. L., Effect of penetration enhancers on the permeation of mannitol, hydrocortisone and progesterone through human skin, *J. Pharm. Pharmacol.,* 39, 535, 1987.
16. Tata, S., Weiner, N., Flynn, G., Relative influence of ethanol and propylene glycol cosolvents on deposition of minoxidil into the skin, *J. Pharm. Sci.,* 83, 1508, 1994.
17. Chatterjee, D. J., Li, W. Y., Koda, R. T., Effect of vehicles and penetration enhancers on the *in vitro* and *in vivo* percutaneous absorption of methotrexate and edatrexate through hairless mouse skin, *Pharm. Res.,* 14, 1058, 1997.
18. Murakami, T., Yoshioka, M., Higashi, Y., Shigeki, S., Ikuta, Y., Yata, N., Topical delivery of keloid therapeutic drug, tranilast, by combined use of oleic acid and propylene glycol as a penetration enhancer: evaluation by skin microdialysis in rats, *J. Pharm. Pharmacol.,* 50, 49, 1998.

19. Carelli, V., Di Colo, G., Nannipieri, E., Serafini, M. F., Effect of vehicles on yohimbine permeation across excised hairless mouse skin, *Pharm. Acta Helv.,* 73, 127, 1998.
20. Arellano, A., Santoyo, S., Martin, C., Ygartua, P., Influence of propylene glycol and isopropyl myristate on the *in vitro* percutaneous penetration of diclofenac sodium from carbopol gels, *Eur. J. Pharm. Sci.,* 7, 129, 1999.
21. Lin, H. H., Hsu, L. R., Wu, P. C., Tsai, Y. H., Increased norfloxacin skin permeability for fatty alcohol propylene glycol (FAPG) ointment by optimized process of preparation: behavior of stearic acid in stratum corneum lipids, *Biol. Pharm. Bull.,* 18, 1560, 1995.
22. Robinson, M. K., Parsell, K. W., Breneman, D. L., Cruze, C. A., Evaluation of the primary skin irritation and allergic contact sensitization potential of transdermal triprolidine, *Fundam. Appl. Toxicol.,* 17, 103, 1991.
23. Hannuksela, M., Allergy to propantheline in an antiperspirant, *Contact Dermatitis,* 1, 244, 1975.
24. Ågren-Jonsson, S., Magnusson, B., Sensitization to propantheline bromide, trichlorocarbanilide and propylene glycol in an atiperspirant, *Contact Dermatitis,* 2, 79, 1976.
25. Cajkovac, M., Oremovic, L., Cajkovac, V., Influence of emulsoid vehicle on the release and activity of allantoin, *Pharmazie,* 47, 39, 1992.
26. Bronaugh, R. L., Congdon, E. R., Scheuplein, R. J., The effect of cosmetic vehicles on the penetration of N-nitrosodiethanolamine through excised human skin, *J. Invest. Dermatol.,* 76, 94, 1981.
27. Lahti, A., Poutiainen, A.-M., Hannuksela, M., Alcohol vehicles in tests for non-immunological immediate contact reactions, *Contact Dermatitis,* 29, 22, 1993.
28. Kinnunen, T., Hannuksela, M., Skin reactions to hexylene glycol, *Contact Dermatitis,* 21, 154, 1989.
29. Goldsmith, L. A., Baden, H. P., Propylene glycol with occlusion for treatment of ichthyosis, *J.A.M.A.,* 220, 579, 1972.
30. Baden, H. P., Alper, J. C., A keratolytic gel containing salicylic acid in propylene glycol, *J. Invest. Dermatol.,* 61, 330, 1973.
31. Gnemo, A., Vahlquist, A., Lamellar ichthyosis is markedly improved by a novel combination of emollients, *Br. J. Dermatol.,* 137, 1017, 1997.
32. Adams, R. M., Maibach, H. I., A five-year study of cosmetic reactions, *J. Am. Acad. Dermatol.,* 13, 1062, 1985.
33. Andersen, K. E., Storrs, F. J., Hautreizungen durch propyleneglykol, *Hautarzt,* 33, 12, 1982.
34. Warshaw, T. G., Herrmann, F., Studies of skin reactions to propylene glycol, *J. Invest. Dermatol.,* 19, 423, 1952.
35. Hannuksela, M., Pirilä, V., Salo, O. P., Skin reactions to propylene glycol, *Contact Dermatitis,* 1, 112, 1975.
36. Fan, W., Kinnunen, T., Niinimäki, A., Hannuksela, M., Skin reactions to glycols used in dermatological and cosmetic vehicles, *Am. J. Contact Dermatitis,* 2, 181, 1991.
37. Meneghini, C. L., Rantuccio, F., Lomuto, M., Additives, vehicles and active drugs of topical medicaments as causes of delayed-type allergic dermatitis, *Dermatologica,* 143, 137, 1971.
38. Hannuksela, M., Kousa, M., Pirilä, V., Allergy to ingredients of vehicles, *Contact Dermatitis,* 2, 105, 1976.
39. Angelini, G., Vena, A., Meneghini, C. L., Allergic contact dermatitis to some medicaments, *Contact Dermatitis,* 12, 263, 1985.
40. Hannuksela, M., Salo, H., The repeated open application test (ROAT), *Contact Dermatitis,* 14, 221, 1986.
41. Uter, W., Schwanitz, H. J., Contact dermatitis from propylene glycol in ECG electrode gel, *Contact Dermatitis,* 34, 230, 1996.
42. Hannuksela, M., Förström, L., Reactions to peroral propylene glycol, *Contact Dermatitis,* 4, 41, 1978.
43. Funk, J. O., Maibach, H. I., Propylene glycol dermatitis: re-evaluation of an old problem, *Contact Dermatitis,* 11, 236, 1984.
44. Faergemann, J., Fredriksson, T., The antimycotic activity *in vitro* of five diols, *Sabouraudia,* 18, 287, 1980.
45. Sugiura, M., Hayakawa, R., Contact dermatitis due to 1,3-butylene glycol, *Contact Dermatitis,* 37, 90, 1997.

46. Faergemann, J., The *in vitro* antimycotic activity of propane-1,2-diol, 2-methyl-2,4-pentanediol, alclomethasone dipropionate cream, and Essex® cream with the addition of propane-1,2-diol against *Staphylococcus aureus, Staphylococcus epidermidis, Candida albicans, Trichophyton rubrum*, and *Pityrosporum orbiculare*. *Curr. Ther. Res.*, 43, 547, 1988.

35 Contact Urticaria

Matti Hannuksela

CONTENTS

35.1 INTRODUCTION

Contact urticaria (CU) is divided into two main types: immunologic (allergic) or IgE-mediated (ICU) and nonimmunologic CUs (NICU). In ICU, the sensitized person synthesizes specific IgE, which, in turn, reacts with IgE receptors on the mast cells, basophils, eosinophils, Langerhans cells, and certain other cells. In this reaction, histamine, leukotriens, and the cells secrete eosinophil peroxide (EPO) and other vasoactive substances. The severity of the reaction varies from a mild local itch and redness to widespread urticaria and anaphylactic shock. We do not know the frequency of such reactions, but we can assume that 20 to 30% of the population has some experience of immediate contact reactions (ICRs) to everyday cosmetics and personal hygiene products. The causes of cosmetic contact urticaria are numerous, with sorbic and benzoic acids and fragrances being the most common among them.

The reaction usually appears within 5 to 15 minutes as local wheals and flare, and a reaction of medium intensity usually disappears in 20 to 30 minutes. Sometimes tiny eczematous vesicles develop within 20 to 30 minutes. They seem to be true eczematous vesicles, and they will subside with slight scaling in a couple of weeks.

The mechanisms underlying NICU are mostly unknown. Prostaglandins are involved in the reaction to at least benzoic (BA) and sorbic acids (SA) and to methyl nicotinate. NICU reactions appear in 15 to 90 minutes and also disappear slightly more slowly than ICU.

A third category is CU of uncertain mechanism. In some instances, e.g., cases with persulfates, the reaction resembles that of ICU, but no IgE can be demonstrated in the patient's serum or in the tissues, suggesting that there are other immunologic mechanisms in addition to the IgE-mediated ones.

Antihistamines, acetylsalicylic acid, and other inhibitors of prostaglandin synthesis, ultraviolet radiation, and heat (infrared radiation) influence the severity of both ICU and NICU.

0-8493-7520-7/00/$0.00+$.50

35.2 OCCURRENCE OF CONTACT URTICARIA REACTIONS

In an open application test, 39% of Caucasian people living in Finland reacted with edema and redness and 19% with redness only to 2.5% sorbic acid in petrolatum.[1] Sixteen out of 26 people reacting to 2.5% sorbic acid in a w/o cream showed CU, and 10 people showed only redness. This finding means that as many as 50% of people may get untoward immediate skin symptoms from a moisturizer containing sorbic acid as the preservative.

Fragrances are also able to produce ICRs. Usual patch test concentrations of cinnamic alcohol, cinnamic aldehyde, geraniol, eugenol, balsam of Peru, anisyl alcohol, benzyl alcohol and coumarin produced wheal and flare reactions or redness only in 36 to 78% of 50 people (31 patch test clinic patients and 19 controls) tested with an open application method.[2] The other ingredients causing immediate reactions included formaldehyde, imidazodinyl urea, bronopol, Kathon CG®, and paraben mixture. No correlation between the open application test result and the cosmetic sensitivity reported by the patients was found.

In another study on fragrance materials, 80 housewives without a history of cosmetic intolerance reacted with erythema to 2% cinnamic aldehyde, 2% sorbic acid, and 2% eugenol in petrolatum in a 20-minute occluded Finn Chamber test.[3] In the same population, 76 (95%) reacted to 2% benzoic acid. Sixteen also showed edema from cinnamic aldehyde and 15 from benzoic acid. The proportion of people who would have reacted to these or other fragrance materials at the concentrations usually present in everyday cosmetics is not known.

The occurrence of ICRs from sunscreens was studied in a random sample of subjects aged over 40 years using sunscreens.[4] One of the 603 people had generalized urticaria of unknown cause, one possibly had contact urticaria with a weakly positive scratch test to the sunscreen used, and one obviously had a NICU reaction without any knowledge of the causative agent. Sunscreens may be present in moisturizers, but their concentration is so low that any immediate contact reactions are rarely expected.

Halpern[5] conducted a study among the subjects attending his dermatological practice on Kauai, the most westerly of the major Hawaiian Islands. Twenty-six percent of the 1020 sequential patients were aware of the substances that elicited immediate symptoms. None of them mentioned moisturizers or cosmetics as a possible cause of such reactions. The mode of questioning may have played a role in the lack of cosmetic intolerance in this particular study, but the abundance of ultraviolet radiation on the Hawaiian Islands may also have prevented ICRs.

35.3 MECHANISMS OF CONTACT URTICARIA REACTIONS TO MOISTURIZERS

35.3.1 Immunolgic Contact Urticaria

35.3.1.1 Sensitization

The route of immunization, the amount of antigen/allergen, and the presence of adjuvant are important factors in determining the tissue response. The parenteral challenge to proteins usually leads to the production of IgG; the gastrointestinal route sometimes leads to an IgA response; and the respiratory route leads to an IgE response. When a low molecular weight chemical reaches the immunologically active cells through the skin, tolerance or contact allergy is the most common consequence. IgE response may also be possible in percutaneous challenge. Great or minimal amounts of allergens may induce tolerance, while relatively small amounts may lead to allergy.

In the mucosa and the skin, Langerhans cells (LCs) or other antigen presenting cells (APCs) present both chemicals and protein allergens to T-cells. In immediate allergy, T-helper 2 (Th2) cells are activated. They produce interleukins (IL), which switch B-cells to produce IgE. IL-4 and IL-13 have been shown to be potent switch factors. However, they seem to induce nonspecific rather than specific IgE production in peripheral B-cells.[6]

35.3.1.2 The Immunologic Contact Urticaria Reaction

Mast cells, basophils, eosinophils, and LCs carry high-affinity IgE receptors. In ICU, mast cells and the substances produced by them are of major importance. Histamine, neutral proteases, exoglycosidases, and proteoglycans are released within some minutes from the granules of the mast cells, resulting in a wheal and flare reaction in the skin. Massive amounts of these substances lead to anaphylaxis.

An immediate allergic reaction also leads to a synthesis of leukotrienes (LTs), prostaglandins (PGs), and platelet-activating factor (PAF) in the cell membranes of the activated mast cells. Together with histamine, they produce mucosal edema and obstruction of the airways. Symptoms of allergic rhinitis and asthma are common complaints reported by ICU patients.

The mast cells also release chemotactic factors, which bring eosinophils and T-cells from the vessels into the dermis. The role of these cells is usually insignificant. In long-lasting antigen exposure they may take part in the development of an eczematous reaction, which is sometimes seen in IgE-mediated allergy. Another possible mechanism for the development of eczematous dermatitis is the binding of IgE molecules to the high-affinity receptors on LCs.[7]

35.3.2 Nonimmunologic Contact Urticaria

Substances capable of producing NICU are usually low molecular weight chemicals which easily cross the horny layer. Men seem to react more readily than women.[1] Most NICU substances are aldehydes or weak acids or their salts, but acidity itself is not essential for producing the reaction. A minor change in the structure of a substance may alter greatly its capacity to produce an NICU reaction.

The NICU reaction usually appears in 1 h, and the edema disappears within 1 h, but redness may still be visible 6 h after the application of an NICU substance. Repeated applications diminish the strength of the reaction, and the effect can be still seen on the following day. Scratching and stripping the skin also weaken the reaction.[1]

Perorally taken acetylsalicylic acid (ASA) and indomethacin,[8-10] as well as topically applied diclofenac and naproxen gels,[11] inhibit the reaction for up to 4 days.[12] Strong corticosteroid creams also diminish the strength of the NICU reaction.[1,9]

Ultraviolet A and B irradiations inhibit the NICU reaction for at least 2 weeks.[13] Ultraviolet irradiation has been shown to have a systemic effect, i.e., to inhibit the reaction even in an area which was sheltered from ultraviolet irradiation.[14] An inhibitory effect on NICU has also been demonstrated from PUVA treatment.[15]

All the previous observations speak in favor of most, if not all, NICU reactions being mediated by prostaglandins. The role of cutaneous nerves has also been studied. The most important pungent substance of Capsicum (red) pepper, capsaicin (trans-8-methyl-*N*-vanillyl-6-nonenamide), releases substance P and other active peptides from the axons of unmyelinated C-fibers of sensory nerves. Pretreatment of the skin with capsaicin diminished the flare and edema reaction from sorbic acid,[9] but did not influence the intensity of the NICU reactions from benzoic acid and methyl nicotinate.[16] Local anesthesia has shown a slight inhibitory effect on the NICU reaction.[1,9,16]

Infrared irradiation increases the intensity of the NICU reaction,[17] and so does pretreatment of the skin with a surface-active agent, sorbitan sesquioleate.[18] A quenching effect of eugenol on NICU reactions to cinnamic aldehyde was seen in 9 out of 23 subjects tested with cinnamic aldehyde alone and with a mixture of cinnamic aldehyde and eugenol.[19]

35.3.3 Unknown Mechanisms

Ammonium and potassium persulfates are further examples of agents producing occasional immediate skin and airway reactions, but without any evidence of IgE-mediated allergy.[20,21] Repeated exposure to formaldehyde is another example of CU of unknown mechanism.[22]

35.4 INGREDIENTS OF MOISTURIZERS CAUSING IMMEDIATE CONTACT REACTIONS

The chemicals and other substances in moisturizers known to cause ICRs are listed in Table 1. Many of the substances listed in the table can cause only nonimmunologic reactions. There is some evidence to suggest that many chemicals may produce immunologic reactions, but the final proof is still lacking. Sorbitan esters, for example, which are used as emulsifiers, are reported to cause widespread acute skin reactions. These reactions might be due to an impurity in the sorbitol anhydrides rather than to the esters themselves.[19] Alcohols (ethanol, butanol, and propanol) have been shown to produce immunologic reactions, and the patients react both to a topical application and to oral intake of these particular alcohols. [45]

In the 1970s and even in the 1980s, sorbic acid was one of the most important ingredients of moisturizers causing CU. Its importance has diminished during recent years because it has lost its popularity as a preservative. Benzoic acid and benzoates are also used very seldom as preservatives in moisturizers.

The technochemical industry has brought an increasing variety of plant and animal products into everyday cosmetics including moisturizers. These substances may contain natural or modified proteins capable of causing IgE-mediated allergy. The concentration of immunologic proteins in commercial products is usually so low that the risk of sensitization cannot be high. Another concern may be due to the natural fragrances present in flowers and their extracts. The concentrations of single separate chemicals are, however, so low that the risk of ICRs is usually minimal.

In addition to the substances presented in Table 1, many other chemicals are able to produce redness of the skin within tens of minutes after the application of the substance to the skin. Such reactions cannot be regarded as NICU, unless at least some of the test persons get contact urticarial lesions.

35.5 FACTORS INFLUENCING THE SEVERITY OF CONTACT URTICARIA REACTIONS

Gollhausen and Kligman[25] applied 2.5 to 5.0% SA and 2.5 to 5.0% BA to various body areas and found the following rank order of diminishing reactivity: face > antecubital space > upper back > upper arm > inner forearm > lower back > leg. Sodium pyrrolidone carboxylate, the most important component of a substance called the natural moisturizing factor, caused redness in the back skin, but not in the face or the neck.[40] Thus, the face seems to be more sensitive than other parts of the body to the common NICU substances, but not to all, as was shown by sodium pyrrolidone carboxylate.

"Quenching" refers to the ability of a substance to reduce the potential of another substance to sensitize or to cause contact urticaria. Eugenol has been shown to reduce the severity of ICRs to BA, SA, and cinnamic aldehyde.[24,25,49,50] This quenching action can be demonstrated by a simultaneous application of eugenol and an NICU substance or by pretreating the skin with eugenol prior to an NICU test.

Pretreatment of the skin for 2 days with a 20:80 mixture of sorbitan sesquioleate and petrolatum increased the skin response to BA applied to the skin in yellow petrolatum.[51] When BA was applied in a mixture of sorbitan sesquioleate and petrolatum, the skin response was significantly weaker than that to BA in petrolatum (ibid). These results also emphasize the importance of other substances used in skin care for the skin reactivity to NICU substances.

TABLE 1
Chemicals and Other Substances in Moisturizers Causing Immediate Contact Reactions

Substance/Chemical	Type of Reaction[a]	References
1. Preservatives		
Benzoic acid	N, I?	1, 19, 23–25
Sorbic acid	N	1, 9, 19, 24–26
Chlorocresol	N, I?	27, 28
Parabens	I?	2, 29
Bronopol[R]	N	2
Kathon CG[R]	N	2
Imidazodinyl urea	N	2
Formaldehyde	I, U	2, 22, 30
2. Fragrance materials		
Balsam of Peru	N, I?	1, 2, 19, 25, 31
Fragrance mix	N	24
Cinnamic aldehyde	N	2, 19, 24, 25, 32
Cinnamic alcohol	N	2, 24
Cinnamic acid	N	1, 19, 25
α-Amyl cinnamic aldehyde	N	2
Coumarin	N	2
Benzyl alcohol	N	2
Anisyl alcohol	N	2
Eugenol	N	2, 24
Geraniol	N	2, 24
Hydroxycitronellal	N	24
Cassia oil	N	26, 33
3. Emulsifiers		
Cetyl alcohol	U	34
Stearyl alcohol	U	34
Sorbitan monolaurate	I?	35
Sorbitan monostearate	I?	36
Sorbitan sesquioleate	I?	37
4. Other substances		
Wool alcohols	U	38
Pyrrolidone carboxylate	N	39
Lecithin	I?	40
Allantoin	I?	40
Aloe gel	I?	40
Chomomile extract	I?	40
Melissa extract	I?	40
Protein hydrolysate	I?	41, 42
Butylhydroxytoluene	I?	43, 44
Ethanol	I, N	45–47
Propanol	I	45
Butanol	I	45
Propylene glycol	N	48

[a] I = immunologic; N = non-immunologic; U = unknown mechanism.

REFERENCES

1. Lahti, A., Non-immunologic contact urticaria, *Acta Derm. Venereol (Stockholm)*, 60, Suppl. 91, 1, 1980.
2. Emmons, W. W., Marks, J. G., Immediate and delayed reactions to cosmetic ingredients, *Contact Dermatitis*, 13, 258, 1985.
3. Safford, R. J., Basketter, D. A., Allenby, C. F., Goodwin, B. F. J., Immediate contact reactions to chemicals in the fragrance mix and a study of the quenching action of eugenol, *Br. J. Dermatol.*, 123, 595, 1990.
4. Foley, P., Nixon, R., Marks, R., Frowen, K., Thompson, S., The frequency of reactions to sunscreens: results of a longitudinal population-based study on the regular use of sunscreens in Australia, *Br. J. Dermatol.*, 128, 512, 1993.
5. Halpern, D. J., The syndrome of immediate reactivities (contact urticaria syndrome). An historical study from a dermatology practice. I. Age, sex, race, and putative substances, *Hawaii Med. J.*, 44, 426, 1985.
6. Dolecek, C., Steinberger, P., Susani, M., Kraft, D., Valenta, R., Boltz-Nitulescu, G., Effects of IL4 and IL-13 on total and allergen specific IgE production by cultured PBMC from allergic patients determined with recombinant pollen allergens, *Clin. Exp. Allergy*, 25, 879, 1995.
7. Bruynzeel-Koomen, C., IgE on Langerhans cells: new insights into the pathogenesis of atopic dermatitis, *Dermatologica*, 172, 181, 1986.
8. Lahti, A., Oikarinen, A., Ylikorkala, O., Viinikka, L., Prostaglandins in contact urticaria induced by benzoic acid, *Acta Derm. Venereol. (Stockholm)*, 63, 425, 1983.
9. Soschin, D., Leyden, J. J., Sorbic acid induced erythema and edema, *J. Am. Acad. Dermatol.*, 14, 234, 1986.
10. Lahti, A., Väänänen, A., Kokkonen, E.-L., Hannuksela, M., Acetylsalicylic acid inhibits non-immunologic contact urticaria, *Contact Dermatitis*, 19, 161, 1988.
11. Johansson, J., Lahti, A., Topical non-steroidal anti-inflammatory drugs inhibit non-immunologic immediate contact reactions, *Contact Dermatitis*, 16, 133, 1987.
12. Kujala, T., Lahti, A., Duration of inhibition of non-immunologic contact reactions by acetylsalicylic acid, *Contact Dermatitis*, 21, 60, 1989.
13. Larmi, E., Lahti, A., Hannuksela, M., Ultraviolet light inhibits nonimmunologic immediate contact reactions to benzoic acid, *Arch. Dermatol. Res.* 280, 420, 1988.
14. Larmi, E., Systemic effect of ultraviolet irradiation on nonimmunologic immediate contact reactions to benzoic acid and methyl nicotinate, *Acta Derm. Venereol. (Stockholm)*, 69, 296, 1989.
15. Larmi, E., PUVA treatment inhibits nonimmunologic immediate contact reactions to benzoic acid and methyl nicotinate, *Int. J. Dermatol.*, 28, 609, 1989.
16. Larmi, E., Lahti, A., Hannuksela, M., Effects of capsaicin and topical anesthesia on nonimmunologic immediate contact reactions to benzoic acid and methyl nicotinate, in *Current Topics in Contact Dermatitis*, Frosch, P. J., Dooms-Goossens, A., Lachapelle, J.-M., Rycroft, R. J. G., Scheper, R. J., Eds., Springer-Verlag, Berlin, 1989, 441.
17. Larmi, E., Lahti, A., Hannuksela, M., Effects of infra-red and neodymium yttrium aluminium garnet laser irradiation on non-immunologic immediate contact reactions to benzoic acid and methyl nicotinate, *Dermatosen*, 37, 210, 1989.
18. Larmi, E., Lahti, A., Hannuksela, M., Effect of sorbitan sesquioleate on non-immunologic immediate contact reactions to benzoic acid, *Contact Dermatitis*, 19, 368, 1988.
19. Safford, R. J., Basketter, D. A., Allenby, C. F., Goodwin, B. F. J., Immediate contact reactions to chemicals in the fragrance mix and a study of the quenching action of eugenol, *Br. J. Dermatol.*, 123, 595, 1990.
20. Calnan, C. D., Shuster, S., Reactions to ammonium persulfate, *Arch. Dermatol.* 88, 812, 1963.
21. Fisher, A. A., Dooms-Goossens, A., Persulfate hair bleach reactions, *Arch. Dermatol* 112, 1407, 1976.
22. Lindskov, R., Contact urticaria to formaldehyde, *Contact Dermatitis*, 8, 333, 1982.
23. Forsbeck, M., Skog, E., Immediate reactions to patch tests with balsam of Peru, *Contact Dermatitis*, 3, 201, 1977.
24. Hjorth, N., Trolle-Lassen, C., Skin reactions to preservative in creams, *Am. Perfum.*, 77, 43, 1962.

25. Gollhausen, R., Kligman, A. M., Human assay for identifying substances which induce non-allergic contact urticaria: the NICU-test, *Contact Dermatitis,* 13, 98, 1985.
26. Rietschel, R. L., Contact urticaria from synthetic cassia oil and sorbic acid limited to the face, *Contact Dermatitis,* 4, 347, 1978.
27. Freitas, J. P., Brandão, F. M., Contact urticaria to chlorocresol, *Contact Dermatitis,* 15, 252, 1986.
28. Goncalo, M., Goncalo, S., Moreno, A., Immediate and delayed sensitivity to chlorocresol, *Contact Dermatitis,* 17, 46, 1987.
29. Henry, H. C., Tschen, E. H., Becker, L. E., Contact urticaria to parabens, *Archives of Dermatology,* 115, 1231, 1979.
30. Gehse, M., Gehring, W., Gloor, M., Berufsbedingte Formaldehyd-Allergie vom Soforttyp, *Dermatosen,* 36, 101, 1988.
31. Temesvári, E., Soos, G., Podányi, B., Kovács, I., Nemeth, I., Contact urticaria provoked by balsam of Peru, *Contact Dermatitis,* 4, 65, 1978.
32. Mathias, C. G. T., Chappler, R. R., Maibach, H. I., Contact urticaria from cinnamic aldehyde, *Arch. Dermatol.,* 116, 74, 1980.
33. Rudzki, E., Grzywa, Z., Immediate reactions to balsam of Peru, cassia oil and ethyl vanillin, *Contact Dermatitis,* 2, 360, 1976.
34. Gaul, L. E., Dermatitis from cetyl and stearyl alcohols, *Arch. Dermatol.,* 99, 593, 1969.
35. Boyle, J., Kennedy, C. T. C., Contact urticaria and dermatitis to Alphaderm®, *Contact Dermatitis,* 10, 178, 1984.
36. Maibach, H. I., Conant, M., Contact urticaria to a corticosteroid cream: polysorbate 60, *Contact Dermatitis,* 3, 350, 1977.
37. Hardy, M. P., Maibach, H. I., Contact urticaria syndrome from sorbitan sesquioleate in a corticosteroid ointment, *Contact Dermtitis,* 32, 114, 1995.
38. von Liebe, V., Karge, H.-J., Burg, G., Kontakturtikaria, *Hautarzt,* 30, 544, 1979.
39. Larmi, E., Lahti, A., Hannuksela, M., Immediate contact reactions to benzoic acid and the sodium salt of pyrrolidone carboxylic acid. Comparison of various skin sites, *Contact Dermatitis,* 20, 38, 1989.
40. West, I., Maibach, H. I., Contact urticaria syndrome from multiple cosmetic components, *Contact Dermatitis,* 32, 121, 1995.
41. Kousa, M., Strand, R., Mäkinen-Kiljunen, S., Hannuksela, M., Contact urticaria from hair conditioner, *Contact Dermatitis,* 23, 279, 1990.
42. Freeman, S., Lee, M.-S., Contact urticaria to hair conditioner, *Contact Dermatitis,* 35, 195, 1996.
43. Roed-Petersen, J., Hjorth, N., Contact dermatitis from antioxidants, *Br. J. Dermatol.,* 94, 233, 1976.
44. Osmundsen, P. E., Contact urticaria from nickel and plastic additives (Butylhydroxytoluene, oleylamide), *Contact Dermatitis,* 6, 452, 1980.
45. Rilliet, A., Hunziker, N., Brun, R., Alcohol contact urticaria syndrome (Immediate-type hypersensitivity), *Dermatologica,* 161, 361, 1980.
46. Kanzaki, T., Hori, H., Late phase allergic reaction of the skin to ethyl alcohol, *Contact Dermatitis,* 25, 252, 1991.
47. Wilkin, J. K., Fortner, G., Ethnic contact urticaria to alcohol, *Contact Dermatitis,* 12, 118, 1985.
48. Funk, J. O., Maibach, H. I., Propylene glycol dermatitis: re-evaluation of an old problem, *Contact Dermatitis,* 31, 236, 1994.
49. Guin, J. D., Meyer, B. N., Drake, R. D., Haffley, P., The effect of quenching agents on contact urticaria caused by cinnamic aldehyde, *J. Am. Acad. Dermatol.,* 10, 45, 1984.
50. Allenby, C. F., Goodwin, B. F. J., Safford, R. J., Diminution of immediate reaction to cinnamic aldehyde by eugenol, *Contact Dermatitis,* 11, 322, 1984.
51. Larmi, E., Lahti, A., Hannuksela, M., Effects of sorbitan sesquioleate on non-immunologic immediate contact reactions to benzoic acid, *Contact Dermatitis,* 19, 368, 1988.

36 Sensitive Skin

Ai-Lean Chew and Howard I. Maibach

CONTENTS

36.1 INTRODUCTION: DEFINITION OF SENSITIVE SKIN

Facial moisturizers frequently produce burning, stinging, itching, and suberythematous irritant dermatitis. Rates occasionally proximate 20%. The subjective symptoms are generally described by consumers as "sensitive skin."

The term "sensitive skin" has become ubiquitous in the world of cosmetology in recent years, yet no formal definition exists. Consumers use the term to describe a variety of adverse skin reactions to cosmetics and other topical products, as well as skin reactions triggered by environmental (e.g., temperature, wind, pollution), lifestyle (e.g., stress, emotion, diet), and hormonal factors (e.g., menstrual cycle).[1] This all-encompassing interpretation includes the spectrum of dry skin; oily or acne-prone skin; tendency to flushing; and nonspecific sensations of burning, stinging, and itching. Dermatologists and cosmetic chemists use the term to express both a situation of facial skin hyperreactivity on contact with a variety of topical agents, as well as the occult dermatoses resulting from or flaring up with topical applications and other exogenous factors.[1,2] Controversy exists over whether the term is reserved purely for visible hyperreactive responses or for susceptibility to chemically induced stinging and other such sensations.[1] Contrary to consumer perception, few conventional medical

0-8493-7520-7/00/$0.00+$.50

assessments of sensitive skin take hormonal or lifestyle factors into account. Thus, sensitive skin remains an imprecise phenomenon. In broad terms, sensitive skin is largely agreed to be a lay term used by individuals who consider themselves more intolerant of topical preparations and environmental conditions than the general population. The onus on the medical practitioner, then, is not merely to label a patient has having sensitive skin, but to diagnose the underlying condition causing his/her symptoms.

Acne-prone skin is often classified under the sensitive skin category by cosmetic consumers. However, as many dermatologists consider it to be a separate clinical entity, acne-prone skin and acneiform eruptions will not be discussed here.

36.2 EPIDEMIOLOGY

Sensitive skin is largely believed to be a widespread phenomenon. Epidemiological studies have shown that as many as one quarter to one half of the adult population consider themselves as having sensitive skin.[1] However, consumer-perceived cutaneous reactions are usually scientifically unconfirmed; self-assessment is not an accurate parameter. Furthermore, estimates of the prevalence or incidence of sensitive skin are problematic as the term "sensitive skin" lacks a consistent definition.

The North American Contact Dermatitis Group has published data on a multicenter study of cosmetic reactions from 1977 to 1983 conducted by dermatologists with a special interest in contact dermatitis.[3,4] They identified patients with cosmetic dermatitis as 5.4% of 13,216 patients with contact dermatitis. Allergic contact dermatitis was identified as the most frequent cause of cosmetic dermatitis, although this may have been a misrepresentation of the population due to the special interests of the dermatologists involved. Irritant dermatitis was thought to be underreported, as it is a diagnosis of exclusion. We feel that although this study serves to alert physicians and consumers to suspect cosmetic reactions, it does not in any way represent the true prevalence of the problem. Individuals with sensitive skin may not have been identified as many experience sensory reactions with no visible inflammation. Frequently, consumers who experience a reaction to a cosmetic product will merely discontinue use of the suspected item, rather than consult a physician. While this action is certainly adequate in treating the symptoms at hand, it hinders both our ability to quantify the percentage of adverse reactions caused by cosmetics, as well as identification of the ingredients which cause these reactions.

In the previous study, 79% of the patients with cosmetic dermatitis were female and 85% were Caucasian. Correspondingly, in a series of skin reactivity studies, Frosch and Kligman concluded that the typical "hyperreactor" had the following characteristics: white, fair skin, high susceptibility to sunburn and poor ability to tan (Fitzpatrick phototype I or II), and blond or red hair.[5] These features were most prominent in people of Celtic lineage. Accordingly, dark skin is commonly thought to resist chemical injury better, presumably because erythema is less discernible.[6] However, in light of recent studies, ethnic skin has been found to play a complex role in sensitive skin — this has been reviewed by Berardesca and Maibach.[6]

36.3 SYMPTOMATOLOGY

Although the differential diagnosis of sensitive skin encompasses a range of possible skin diseases, the types of complaints reported are very similar. Burning, itching, stinging, or a tight feeling (due to associated dry skin) are frequently reported symptoms.[2,7] These symptoms vary in intensity from mild to severe and may be intermittent or continuous throughout the day. Onset or exacerbation of symptoms correlates to application of the offending topical product(s). Clinical signs are usually minimal — even though erythema and edema may be evident, these inflammatory changes are often transient and have no long-term clinical sequelae. The lack of objective signs and overall similarity in clinical symptoms poses a challenge to the clinician's diagnostic acumen.

The face is the most common site for cosmetic reactions, particularly in the eyelid area.[3,4,8] Facial skin is highly permeable, due to a thinner stratum corneum and a greater density of

TABLE 1
Etiology of Sensitive Skin: Differential Diagnosis[8]

Exogenous	
Subjective irritation	Common; acute onset; burning, stinging, itching within minutes of application
Objective irritation	Common; morphologically difficult to differentiate from ACD, diagnosis by exclusion
Suberythematous irritation	Burning, stinging, itching. Squamometry may show protein abnormality
Allergic contact dermatitis	Uncommon; diagnostic patch test essential
Photoallergic contact dermatitis	Uncommon; diagnosis by photopatch testing
Contact urticaria	Query patient about burning, stinging, itching. Diagnosis by immediate-type testing for wheal-and-flare reaction
Endogenous	
Seborrheic dermatitis Rosacea Psoriasis Atopic dermatitis	Common diagnoses, but small percentage have atypical morphology → difficult diagnosis
Dysmorphophobia	Rare; diagnosis of exclusion

appendages (e.g., sweat glands, hair follicles). Moreover, facial skin contains an elaborate network of sensory nerves. The frequency of cosmetic application is also increased at this body site. Although mild inflammatory changes are often masked on the face, in the event that eruptions do occur, they are readily noticed by the consumer.

36.4 CLASSIFICATION AND ETIOLOGY

Skin reaction to moisturizers and other cosmetic products have a varied differential diagnosis, challenging the clinician's ability to pinpoint the underlying cause. Indeed, sensitive skin is often regarded as a complex multifactorial syndrome, rather than a single entity. Maibach and Engasser coined the term "cosmetic intolerance syndrome" to describe this heterogeneous syndrome, whereby certain susceptible individuals cannot tolerate a wide range of cosmetic products.[8,9]

Fisher coined the term "status cosmeticus," a condition in which every cosmetic product applied to the face produces itching, burning, or stinging, rendering the sufferer incapable of using any cosmetic product.[10] The patient with status cosmeticus typically has a clinically unremarkable presentation. They may have a mild malar erythema with slight edema of the eyelids. Sometimes this is accompanied by a follicular eruption. The mild clinical picture usually contrasts vividly with the patients' bitter complaints of burning or stinging sensations. The history usually includes "sensitivity" to innumerable cosmetics, while patch test and "use" test results using various implicated products will be negative. Status cosmeticus may be considered to be at the extreme end of the spectrum of sensitive skin. In practice, the term "status cosmeticus" is only applied to a patient who has undergone a thorough workup and other diagnoses have been excluded.

When dealing with patients with sensitive skin, the following differential diagnoses have to be considered (see Table 1), thus permitting a rational approach.

36.4.1 Exogenous Causes

36.4.1.1 Subjective Irritation

Subjective or sensory irritation is defined as chemically induced burning, stinging, or itching sensations without detectable visible or microscopic changes.[2,8] This reaction commonly appears within an hour of application in certain susceptible individuals (known as "stingers") and is usually transient, lasting minutes. Ingredients which cause this reaction may not generally be considered objective irritants and will not cause abnormal responses in non-susceptible persons ("nonstingers"). This nonspecific reaction is probably grossly underreported, due to its transient nature. Furthermore, in specialized skin sites, such as the face and scalp, subtle inflammatory changes are often masked.

Subjective irritation is believed to be the most common cause of sensitive skin and cosmetic reactions.[2] Propylene glycol, butylene glycol, and hydroxy acids are examples of subjective irritants present in modern-day cosmetics.[2,11] Alcohol is also capable of causing subjective irritation, but is not commonly known to cause objective irritation, whereas SLS, a strong objective irritant, does not usually cause stinging.[2] This suggests that subjective irritation is not just a mild form of objective irritation.

The precise mechanism of subjective irritation has yet to be determined. Insights concerning the mechanism of subjective irritation may be gleaned from the fact that local anesthetics block the response,[2] and stingers respond more vigorously to vasodilators.[12] Recent studies utilizing quantitative sensory testing methods, such as the thermal sensory analyzer (TSA), on anti-inflammatory agents have provided insight into their action of cutaneous sensation.[13,14] Such studies with sensory irritants and their inhibitors may provide similar insight into the pathophysiology of subjective irritation.[2]

Before confirming a diagnosis of subjective irritation, patients must be patch tested and open tested to exclude allergic contact dermatitis and contact urticaria, respectively. Subclinical contact urticaria, in particular, mimics sensory irritation.

36.4.1.2 Objective Irritation and Nonerythematous Irritation

Objective irritation is defined as nonimmunologically mediated, localized inflammation of the skin, usually resulting from contact with a substance that chemically damages the skin.[2,8] The exact mechanism is unknown, and it is likely that both endogenous and exogenous factors are involved. *In vivo* predictive testing in animals (e.g., modified Draize test, repeated application patch tests, guinea pig immersion test) and humans (e.g., cumulative irritation assay, chamber scarification test) can detect moderate to strong irritants, allowing manufacturers to eliminate these potential hazards prior to marketing a cosmetic.[15] Mild irritants, however, are more difficult to identify and are sometimes missed. Although irritation normally causes an erythematous reaction, dermatologists may have difficulty identifying low-grade inflammatory changes in the face. Careful examination of the facial area, aided by slight magnification, may be useful in unmasking the diagnosis. Patch testing to rule out allergic contact dermatitis is obligatory. Photoirritation or phototoxicity should also be considered. Some cosmetic products which cause irritant contact dermatitis are soaps and detergents, deodorants and antiperspirants, eye makeup, shampoo, permanent hair-waving products, and moisturizers.[8] It should be noted that many moisturizers contain surfactants and emulsifiers that are cumulative irritants, i.e., mild irritants that produce inflammation only after repeated application.[8] This fact is frequently overlooked as moisturizers are commonly used in the treatment and prevention of irritant dermatitis.

Nonerythematous or *suberythematous irritation* is defined as a state in which the clinical observer sees no abnormality; the patient knows that there is something wrong and may describe it as burning, stinging, or itching. Charbonnier et al. have shown that objective alterations are present and are readily demonstrable by the technique of squamometry.[16] The latter utilizes protein staining and microscopic examination of stratum corneum tape strippings. The greater the protein abnormality, the greater the irritation. This is more discriminating than visual examination and current bioengineering technology.

Management of these patients is difficult as almost any chemical can be an irritant, depending on a host of factors, such as the concentration of the chemical, the mode of exposure, other chemicals in the formulation, and other environmental and constitutional factors.

36.4.1.3 Allergic Contact Dermatitis

Allergic contact dermatitis is dermatitis caused by prior exposure to an allergen leading to specific cell-mediated sensitization. It is classified as delayed-type hypersensitivity, as inflammation develops after a relatively long time interval following the exposure. Clinically, it manifests as a pruritic erythematous eruption, with papules and vesicles at the site of exposure. This is the simplest cause of sensitive skin, in terms of diagnosis and management. Patch testing is the diagnostic gold standard; all the patient's cosmetics and skin care items should be included in the patch testing procedure — it is not sufficient to patch test with the routine series.[8] As the most common cosmetic allergens are fragrances and preservatives, patch testing with the fragrance and preservatives series is imperative.[3,4] Lanolin, a naturally occurring wax emollient, is an uncommon albeit important cause of cosmetic allergy. Note that many allergenic cosmetics are mild irritants under occlusion — this is a potential cause of false-positive patch test results.

Management of cosmetic allergy is relatively straightforward since the advent of cosmetic ingredient labeling. "Hypoallergenic" formulations of cosmetic products seem to be in vogue at present. Fragrance-free formulations are also available for the fragrance allergic — these are useful, as fragrance allergies are complex and difficult to isolate.

36.4.1.4 Contact Urticaria Syndrome

Most people think that the most common part of sensitive skin is sensory irritation. Contact urticaria syndrome (CUS) comprises a presumably smaller part and is a heterogeneous group of inflammatory reactions characterized by burning, tingling, itching, and a wheal-and-flare response that usually appear within minutes after contact with the eliciting substance.[17] These reactions are transient, disappearing within 24 h, with the majority fading within a few hours. In its more severe forms, generalized urticaria and extracutaneous manifestations, such as respiratory or gastrointestinal symptoms and even anaphylaxis, may be experienced.[17]

Three mechanisms are implicated in CUS: immunologic (ICU), nonimmunologic (NICU), or uncertain mechanism.[17] ICU is a type I hypersensitivity reaction that is IgE mediated and is associated with atopy. NICU is the more common variety of CUS. NICU due to cosmetics is most commonly caused by fragrances (e.g., cinnamic aldehyde) and preservatives (e.g., benzoic acid and sorbic acid).[2] Parabens have been documented by passive transfer to cause ICU.[18]

Muizzuddin et al. recently studied contact urticaria in an attempt to define sensitive skin objectively.[19] Skin responsiveness was assessed using balsam of Peru, which induces NICU. They found that individuals with self-assessed sensitive skin were more susceptible to NICU. This group was also more susceptible to stinging induced by lactic acid and stratum corneum barrier removal using tape stripping.

Diagnosis of CUS involves a high index of suspicion and appropriate open testing for "immediate" onset lesions. These are easily missed on the face, and careful observation is required.

36.4.1.5 Photosensitivity Reactions

Photosensitivity reactions are adverse cutaneous responses to the synergistic actions of a chemical agent and ultraviolet light.[21] Photosensitivity reactions may be broadly categorized into phototoxic reactions and photoallergic reactions. Phototoxic reactions may be experienced by any individual under appropriate conditions (i.e., appropriate wavelength of ultraviolet radiation and sufficient concentration of phototoxic chemical), while photoallergic reactions are delayed-type immunologic reactions requiring a period of sensitization.[20,21] Photopatch testing is an invaluable diagnostic tool for photoallergic contact dermatitis. This is a modification of the basic patch test procedure — patch test sites of the suspected substance(s) are applied in duplicate; one site is irradiated with ultraviolet light, and the results are compared to the nonirradiated site. A stronger reaction in the irradiated site suggests photoallergy.

Cosmetic products that are photoallergenic include fragrances, such as musk ambrette and 6-methylcoumarin, and sunscreens (e.g., para-aminobenzoic acid and its derivatives, benzophenones, dibenzoylmethanes).[15] Oil of bergamot, previously a popular ingredient in fragrances, has now been eliminated from most perfumes due to its phototoxic properties.[20]

36.4.2 Endogenous Causes

These include atypical or subtle manifestations of dermatologic conditions such as seborrheic dermatitis, rosacea, psoriasis, atopic dermatitis, and ichthyosis. Classic manifestations of such diseases are diagnosed with relative ease. However, diagnostic difficulty arises in the presence of atypical morphology, lesions masked by topical therapy (e.g., corticosteroids), or exacerbations due to other topical agents (e.g., skin care products).[2,9]

A thorough clinical review sometimes directs the clinician to the correct diagnosis. In other cases, time is required for other stigmata to surface. Appropriate diagnostic testing and a prolonged cosmetic elimination program should be implemented in the first instance, but if all else fails, therapeutic trials may be indicated. Topical corticosteroids may sometimes prove useful to break a cycle of cosmetic intolerance syndrome.[9]

Another factor to consider is that patients with endogenous skin disease are frequently more susceptible to cosmetic reactions. One reason is that patients with preexisting skin disease may have skin barrier dysfunction, with consequent increased permeability. Skin hyperreactivity in atopic patients, particularly, has been gathering interest in recent years. Epidemiologic associations between atopic dermatitis and irritant dermatitis are now supported by skin bioengineering data.[22]

Certain substances have been reported to affect eczematous skin, but not normal skin. One example is parabens, a popular preservative that may sensitize eczematous skin, but rarely causes reactions in normal skin.[15] Fisher has termed this phenomenon the "paraben paradox."[10] Likewise, lanolin, a popular emollient, is an important sensitizer when applied to eczematous eruptions, particularly stasis dermatitis, but rarely affects individuals with normal skin.[15]

36.4.3 Dermatologic Nondisease

Cotterill used the term "dermatologic nondisease" to describe a group of patients who presented with significant skin symptomatology, but no significant objective skin pathology on examination.[23,24] In his experience, the majority of patients were female and middle-aged. Burning, itching, or discomfort were the most frequent complaints, and these were most often experienced in the face, scalp, and perineum. Other features which may be present include a preoccupation with imagined excessive facial hair, imagined excessive hair loss, and orodynia. Cotterill found that these patients were commonly depressed, sometimes with suicidal ideation, and often suffered from dysmorphophobia or a disturbed psychological body image. Management of these patients is a delicate matter, as they often react badly to referral to a psychiatrist. These patients also largely fail to respond to any topical or oral therapy, and a placebo response is never seen. When associated with depression, systemic antidepressant treatment may be attempted, but is generally ineffective.

36.5 DIAGNOSTIC TESTS FOR SENSITIVE SKIN

Measurement of differences in skin reactivity or "sensitivity" among individuals plays an important role in the workplace, as well as in the manufacture of safe topical therapeutics and cosmetics. Outlined in the following sections are objective and subjective methods of quantifying the reactivity of human skin to chemicals, which are potential irritants.[5] The experimental basis of such testing is to quantify the differences among individuals to chemicals that produce characteristic responses using a standard reproducible procedure. Individuals classified as hyperreactors (sensitive skin) and hyporeactors can then be identified.

36.5.1 Objective Methods

1. Ammonium hydroxide blistering time[5] — This test measures the permeability of the stratum corneum barrier, the rationale being that the time taken to raise a blister is a function of the number of cell layers in the horny layer. An aqueous dilution of concentrated ammonium hydroxide is placed in a small plastic well, which is subsequently covered with a glass slip. Careful observation using a magnifying lens is then carried out until a tense blister forms in the well. Tiny vesicles initially appear, and formation of a full blister usually takes a few minutes; the time taken for the full blister to form is known as minimal blistering time (MBT). Lower values of MBT correspond to skin that is more reactive.
2. Dimethyl sulfoxide (DMSO) test[5] — This test measures the diffusional resistance of the horny layer. Equal quantities of three different concentrations of DMSO are applied to three plastic wells for 5 minutes. DMSO provokes whealing in human skin. The wheals are scored 10 minutes after removal of the test fluid using a scale. Individuals with high reactivity are those susceptible to whealing with the lowest concentration of DMSO.
3. Sodium lauryl sulfate (SLS) test[5] — SLS attacks the horny layer, making it more penetrable to chemicals and also causing inflammation. Thus, it measures both the horny layer barrier and tissue reactivity to toxic substances. Aluminum chambers are filled with 0.1 ml of 1 and 2.5% aqueous solutions of SLS. The chambers are then applied to the ventral forearm for 24 h. The reactions are scored 3 h after removal of the chambers on a scale. Those reacting strongly to the lower concentration of SLS are deemed more reactive or sensitive.

36.5.2 Subjective Methods

Subjective responses are nerve-mediated sensory responses such as burning, stinging, itching, or pain that may be experienced in varying intensities, but do not induce visible changes that can be perceived by an outside observer. Semiquantitative methods of assessment have been devised to measure such responses.

1. Chloroform-methanol pain threshold[5] — A 0.1-ml solution of equal parts chloroform and methanol (CM) is placed in a plastic well. This mixture rapidly induces sharp pain. As soon as the subject perceives this pain, the fluid is removed and the elapsed time is recorded. Highly sensitive individuals experience pain induced by CM more rapidly than less sensitive individuals.
2. Lactic acid sting test[5] — This test, devised by Frosch and Kligman in 1977,[25] utilizes the subjective irritant, lactic acid, and remains the most popular test for subjective irritation. Lactic acid, as well as a number of other substances, will induce a sharp stinging sensation without overt inflammation in a number of susceptible individuals, known as stingers. Stinging potential of a substance is not strictly related to its objective irritancy. The subject is placed in a hot, humid environmental chamber until profuse sweating is achieved. Then a 5% solution of lactic acid is rubbed over the nasolabial folds and cheeks with a cotton-tipped applicator. The stinging sensation is scored on a scale at 10 seconds, 2.5 minutes, and 5 minutes.

The methods for assessing reactivity previously outlined are simple, convenient, inexpensive, and noninvasive or minimally invasive.[5] However, cutaneous reactivity depends on many factors. None of the previous methods give a full picture of the characteristics of sensitive skin, only susceptibility of skin to irritants. Subtle manifestations of endogenous cutaneous conditions must still be clinically

TABLE 2
Bioengineering Methods and Biophysiological Parameters in Sensitive Skin Research[30]

Method	Biophysiological Parameter
Evaporimetry	Transepidermal water loss (TEWL)
Colorimetry/Chromametry (CIE system)	L*: skin reflectance a*: red/green axis b*: blue/yellow axis
Laser Doppler velocimetry	Skin blood flow
Ultrasound	Skin thickness (edema formation)
pH meter	Skin pH
Corneometer (electric capacitance)	Stratum corneum hydration
Sebumeter	Sebum excretion

excluded. Exclusion of allergic contact dermatitis must still be performed by patch testing, exclusion of contact urticaria by open tests or PUT/ROAT, and exclusion of photoallergy by photopatch testing.

36.6 PATHOPHYSIOLOGY

As the definition of sensitive skin is controversial and its etiology is thought to be heterogeneous, it follows that the pathophysiology of sensitive skin is thus far incompletely defined and probably embraces an array of mechanisms. Clinical manifestations such as contact dermatitis in a hyperreactor probably have the same mechanisms as in a "normal" person with the same dermatoses. However, some general features causing enhanced reactivity have been identified in individuals with sensitive skin. Increased susceptibility to irritation from exogenous substances may be due to inherent structural features of the skin, for instance, hyperreactors may have a thinner stratum corneum with a reduced corneocyte area,[26] thus allowing a higher transcutaneous penetration of water-soluble chemicals.[27] A heightened neurosensory input in subjects with sensitive skin, corresponding to an augmented response to cutaneous stimulation, may also lower the threshold to irritant stimuli.[28] Release of a different makeup of inflammatory mediators, which may alter the inflammatory response, has also been implicated in individuals with sensitive skin.[29] A great deal of work remains to be done in this field.

36.7 SKIN BIOENGINEERING AND SENSITIVE SKIN

Studies on sensitive skin are often performed using subjective self-assessment — this naturally yields results of variable reliability. The current trend is striving toward identification of more objective biophysiological measures of skin sensitivity. Today, skin bioengineering studies are employed to investigate the correlation of various biophysiological parameters with skin reactivity, thereby also conveying some insight into its mechanisms.[30] The advantages of bioengineering instruments are that they are quantitative, noninvasive, and detect subtle changes that would otherwise be undetectable to the naked eye.[31] Examples of bioengineering techniques used to evaluate the pathophysiology of skin reactivity include transepidermal water loss, skin conductance, resistance, impedance, blood flow velocity, and skin pH (Table 2).[15] Descriptions of these methods may be found in the textbooks of Berardesca et al.[32] and Elsner et al.[33]

Determination of basal biophysiological parameters may identify subjects with sensitive skin. Earlier studies have shown that increased skin susceptibility has been correlated with an increased basal transepidermal water loss (TEWL),[34-36] skin surface pH,[37] and fair skin complexion (measured by chromametric L* values),[38] whereas no relationship was shown for basal skin thickness, skin

TABLE 3
Management of Sensitive Skin[8]

1. Clinical review: history and physical examination
2. Examine every cosmetic and skin care product
3. Patch test and photopatch test — to rule out contact and photocontact allergy
   Immediate-type testing — to rule out contact urticaria
4. Avoid causative ingredient, if identified by testing.
5. Treat any endogenous inflammatory disease.
6. Cosmetic elimination program — 6 to 12 months.
   Avoid all cosmetics apart from:
   - Lip cosmetics
   - Eye cosmetics
   - Face powder
   - Glycerin and rose water

   After 6 to 12 months, gradually reintroduce one product every 1 to 2 weeks
7. Be alert to depression and other neuropsychiatric conditions

blood flow, sebum excretion, and skin hydration.[30] However, a recent study by Seidenari et al. utilizing multiple bioengineering techniques showed significant correlations only for capacitance and colorimetric a* values.[39]

Individuals with sensitive skin often have associated dry skin. In a recent study of subjects with sensitive hands, no difference in skin hydration was seen macroscopically between normal subjects and sensitive hand subjects (who had self-perceived dry skin). However, measurement with the corneometer confirmed reduced skin surface moisture in the group with sensitive hands, and D-squame analysis showed greater loss of cohesiveness between corneocytes harvested from the sensitive hands group.[40] In this study, no correlation was found between sensitive hands and TEWL or skin redness.

The results of the latter two studies described contradict earlier data. Up to this point, an elevated TEWL had been the most widely accepted biophysiological parameter associated with sensitive skin, due to impairment of the skin barrier function or composition. That further studies are imperative to create a consistent and objective operational definition for "sensitive skin" is affirmed by these conflicting results.

36.8 MANAGEMENT OPTIONS

The first step in management is to identify the causative ingredient(s), as well as the causative mechanism, if possible. As sensitive skin is often multifactorial, the approach to the patient should cover the range of differential diagnoses. Thus, starting with a complete history and examination, clues derived from clinical suspicion should aid in devising a plan for diagnostic testing (Table 3).

A thorough history for burning, stinging, and itching identifies sensory irritation and possible CUS. The history should include careful questioning of all topical products applied, as well as the time of onset in relation to exposure. Personal and family history of atopy should be actively sought, as should other skin conditions such as psoriasis and rosacea. A meticulous physical examination may identify other stigmata of atopic dermatitis, psoriasis, or other skin disease.

Patch testing (and photopatch testing) should document the few cases due to allergic contact dermatitis. Apart from the routine battery, testing should be performed with the fragrance and preservative series, as well as any cosmetic or skin care product that the patient uses. Immediate-type testing should be performed if indicated by the history. If systemic symptoms were present, perform only in the presence of emergency resuscitative facilities.

If an ingredient is identified as the causative agent, then avoidance of the ingredient is advised. If, however, no substance is identified or the patient reacts to a wide range of substances, then a prolonged cosmetic elimination program may be considered.[8,9] The patient will be barred from using most cosmetic products for a period of 6 to 12 months. For the duration of the cosmetic elimination program, no soaps or detergents or moisturizers are allowed. Glycerin and rose water may function as a substitute for commercial moisturizers. Lip and eye cosmetics may be used freely if no problems are identified in these areas. Face powder may also be used. After the allotted time, gradual reintroduction of one cosmetic product will be instituted periodically, for instance, one product every 2 weeks, so that in the end, a simple skin care regime is devised for the patient.

36.8.1 Hypoallergenicity

Because up to 40% of the population claim to possess sensitive skin,[41] numerous cosmetic and skin care items have been formulated to be "hypoallergenic" or literally "reduced allergy." These are products designed for the individual with sensitive skin. Marketing claims for hypoallergenicity are based on objective tests performed on these products, such as the guinea pig maximization test, repeat insult patch test, cumulative irritancy test, chamber scarification test, photopatch test, and facial sting test (lactic acid test), as well as postmarketing surveillance programs.[42] However, no formal criteria exist for evaluation of hypoallergenic products. Draelos and Rietschel demonstrated the ambiguity of the term "hypoallergenicity" in a recent study.[42] Although 75% of dermatologists believed that the concept was relevant to their clinical practice, dermatologists' perceptions of the hypoallergenicity claim was varied. Most believed that hypoallergenicity embodied skin irritation (72.6%) and contact allergy (87.9%), while opinions were divided over subjective irritation (59.8%), contact urticaria (46.4%), photomediated responses (31.5%), and acne (23.4%). A similar ambiguity exists among cosmetic manufacturers: some hypoallergenic products are low in certain allergens, others are low in certain irritants; some are preservative free; some are fragrance free — the diversity is potentially endless. This is an issue which clearly needs to be addressed.

36.8.2 Anti-Irritants

Goldenberg and Safrin suggested that the sensory effects of topical irritants may be neutralized by "anti-irritants."[43] They proposed three possible mechanisms of action of anti-irritants: complexing of the irritant, blocking the reactive sites in the skin, and preventing physical contact with the skin. The main anti-irritant cosmetic chemicals are imidazole, hydroxy, and carboxyl compounds. Studies of the safety and efficacy of these anti-irritants in cosmetics are ongoing.[10]

36.9 SUMMARY

Sensitive skin is not a single entity, but a heterogeneous syndrome, puzzling both consumer and clinician alike. The definition remains obscure, and so it follows that prevalence and pathophysiology are as yet undetermined. Innovative skin bioengineering techniques have opened up new avenues for sensitive skin research. Such studies are still in their infancy and continue to be published — this will undoubtedly shed new light on the topic.

REFERENCES

1. Morizot, F., Le Fur, I., Tschachler, E., Sensitive skin: definitions, prevalence and possible causes, *Cosm Toiletries*, 113, 59–66, 1998.
2. Amin, S., Engasser, P., Maibach, H. I., Sensitive skin: what is it? in *Textbook of Cosmetic Dermatology*, 2nd edition, Baran, R. and Maibach, H. I., Eds., Martin Dunitz Ltd., London, 1998, ch. 28, 343–349.

3. North American Contact Dermatitis Group and Food and Drug Administration, Prospective study of cosmetic reactions: 1977–1980, *J Am Acad Dermatol*, 6, 909–917, 1982.
4. North American Contact Dermatitis Group, A five-year study of cosmetic reactions, *J Am Acad Dermatol*, 13(6), 1062–1069, 1985.
5. Frosch, P. J. and Kligman, A. M., Recognition of chemically vulnerable and delicate skin, in *Principles of Cosmetics for the Dermatologist*, Frost, P. and Horwitz, S. N., Eds., C. V. Mosby Company, St. Louis, 1982, ch. 36, 287–296.
6. Berardesca, E. and Maibach, H. I., Sensitive and ethnic skin: a need for special skin-care agents? *Dermatologic Clinics*, 9(1), 89–92, 1991 Jan.
7. Mills, O. H. and Berger, R. S., Defining the susceptibility of acne-prone and sensitive skin populations to extrinsic factors, *Dermatologic Clinics*, 9, 93–98, 1991.
8. Maibach, H. I. and Engasser, P. G., Dermatitis due to cosmetics, in *Contact Dermatitis*, 3rd edition, Fisher, A. A., Ed., Lea and Febiger, Philadelphia, 1986, ch. 21, 368–393.
9. Maibach, H. I. and Engasser, P. G., Management of cosmetic intolerance syndrome, *Clinics in Dermatology*, 6, 102–107, 1988.
10. Fisher, A. A., Cosmetic actions and reactions: therapeutic, irritant, and allergic, *Cutis*, 26, 22–29, 1980.
11. Engasser, P. G. and Maibach, H. I., Cosmetics and skin care in dermatologic practice, in *Fitzpatrick's Dermatology in General Medicine,* 5th edition, Freedberg, I. M., Eisen, A. Z., Wolff, K. et al., Eds., McGraw-Hill, New York, 1998, ch. 251, 2772–2782.
12. Lammintausta, K., Maibach, H. I., Wilson, D., Mechanisms of subjective (sensory) irritation. Propensity to non-immunologic contact urticaria and objective irritation in stingers, *Derm Beruf Umwelt*, 36, 45–49, 1988.
13. Yosipovitch, G., Szolar, C., Hui, X., Maibach, H. I., Effect of topically applied menthol on thermal, pain and itch sensation and biophysical properties of the skin, *Arch Dermatol Res,* 288, 245–248, 1996.
14. Yosipovitch, G., Ademola, J., Liu, P., et al., Topically applied aspirin rapidly decreases histamine-induced itch, *Acta Derm Venereol* (*Stockh.*)*,* 77, 46–48, 1997.
15. Toro, J. R., Engasser, P. G., Maibach, H. I., Cosmetic reactions, in *Dermatotoxicology*, 5th edition, Marzulli, F. N. and Maibach, H. I., Eds., Taylor and Francis, Washington, D.C., 1996, ch. 47, 607–642.
16. Charbonnier, V., Morrison, B. M., Jr., Paye, M., Maibach, H. I., Open application assay in investigation of subclinical irritant dermatitis induced by sodium lauryl sulfate (SLS) in man: advantage of squamometry, *Skin Res Tech*, 4, 244–250, 1998.
17. Amin, S., Lahti, A., Maibach, H. I., Eds., *Contact Urticaria Syndrome*, CRC Press, Boca Raton, FL, 1997.
18. Henry, J. C., Tschen, E. H., Becker, L. E., Contact urticaria to parabens, *Arch Dermatol*, 115, 1231–1232, 1979.
19. Muizzuddin, N., Marenus, K. D., Maes, D. K., Factors defining sensitive skin and its treatment, *Am J Contact Dermatitis*, 9, 170–175, 1998.
20. Marzulli, F. N. and Maibach, H. I., Photoirritation (phototoxicity/phototoxic dermatitis), in *Dermatotoxicology*, 5th edition, Marzulli, F. N. and Maibach, H. I., Eds., Taylor and Francis, Washington, D.C., 1996, ch. 16, 231–237.
21. Rietschel, R. L. and Fowler, J. F., Jr., *Fisher's Contact Dermatitis*, William & Wilkins, Baltimore, MD, 1995, ch. 23, 524–543.
22. Seidenari, S., Skin sensitivity, interindividual factors: atopy, in *The Irritant Contact Dermatitis Syndrome*, Van der Valk, P. G. M. and Maibach, H. I., Eds., CRC Press, Boca Raton, FL, 1996.
23. Cotterill, J. A., Dermatological non-disease: a common and potentially fatal disturbance of cutaneous body image, *Br J Dermatol*, 104, 611–619, 1981.
24. Cotterill, J. A., Clinical features of patients with dermatologic nondisease, *Seminars in Dermatology*, 2(3), 203–205, September 1983.
25. Frosch, P. and Kligman, A. M., A method for appraising the stinging capacity of topically applied substances, *J Soc Cosmet Chem*, 28, 197–209, 1977.
26. Hamami, I. and Marks, R., Structural determinants of the response of the skin to chemical irritants, *Contact Dermatitis*, 18, 71–75, 1988.
27. Berardesca, E., Cespa, M., Farinelli, N., et al., *In vivo* transcutaneous penetration of nicotinates and sensitive skin, *Contact Dermatitis*, 25, 35–38, 1991.

28. Rietschel, R. L., Stochastic resonance and angry back syndrome: noisy skin, *Am J Contact Dermatitis*, 3, 152–154, 1996.
29. Frosch, P. J., Irritant contact dermatitis, in *Current Topics in Contact Dermatitis*, Frosch, P. J. et al., Eds., Springer-Verlag, Heidelberg, 1989, 385–398.
30. Agner, T., Bioengineering and sensitive skin, in *The Irritant Contact Dermatitis Syndrome*, Van der Valk, P. G. M. and Maibach, H. I., Eds., CRC Press, Boca Raton, FL, 1996.
31. Van Neste, D. and de Brouwer, B., Monitoring of skin response to sodium lauryl sulfate: clinical scores vs. bioengineering methods, *Contact Dermatitis*, 27, 151–156, 1992.
32. Berardesca, E., Elsner, P., Wilhelm, K., Maibach, H. I., *Bioengineering of the Skin: Methods and Instrumentation*, CRC Press, Boca Raton, FL, 1995.
33. Elsner, P., Berardesca, E., Maibach, H. I., *Bioengineering of the Skin: Water and the Stratum Corneum*, CRC Press, Boca Raton, FL, 1994.
34. Muruhata, R., Crove, D. M., Roheim, J. R., The use of transepidermal water loss to measure and predict the irritation response to surfactants, *Int J Cosm Sci*, 8, 225–231, 1986.
35. Tupker, R. A., Pinnagoda, J., Coenraads, P. J., Nater, J. P., The influence of repeated exposure to surfactants on the human skin as determined by transepidermal water loss and visual scoring, *Contact Dermatitis*, 20, 108–114, 1989.
36. Tupker, R. A., Coenraads, P. J., Pinnagoda, J., Nater, J. P., Baseline transepidermal water loss (TEWL) as a prediction of susceptibility to sodium lauryl sulfate, *Contact Dermatitis*, 20, 265–269, 1989.
37. Wilhelm, K. P. and Maibach, H. I., Susceptibility to irritant dermatitis induced by sodium lauryl sulfate, *J Am Acad Dermatol*, 23, 122–124, 1990.
38. Agner, T., Basal transepidermal water loss, skin thickness, skin blood flow and skin colour in relation to sodium-lauryl-sulfate-induced irritation in normal skin, *Contact Dermatitis*, 25, 108–114, 1991.
39. Seidenari, S., Francomano, M., Mantovani, L., Baseline biophysical parameters in subjects with sensitive skin, *Contact Dermatitis*, 38, 311–315, 1998.
40. Paye, M., Dalimier, Ch., Cartiaux, Y., Chabassol, C., Consumer perception of sensitive hands: what is behind it? *Skin Res Tech*, 5, 28–32, 1999.
41. Jackson, E. M., The science of cosmetics, *Am J Contact Dermatitis*, 4, 108–110, 1993.
42. Draelos, Z. D. and Rietschel, R. L., Hypoallergenicity and the dermatologist's perception, *J Am Acad Dermatol*, 35, 248–251, 1996.
43. Goldenberg, R. L. and Safrin, L., Reduction of topical irritation, *J Soc Cosmet Chem*, 28, 667, 1977.

Index

A

B

C

D

E

N

O

P

Q

R

S

T

U

V

W

X

Z